Clinical Physiology

Dr. Keith E. Evans.

[London Chest Hospital, 1970.]

Clinical Physiology

edited by

E. J. MORAN CAMPBELL

B.Sc. Ph.D. M.D. F.R.C.P.

R. Samuel McLaughlin Professor and
Chairman of the Department of Medicine
McMaster University,
Hamilton, Ontario, Canada

C. J. DICKINSON

B.Sc. M.A. D.M. F.R.C.P.

Physician, University College Hospital
Senior Lecturer
University College Hospital Medical School

and

J. D. H. SLATER

M.A. M.B. M.R.C.P.

Physician, The Middlesex Hospital
Senior Lecturer
The Middlesex Hospital
Medical School, London

THIRD EDITION
SECOND PRINTING

BLACKWELL SCIENTIFIC PUBLICATIONS
OXFORD AND EDINBURGH

SBN 632 00740 0

FIRST PUBLISHED MARCH 1960
REVISED REPRINT FEBRUARY 1961
SECOND EDITION MARCH 1963
REVISED REPRINT MARCH 1965
THIRD EDITION APRIL 1968
REPRINTED FEBRUARY 1970

E.L.B.S. EDITION
FIRST PUBLISHED 1969
REPRINTED 1970

Printed in Great Britain by
ADLARD AND SON LTD
BARTHOLOMEW PRESS, DORKING
and bound by
THE KEMP HALL BINDERY, OXFORD

Contents

Contributors

G. M. BERLYNE M.D. M.R.C.P. Senior Lecturer, University of Manchester
The Kidney

A. J. BULLER B.Sc. M.B. B.S. Professor of Physiology, University of Bristol
The Nervous System in the Control of Movement

E. J. M. CAMPBELL B.Sc. Ph.D. M.D. F.R.C.P. R. Samuel McLaughlin Professor and Chairman of the Department of Medicine, McMaster University, Hamilton, Ontario, Canada
Respiration; Hydrogen Ion (Acid : Base) Regulation

T. M. CHALMERS M.A. M.D. F.R.C.P. Physician, United Cambridge Hospitals
The Pituitary Gland

M. d'A CRAWFURD M.B. B.S. M.C.Path. Senior Lecturer, Department of Genetics, University of Leeds
Genetics

C. J. DICKINSON B.Sc. M.A. D.M. F.R.C.P. Physician, University College Hospital; Senior Lecturer, University College Hospital Medical School, London
Heart and Circulation

R. L. HIMSWORTH M.B. M.R.C.P. Lecturer, University College Hospital, London
Energy Sources and Utilization

C. D. HOLDSWORTH M.D. M.R.C.P. Senior Lecturer, St Bartholomew's Hospital; Physician, St Leonard's Hospital, London
The Gut

N. C. HUGHES JONES M.A. D.M. Ph.D. Senior Lecturer, Department of Haematology, St Mary's Hospital, London
Formed Elements of Blood and Haemostasis: Immune Mechanisms

D. S. MUNRO M.D. F.R.C.P.   Professor of Clinical Endocrinology, University of Sheffield
The Thyroid Gland

B. L. PENTECOST M.D. M.R.C.P.   Physician, General Hospital, Birmingham
Heart and Circulation

J. D. H. SLATER M.A. M.B. M.R.C.P.   Physician, the Middlesex Hospital; Senior Lecturer, The Middlesex Hospital Medical School, London
The Body Fluids; Bone; The Adrenal Glands; Sex and Reproduction

P. K. THOMAS B.Sc. M.D. F.R.C.P.   Neurologist, Royal Free and Royal National Orthopaedic Hospitals; Senior Lecturer, Institute of Neurology, London
Skeletal Muscle

J. G. WALKER M.B. M.R.C.P.   Senior Registrar, Department of Gastroenterology, The Central Middlesex Hospital, London
The Liver

Foreword to the First Edition

BY SIR ROBERT (NOW LORD) PLATT

The fascination of the Medicine of my time, which has made it so exciting to have witnessed the last forty years, has been twofold: first, the rational understanding of the phenomena of disease in terms of physiology, and second, the therapeutic triumphs which although sometimes seeming to arise by chance were only possible on the new background of clinical science.

As a natural and essential accompaniment to these advances there has grown up a generation of younger physicians whose thinking and outlook on illness is essentially physiological. What is more, many of the men who might have been the pure physiologists of this generation went into medicine instead, feeling that the emphasis and interest was shifting from the crude procedures of experimental physiology to the more subtle experiments of nature as witnessed at the bedside, and in the pursuit of their clinical studies it is perhaps not going too far to say that they have in the last twenty years contributed as much, or more to the study of physiology as have the physiologists to medicine.

This book is written by men of this generation. Instead of the physiologist picking out those aspects of his subject which he deems to be of interest to physicians, here is the clinician himself speaking mainly of his own contributions to physiology.

The book is long overdue, for the processes which have led up to it have been going on now for many years. It is high time that the fruits of this most fruitful period of clinical science were presented in readable form for the student, the postgraduate and, perhaps above all, for the established physician who realizes that the younger men have been getting ahead of him.

Here it is, and I wish it the success it deserves. I have in the past declined to write forewords and must therefore explain this lapse on my part. This was a venture in which I believed so much, I could not resist the temptation to be associated with it.

Preface to the Third Edition

Most chapters have been re-written, all have been revised and two new ones have been added. Dr Hughes Jones has written an account of Immunological Mechanisms and Dr Crawfurd has expanded the account of Genetics, previously included in the chapter on Reproduction, to form a chapter on its own. We welcome eight new contributors, recruited in the policy of keeping this a book not only for but also by the younger generation. This edition has only 50 more pages than the last and the basic design of the book has been preserved. As in the first edition, the emphasis throughout is on the physiological knowledge which we actually use in clinical practice. Although the style is didactic and the scientific pretensions are slight, we hope that the book will promote rational medicine by encouraging reference to the basic sciences and acceptance of their critical approach. Despite the tendency to be dogmatic in order to be clear, we have tried to emphasize important areas of controversy. But we must again stress that this is not a textbook of physiology. It does not cover any syllabus and it deals with physiology as part of the practice of medicine rather than in the restricted sense of the science of normal function—an expansion of meaning justified by usage.

In the hope of improving feedback from our readers, we are trying the experiment of including a questionnaire in a sample number of copies. We hope those who receive these will help us by returning them so that we can base our future revisions on them, as well as on our own hunches.

ACKNOWLEDGEMENTS

We are grateful to our contributors both past and present for their co-operation. We also thank Mrs D. Blake for preparing the index, the medical art and photographic departments of the Middlesex and

xi

University College Hospitals and of the Royal Postgraduate Medical School and University College for preparing new illustrations, and the authors and publishers of illustrations reproduced and acknowledged in the text. As editors we are again particularly indebted to Mr Per Saugman and Mr John Robson of Blackwell Scientific Publications for their help and forbearance.

MORAN CAMPBELL
JOHN DICKINSON

March, 1968   WILLIAM SLATER

Preface to the First Edition

One of the most striking changes in medicine in recent years has been the increasing use of physiology and biochemistry, not only to provide greater diagnostic accuracy, but also to guide treatment. In return, clinicians are making extensive use of their unique opportunities to observe disordered function in disease, and are thereby advancing basic physiological knowledge. For these and other reasons the contributors to this book believe that a good knowledge of physiology is becoming increasingly important in the practice of medicine. Applied physiology and functional pathology have, as yet, little place in teaching, and although there are many good textbooks of clinical biochemistry, there are few dealing with clinical physiology. This book, written by practising clinicians, is an attempt to fill the gap. We have not tried to cover the entire subject but have chosen rather to discuss those aspects which can profitably be presented from a more clinical stand-point than that of the academic physiologist, having in mind the interests of the senior student and postgraduate. Reluctantly, and only after much consultation, we decided not to include a chapter on neurology. This branch of medicine is, of course, firmly based on physiology, and neurophysiology is rapidly expanding in many directions. Unfortunately the time has not yet come when the newer knowledge can be encompassed in a short account designed for the general reader.

Each chapter is divided into four sections. The first and second sections deal with normal and disordered function. The third is an account of the physiological principles underlying tests and measurements used in modern practice. The fourth section, 'Practical Assessment', is essentially a summary of the three preceding sections, to show how the information can be used in diagnosis and assessment. We hope that this section will prove useful in clinical practice by showing how evidence can be built up starting with clinical information and then proceeding to generally available procedures and, if necessary, to special techniques. In some chapters the connection between physiology and practice is so clear that it has been possible to summarize

'Practical Assessment' in almost tabular form. Technical details of tests have not been included, because this book does not pretend to be a manual of 'function testing'. One of the happy results of increased physiological knowledge is that many symptoms, signs and tests which were formerly empirical can now be rationally explained, thereby increasing the reliance that can be placed on clinical evidence and often decreasing the need for laboratory investigations.

References have not been included in the text. A selection of monographs, reviews and key papers is given at the end of each chapter. We share the belief that students should be encouraged to use the library and we realize also that some more experienced readers will be irritated not to have some statements supported by references in the text. It is unfortunately not practicable to document the text to a degree suitable for both the beginner and the expert. The beginner will find plenty of further reading in the references and the expert should have little difficulty in tracing the source of any point. The style of presentation of the references has been chosen to help both types of readers, the title and length of all works being stated.

Although each contributor has been responsible for the preliminary writing of the section dealing with his special interest, there has been extensive consultation between contributors and editors.

ACKNOWLEDGEMENTS

We are grateful to all those who read the manuscript and who advised us about the style and content of the book. On behalf of the contributors we also thank friends and colleagues for their help. Many people have helped in the preparation; among them we would particularly like to acknowledge the following: the staff of the photographic and medical art departments of the Middlesex Hospital who prepared many of the illustrations; Mr T. F. Howarth, who checked the references; Mr L. T. Morton who compiled the index. We are grateful to the authors and publishers of illustrations reproduced and acknowledged in the text. As editors, we thank Mr Per Saugman of Blackwell Scientific Publications for his help in many ways during the publication, and the contributors for tolerating so much editorial interference.

Sir Robert Platt has always been an inspiration to clinical scientists in this country, and we are very grateful to him for writing a foreword to introduce this book.

The Middlesex Hospital   MORAN CAMPBELL
February, 1960   JOHN DICKINSON

The Body Fluids

Normal function

DISTRIBUTION AND COMPOSITION

Almost two-thirds of the body consists of water. It can be regarded as a continuous aqueous phase in which the concentration of osmotically-active particles is everywhere the same. Subdivisions can be distinguished by their chemical composition and anatomical location; these make up the body fluids. Active processes and physicochemical properties maintain differences of composition which determine the distribution of water into its different compartments. These may or may not coincide with anatomically identifiable boundaries.

The body water is both intracellular and extracellular. Extracellular fluid is further divided into interstitial fluid and plasma. These conventional subdivisions imply a homogeneity in each compartment which does not exist. For example, most of the space into which tracer substances equilibrate rapidly consists of the plasma, interstitial fluid and the lymph. Within the extracellular fluid space there is, however, additional fluid with which some tracer substances do not equilibrate at all, whilst others do so only slowly. Some of this is the fluid of dense connective tissue and cartilage; it also includes inaccessible water in bone. Some is the water of secretions, such as cerebrospinal fluid and digestive juices, which are extracellular in site but depend on glandular activity for their composition. These secretions are sometimes referred to as transcellular fluid (Fig. 1). Intracellular water almost certainly has similar but more complex subdivisions but it is not yet possible to treat it as more than one uniform compartment.

An average 70 kg man contains about 40–45 l. of water. Except for bone, tissues which do not contain fat (called the 'lean body mass') consist of 60–85 per cent water. Muscle and the grey matter of brain are the wettest tissues of the body (70–85 per cent water) whilst connective

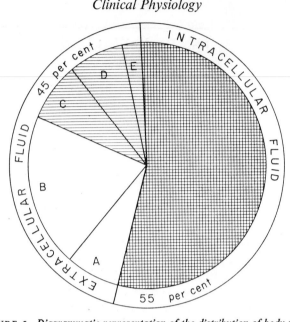

FIGURE I. *Diagrammatic representation of the distribution of body water.*
The extracellular fluid does not consist of a single functional unit. Most
of the ECF (plasma+interstitial+lymph water) is readily accessible, and
tracer substances equilibrate rapidly. The remainder of the ECF is relatively
inaccessible. Future studies may well show similar subdivisions in the ICF.

A	Plasma water	7·5 per cent
B	Interstitial and lymph water	20·0 per cent
C	Dense connective tissue water	7·5 per cent
D	Inaccessible bone water	7·5 per cent
E	Transcellular water	2·5 per cent

tissue and erythrocytes are the driest non-adipose tissues (60 per
cent water). Fat (or adipose) tissue, on the other hand, contains only
20 per cent water. A small amount of fat is a structural component of all
cells but most of it is not essential and varies from person to person.
Therefore a fat person contains, by weight, proportionately less water
than a thin one. In a normal adult man about 60 per cent of the body
weight consists of water but in obese individuals the figure falls to nearer
40 per cent. In general, women contain more fat than men so that the
water content of women is relatively less than that of men. The water
content of the body is relatively high in infancy, it falls to adult levels in
late childhood, and then falls slightly but progressively with age: the sex
difference develops at puberty and remains throughout life.

Intracellular water constitutes some 55–60 per cent of the total body water. Extracellular fluid water makes up the difference so that for an average man it amounts to about 15 l. or 20–25 per cent of the body weight. The extravascular or interstitial fluid space accounts for about 12 l. of the extracellular fluid and only 3 l. are present as plasma within the circulation. In an average man the total blood volume is about 6–8 per cent of the body weight and therefore amounts to about 70 ml/kg, which gives absolute figures for blood and plasma volumes of 5·0 l. and 3·0 l. respectively.

CELL *ECF*

$K^+ Mg^{++}, PO_4', P_r'$ $Na^+ Cl' HCO_3'$

COMPOSITION

Potassium is the main cation of intracellular fluid but magnesium is also present in smaller amounts; phosphate and protein are the principal anions. In contrast, sodium is the main cation of extracellular fluid; chloride and bicarbonate are the principal anions. Within the extracellular fluid the concentration of osmotically-active particles is identical except for slight but important modifications due to the presence of protein in the plasma.

The potassium content of the average-sized person is about 3400 m-equiv of which 90 per cent is in a freely exchangeable form (p. 35). Over 95 per cent of this, the total exchangeable potassium (K^e), is in the intracellular fluid at a concentration of about 150 m-equiv/l. whilst the remainder (less than 5 per cent) is in the extracellular fluid at a concentration of about 4 m-equiv/l. *ie. 95% K^e is in cells ; 5% = 4m-eq/l.*

The total amount of sodium in the body, as determined by carcass analysis, is about 4000 m-equiv of which 40 per cent is in bone. However, much of this bone sodium is not freely exchangeable so that the total exchangeable sodium (Na^e) represents only about 70 per cent of the total body sodium. About 3 per cent is present in the intracellular fluid, at a concentration of about 4 m-equiv/l., whilst 97 per cent is in the extracellular fluid, at a concentration of 136–144 m-equiv/l.; 57 per cent is readily accessible in the plasma, interstitial and lymph fluids and 40 per cent is present in the transcellular fluid, dense connective tissue and bone.

Magnesium behaves in an intermediate fashion because, although it is selectively concentrated within cells to a concentration of about one-third that of potassium, i.e. 45 m-equiv/l., it is also stored in bone. The total exchangeable magnesium is about 2000 m-equiv but about half of it is not freely exchangeable and this includes most of the magnesium in bone. In the plasma the concentration of magnesium is remarkably constant (1·5–1·8 m-equiv/l.) and, like calcium, about 40 per cent is protein-bound.

Cell membranes are freely permeable to water and there is a constant exchange (or 'flux') of sodium and potassium across them. This means that an active, energy-requiring process is required to maintain potassium inside and sodium outside the cell against their respective concentration gradients. The observed sodium-potassium distribution can be adequately explained by the active extrusion of sodium which creates an electro-chemical gradient of some 90 mV (positive charge outside, negative inside) opposing the outward diffusion of potassium. In some situations, this so-called sodium 'pump' may be more in the nature of an active sodium-potassium exchange.

This process of active ion transport enables the cell membrane to behave as if it were semi-permeable so that, as indicated above, changes of water content within the cell occur by passive transfer to eliminate osmotic gradients.

There is no good evidence for the idea of an active water 'pump' in mammals. The question of whether there is strict osmotic equality of intracellular and extracellular fluid is difficult to resolve because the osmolality within the cytoplasm of cells must fluctuate with its metabolic activity. On the other hand, cells do behave volumetrically as if they were osmometers.

Unlike unicellular organisms which are surrounded by a limitless fluid environment, the cells of mammals are surrounded by an extra-cellular fluid whose volume is small (15 l.) in relation to the quantity of cells it holds (45 kg). In addition, the cells of higher organisms are intolerant of changes in the temperature or composition of the fluid surrounding them. The extracellular fluid is the 'milieu intérieur' of Claude Bernard who recognized that the maintenance of a constant composition of the extracellular fluid was essential to the life of complex organisms. Respiration, absorption and selective renal excretion are all examples of special mechanisms which have evolved to maintain this constancy; these processes depend, in turn, on the circulation which keeps the extracellular fluid stirred and smooths local alterations in composition or temperature.

Since sodium ions and their equivalent anions are responsible for over 90 per cent of the osmolality of the extracellular fluid, they are the dominant variable influencing the volume of both the intracellular fluid and the extracellular fluid. All losses and gains occur through the extracellular fluid so that sodium is of central importance. Whilst losses of the main anion, chloride, can be rapidly replaced by bicarbonate no ion can replace sodium in the extracellular space. For example, a loss of sodium from the body causes a fall in the concentration of sodium within the extracellular fluid if water-drinking is continued. Osmolality is restored largely by an increased output of water from the kidneys but also by an osmotic shift of water into the cells. Both of these processes lead to a diminution in the size of the extracellular space. Similarly, if the extracellular concentration of sodium becomes raised, as in water deficiency, there is an increase in the extracellular fluid volume partly because water loss in the urine is reduced and partly because there is an osmotic transfer of water from the intracellular fluid. Therefore variations in the sodium concentration of the extracellular fluid cause profound alterations in the volume of both the extra- and intracellular fluid spaces.

EXCHANGES BETWEEN EXTRA- AND INTRAVASCULAR COMPONENTS OF THE EXTRACELLULAR FLUID

Within the extracellular space the distribution of fluid between its extra- and intravascular components depends on the forces which act across the capillary membrane. All molecules and ions smaller than proteins exchange across the capillary wall very rapidly. Water exchanges at approximately double the rate of inorganic ions. In fact the overall flux is so great that about three-quarters of the plasma exchanges with the interstitial fluid every minute. These fluxes are nearly equal in each direction so that the net exchange is very small but it is these net exchanges which matter. Net exchanges do not involve active transport and, according to the Starling concept, they depend on the hydrostatic pressure provided by the arterial blood pressure and hence the heart. This hypothesis holds that the capillary membrane is a kind of sieve which allows exchange only through the pores by ultrafiltration. Equilibrium depends on balancing hydrostatic pressure against the colloid osmotic (or oncotic) pressure of the plasma proteins. This is made up partly by the osmotic pressure of the colloid particles themselves and partly by the osmotic pressure of the extra sodium held by their ionic charges (Donnan effect). At the arterial end of the capillary the hydrostatic pressure is higher than the protein oncotic pressure so that the net flux is outwards; at the venous end the balance of pressures is reversed so that the net flux is inwards. Estimates of the magnitude of the forces concerned may now need modifying because it now seems likely that the hydrostatic pressure in the extravascular fluid is sub-atmospheric. Another possibility is that the constituents of plasma diffuse across the whole surface of the capillary endothelium according to their chemical 'activity' and co-efficient of diffusion. These forces are also influenced by hydrostatic pressure so both mechanisms may give somewhat similar results. The net result of the various forces acting across the capillary endothelium must differ, however, from tissue to tissue. Where the blood flow is sluggish diffusion may predominate but, where it is rapid hydrostatic and osmotic forces may be the main mechanism of exchange. In the lung, the hydrostatic pressure at the arterial end of the capillary is very low, so that the hydrostatic pressure difference across the endothelium is well below the colloid osmotic pressure of the plasma. Thus the conditions do not favour ultrafiltration, which would otherwise waterlog the alveoli.

Some protein inevitably escapes from the capillaries into the tissues; it must be removed because otherwise fluid would not re-enter the circulation. The terminal ends of the lymphatic vessels are freely permeable to protein. This is transported, by bulk flow, along the pressure gradient created by the low intrathoracic pressure in the thoracic duct. It is assisted by intermittent compression of lymphatics by muscular contraction. Lymphatic valves prevent retrograde flow.

EXCHANGE AND LOSS WITH THE ENVIRONMENT

The lumen of the gastro-intestinal tract, the renal excretory ducts (including the renal tubules), the sweat ducts, and the lungs can be regarded as invaginations of the external environment into the organism; fluid exchanges with the outside world take place across them because it is only in these regions that the extracellular fluid faces the environment. The size of these exchanges is very great; for example, some 170 l. of glomerular filtrate is formed each day and the digestive glands secrete about 8 l. of fluid into the alimentary tract—yet normally only 1–2 l. of all this is lost from the body each day; the remainder is reabsorbed (in the renal tubules and intestine respectively).

Routes of water loss

Internal exchanges of fluid appear to be finely controlled and the amount of free water (p. 186) lost through the kidney is strictly regulated to the body's needs (*vide infra*). In contrast, loss of water through the skin and the lungs is uncontrolled; it depends only on the humidity and temperature of the surrounding air and on the body's need to regulate its temperature. Similarly, a proportion of the water excreted as urine is osmotically inevitable and depends largely on the intake of sodium, potassium and protein (which is then broken down into urea). It is therefore impossible to define the 'normal' intake; in addition most people have drinking habits which are excessive in terms of physiological need. It is possible, however, to define the irreducible minimum beneath which the body's compensatory mechanisms become inadequate.

Normally there are four routes of water loss.

Skin. Although the outer layers of the skin are almost waterproof, the surface is moist. Water is lost continuously as vapour and is then replenished by diffusion from the deeper layers of the skin. The rate of this depends on the skin temperature, which fixes the vapour pressure, and on the humidity of the air immediately in contact with the skin. In temperate climates 300–500 ml/day are lost by evaporation and the body loses 200–300 calories of heat in the process as the latent heat of vaporization.

The skin is pierced by the ducts of the sweat glands and the amounts of water and sodium chloride, the principal sweat solute, lost as sweat are governed by the activity of the autonomic nervous system. This, in turn, is usually governed by the body's need to dissipate heat, but it may also be influenced by emotional factors. Sodium chloride is secreted actively and its concentration in sweat is usually less than half that of plasma. In temperate climates only about 5 m-equiv of sodium and less than 100 ml of water are lost through the sweat each day but these sodium chloride losses can greatly increase in hot climates, in prolonged exercise and in fevers. For example, the rate of water loss by sweating can exceed 10 l. per day. During acclimatization to a hot climate the sodium concentration in the sweat falls so that sodium loss per unit of heat loss becomes considerably less.

A distinction between sweat and 'insensible' perspiration is often made but sweat may be 'insensible' if it evaporates as fast as it is formed. It is simpler to consider losses through the skin as either pure water as vapour (sometimes called transpiration) or as a specific watery secretion containing sodium chloride which may or may not subsequently evaporate (sweat).

The lungs. Like transpiration through the skin, water loss in the expired air is inevitable. It is accompanied by the heat of vaporization. During inspiration the air is warmed to 37° and fully humidified in the respiratory tract. During expiration the air cools to 33° at the mouth and by this process returns about one-third of the water to the mucosa. Therefore, the respiratory tract operates as a heat and water exchanger with, normally, a turnover of about 1000 ml of water per day, and a net loss of 700 ml. When ventilation is greatly increased the loss of water and heat through the lung may become important.

The alimentary tract. Of about 8 l. of digestive juices secreted into the gastro-intestinal tract each day (Table I), all but about 200 ml are reabsorbed. This reabsorption of water is thought to take place passively along concentration gradients created by the active absorption of intestinal solutes. The water absorption by the bowel in excess of that needed to maintain isotonicity is not under physiological control: the amount taken by mouth is totally absorbed irrespective of need, and water intoxication can be produced. The body therefore appears to depend on the thirst mechanism to regulate the amount ingested rather than regulating the amount absorbed. Although, normally, only 100–200 ml of water are lost in the faeces each day, losses of water and electrolytes can be enormous in severe diarrhoea, especially cholera.

TABLE I. The normal daily volume, in an adult, of the various secretions into the alimentary tract
(From Gamble, J. L., 1954)

Source	Volume
Saliva	1500 ccs.
Gastric secretion	2500 ccs.
Bile	500 ccs.
Pancreatic juice	700 ccs.
Secretion of intestinal mucosa	3000 ccs.
Total	8200 ccs.
Normal plasma volume	3500 ccs.

The kidney. The kidneys control the losses of water and solutes from the extracellular fluid and so adjust both the composition and the volume of the principal fluid compartments of the body. Their main function is an active absorption of the glomerular filtrate from the tubular lumen to the blood, as in the case of the gastro-intestinal tract.

The kidney can produce a urine with a solute concentration which differs greatly from that of the plasma from which it is derived. Despite wide fluctuations of water intake and extrarenal water losses, the kidneys maintain the solute concentration and the volume of the extracellular fluid within very narrow limits. However, the human kidney cannot concentrate urine beyond 1400 m-osmols/kg. which represents a specific gravity of about 1·035. It is limited by the need to excrete excess electrolytes and end products of metabolism such as urea. There is, therefore, an obligatory volume of urine which depends on the solute intake and on the rate of urea production (Fig. 2). If the amount of water available for excretion is inadequate, then the blood urea concentration rises; similarly, if solute or protein intake is increased then a greater volume of urine is needed to prevent a rise in blood urea concentration. For example, following an acute bleed into the bowel the combination of hypovolaemia and increased protein intake is associated with a rapid rise of blood urea concentration.

The capacity of the kidney to produce a dilute urine is greater than the capacity of the kidney to produce a concentrated one. Urine can be diluted to about 30 m-osmole/kg. which is over 10 times less than the osmolality of plasma water; it can be concentrated to 1400 m-osmole/kg.

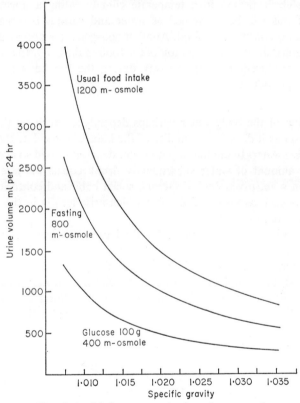

FIGURE 2. *The relationship between maximal renal concentrating power and minimal obligatory urine volume at three different solute loads.*

The upper curve is for a normal dietary intake which provides about 1200 mOsm. to be excreted daily. Breakdown of tissue protein under fasting conditions (middle curve) produces 800 mOsm. daily. Provision of calories in the form of glucose spares protein breakdown and the solute load is reduced to 400 mOsm. The minimal obligatory urine volume is increased by a fall in the concentrating power or a rise in the solute load.

(Modified from Gamble, 1954.)

which is only about 4 times more than the osmolality of plasma water. In fact the main function of vasopressin (antidiuretic hormone) is to prevent over-dilution of the urine and the water saved by not excreting a dilute urine is many times greater than the water saved by excreting a maximally concentrated one.

To remain in water balance, the intake of water must, of course, at least equal the water lost by all routes. The precise minimum daily water intake is necessarily variable but will range from 500 to 1000 ml/day for an afebrile person in a temperate climate eating a normal diet. Some of this will be consumed as water and various beverages, but about half is consumed as food. Another 200–300 ml is provided by the water formed during the oxidation of the food in the body. In starvation water is produced in a similar way during the breakdown of body tissues to provide energy.

Thirst

Regulation of the body water perhaps depends as much on the thirst mechanism as it does on the ability of the kidney to regulate the excretion of free water. In animals a pure water deficit is sensed so accurately that the amount of water subsequently drunk equals the size of the deficit. In man, psychological factors, social habit and confusion over sensations such as taste and dryness which arise locally in the mouth, often obscure this mechanism.

Hypertonicity of the extracellular fluid does not, *per se*, stimulate water-drinking. In uraemia, for example, the plasma osmolality may be greatly increased but thirst is not a prominent symptom. If, on the other hand, the osmolality of the extracellular fluid is increased by the administration of hypertonic saline then intense thirst ensues. Urea crosses cell membranes readily so that there is no osmolar disequilibrium between the fluid inside and that outside the cells but sodium chloride does not, so the cells shrink. Intracellular dehydration is not the only stimulus to water-drinking because contraction of the extracellular fluid, as when isotonic fluid is lost from the body in severe diarrhoea or haemorrhage, is associated with a feeling which, for most people, is indistinguishable from that of thirst. The fact that the plasma sodium concentration tends to fall in hypovolaemia probably reflects this stimulus to increased water-drinking which still occurs when the extracellular osmolality is low rather than high.

EXCHANGE AND LOSS OF SODIUM CHLORIDE

In contrast to water where the main problem facing the body is conservation, the inevitable losses of sodium from the body are normally so small that sodium balance can be preserved almost indefinitely on a diet as low in sodium as the dietician's ingenuity can fashion. In the absence of visible sweat or diarrhoea, sodium losses occur exclusively through the kidney which has such remarkable powers of sodium conservation that the urine may contain no more sodium than tap water. Even with a greatly reduced intake of sodium, say 10 m-equiv/day, equilibration with intake occurs within 3–6 days, depending on the initial sodium intake. The total loss of sodium from the body is only about 200 m-equiv—or less than 10 per cent of the total exchangeable sodium. In man, this is brought about mainly by an increase in the rate of sodium reabsorption by the kidney, particularly by the proximal tubules. Usually, however, dietary intake is unnecessarily large in relation to need. Western diets usually contain between 100 and 300 m-equiv of sodium so that in the overall economy of the body the problem is not one of conservation, like water, but one of the excretion of an excess. Nevertheless, so far as the kidney is concerned, the problem is one of conservation. About 24,000 m-equiv of sodium are filtered each day at the renal glomeruli—or approximately 10 times the total exchangeable sodium in the body—yet all but about half per cent of this is normally reabsorbed by the renal tubules. The energy required for this process accounts for most of the oxygen consumed by the kidney.

REGULATION OF FLUID BALANCE
Because of the need to maintain the volume of the circulating blood and hence an adequate rate of perfusion of vital organs, the regulation of the body fluids is dominated by the factors regulating the volume and composition of the extracellular fluid. Although closely interrelated, regulation of the volume and regulation of the composition of the extracellular fluid are best considered separately because the mechanisms are different.

Regulation of the osmotic composition
Sodium chloride makes up over 93 per cent of the osmotic pressure of the extracellular fluid and hence of the plasma. In health, the osmolality within this space is remarkably constant and varies by less than 1 per cent despite wide fluctuations in the solute intake. This is carried out by changes in the rate of free water clearance by the kidney (p. 186) under the delicate control of vasopressin secreted by the hypothalamic osmoreceptor-posterior pituitary mechanisms (p. 514). Sodium concentration in the extracellular fluid is therefore controlled over short periods more by changes of the volume of the extracellular fluid than

by changes of its total sodium content. However, in many clinical situations quite large alterations of the concentration of sodium chloride in the extracellular fluid are tolerable, and factors other than osmolality can become important influences on the rate of vasopressin release. Blood volume is an important influence, possibly acting through receptors in the left atrium. For example, a rapid infusion of isotonic saline may be followed by a pure water diuresis of the type associated with inhibition of vasopressin. Emotion, exercise and various drugs such as barbiturates and morphine enhance the rate of vasopressin secretion; ethanol depresses it.

Control of the volume of the extracellular fluid

Although the osmolality in the extracellular fluid is largely controlled by relatively quick changes of the rate of renal excretion of osmotically free water via the vasopressin mechanism, the factors controlling the volume of the extracellular fluid are less well understood. One reason for this is that, unlike measurements of osmolality, measurements of the volume of the extracellular fluid are notoriously imprecise. They depend on the volume of distribution of appropriate substances and are liable to errors of equilibrium and representative sampling as well as to errors of chemical estimation (p. 34). However, since sodium and its equivalent anions are the main osmotically-active constituents of the extracellular fluid, the problem resolves itself into the factors controlling that portion of the total body sodium which is physiologically effective. Since the sodium concentration of the extracellular fluid is normally kept within narrow limits, the total sodium content of the extracellular fluid must govern its overall volume. Extrarenal sodium losses are normally negligible in the absence of sweating, so that the rate of sodium excretion by the kidney determines the volume of the extracellular fluid.

As mentioned above, the way in which the kidney monitors the extracellular fluid volume must be very sensitive indeed. Any manoeuvre which reduces the physiologically effective volume of plasma such as haemorrhage or pooling of blood in the legs (by cuffing of the thighs, tilting or quiet standing) also reduces the rate of sodium excretion in the urine; conversely, manoeuvres which increase the plasma volume, such as infusions of isotonic sodium chloride, increase the rate of sodium excretion in the urine. Although changes of the rate of the glomerular filtration are probably important in mediating rapid exchanges of sodium excretion, changes in the rate of tubular sodium reabsorption are more important, at least in man, in mediating more prolonged changes. How this is done is controversial. Eighty-five per cent of the filtered sodium chloride is reabsorbed isotonically in the proximal tubule. This is an active process but is probably influenced by hydro-static forces. It has been termed 'obligatory' and this carries with it the implication that changes in the rate of tubular sodium reabsorption to meet the needs of the body are not mediated via the proximal tubule. About 15 per cent of the filtered sodium is reabsorbed in the distal tubule; this process is also an active one and it consists partly of sodium reabsorbed together with chloride and partly of sodium reabsorbed in exchange for potassium and hydrogen. It has been termed 'facultative' because the rate of sodium reabsorption by the distal tubule is detectably related to the needs of the body. Just how the rate of tubular sodium reabsorption is geared to the volume of the extracellular fluid is debatable but it seems likely that there are receptors sensitive to some function of the circulating blood volume which provide the afferent stimulus. The efferent stimulus is probably humoral and here the role of the adrenal cortex is important.

Cortisol, from the adrenal fasiculata-reticularis, does have some mineralocorticoid activity but only about 10–20 per cent of the total mineralocorticoid activity in the adrenal venous blood can be ascribed to it. It does, however, sustain a normal rate of glomerular filtration and is necessary for the normal renal response to a water load. Aldosterone, from the adrenal glomerulosa, is the principal mineralocorticoid and is an important influence on the rate of exchange of sodium for potassium and hydrogen in the distal tubule. Without it sodium depletion occurs if the sodium intake is not increased considerably. Unlike cortisol, which is governed by the pituitary gland, the rate of aldosterone secretion is a close inverse function of the volume of the plasma and extracellular fluid: salt loading depresses it and salt depletion increases it.

Other humoral factors, apart from adrenocortical hormones, are also important in the control of the rate of sodium excretion by the kidney. For example the renin-angiotensin system (p. 165) potentially provides a way by which the kidney could sense the degree of filling on the arterial side of the circulation and at the same time provide an effector mechanism to influence it. Renin is produced by specialized cells in the wall of the afferent arteriole (p. 149) and its rate of secretion may be inversely related to the degree of distension of these vessels. Renin produces angiotensin II which stimulates aldosterone production and also directly influences the rate of sodium excretion by the kidney. A slow rate of infusion of angiotensin promotes sodium retention in man, and most animals; rapid rates of infusion cause a sodium and water diuresis. The diuretic effect of angiotensin in some patients with cirrhosis of the liver is probably related to the initially high plasma concentration. Whether the rôle of the renin-angiotensin system in the control of salt is analogous to that of vasopressin in the control of water remains to be seen. Recent experiments suggest that the increased rate of sodium excretion which follows a rapid saline infusion depends on some humoral mechanism other than angiotensin or aldoterone but the nature and site of production of the hormone are not yet established.

CONTROL OF POTASSIUM

The factors controlling the amount of potassium in the body are largely independent of those controlling the amount of sodium and water. They are, however, related. The rate of potassium excretion in the urine depends on the activity of the sodium/potassium exchange mechanism and on the rate of hydrogen ion secretion in the distal tubule. The rate of sodium/potassium exchange depends on the aldosterone concentration acting on the renal tubular cell and also on the amount of sodium available for exchange in the distal tubule. For example, rapid sodium loading increases potassium excretion and depresses the level of potassium in the plasma; sodium depletion reduces the rate of potassium excretion and increases the level of potassium in the plasma. All but about 10 per cent of the ingested potassium is excreted in the urine by tubular secretion; the filtered potassium is almost wholly reabsorbed. Therefore, under most circumstances the rate of urine excretion of potassium is poorly related to the concentration of potassium in plasma but correlates much better with what may be inferred to be the potassium concentration inside cells. For example, when the intake of potassium is reduced, the rate of urinary potassium excretion takes much longer to fall compared with the rate at which the body comes into equilibrium with a reduction of sodium intake. The concentration of potassium in the plasma is therefore related to excretion only in so far as there is a relationship between the plasma potassium concentration and the concentration of potassium within the cells. This relationship is closely dependent on the relative hydrogen ion concentrations inside and outside the cells. Extracellular alkalosis increases the gradient of potassium across the cell membrane and extracellular acidosis reduces it. Conversely, potassium depletion is associated with an intracellular acidosis and an extracellular alkalosis. Because of these intimate interrelationships between potassium and the hydrogen ion, the urine may be acid despite an extracellular alkalosis (p. 212).

The amount of potassium in the body cells appears, superficially, to be quite delicately controlled by some homeostatic mechanism. For example, a moderate load of potassium (say 60 m-equiv) is accurately and promptly (within 2 hr) excreted in the urine. Whether this means that there is a true physiological control mechanism is uncertain because it may simply be the result of an increased potassium concentration in the body cells, particularly those of the renal tubules. Dehydration, which increases intracellular potassium concentration by a different mechanism, also promotes potassium excretion. On the other hand, a control mechanism via aldosterone may operate. Aldosterone promotes potassium loss from both renal tubular cells and the mucosa of the large bowel. But the rate of aldosterone production, and hence the probable activity of aldosterone on the renal and intestinal cells, itself varies directly with the plasma potassium concentration, and hence, in most situations, with the intracellular potassium concentration.

CONTROL OF MAGNESIUM

Little is known about the control of magnesium but it is probably linked with the control of potassium and calcium. Magnesium and calcium may share a common transport system in the renal tubule because the rate of tubular reabsorption of magnesium tends to vary inversely with that of calcium. The same may be true in the intestine because the rate of magnesium excretion in the faeces, which is normally about two-thirds of the magnesium intake, falls when dietary calcium is reduced.

Disordered function

BODY FLUID DEPLETION

Depletion of body fluid occurs either because the intake of water is not enough to correct the inevitable losses of water (p. 6) or because there is an abnormal loss of fluid from the body. Fluid losses nearly always consist of extracellular fluid or minor modifications of it. Both water and electrolytes are lost; either without protein, as in diarrhoea and vomiting, or with protein, as in haemorrhage or burns. The situation is dominated by the effects of sodium loss because this ion controls the volume of the extracellular fluid and hence the plasma. Losses of isotonic fluid are therefore spoken of as leading to salt depletion but the clinical condition itself is often called 'dehydration'. This is loose terminology because the clinical effects of pure water deficiency and pure sodium deficiency are different. Often, however, there is a net water deficit in addition to loss of isotonic fluid so that a mixed picture of water and salt depletion results. In addition, deficits of potassium and disturbances of hydrogen ion regulation may complicate the issue. For the sake of clarity, however, the different types of depletion will be considered separately.

WATER DEPLETION

In contrast to sodium depletion, water depletion is usually caused by an inadequate intake. Water depletion from an excessive rate of water loss is rare, even if the vasopressin mechanism is defective, because thirst, a compelling symptom, develops early. Water is first lost from the extracellular fluid where the osmolality rises. Water is drawn out of the cells to maintain osmotic equilibrium so that the main result is cellular dehydration with a relatively small contraction of the extracellular fluid volume. Genuine thirst is intense and the blood pressure is maintained until relatively late. The urine is highly concentrated and its volume low owing to an increased rate of secretion of vasopressin. The blood urea concentration rises relatively early, not so much because there is a fall in the renal blood flow but because urea reabsorption by the renal tubules increases when the rate of urine formation is low (p. 162). Contraction of the extracellular fluid and plasma volumes with haemo-concentration only occur late so that apart from a dry mouth there are few physical signs. In confused or comatose patients who are unable to describe their symptoms, this may cause diagnostic difficulties. Fever may be due to water deficiency alone, particularly in infants. The concentration of all the constituents of plasma tends to increase. This is particularly obvious (and relevant) with sodium because the plasma sodium concentration normally varies so slightly (p. 29). Although the concentration of plasma proteins is increased, the haematocrit (packed cell volume) is not because, in contrast to sodium depletion, loss of fluid from the plasma is matched by a corresponding loss from the erythrocytes.

Pure water deficiency is particularly prone to develop when the powers of water conservation by the kidney are impaired either because vasopressin is not produced as in pituitary diabetes insipidus, or because the effect of vasopressin on the renal tubules is weakened, as in nephrogenic diabetes insipidus, in infancy, and in the renal lesion of sickle-cell anaemia. It is also common when the thirst mechanism is impaired as in patients with intracranial lesions.

SODIUM DEPLETION

The kidneys' powers of sodium conservation are so good that it is impossible to develop serious sodium depletion by a reduction of intake alone. There is very little obligatory loss of sodium from the body so that in contrast to water deficiency, which is commonly caused by an inadequate intake, clinically recognizable sodium depletion is virtually synonymous with an excessive rate of sodium loss. This almost always takes place as a loss of isotonic extracellular fluid from the circulation as in haemorrhage, from the interstitial fluid as in sweating, diarrhoea and vomiting, or, more subtly, by a reduction of the rate of isotonic sodium chloride reabsorption in the proximal tubules of the kidney as in the osmotic diuresis of diabetic ketosis. The renal mechanism of isotonic fluid loss is illustrated nicely by the response to a simple reduction of salt intake. Since, as a first approximation, the amount of fluid held in the extracellular space depends on the amount of sodium in the body, a reduction of sodium intake leads initially to a loss of isotonic fluid in the urine so that it remains relatively dilute as compared with the concentrated urine of water deficiency. In teleological terms, the serum osmolality is maintained at the expense of volume. Soon, however, the resulting hypovolaemia stimulates vasopressin release; water loss lessens and, provided water drinking continues, there is dilution of the extra-cellular fluid. To restore osmotic equilibrium some water is lost, not through the kidneys, but into the cells which therefore swell.

Within the extracellular fluid the diminution of volume is not evenly distributed between its intra- and extravascular components because the osmotic pressure of the plasma proteins tends to maintain the plasma volume at the expense of the interstitial cell volume. This mechanism is good protection when the loss of extracellular fluid is slight and slow but if the loss is considerable and rapid it is easily overwhelmed and the circulatory volume falls. For example, sodium losses of 200–300 m-equiv may be difficult to detect clinically but with a relatively small further loss the blood pressure may drop swiftly. The depletion of plasma volume leads to an increase of haematocrit and plasma protein concentration. The low plasma volume is reflected by a low central venous pressure, diminished cardiac output, a narrow pulse pressure and, later, arterial hypotension. Selective vasoconstriction diminishes the blood flow to the skin which becomes cold. The superficial veins are empty and they fill slowly. Inelasticity of the skin and reduction of intraocular tension reflect interstitial fluid depletion and so are early signs. Arterial hypotension induces weakness, postural faintness, and tachycardia. Other effects of sodium depletion, such as anorexia, vomiting and muscle cramps do not depend on hypovolaemia. Since they are also seen in water intoxication, they may be the result of the increased intracellular fluid volume and cellular hypotonicity.

As the circulating volume becomes further reduced, vasoconstriction involves the kidneys; perfusion of the glomeruli becomes inadequate and the blood urea rises, causing 'prerenal' uraemia (p. 172).

The clinical picture of sodium depletion varies with the size of the deficit and the time over which it has developed. Mild states are associated with a deficit of 100–150 m-equiv but alimentary losses and urine losses (as in the osmotic diuresis of severe diabetic ketosis) may cause deficits of 1500 m-equiv or more.

The condition of sodium depletion is often referred to as salt depletion. This implies an equal deficit of sodium and chloride. Sodium and chloride are usually lost roughly in the proportion of 3:2, which is their concentration ratio in the extracellular fluid. In vomiting of gastric contents or in the excess urinary chloride loss produced by some diuretics, the relative deficits of the two ions are, however, dissimilar so that changes of chloride concentration (in the urine, for example) are a poor index of changes of sodium balance. When sodium is lost, the volume of the extracellular fluid falls but when chloride is lost, even in large amounts, ECF volume hardly changes, although its composition is altered.

POTASSIUM DEPLETION

The kidney cannot conserve potassium as readily as it conserves sodium. Potassium depletion may develop, therefore, because the intake of potassium is reduced, as in anorexia or prolonged intravenous fluid therapy. Nevertheless considerable potassium depletion usually means abnormal losses. These occur through the gastro-intestinal tract, through the kidneys, or through both. For example, gastric juice contains about the same concentration of potassium as plasma and intermittent vomiting of gastric contents with an otherwise normal intake is not an important cause of potassium depletion, but when vomiting is severe and associated with hypovolaemia and semi-starvation, as in pyloric stenosis, then considerable potassium depletion may occur. The reason is not simply loss of potassium in the vomit (even 2 l. of gastric juice only contain about 10 m-equiv of potassium) but because there is a secondary increase of potassium loss in the urine. The reduction of volume of the extracellular fluid increases the rate of aldosterone secretion which, if enough sodium reaches the distal tubule (see below), promotes tubular Na/K exchange; and the extracellular alkalosis also promotes potassium secretion in the distal tubule by increasing the concentration of potassium within its cells (p. 165). Furthermore, lost tissue protein will carry potassium with it.

Potassium depletion may occur as a specific event but whenever a patient is breaking down tissue protein, loss of potassium is inevitable. It is fixed by the extent of the negative nitrogen balance; for each gram of nitrogen excreted in excess of intake, 2·7 m-equiv of potassium goes with it. Therefore the potassium 'deficiency' so induced is not inappropriate when body potassium content is expressed in units of lean body mass.

An important source of potassium loss is through the large bowel. In the upper intestinal juices the ratio of Na/K, like plasma, is about 20:1 but in the stools the ratio is nearer 1:2 and in diarrhoea potassium losses become even more disproportionate to sodium losses. Although undue sodium loss does not occur in a formed stool, significant potassium losses can occur in bulky solid stools, as in steatorrhoea and excessive purgation.

Excess potassium loss through the kidneys may be part of a general process of discharge of potassium from cells; it may be the result of a high concentration of aldosterone or other factors influencing the ion exchange process in the distal tubule (p. 163); or, rarely it may be caused by a primary defect of tubular potassium secretion, as in some renal tubular lesions.

Since the intracellular potassium concentration diminishes as the extracellular concentration of hydrogen-ion rises, acidaemia, as in diabetic ketosis, causes a redistribution of potassium so that there is relatively more outside cells. An extracellular alkalosis does the reverse and since the rate of potassium secretion by the renal tubules depends partly on the potassium concentration within them, the rate of potassium excretion increases.

Starvation produces potassium depletion both by inducing a negative nitrogen balance and by the fact that intracellular potassium concentration is influenced by the rate at which glucose enters cells. When this is slow, there is a diminution of the efficiency of the active process which maintains the potassium gradient across the cell membrane so that potassium tends to leak out along its concentration gradient.

The rate of ion-exchange in the distal tubule is the dominant intra-renal mechanism which determines the rate of potassium loss in the urine. It is enhanced, not only by the activity of aldosterone and other agents having mineralo-corticoid actions, but also, more intimately, by the amount of sodium available for exchange which is delivered to the distal tubule. Therefore any factor, such as the action of most diuretics, osmotic or otherwise, which inhibits sodium reabsorption proximal to the site of Na/K exchange, will tend to enhance potassium loss in the urine. Potassium depletion produced by abnormal losses through the kidney is therefore seen in the hyperaldosteronism of adrenal glomerulosa tumours and malignant hypertension, and also following the use of diuretics which act chiefly on the rate of sodium reabsorption in the more proximal portions of the nephron.

Excessive external loss of potassium reduces its concentration inside cells. To maintain intracellular osmolality, potassium is replaced by hydrogen ion, sodium, and cationic amino-acids from the extracellular fluid. The cells become more acid and there is an extracellular alkalosis. This remains largely uncompensated possibly because pulmonary ventilation and hence the arterial Pco_2 is determined by the hydrogen-ion concentration inside the cells of the medullary control mechanism which are, if anything, more acid than normal (p. 211).

Potassium deficits of up to about 10 per cent of the total exchangeable potassium are usually well tolerated but if there is an associated sodium and water depletion, small deficits may cause symptoms, particularly if they occur rapidly. These are largely determined by the effect of potassium on muscle and renal function. Smooth muscle is particularly vulnerable to the effects of potassium depletion. In the heart, arrythmias and myocardial inefficiency with hypotension are common. The heart may stop in diastole. The electrocardiogram shows depression of the S-T segments, prolongation of the Q-T interval, T-wave flattening, and the appearance of U-waves. The direct myocardial effects of digitalis are enhanced. In the gastro-intestinal tract, abdominal distension and constipation may be features of chronic potassium deficiency but acute depletion may precipitate paralytic ileus. Skeletal muscles are usually weak, flaccid, and respond poorly to the deep tendon reflexes; less commonly, carpo-pedal spasm with hyper-reflexia may result. Many undefined factors influence the effect of potassium deficiency on skeletal muscle function but they must include the actual gradient of potassium across cell membranes because this determines the threshold for depolarizing stimuli. In potassium depletion, this gradient can clearly be high or low, depending on other factors which influence the distribution of potassium across the cell membrane.

In the kidney, potassium depletion causes a specific renal tubular lesion characterized functionally by an inability to concentrate the urine normally and an increased susceptibility to infection (p. 175).

MAGNESIUM DEPLETION

Magnesium depletion is probably more common than usually recognized, and occurs in situations similar to those in which potassium deficiencies arise, and also when the concentration of calcium in the plasma is abnormal. Thus, it can be important in malabsorption syndromes, in primary hyperaldosteronism, in renal tubular defects, in cirrhosis of the liver, and after diuretic therapy. It may also be produced in patients losing gut fluids after surgical operations, unless magnesium supplements are given.

Magnesium deficiency is recognized by a plasma magnesium concentration of less than 1·4 m-equiv/l. Most of the clinical manifestations are non-specific, e.g. tremor, ataxia, irritability, weakness: most important, however, are convulsions, which can be fatal. Carpopedal spasm does not occur without hypocalcaemia but Chvostek's sign may be present.

In all species of animals studied, magnesium deficiency tends to produce hypercalcaemia and the rapid development of nephrocalcinosis. It is not known whether the same is true of man.

There is an invariable fall of plasma magnesium concentration following removal of a functioning parathyroid tumour, presumably because of the rapid sequestration of magnesium in bone.

BODY FLUID EXCESS

The effects of an excess of fluid in the body depend on which of the body fluid compartments is particularly affected. A fluid which contains protein or some other material, such as dextran which exerts a colloid osmotic pressure, is initially largely confined to the circulation. The central venous pressure rises and cardiac embarrassment with pulmonary and peripheral oedema commonly develop secondarily if the amount and rate of administration are excessive. A fluid which contains sodium, but no colloid material, diffuses freely throughout the whole extracellular fluid space so causing oedema directly as well as overfilling the circulation. Water (or a fluid containing solute, such as glucose, which is removed metabolically) is distributed throughout the body cells as well as the extracellular fluid. Overfilling of the circulation and some oedema do result but the effects of water intoxication are dominated by the consequences of swelling of the brain cells. This is commonly called cerebral 'oedema' despite the fact that the excess fluid is inside rather than outside the cells.

WATER INTOXICATION

This only develops when there is some impairment of the ability of the kidney to excrete water. It may be due to an inappropriately high rate of vasopressin release (i.e. inappropriate for the prevailing plasma osmolality), or it may be due to intrinsic renal disease. An irritative lesion of the supra-optico-hypophysial tract may release vasopressin irrespective of the body's needs and a tumour, commonly of bronchial origin, may also produce, autonomously, an antidiuretic material indistinguishable from vasopressin. In other situations, the vasopressin-releasing mechanism may be normal but the stimulus of hypovolaemia overcomes the inhibiting effect of hypo-osmolality. For example, sodium depletion, *per se*, impairs the ability to excrete a water load probably because contraction of the extracellular fluid volume stimulates vasopressin release despite the fall of plasma osmolality. A similar mechanism probably explains the hyponatraemia which is so common in patients with hypoproteinaemic oedema, particularly when it is due to cirrhosis of the liver. Although there is clearly a gross excess of total body sodium, the physiologically effective plasma volume is reduced, so maintaining vasopressin secretion. The tendency to water retention seen after surgical trauma is probably due to the combined effects of anaesthesia, emotion and hypovolaemia which provoke a discharge of vasopressin.

More commonly, water intoxication is caused by intrinsic renal disease. In acute renal failure, severe oliguria clearly predisposes to water intoxication and the regulation of water intake is a major feature of its treatment. In chronic renal failure, there is also an inability to excrete a water load at a normal rate, despite the presence of polyuria (p. 188).

The main symptoms of water intoxication are headache, nausea and confusion; later, convulsions and coma occur. They are caused by cerebral 'oedema'. The face may be puffy and the central venous pressure elevated. The peripheral vessels are full. The plasma constituents are disturbed; this is particularly noticeable in the sodium concentration which falls well below its normally narrow range. Paradoxically, the urine is usually of low volume (or at least lower than it should be) and its osmolality may be higher than that of the plasma, particularly after surgical trauma. It reflects, therefore, the cause rather than the result of water intoxication. The rate of sodium excretion in the urine varies according to the cause but, in general, it tends to be high because the rate of aldosterone secretion is depressed by expansion of the extracellular fluid. This is particularly obvious in the 'salt wasting' syndrome seen in patients with chronic water intoxication due to inappropriate vasopressin secretion.

MECHANISMS OF OEDEMA FORMATION

Excess fluid between the cells (interstitial fluid) produces clinically recognizable oedema if it exceeds 10 per cent of its normal volume. It occurs whenever there is a disruption of the normal exchanges across the capillary endothelium. Increased colloid osmotic pressure of the interstitial fluid results when protein leaks through excessively permeable capillaries as in urticaria, inflammation or angioneurotic oedema; or when the normal amount of protein which leaks through capillary walls cannot be removed, as in lymphatic obstruction. Increased pressure at the venous end of the capillaries, caused by an obstructed venous return; or a decrease of tissue tension may also cause oedema. Lax tissues encourage the accumulation of oedema around the eyes when lying flat, as in acute nephritis. With hypoproteinaemic syndromes, such as the nephrotic syndrome, cirrhosis of the liver and protein-losing enteropathy, increased fluid transudation will tend to occur in all capillaries due to the fall of plasma colloid osmotic pressure. It is most obvious in capillary beds subject to the effect of gravity. If fluid transudation is extensive enough, the plasma volume falls. The kidney senses this so quickly that by reducing the rate of sodium and water loss in the urine, the reduction of plasma volume is usually made good.

In other oedematous conditions, the first event is an inability of the kidney to excrete sodium rather than increased fluid loss through capillaries. This tends to happen whenever the rate of glomerular filtration is primarily reduced. This may be due to reduced renal perfusion, as in some patients with cardiac failure, or it may be due to glomerular damage, as in chronic renal failure.

When the primary event is fluid loss by extensive capillary transudation, as in the hypoproteinaemic syndromes, the resulting fall in plasma volume stimulates potent renal sodium retaining mechanisms. These may be glomerular or tubular in nature and some component of the renin-angiotensin system is probably involved. Although the rate of glomerular filtration, which is a major influence on the rate of renal sodium loss, is a sensitive function of the effective plasma volume, hypoproteinaemia will tend to counteract any fall of the rate of glomerular filtration by reducing the colloid osmotic pressure which normally limits it; some of the highest rates of glomerular filtration recorded in man have been observed in the nephrotic syndrome. Therefore, at least in man, tubular factors are dominant. Among these, the best known is aldosterone (p. 522) which is produced at very high rates in hypoproteinaemia. The concentration of aldosterone in the plasma is almost always a direct function of its rate of secretion which is specifically increased by a reduction of plasma volume, even though the volume of the interstitial cell fluid rises. The result is sodium retention. However, this simple and comfortable concept ignores two important facts. Firstly, the sodium retention in hypoproteinaemia is not usually associated with obvious hypokalaemia, as would be expected if aldosterone were exerting its well-known function of accelerating the Na/K exchange process in the distal tubules. In fact the increased sodium reabsorption takes place in the proximal tubule rather than the distal one, and the absence of much potassium deficiency (in the absence of diuretic therapy) is explained by inadequate delivery of sodium to the site of distal Na/K exchange (p. 163). Whether this means that hypoproteinaemia enables aldosterone to have a dominant action on the proximal tubule or whether, as is generally believed, there is some other process which enhances proximal tubular sodium reabsorption is not known (p. 13). Secondly, the existence of another major factor which promotes sodium retention in hypoproteinaemic oedema is illustrated by the fact that hyperaldosteronism caused by a tumour of the zona glomerulosa (p. 533) or by malignant hypertension (p. 69) is not characterized by oedema unless hypertensive heart failure is present. In addition, if large doses of aldosterone are given to normal people repeatedly, a paradoxical increase of sodium excretion takes place in about 10 days. The mechanism of this 'escape' phenomenon is obscure but the faster the rate of expansion of the extracellular fluid, the earlier it happens.

In contrast to hypoproteinaemic oedema, the rate of aldosterone production is not enhanced when the primary event is increased sodium retention by the kidney because the plasma volume is increased rather than decreased. In cardiac failure, for example, hyperaldosteronism is inconspicuous unless hypoproteinaemia is present.

HAEMORRHAGE

The immediate response to a rapid loss of, say, 10 per cent of the total blood volume (500 ml) is probably a reduction in the capacity of the circulation by reflex constriction of the veins. This is mediated by low pressure receptors in the large veins. Somewhat later, when the arterial pulse pressure falls, the mechanoreceptor reflex mechanisms in the carotid body and aortic arch (p. 42) provoke peripheral vasoconstriction of the resistance vessels, with discharge of noradrenaline from sympathetic nerve endings. This is most obvious in the circulation of tissues such as the skin, the splanchnic area and the kidneys, where the calibre of the resistance vessels (p. 45) is largely controlled by the adrenergic activity of the sympathetic system. It is minimal in the circulation of tissues such as the brain and myocardium, where local factors rather than sympathetic tone are dominant in controlling the calibre of the resistance vessels. The result is a pale, cold, clammy skin, slow capillary filling, tachycardia, and oliguria. The cardiac output may or may not fall although the central venous pressure is reduced. Different individuals vary greatly in their ability to compensate for blood loss but, in general, compensatory mechanisms are most active in the young and fit and least active in the old and debilitated. In young people the heart rate increases early and the blood pressure may barely fall, whereas in old people the blood pressure may fall early without tachycardia.

Because the capillary perfusion pressure falls after haemorrhage, the equilibrium of the various forces acting across the capillary membranes is disturbed so that protein-free tissue fluid is drawn into the circulation. This process is limited both because the colloid osmotic pressure of the plasma falls and also because the hydrostatic pressure in the interstitial fluid falls considerably. However the rapid increase in the rate of albumin synthesis by the liver offsets these limitations so that this mechanism, as well as the associated oliguria, probably explains why, after a loss of, say, 500 ml of blood, the plasma volume is made up within hours. It takes weeks for the loss of erythrocytes to be replaced. Changes of haematocrit reflect the rates of these various processes; at first, there is little change but within a few hours the haematocrit falls and then rises slowly.

Sometimes a different reaction occurs despite a relatively small haemorrhage, because the patient faints (vasomotor syncope). This phenomenon was formerly called 'primary shock'. The faint, which is associated with a sudden fall of blood pressure, pronounced bradycardia and sweating, is due to sudden vasodilatation in muscle, mediated by cholinergic vasomotor nerves (p. 63).

SHOCK

When a haemorrhage is too large compensation fails. A state of 'shock' or peripheral circulatory failure is then said to exist. This is characterized clinically by an exaggeration of the response to a smaller bleed; the arterial pressure is low, the pulse is weak and rapid, the extremities are pale, cold and sweaty, and the peripheral veins are empty. The patient is weak, restless, apprehensive and often disorientated with deep, sighing respirations. At this stage the cardiac output is characteristically low and the peripheral resistance unchanged or higher than before. Tissue perfusion falls and oxidative metabolism is compromised, causing lactic acidosis. Cells die and their enzymes are released into the blood stream. Capillary stagnation leads to further reduction of the effective circulating volume by peripheral sequestration. This may be aggravated by agglutination of the erythrocytes or by haemoconcentration, as seen after extensive trauma or severe burns.

The clinical syndrome of shock can also occur after acute myocardial infarction or pulmonary embolism. The existence of this so-called cardiogenic shock lends support to the idea that the syndrome of shock following haemorrhage is also primarily due to a failure of cardiac output.

Sometimes shock cannot be corrected by apparently adequate replacement of blood volume. This state of so-called 'irreversible' shock is commonly due to an underestimation of the volume of the blood loss but after prolonged and severe blood loss the blood pressure may only be maintained at the expense of a progressively increasing central venous pressure. In animals irreversible shock is associated with the accumulation of bacterial endotoxins. These may permeate into the blood stream through intestinal mucosa damaged by anoxia, or splanchnic vasoconstriction may so damage the liver that it fails to destroy normally absorbed endotoxins. In man there is no evidence of this but it is certainly true that sepsis potentiates shock.

Irreversible shock is also caused by acute adrenal insufficiency (p. 526). Unless this is present, shock, whether hypovolaemic or cardiogenic, is associated with greatly increased levels of cortisol in the blood. Nevertheless, heroic doses of cortisol may help clinically by increasing tissue blood flow.

METABOLIC RESPONSE TO INJURY

After any injury there is a metabolic response which is, in general, proportional to the degree of trauma. It is characterized (i) by a very low output of concentrated urine for 24–36 hr. This is due to an increased rate of production of vasopressin, probably stimulated by hypovolaemia, pain, and anaesthesia (p. 514). Excess loads of water cannot be excreted; (ii) immediate reduction of sodium excretion which lasts for 3–5 days. This may be due to increased secretion of aldosterone from the adrenal glomerulosa because it is associated with a loss of potassium in the urine in excess of nitrogen, particularly in the first 2–3 days; and (iii) a negative nitrogen balance, the so-called catabolic phase. This is presumably due to a combination of starvation and tissue breakdown, both due to the injury and to an increased rate of adreno-corticotrophic hormone release (and hence secretion of cortisol) which occurs in the first 24 hr.

In addition, injury is associated with a movement of sodium into cells and a movement of potassium out of them. The plasma sodium concentration falls (contributing to the dilution hyponatraemia often observed) and the plasma concentration of potassium may rise. These changes indicate a temporary disturbance of selective membrane permeability.

Principles of tests and measurements

PACKED CELL VOLUME (PCV)

The packed cell volume (or haematocrit) gives an index of the concentration of erythrocytes in a sample of blood. It is the height of the column of erythrocytes after centrifugation in a graduated tube, expressed as a percentage of the total height of the column of liquid. The PCV is influenced by the shape and size of the erythrocytes and by the volume of plasma which is inevitably trapped between them. Therefore the PCV is only meaningful if the conditions of centrifugation are standardized and if the anti-coagulant used (normally heparin) does not alter the size and shape of the cells. Under optimal conditions the volume of trapped plasma should not exceed 1 per cent.

The PCV of a specimen of blood collected from a peripheral vein is not the same as the erythrocyte concentration in the whole body. Local stasis can cause large errors and the PCV in peripheral blood is about 10 per cent higher than the so-called whole body haematocrit, which is calculated from the total red cell volume and the plasma volume (p. 224).

Changes of the PCV reflect either changes of red cell mass or changes of plasma volume. Anaemia lowers the PCV (relatively more if the cells are small rather than large) and polycythaemia raises it; increased plasma volume lowers it and loss of extracellular fluid raises it. Therefore in individual patients the absolute value of the PCV is difficult to interpret. For example, vomiting in an anaemic patient may raise the PCV into the normal range, and after an acute bleed, there is no change of PCV for at least 2 hr (p. 25). On the other hand, in the absence of bleeding, rapid changes of PCV reflect changes of plasma volume. With appropriate adjustment for changes of red cell volume, the PCV can provide a useful index of the changes of plasma volume over a matter of hours or days.

*

Changes of pure water balance do not, *per se*, alter the PCV because the red cells shrink or swell with changes of the tonicity of the extracellular fluid. Pure water deficiency does not raise the PCV nor does water intoxication lower it unless the measurement is made before equilibration across cell membranes has taken place.

HAEMOGLOBIN CONCENTRATION

The haemoglobin concentration is a function of the number of circulating erythrocytes and the amount of haemoglobin in each erythrocyte. Like the PCV it can be used as an index of haemoconcentration and haemodilution but, generally, it is not such an accurate estimation. The ratio of the haemoglobin concentration and the PCV gives the mean corpuscular haemoglobin concentration (MCHC), rapid changes of which can be used to represent changes of cell volume.

PLASMA PROTEIN CONCENTRATION AND PLASMA SPECIFIC GRAVITY

In acute changes of fluid balance changes of total plasma protein concentration can be used as an index of plasma volume in the same way as the PCV or haemoglobin. They are not so reliable, however, because the liver increases the rate of albumin synthesis within hours whenever protein is lost, as, for example, in severe burning.

The concentration of plasma proteins is often measured as the specific gravity (or density) of plasma. This is the mass per unit volume relative to that of water. 100 ml of plasma contains roughly 93 g of water, 6 g of protein, and 1 g of salt. Therefore with plasma, the protein concentration is the dominant factor which influences the specific gravity whereas, with urine, it is the salt and urea concentration.

Because albumin is a relatively small molecule, the plasma albumin concentration usually accounts for over 90 per cent of the plasma colloid osmotic pressure although it only makes up about 60 per cent of the total protein mass. Occasionally, however, the colloid osmotic pressure can be maintained by low molecular weight globulins. This happens in some cases of congenital analbuminaemia when oedema may be inconspicuous and it may explain the capricious relationship between plasma albumin concentrations and the appearance of oedema in more common clinical situations, such as malnutrition. A high plasma protein concentration usually means dehydration, excessive stasis during venesection, or a disorder of protein synthesis, such as myelomatosis. A low plasma protein concentration usually means overhydration, a reduced rate of albumin synthesis, as in liver disease and malnutrition, or an increased rate of protein loss, as in the nephrotic syndrome and protein-losing enteropathy.

BLOOD UREA CONCENTRATION

The concentration of urea in the blood is determined by the rate of urea production by the liver and by the rate of urea excretion by the kidneys. It is measured either as urea itself or as urea nitrogen which is 48.5 per cent of the urea concentration. Urea comprises about half the non-protein nitrogen of blood; the rest is mainly the nitrogen of uric acid and free amino-acids. In the absence of liver disease, the rate of urea production depends on the protein load. The blood urea rises when more protein is eaten and it also rises if there is bleeding into the gastro-intestinal tract or an increased rate of tissue breakdown. The extent to which the blood urea falls with a reduction of protein intake depends on the nature of the protein eaten and the existence or otherwise of a co-existing increased rate of tissue destruction. For example the blood urea concentration may rise with severe protein restriction but if the protein eaten contains enough essential amino-acids to spare endogenous protein breakdown, then the blood urea will fall.

The rate of urea excretion depends on the rate of glomerular filtration and the rate of tubular reabsorption. The latter is increased when the urine flow slows so that in dehydration with oliguria the blood urea will rise for this reason alone.

Thus, a high blood urea concentration means an increased protein load or a reduced rate of glomerular filtration. A low urea concentration means liver disease, a reduced protein intake, or malabsorption. Usually, however, the dominant determinant of the blood urea concentration is the capacity of the kidney to excrete urea. The renal excretion of urea is discussed further on p. 181.

PLASMA SODIUM CONCENTRATION

The plasma sodium concentration usually varies between the narrow limits of 136–144 m-equiv/l. or ± 3 per cent of 140 m-equiv/l. Changes in plasma sodium concentration reflect the water content of the extra-cellular fluid. Probably even severe sodium depletion only produces hyponatraemia indirectly by increasing the rate of vasopressin release (p. 17).

A low plasma sodium concentration indicates, therefore, a relative excess of water which may or may not be associated with a reduction of the total amount of sodium in the extracellular fluid. When the total body sodium is low, the development of hyponatraemia probably depends largely on whether water-drinking continues and severe sodium depletion may be associated with a normal plasma sodium concentration. Usually, however, some hyponatraemia does develop even if water deficiency co-exists. This presumably means that the demands for volume regulation over-ride those for osmolar regulation.

When associated with a normal or high total body sodium, a 'dilution hyponatraemia' is said to exist. It occurs whenever the secretion of vasopressin continues despite a fall of plasma osmolality. The rate of vasopressin release may be 'appropriate' when the stimulus of hypo-volaemia is dominant or 'inappropriate' when vasopressin is produced autonomously (p. 515). Dilution hyponatraemia may develop without an excess of body water whenever there is a breakdown of the energy-supplying process which maintains the gradient of sodium and potassium across cell membranes. For example, in prolonged illnesses, the intra-cellular sodium concentration may rise at the expense of the extra-cellular sodium. Vasopressin secretion continues, despite the resulting hyponatraemia, because the cells of the osmoreceptor mechanism in the hypothalamus are themselves affected similarly.

Finally, hyponatraemia can be an artifact. The concentration of sodium is measured flame-spectrophotometrically as milli-equivalents per unit volume of whole plasma. Plasma usually consists of 94 per cent water so that the concentration of sodium in whole plasma will be an underestimate of the concentration in plasma water by about 6 per cent. Sometimes there is so much lipid material, as in primary biliary cirrhosis or the nephrotic syndrome, or so much protein, as in myelomatosis, that the plasma contains considerably less than 94 per cent water by volume. Because the concentration of sodium in the plasma water remains unchanged, the 'hyponatraemia' is false.

A high plasma sodium concentration, like a low one, most commonly reflects the state of water rather than sodium balance. Persistent underhydration, as in comatose patients, readily produces an increase of plasma sodium concentration. This may be so pronounced (up to 180 m-equiv/l.) that attempts are periodically made to use this fact to support the idea of a sodium sensitive receptor in the brain. Largely because precise metabolic measurements in confused or comatose patients are so difficult, the evidence that so-called cerebral hyper-natraemia is anything more than the effects of dehydration remains unconvincing, especially as diabetes insipidus from damage to the supra-optico-hypophysial system often co-exists. A primary excess of sodium without a corresponding retention of water only occasionally leads to an increase in the concentration of sodium in the plasma. This may be seen in the hyperaldosteronism of adrenal glomerulosa tumours but even then the plasma sodium concentration is not usually above the upper limit of normal.

PLASMA OSMOLALITY AND OSMOLARITY

One osmole is the mass of a solute (or mixture of solutes) which when dissolved in 1 l. gives a solution which has an osmotic pressure of 22·4 atmospheres at 0° C. Osmolar concentrations are generally determined indirectly by measuring the changes of some other physical function of solutions, such as the depression of freezing point below that of water. Measured like this, the osmolality (or osmoles/1000 g of plasma water) is obtained and it is this term, rather than the commonly misused term osmolarity (or osmoles/l. of whole plasma), which is appropriate when considering osmotic relationships physiologically. The osmolality of plasma is not necessarily equal to the sum of the molar concentration of the individual osmotically-active particles in plasma, whether dissociated or undissociated. In very dilute solutions osmolality and osmolarity are practically identical, but at higher concentrations, such as those seen in plasma, the difference between them increases because the specific volume of dissolved solutes (such as proteins) form an increasingly high proportion of the total volume. Moreover, interionic forces in concentrated solutions of sodium chloride (and other salts) have an effect which simulates incomplete dissociation. Therefore the sum of the molar concentrations of all the osmotically-active constituents of plasma approximates to, but is not the same as, the plasma osmolality.

In practice, plasma osmolality mainly reflects the plasma sodium concentration since sodium and its main anions, chloride and bicarbonate, usually make up over 93 per cent of the plasma osmolality. It may, however, be considerably increased by a high concentration of glucose or urea. Normally glucose and urea only contribute about 5 m-osmole/l. each to the total plasma osmolality. If, however, the glucose concentration rises to 1000 mg/100 ml, as it may do in diabetic coma, then it will contribute a further 50 m-osmole/l. Since glucose is predominantly extracellular, cell shrinkage and coma may occur even without ketosis. Likewise, if the blood urea concentration rises to 500 mg/100 ml, this will contribute a further 78 m-osmole/l. to the plasma osmolality. Since urea is freely diffusible across cell membranes, no osmotic effects develop after equilibration. However, equilibration to rapid changes of blood urea concentration is relatively slow and transient osmotic disequilibrium may, for example, account for the cerebral 'oedema' sometimes seen following haemodialysis when the plasma urea concentration falls quickly.

PLASMA POTASSIUM CONCENTRATION

In contrast to plasma sodium, the plasma potassium concentration varies over a comparatively wide range. Values of 3·5–5·5 m-equiv/l. or ± 22 per cent of 4·5 m-equiv/l. are within normal limits. Apart from variations due to changes of the water content of extracellular fluid, plasma potassium concentrations are influenced by the total body potassium, the gradient of hydrogen ion across cell membranes, the rate of glucose entry into cells, and the ability of the kidney to excrete potassium. A low plasma potassium concentration may indicate potassium depletion but extracellular potassium is such a small fraction of cellular potassium and so many factors affect the gradient of potassium across cell membranes, that the relationship between total body potassium and plasma potassium concentration is poor. For example, extracellular acidosis raises the plasma potassium concentration disproportionately in relation to the total body content and extracellular alkalosis lowers it disproportionately. An increase in the rate of glucose entry into cells, as in recovery from diabetic ketosis or in familial periodic paralysis, lowers the plasma potassium concentration despite a normal or increasing total body content. Loss of potassium from the extracellular fluid, as in gastrointestinal fluid loss, or loss in the urine, as in starvation or primary hyperaldosteronism, generally leads to a proportionately greater fall in plasma potassium concentration than in total body potassium. This happens partly because the primary event is loss from the extracellular fluid and partly because potassium depletion itself causes an extracellular alkalosis which favours a high gradient across cell membranes.

A low plasma potassium concentration therefore suggests potassium depletion, extracellular alkalosis, overhydration, or a rapid rate of glucose uptake by the cells. A high plasma potassium concentration suggests potassium overloading, dehydration, extracellular acidosis or renal failure.

Apart from providing a rough guide to the total body potassium, the concentration of potassium in the plasma is important in itself because the cardiac effects of hypo- or hyperkalaemia (p. 80) are more closely related to plasma levels than to total body content.

PLASMA MAGNESIUM CONCENTRATION

Like calcium, the normal range of plasma magnesium concentrations is narrow, from 1·5–1·8 m-equiv/l. Factors influencing it are complex because the plasma magnesium varies both with the plasma calcium and the plasma potassium concentration. Hypomagnesaemia is seen after treatment with potassium-losing diuretics and in primary hyper-aldosteronism. It is common in malabsorption syndromes when both calcium and potassium concentrations are low. Hypomagnesaemia may also be present in hyperparathyroidism when the plasma calcium concentration is high and magnesium balance is usually negative in this condition. More regularly, however, the plasma magnesium concentration falls after removal of a parathyroid adenoma. Finally, the plasma magnesium concentration appears to be rather specifically depressed in chronic alcoholism.

URINE VOLUME

This is determined by the circulating levels of vasopressin and the quantity of osmotically-active solute filtered at the glomeruli. Vaso-pressin secretion is influenced by the state of the body's fluid balance and by intrinsic abnormalities of the secreting mechanism; the quantity of osmotically-active solute filtered is influenced by the rate of glomerular filtration and by the quantity excreted. Therefore, the urine volume in disease broadly reflects disturbances of fluid balance, disturbances of the vasopressin mechanism, and disturbances of renal function. A low urine volume suggests dehydration, acute renal failure, or avid sodium retention; a high one suggests overhydration, chronic renal disease, diabetes insipidus, or an osmotic diuresis, as in diabetes mellitus.

URINE SPECIFIC GRAVITY AND OSMOLALITY

The specific gravity of a solution is its density in relation to that of water; it depends only on the weight of dissolved substances per unit volume. Therefore, although there is a rough relationship between specific gravity and osmolality (p. 8), a high proportion of light particles gives a misleadingly low specific gravity whilst the same high proportion of heavy particles (e.g. glucose) gives a misleadingly high figure. The specific gravity of the glomerular ultrafiltrate (about 1·010) approximates to the osmolality of plasma water, i.e. 330 m-osmole/l., whereas that of plasma (about 1·026) reflects the concentration of plasma proteins.

Urine osmolality is largely governed by alterations of water content as determined by vasopressin activity (p. 8). A high concentration of osmotically-active particles in the glomerular ultrafiltrate produces an osmotic diuresis which is characterized by the fact that the osmolality of the urine approaches that of plasma water whether the urine is initially dilute or initially concentrated (p. 166). In uncontrolled diabetes or chronic renal failure, the urine osmolality approaches plasma osmolality whatever the state of hydration but because glucose and urea are relatively heavy, an increasing osmotic diuresis in these conditions always increases the urine specific gravity.

BODY FLUID SPACE MEASUREMENTS

The volumes of the various body fluid compartments can only be measured by dilution. A known quantity of an appropriate substance, thought to be largely confined to the space whose volume is required, is injected intravenously (or taken by mouth if intestinal absorption is complete) and its concentration measured in the plasma (or preferably the plasma water) when full equilibration has occurred. Theoretically, multiple samples of plasma should be assayed to determine the equilibrium concentration when all the mixing processes are complete but in practice somewhat arbitary equilibration periods are generally taken, depending on the space being measured. The volume of distribution is given by the amount of indicator remaining in the body (i.e. the amount given minus the amount that has left the body during the period of equilibration) divided by the equilibrium concentration.

Plasma is the only body fluid space that can be sampled directly so that only the volume of the plasma, extracellular fluid and total body water can be measured directly; the volumes of the interstitial cell fluid and the intracellular fluid have to be assessed by subtraction. The dilution principle only measures a body fluid space if mixing is complete at the time of sampling and if the substance chosen is confined to the space under study. An inadequate equilibration period tends to produce an underestimation of the volume, and leakage out of the space in question tends to produce an overestimation. Uneven distribution usually produces an overestimation because large particles, such as inulin, may be partly sequestrated at high concentration at some inaccessible site, such as the reticulo-endothelial system. When all losses during the period of equilibration cannot be measured, the volume of distribution may be obtained by extrapolation from the slope of the plasma concentrations after mixing is complete. This makes the additional assumption that losses are taking place at a steady rate and there are the inherent difficulties of determining the precise slope.

Total body water is generally measured from the volume of distribution either of tritiated water (H_3O) which is radioactive or of heavy water (D_2O). Urea, ethanol and antipyrine can also be used.

Approximations to the extracellular fluid volume can be made from the volume of distribution of thiocyanate, inulin, bromide, or radioactive sodium. Inulin, a relatively large molecule, only penetrates into transcellular spaces and dense connective tissue with difficulty so that the values obtained underestimate the ECF volume; sodium and bromide inevitably penetrate across cell membranes to some degree so their volumes of distribution overestimate the ECF volume.

The blood volume can be measured either from the volume of distribution of albumin (labelled with a dye such as Evans' blue or with radioactive iodine), or from the volume of distribution of suitably labelled erythrocytes (usually labelled with radioactive chromium). The former gives the plasma volume and the latter the red blood cell volume. In either case the blood volume is obtained from the peripheral haematocrit corrected for the difference between this and the whole body haematocrit (p. 224). Alternatively, both the erythrocyte volume and the plasma volume can be measured simultaneously. Because there is inevitably a small leak of protein from the vascular system, the use of labelled red cells is probably more accurate.

TOTAL EXCHANGEABLE ELECTROLYTE CONCENTRATION

These are measured by the same principles of dilution used for body space measurements except that the quantity of marker in the body at equilibration is divided by the ratio of labelled to unlabelled electrolyte (i.e. the so-called specific activity), instead of the ratio of labelled indicator to water (i.e. the concentration). The same limitations apply. Total exchangeable sodium is best measured from the specific activity (e.g. $^{24}Na/^{23}Na$) in the plasma and the total exchangeable potassium from the specific activity (e.g. $^{42}K/^{39}K$) in the urine. Since potassium is secreted by the renal tubules, the urine potassium is more likely to be representative of the specific activity of intracellular potassium.

EXTERNAL BALANCE STUDIES

Metabolic balance studies require painstaking accuracy if they are to be meaningful over any length of time. The intake and output must be measured accurately because, for example, a systematic error of intake by even a small amount will tend in time to a progressively greater positive or negative 'balance' which is bogus. This limitation, together with the difficulty of collecting faeces reliably over specified periods, means that, except over short periods of time for substances such as sodium, external balance studies remain a research tool.

Practical assessment

HAEMORRHAGE AND SHOCK
Clinical observations
Loss of less than 10 per cent of blood volume: no definite signs. Increasing losses cause, in roughly the following sequence: pale, cold skin; postural hypotension; empty veins; tachycardia; small pulse pressure; hypotension even when lying flat; sweating; restlessness; irregular, rapid breathing; mental confusion. Best index of the size of the haemorrhage is the pulse rate but in older people the supine blood pressure drops early, sometimes before tachycardia is obvious. With shock, peripheral blotchy cyanosis.

Routine methods
Immediately after haemorrhage: no changes. Within a few hours: falling PCV and Hb; rising blood urea, particularly with blood loss into the bowel. With shock, PCV and Hb may be raised, especially with burns. Central venous pressure reduced.

Special techniques
Volume of distribution of ^{131}I-albumin or Evans' Blue (plasma volume); cardiac output; peripheral resistance.

WATER DEPLETION
Clinical observations
Thirst; dry mouth; oliguria. Later coma when it may be difficult to distinguish cause from effect. No physical signs until late. Then, loss of skin turgor; tachycardia; hypotension; fever (particularly in infants).

Routine methods
Concentrated urine (specific gravity > 1015); raised blood urea; hypernatraemia. No change in PCV or Hb.

Special techniques
Total body water (e.g. H_3O space).

SODIUM DEPLETION
Clinical observations
Lethargy; inelastic subcutaneous tissues. Later, signs of circulatory failure, often with vomiting.

Routine methods
Raised PCV and Hb; rising blood urea; plasma sodium concentration normal at first but falls later. Unless water deficiency also prominent, urine volume not obviously reduced but urine concentration of sodium and chloride very low (<10 m-equiv/l.). Sodium depletion cannot be reliably estimated from urine chloride concentration (p. 18).

Special techniques
Total exchangeable sodium; balance studies; plasma volume; ECF volume (e.g. bromide or inulin space).

POTASSIUM DEPLETION
Clinical observations
Weakness and reduced tone of limb muscles; cardiac arrhythmia; constipation; paralytic ileus. Sometimes carpo-pedal spasm (or positive Trousseau sign).

Routine methods
Plasma potassium concentration often, but not necessarily, low; raised plasma bicarbonate concentration. ECG may be pathognomic.

Special techniques
Total exchangeable potassium; balance studies; tests for renal lesion of potassium depletion (p. 176).

MIXED BODY FLUID DEPLETION
Clinical observations
Symptoms and signs develop with fluid loss greater than 6 per cent of usual weight when those of salt depletion predominate. Thirst may be minimal despite large intracellular deficit.

Routine methods
Findings variable but usually urine sparse and concentrated with a low concentration of sodium and chloride. PCV and Hb raised unless there is bleeding; raised blood urea; high, normal or low plasma sodium concentration depending on relative deficits of sodium and water; plasma potassium concentration often normal, despite overall deficit. Changes of body weight useful, especially with infants.

Special techniques
See under individual components.

BODY FLUID EXCESS
Clinical observations
Overloading with blood, plasma, or saline: raised central venous
pressure; pulmonary and peripheral oedema. Overloading with water:
restlessness; nausea; epileptic fits; coma.

Routine methods
PCV and Hb unchanged, then raised with blood; lowered with plasma,
saline or water. Plasma electrolyte concentration only lowered with
water overloading (lowered sodium concentration most obvious).

Special techniques
As for body fluid deficits.

TABLE 2 Normal values

Body fluid spaces (approx.)	Total body water	45 l.
	Intracellular water	25–30 l.
	Extracellular water	12–15 l.
	Interstitial water	9 l.
	Plasma volume	3 l.
	Blood volume	5 l.
Total exchangeable electrolytes	Sodium approx.	40 m-equiv/kg
	Potassium approx.	45 m-equiv/kg
Packed cell volume (PCV)	Men	40–54 per cent
	Women	38–46 per cent
Haemoglobin concentration	Men	13·0–17·5 g/100 ml
	Women	12·4–16·0 g/100 ml
Plasma protein concentration		6·0–8·0 g/100 ml
Blood urea concentration		15–40 mg/100 ml
Plasma electrolyte	Sodium	136–144 m-equiv/l.
concentration	Potassium	3·5–5·5 m-equiv/l.
	Magnesium	1·5–1·8 m-equiv/l.
	Chloride	97–107 m-equiv/l.
Urine specific gravity		1·000–1·032
Urine osmolality		30–1400 m-osmole/kg
Urine electrolyte concentration	Concentration of Na, Cl and K normally above 25 m-equiv/l.	See text

References

BODY FLUID DISTRIBUTION: DISTURBANCES OF WATER AND
    ELECTROLYTE BALANCE
EDELMAN I.S. & LEIBMAN J. (1959) Anatomy of body water and electrolytes. *Amer.
    J. Med.* **27**, 256–277.

STRAUSS M.B. (1957) *Body Water in Man.* London: Churchill.
GAMBLE J.L. (1954) *Chemical Anatomy, Physiology and Pathology of Extracellular Fluid.* (6th ed.). Cambridge, Mass.: Harvard Univ. Press.
BLACK D.A.K. (1967) *Essentials of Fluid Balance.* (4th edn.). Oxford: Blackwell.
LE QUESNE L.P. (1957) *Fluid Balance in Surgical Practice.* (2nd edn.). London: Lloyd-Luke.
ROBINSON J.R. (1960) Metabolism of Intracellular Water. *Physiol. Rev.* **40**, 112–149.
MOORE F.D. (1959) *Metabolic Care of the Surgical Patient.* Philadelphia & London: Saunders.
BAULIEU E.E. & ROBEL P. (ed.) (1964) *Aldosterone: a symposium.* Blackwell, Oxford.
CREESE R. (ed.) (1964) *Recent Advances in Physiology.* 8th edn. London: J. & A. Churchill.
COMAR C.L. & BRONNER F. (ed.) (1960) *Mineral Metabolism: an advanced treatise.* Vol. I, part A. New York and London: Academic Press.
SLATER J.D.H. (1964) The Hormonal Control of Body Sodium. *Post. Grad. Med. J.* **40**, 479–96.

BLOOD VOLUME, HAEMORRHAGE AND SHOCK
MOLLISON P.L. (1967) *Blood Transfusion in Clinical Medicine.* (4th edn.). Oxford: Blackwell.
HEYMANS C. & NEIL E. (1958) *Reflexogenic areas of the Cardiovascular System.* London: Churchill.
GREGERSEN M.I. & RAWSON R.A. (1959) Blood volume. *Physiol. Rev.* **39**, 307–342.
BOCK K.D. (ed.) (1962) *Shock: an international symposium held at Stockholm, 1961.* Berlin: Springer-Verlag.

2

Heart and Circulation

Normal Function

THE HEART

All cardiac muscle has the intrinsic capacity for rhythmic excitation. This is most highly developed in the nodal tissue. Normally the pace of the heart is set by the sino-atrial node, whence excitation spreads across the atrium to the atrioventricular node and to the ventricles by the specialized conducting tissues. The processes of excitation by depolarization, coupling by entry of calcium ions, contraction itself, and the energy pathways are essentially similar to those described elsewhere for skeletal muscle (p. 338).

In a young adult, the heart whose nervous connections and response to circulating catecholamines has been blocked by drugs contracts about 110 times/min, but this intrinsic rate falls with age and is about 80 beats/min at the age of 70 years. The intrinsic rate is modified by the central nervous system, which can slow the heart by means of impulses transmitted in the vagi, and speed it up by impulses in the sympathetic cardioaccelerator nerves and by adrenaline released from the adrenal medulla. In a supine young adult at rest the heart is under predominantly vagal influence and contracts about 70 times/min.

The healthy heart obeys Starling's Law, which states that the force of cardiac contraction increases with increasing diastolic stretch of the cardiac muscle fibres. The volume of blood expelled from the heart at each beat (the stroke volume) therefore depends in the first instance on the degree of cardiac filling. At a heart rate of 70 beats/min in a young adult at rest, each ventricle contains at the end of diastole about 120 ml of blood, 70 ml of which is expelled at each systole. The resting cardiac output is therefore approximately 5 l./min.

The force of cardiac contraction is continuously modified by the ionic environment, especially by the concentrations of potassium and calcium in the blood. Vagal inhibitory nerve impulses reduce heart rate and also slightly reduce the force of contraction, whereas circulating adrenal catecholamines and sympathetic cardioaccelerator nerve activity increase heart rate and can greatly increase the force of cardiac contraction. However, the cardiac output can only be increased some 10 per cent even by maximal activation of the sympatho-adrenal system unless venous return is augmented at the same time. Venous return, in the absence of skeletal muscle contraction, is essentially a passive process, and depends on the difference between the mean pressure filling the circulation (about 7 mmHg in a supine subject at rest) and mean right atrial pressure (about −4 mmHg).

Pulmonary capillary pressure probably approximates to alveolar pressure, which in a normal subject during inspiration is not more than 2 mmHg below atmospheric, and at end inspiration is atmospheric (i.e. 0 mmHg). At this time the right heart must therefore raise the pressure from −4 to 0 to make blood flow into the pulmonary capillaries. The mean pulmonary artery pressure is about +11 mmHg, and the excess pressure is dissipated in the pre-capillary pulmonary resistance. Most of the work of the right heart is done by the ventricle, but atrial contraction, as on the left side, makes a small contribution to ventricular output.

Because of the small pressure gradient available to fill the heart, changes in intrathoracic pressure have a big influence on venous return and hence on cardiac filling and cardiac output. During a deep inspiration the intrathoracic pressure may be −25 mmHg, and during diastole most of this pressure is transmitted to the lax right ventricle, which sucks blood in. The diastolic volume of the right ventricle therefore increases and the ventricle has to raise a greater amount of blood to a greater effective pressure during a deep inspiration. Expiration, on the other hand, squeezes blood out of the lungs so that the output from the left heart increases. Right ventricular contraction begins before left but finishes later, so that the pulmonary second sound (marking pulmonary valve closure) follows the aortic second sound (marking aortic valve closure). During inspiration the increase in right ventricular volume prolongs the time taken for the right ventricle to expel its contents. Thus the gap between aortic and pulmonary second sounds gets wider.

The first sound is associated with atrioventricular valve closure, although its origin remains in some dispute. The tricuspid and mitral components of the sound may be heard separately, especially in the presence of bundle branch block.

REGULATION OF CARDIAC OUTPUT

Some 5 l. of blood fill the heart and circulation at a mean pressure of about + 7 mmHg, this being the pressure which would be present everywhere if the heart stopped and all pressures were immediately equalized. Approximate calculations for man indicate that removal of one pint of blood (about 600 ml) would reduce mean circulatory pressure to 0 (i.e. atmospheric), and that addition of one pint would raise it to +14 mmHg. In the absence of compensatory factors such manoeuvres would change venous return, and hence cardiac output, over the range of about 2 to 8 l./min. In practice cardiac output is stabilized by a number of mechanisms, which may be listed in order of rapidity of action, though not necessarily in order of importance.

The sympatho-adrenal system

Receptors in the great veins and atrial walls detect the degree of filling and stretch of these organs. Ventricular wall tension can also probably be detected by mechanoreceptors in the inner surface of the ventricular wall. In addition, a primary change in cardiac output inevitably changes systemic arterial pressure, which can be detected by other stretch receptors in the walls of the large arteries and carotid sinuses. A fall in blood volume decreases central venous pressure, cardiac filling, and systemic arterial pressure, and nervous reflexes mediated through the hind brain and sympatho-adrenal system rapidly decrease the capacitance of those parts of the circulation (the veins) which hold the greater part (about 60 per cent) of the blood, thus minimizing the fall in mean circulatory pressure. Venous constriction is brough about both by sympathetic nervous activity and by circulating noradrenaline, although it may later be maintained by an intrinsic mechanism in the vein walls (see below).

Capillary fluid exchanges

The circulation normally contains some 3 l. of fluid (as plasma) and there are about 9 l. in the interstitial space (p. 3). The partition of this extracellular fluid depends on a dynamic equilibrium at the capillaries:

Mean capillary pressure + Colloid osmotic pressure
                                                  of interstitial fluid

= Mean interstitial fluid   + Colloid osmotic pressure
        pressure   of plasma proteins

Any loss of blood, which must initially reduce the mean capillary pressure, tends to disturb the equilibrium and sucks fluid from the interstitial space into the circulation. Quantitatively this mechanism is probably not very important, because the compliance of the interstitial space is normally very low: i.e. removal of a small volume of fluid lowers interstitial pressure greatly. After the loss of 600 ml of blood from the circulation, for example, approximate calculations suggest that at best only about 250 ml of fluid could be transferred from the interstitial space into the blood stream before a new equilibrium was established at a more negative interstitial pressure. Thus this mechanism could immediately correct only about one-third of any blood volume deficit. Further replenishment of fluid comes either from fluid ingestion or from intracellular water.

Stress relaxation of veins

Veins possess an intrinsic ability to maintain a more or less constant degree of wall tension despite changes in diameter. This mechanism is independent of circulating catecholamines and sympathetic nervous activity; but it is slow and takes about 10 min for each 1 per cent change in blood volume to be fully compensated.

Renal regulation of cardiac filling

The kidney plays a central role in cardiac output regulation, because it is the final arbiter of sodium and water excretion rate, and hence of extracellular fluid volume and circulatory filling.

Regardless of other nervous or hormonal mechanisms, any reduction of renal perfusion pressure which might initially result from a fall of cardiac output reduces the volume and sodium concentration of the urine, thus conserving extracellular fluid. Afferent arteriolar constriction mediated by the sympatho-adrenal system has a similar effect, and probably plays a most important part in conserving extracellular fluid. It is notable that renal blood flow falls sharply after even slight blood loss, though there may be scarcely any change in systemic arterial pressure. In addition to the intrinsic and nervous mechanisms, a fall in venous return and cardiac output resulting from haemorrhage is a powerful stimulus to the release of vasopressin from the posterior pituitary gland (p. 26) and hence to the conservation of water. This stimulus can overrule the normal control of vasopressin secretion rate in accordance with plasma osmolality (p. 22).

It is obvious that these renal mechanisms can compensate for an increase in cardiac output by increasing sodium and water excretion;

but they cannot in themselves compensate for reduced cardiac output. They can only prevent it getting worse by making the kidney hold on to the fluid still in the body. However, thirst increases after haemorrhage (p. 10), and increased fluid ingestion in association with diminished renal excretion can eventually replace any fluid loss.

Another renal mechanism which helps to protect cardiac output is the renin-angiotensin system. A fall in cardiac filling provokes the release of renin from the kidneys. Recent work suggests that the stimulus for the release of renin is not the fall in systemic arterial pressure, which may be scarcely measurable in the presence of intact vasomotor nervous reflexes, but rather a sympathetic nervous action on the kidneys. There is a (presumably) sympathetic innervation of the juxta-glomerular apparatus, which is the site of renin storage. In addition, the renal nerves may act indirectly by bringing about afferent arteriolar vaso-constriction and a fall of glomerular perfusion pressure. It is generally believed that this pressure, or some function of it, controls the rate of renin secretion. Renin catalyses the production of angiotensin (p. 48), which is a powerful vasoconstrictor, acting not only directly on arterioles, but also, indirectly through the nervous system, constricting veins. Over much longer periods of time, the stimulation of aldosterone secretion by angiotensin (p. 526) will contribute to renal sodium reten-tion, and in yet another way help to prevent plasma volume depletion.

THE PERIPHERAL SYSTEMIC CIRCULATION

The systemic vasculature comprises the aorta and central arteries; the peripheral arteriolar tree (arteries of 10–150μ internal diameter); the capillary bed; and the veins.

Aorta and central arteries

The left ventricle ejects about two-thirds of its stroke volume in the first third of systole. In diastole, after a momentary retrograde flow, the aortic wall recoils, releasing the potential energy created by its distension in systole, and accelerating the forward flow of blood. The process is continued in the larger muscular arteries such as the iliac and brachial, and these arteries also contribute a small amount to the total peripheral arterial resistance when flow is greatly increased, e.g. during muscular exercise.

Arterioles

Arterioles have muscular walls which are thick in comparison with their lumens (although standard methods of histological fixation cause vascular contracture and give a completely false impression of the true thickness of arteriolar walls in life). The arterioles contribute virtually all the systemic vascular resistance, and recent work suggest that they behave as miniature waterfalls. Once the intraluminal pressure exceeds the effective transmural pressure the lumen opens and the vessel presents little resistance to flow. The rate of flow appears to be almost independent of pressure at the distal (capillary) end, provided that this is less than tissue pressure (Fig. 3). It is likely that the number of arterioles open at any one time, rather than the average calibre of all the arterioles governs the vascular resistance offered by any tissue.

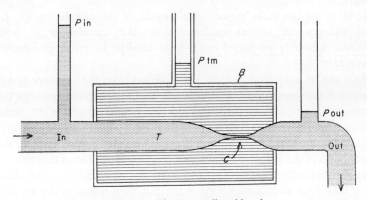

FIGURE 3. *Flow in a collapsible tube.*

T is a collapsible tube, representing an arteriole, conveying blood from input (in) to output (out). The tube is contained by a rigid fluid-filled box (B). P_{in} represents input pressure and P_{out} output pressure. According to the traditional view, the total resistance (R) to flow can be calculated from the formula:

$$R = \frac{P_{in} - P_{out}}{\text{Rate of flow}}$$

However, because of the collapsible nature of tube T, there is effectively a break at point C where the tube collapses. The flow rate is thus independent of P_{out} until P_{out} exceeds P_{tm} (the effective transmural pressure tending to close the tube). In an arteriole, P_{tm} is given by the sum of intrinsic wall tension and interstitial pressure. The resistance to flow through the system is given by

$$R = \frac{P_{in} - P_{tm}}{\text{Rate of flow}}$$

and the internal distending pressure in segment C is equal to P_{tm}.

Capillaries

The total cross-sectional area of the capillary bed is more than 600 times that of the aorta; but not all capillaries are open at any one time. In skeletal muscle at rest only 2 or 3 capillaries may be open in each cmm of tissue, whereas this may go up to 200 to 300 during exercise. Capillaries have no power of independent contraction, and are either fully open or fully closed according to the state of arterioles feeding them (see above). In many tissues, notably skin, there are contractile arteriovenous anastomoses which allow a variable amount of blood to by-pass the capillary bed altogether. Some blood normally passes along these channels during rest, playing no known physiological role except in the case of the skin, in which it controls heat loss.

Veins

The veins are the main 'capacitance' vessels of the circulation (p. 42) and changes in venous calibre allow the circulation to hold different amounts of blood with little change in mean circulatory pressure.

In a supine subject at rest, return of blood from the capillary bed is entirely a passive process, and depends on the difference between the mean capillary pressure (probably 10 to 15 mmHg) and right atrial pressure (about −4 mmHg). In an erect subject whose mean circulatory pressure was normal (+7 mmHg) the passive distension of veins in the lower parts of the body would accommodate so much blood that cardiac filling would almost cease. Venous return during standing is sustained by at least four mechanisms. One is the pumping action of the muscles which compresses segments of peripheral veins isolated by valves, and propels blood towards the heart. A second is the increase of mean circulatory pressure brought about by reflex sympatho-adrenal constriction of the venous reservoirs. A third is the intrinsic, as well as reflex, shutting down of pre-capillary arteriolar sphincters in dependent limbs, which greatly reduces the rate of flow of blood into the limbs. A fourth, recently identified, mechanism is the increase in mean circulatory volume brought about by closing of arterioles supplying the splanchnic area, which has a high compliance.

SYMPATHO-ADRENAL VASCULAR RECEPTORS

The main peripheral systemic vascular resistance lies in the arterioles (see above) whose innervation is mainly sympathetic, adrenergic and vasoconstrictor, although the arterioles of limb muscles also receive a cholinergic vasodilator innervation whose physiological function remains somewhat obscure. Most circulatory reflexes, except the faint reaction, appear mainly to involve changes in sympathetic adrenergic vasoconstrictor activity, though there is increasing evidence of activation of the cholinergic vasodilator system at the same time in emotional reactions, muscular exercise, and on standing up.

The sympathetic receptors responsible for arteriolar constriction can be stimulated by noradrenaline, which is the normal chemical transmitter at the endings of postganglionic sympathetic nerves; and the vasoconstrictor action on skeletal muscle brought about by locally infused noradrenaline can be blocked by substances such as phentolamine and and phenoxybenzamine, which are described as α-blocking agents. Probably because noradrenaline is released from nerve terminals applied extremely close to the cell membrane, no locally infused blocking agent can completely prevent the vasoconstrictor response to adrenergic nerve stimulation.

By contrast, the local infusion of adrenaline into the arterial supply of a skeletal muscle results in vasodilatation, which can be prevented by a different type of drug such as propranolol, which is described as a β-blocking agent. The adrenergic receptors responsible for sympathetically mediated increases of rate and force of cardiac contraction can also be blocked by β-blocking drugs.

Because both adrenaline and noradrenaline possess both α- and β-stimulating activity, which varies in different species and in different organs of the same species, it is more satisfactory to define the nature of a receptor as α- or β- in terms of the effects upon it of α- and β-blocking drugs rather than in terms of its response to noradrenaline and adrenalin.

Veins, like most arterioles, possess an adrenergic vasoconstrictor innervation and constrict to noradrenaline; but they too can dilate in response to circulating adrenaline. The vasodilation which can be shown in skeletal muscles when their sympathetic nerves are stimulated after complete α-blockade by drugs is due to stimulation of the cholinergic vasodilator innervation. This response can be blocked by atropine.

The total effect of a massive discharge of sympathetic nervous impulses and catecholamine release is to bring about a redistribution of blood flow, which is reduced in the skin and splanchnic regions, and increased in skeletal and cardiac muscle and in the brain. In animals deprived of their adrenal medullas the cardiovascular adjustments involving sympathetic hyperactivity (e.g. muscular exercise) are impaired, and in such animals cardiac output does not rise to a normal extent on exercise.

FACTORS MODIFYING SYSTEMIC ARTERIAL PRESSURE

Sympatho-adrenal activity

Alterations in sympathetic nervous activity play an important part in controlling systemic arterial pressure. The well known systemic arterial baroreceptors in the large arteries form the afferent limb of a feedback loop whose integrating centres lie in the medulla oblongata. Sympathetic activity is also influenced by higher centres, especially in the hypothalamus, and by the general level of activity in the reticular activating system. Decreased sympathetic nervous activity together with vagal inhibition are mainly responsible for the fall of blood pressure during sleep. The tonic action of the sympathetic nervous system also depends on the chemical environment of the medulla, and in some species on the spinal cord as well. Normally the cerebral blood flow is held constant (p. 50) and the chemical environment of the central nervous system does not change; but severe medullary ischaemia causes a massive sympatho-adrenal discharge which may act as a last ditch defence of the blood supply to vital centres.

Angiotensin

Arteriolar resistance can be altered by several vaso-active materials conveyed by the blood stream. The precise role of many of them is not fully known. This even applies to angiotensin, the most powerful vaso-constrictor material known. Recent work suggests that the normally circulating concentrations of angiotensin do exert a small vasoconstrictor effect. The concentration of angiotensin increases rapidly if the renal perfusion pressure falls. It seems likely that the initial rise of systemic arterial pressure after putting a constricting clip on the main renal artery of an animal is due largely to the release of renin, liberating angiotensin in the blood stream. However, the long term operation of this mechanism is unknown (p. 68).

Blood volume

The state of filling of the circulation has an important part to play in regulating cardiac output and hence potentially in controlling systemic arterial pressure. Subjects given sodium-retaining steroids for a long period initially expand their plasma volume and cardiac output. After a few weeks the cardiac output tends to fall towards normal and at the same time the systemic arterial pressure rises. Roughly opposite changes occur after the long-term administration of diuretic agents which remove sodium and water from the body. These and other observations suggest that the control of sodium and water excretion by the kidney may influence long term regulation of systemic arterial pressure. Although there is no doubt about the important role of the systemic arterial baroreceptors in the control of systemic arterial pressure over short periods of time, it seems unlikely that they exert any important influence on long-term stability of blood pressure. There is so far no general agreement about the means by which blood pressure is stabilized over long periods of time, although most investigators give the kidney a dominant role, because of its ability to regulate sodium balance.

REGULATION OF TISSUE BLOOD FLOW

The regulation of blood flow to special tissues such as the heart, brain and lungs will be considered separately; but it seems that almost all organs except the skin possess some intrinsic ability to control their blood flow in accordance with metabolic needs. In a general sense this property is known as 'autoregulation'. Most organs maintain stability of blood flow despite changes in perfusion pressure and strictly speaking the term 'autoregulation' was first coined to describe this phenomenon. However, it is very likely that similar mechanisms govern the adjustment of tissue blood flow both to metabolic needs and to changes of arterial perfusion pressure. In organs such as the kidney, which have a constraining capsule, autoregulation could be to some extent a passive process; but in most other situations the calibre of arterioles in an organ is probably governed mainly by its metabolic needs and its perfusion pressure. Even powerful extrinsic vasoconstrictor influences such as those of the sympatho-adrenal system cannot indefinitely reduce the blood flow to most organs, whose autoregulatory mechanisms eventually overrule the extrinsic system which provides only short term control. In some situations, changes in perfusion pressure alone can alter arteriolar calibre, apparently by a local myogenic response of arteriolar smooth muscle; but in most organs some metabolite used or produced by the tissue appears to exert a controlling role. In skeletal muscle oxygen supply is the most important factor, and anoxaemia powerfully dilates muscle vessels independently of any nervous connections to the tissue and of changes in circulating vasoactive substances. In the cerebral circulation (p. 50), carbon dioxide tension is probably the main determining factor. Thus different vascular beds may depend on different control systems. However the general effect of all is to preserve tissue blood flow despite changes in systemic arterial pressure, and also automatically to reduce local vascular resistance, and thus increase blood flow, if tissue metabolic rate increases.

Flow through some organs may be more dependent on nervous and circulatory chemical stimuli than on local metabolic influences. In particular the kidneys and skin have in common a vascular control system which is largely independent of metabolic needs. Indeed, the kidney appears to adjust its metabolic rate to its blood flow and the skin may do the same. In both cases the normal blood flow must be enormously in excess of the minimal metabolic needs, thus enabling the kidney to operate flexibly in the control of water and electrolyte excretion, and the skin to regulate body temperature (p. 54).

THE CORONARY CIRCULATION

Blood flow through the coronary arteries is continuous throughout the cardiac cycle, two-thirds occurring during diastole. The coronary sinus drains 90 per cent of the venous blood from the left ventricular muscle. Blood from the right ventricle drains into the cardiac veins. The proportion of oxygen extracted by the heart muscle is remarkably constant at the relatively large value of around 150 ml O_2/l. of blood flow. The volume of oxygen consumed at rest by the heart is 40 ml/min or 15 per cent of the total body oxygen consumption, and the normal coronary flow is about 250 ml/min or 5 per cent of the resting cardiac output. The main determinant of coronary flow is oxygen consumption of the myocardium, which is directly related to the development of tension by the myocardium.

Sympathetic nerve stimulation probably has a slight vasoconstrictor effect on the coronary vessels and the increased coronary blood flow produced by increased sympathetic nervous tone is mainly due to stimulation of the myocardium and the resulting increase in cardiac work. Vagal stimulation has no direct effect on the coronary vasculature; angiotensin and vasopressin are the only known naturally occurring substances having a vasoconstrictor action on the coronary arteries. Adrenaline has a slight β-stimulating dilator effect.

THE CEREBRAL CIRCULATION

The cerebral blood flow of man is normally about 54 ml/100 g brain/min, which for a brain of 1400 g gives a total cerebral blood flow of about 750 ml/min, i.e. 15 per cent of the resting cardiac output. Consciousness is lost at cerebral blood flows sustained at less than about 32 ml/100 g/min, and irreversible damage occurs at values less than 10 ml/100 g/min. All general anaesthetics reduce cerebral blood flow, in proportion to their depression of cerebral metabolic rate.

The cerebral circulation in some ways resembles the pulmonary circulation, in that there is little autonomic control of the cerebral vessels. Some nervous vasoconstriction can be demonstrated, though with difficulty. However, it is now established that at systemic arterial pressures greater than about 75 mmHg, the brain has the ability to regulate its intrinsic vascular resistance in such a way that blood flow remains almost constant despite changes in systemic arterial pressure. It probably does this partly by virtue of its enclosure within a rigid box, because patients with large skull defects are liable to faint when standing up. There is probably also some degree of myogenic autoregulation; i.e. changes in vascular calibre induced by changes in distension pressure of the resistance vessels. However, stability of cerebral blood flow is probably achieved mainly by control of vascular calibre by carbon dioxide tension. If cerebral blood flow begins to fall, carbon dioxide accumulates and the increased Pco_2 brings about compensatory cerebral vasodilation. In the presence of high arterial Pco_2 almost all auto-regulative capacity disappears.

Not only has the brain itself this intrinsic ability to control its own blood flow: the carotid and arterial baroreceptors lie on the path of blood from heart to brain, and their reflex action tends to maintain the systemic blood pressure fairly constant over short periods of time, thus protecting the brain from acute changes in perfusion pressure.

THE PULMONARY CIRCULATION

The pulmonary arterial tree is perfused at a lower pressure than the systemic so that the effects of gravity are proportionally greater. In the erect posture the arterial pressure in the lung increases below the level of the hilum and decreases from the hilum towards the apex. Pulmonary capillary blood flow depends on the relative values of the alveolar, arteriolar and pulmonary venous pressures. At the apex of the lung the arteriolar pressure is reduced and the pulmonary capillaries are collapsed by the surrounding alveolar pressure. At the base of the lung the arteriolar and venous pressures exceed the alveolar pressure and the capillaries are patent throughout their length. In the midzone arteriolar pressure exceeds alveolar pressure. However, alveolar pressure exceeds the local venous pressure, so that the arteriolar end of the capillary is open and the venous end closed. Blood flow measurements in the human lung show a progressive reduction of blood flow per unit of lung tissue from the base of the lung to the apex. This difference is reduced on exercise and abolished on lying down. Pulmonary hypertension or a large left to right shunt of blood through the lungs also alters the

3

usual pattern and flow in the lower parts of the lungs is reduced.

The principal function of the pulmonary circulation is gas exchange, and it has an appropriately large capillary surface area which contains approximately 20 per cent of the 400 ml blood which constitutes the pulmonary blood volume. Local reduction in alveolar oxygen tension with or without hypercapnia appears to cause local vaso- and broncho-constriction. This process tends to redistribute both blood and gases to more appropriate areas. Systemic anoxaemia produces generalized pulmonary vasoconstriction. This has no obvious role in the adult but in the foetus diverts blood into the systemic circulation and hence to the placenta via the ductus arteriosus.

The pulmonary circulation nourishes the alveolar walls, and in the event of pulmonary arterial occlusion there is inactivation of the sur-factant lining material which normally prevents alveolar collapse (p. 96). Consequently, atelectasis commonly follows pulmonary arterial occlusion.

The pulmonary circulation also filters particles from the mixed venous blood and in addition acts as a reservoir of blood, particularly during changes of posture.

LYMPHATIC CIRCULATION

Albumin molecules and other protein and lipid substances leaked from the capillaries are recovered from the extravascular tissues and returned to the systemic circulation by the lymphatics. The thoracic duct lymph flow in 24 hours is approximately equal to the blood volume and over the same period more than half the total circulating plasma proteins is returned to the central veins through the thoracic duct. Although all protein and lipid components of the blood may be identified in lymph the detailed composition of the fluid varies with the region drained. Hepatic lymph is protein-rich and protein synthesis in the liver plays an important role in the maintenance of normal concentrations of most of the plasma proteins. Lymphatic capillaries are either open-ended or very permeable, allowing the free entry of macromolecules. Larger lymphatics have walls impermeable to substances of molecular weights greater than 6000, thus preventing loss of macromolecules. The pumping mechanisms of skeletal muscle contraction, arterial pulsation, and respiration determine lymph movement and the vessels (like the veins) contain valves which prevent retrograde flow. Although peripheral lympho-venous communications may be demonstrated they have little signifi-cance in health. Foreign particles removed from the extravascular tissue are filtered off by the lymphatic nodes.

GENERAL CARDIOVASCULAR RESPONSES
Exercise

At the onset of exercise, the increased metabolic needs of the muscles are largely met by anaerobic mechanisms, but there is a rapid increase in blood flow to the active muscles and after 30 to 60 sec aerobic mechanisms predominate. At rest the mixed venous blood is about 70 per cent saturated with oxygen, but during severe exercise the saturation may fall as low as 25 per cent and the total oxygen consumption may increase 20-fold (see also p. 110). In health the cardiac output may increase during severe exercise to 30 l/min, with a heart rate of about 190 beats/min and a stroke volume of over 150 ml/beat. The systemic arterial blood pressure only increases moderately and it is therefore obvious that peripheral resistance falls. However, the decreased resistance only occurs in active muscle. The peripheral resistance in inactive limbs and in the splanchnic vasculature rises and blood flow to these regions falls.

As the heart rate goes up, diastole gets shorter, but the heart also completes its contraction more rapidly. This, and the increased venous filling pressure (p. 42) compensate for the reduction in filling time.

In health, the peak flow to the exercising limb occurs during the period of activity, with a rapid return to pre-exercising flow values in the recovery period. The magnitude of the post-exercise hyperaemia in a limb is directly proportional to the severity and duration of the preceding exercise up to a certain point, after which there is no further increase in flow. Physical training reduces the post-exercise hyperaemia probably by more effective capillary perfusion of the muscles during exercise.

Posture

Sudden changes in posture affect the cardiac output by changing the filling pressure of the heart, and the circulatory reflexes normally react to restore the situation towards normal. On tipping a subject from the horizontal to the vertical position there is an immediate pooling of about 800 ml of blood in the veins of the lower limbs. The cardiac output falls and there is increased peripheral vasoconstrictor activity in arterioles, preventing a reduction in blood pressure and protecting the capillary beds of the lower limb from the increased hydrostatic pressure which would otherwise result in massive transudation of fluid at capillary level. The veins also constrict and minimize the volume of pooled blood. Vasoconstriction is probably brought about by signals from receptors in the great veins and atria and also from systemic arterial baroreceptors. Active standing or tensing the leg muscles on tipping reduces the volume of blood pooled in the lower limbs and there is less reduction in cardiac output and a smaller increase in heart rate. After a very short time sympathetically-mediated venoconstriction dimishes, and it is not yet clear what takes its place.

Temperature regulation

The skin circulation is under the control of temperature-regulating centres in the hypothalamus. In a hot environment the skin blood vessels dilate, the blood flow through them increases and heat is lost. The circulation through the skin can be so rapid as to be acting virtually as an arteriovenous fistula, so that the blood in the superficial veins may become almost fully 'arterialized' if the arm is placed in hot water. The cardiac output, pulse pressure and heart rate all increase to meet the demand for increased flow in response to heat, and the extra load on the heart is comparable to that in mild exercise.

In a cold environment there is peripheral vasoconstriction and the skin flow decreases. Provided that increased muscular activity, in the form of shivering, does not occur, the cardiac output falls. The environmental temperature must be taken into account in attempting to assess the cardiac output clinically, for in a warm room the output may well be twice the lowest resting value.

Oxygen and carbon dioxide

The effect of moderate anoxia on the circulation as a whole is to cause a rise in blood pressure and a rise in cardiac output; if severe it eventually causes circulatory collapse. Moderate carbon dioxide excess increases cardiac output usually with little change in blood pressure. The modes of action of anoxia and carbon dioxide excess are complex. Both cause dilatation of most blood vessels by a direct local action, but also cause an increase in nervous vasoconstrictor tone. Anoxia achieves this by stimulating the vasomotor centre reflexly through the sinoaortic chemoreceptors: carbon dioxide stimulates the vasomotor centre both reflexly and directly.

The effects, therefore, of anoxia and carbon dioxide on the local blood flow in any organ and on the peripheral resistance as a whole are variable and depend on the balance between local and central actions.

Disordered function

HEART FAILURE

Heart failure might be defined in physiological terms as a failure of the heart to pump blood normally. It would be difficult, though not impossible, to establish standard conditions of measurement of, say, a

Starling curve relating filling pressure to cardiac output, and then to establish a normal range of variation in the population. One might then define heart failure as a condition in which this measure of cardiac performance fell short of some arbitrary criterion of normality, such as the lower 1 or 5 percentile for the population. This definition has the advantage of bringing heart failure into line with, for example, renal failure or respiratory failure, which can be specified in terms of deviations of blood urea concentration, or blood oxygen and carbon dioxide concentrations, from an agreed though arbitrary range.

This is not what the physician means by heart failure. He uses it as a shorthand term to describe *oedema of the systemic or pulmonary vascular beds, or both, associated with a raised central venous pressure, on either side of the heart; not due either to excess fluid administration exceeding renal excretory capacity or to diminished renal excretory capacity resulting from renal disease.*

This definition sounds clumsy, and is; but it recognizes that many different conditions which cause failure of the heart to expel its contents adequately result in a common and easily recognizable clinical syndrome. The definition embraces cases in which all the clinical features of heart failure coexist with a cardiac output which may be normal or even greater than normal at rest, and which may rise normally with exercise. Some cases of severe anaemia, thyrotoxicosis, cor pulmonale (p. 120), beri-beri and arteriovenous fistula fall into this category. Admittedly the definition implies, or at least suggests that the symptoms and signs of heart failure are brought about by the same mechanism, regardless of whether the primary failure lies with the heart as a pump, or whether the needs of the tissues for blood are so much increased, as in severe anaemia, for example, that even a normal heart cannot keep up with them. However, the proposal of different mechanisms operating in high and low output states is not attractive, and seems needlessly complicated.

When oedema occurs predominantly in the lungs and when left atrial pressure is raised, the heart failure is often described as 'left-sided'; when it occurs in the systemic circulation it is described as 'congestive' or 'right-sided'. The distinction is in one sense trivial, because the fundamental disturbance is in the regulation of extracellular fluid volume, which is increased in all kinds of heart failure. The site at which oedema first appears, usually either at the lung bases or at the ankles of an erect subject, depends on the relative degrees of impairment of contraction of the two ventricles, and on the relative mechanical hindrances to the flow of blood in different parts of the central circulation. There are certain special problems about pulmonary oedema, which will be discussed more fully in a later section (p. 59).

Heart failure used to be discussed in terms of inadequate 'forward flow' and too much 'back pressure'. These are naive concepts, and the syndrome is better considered as a pathological retention of sodium and water by the kidneys. There is no mystery about the initial expansion of intravascular volume which is so characteristic of heart failure. Since the mean pressure within the circulation is 7 mmHg it follows that complete cessation of heart pumping will bring all pressures within the circulation to that value. Normal mean capillary pressure is probably 10 to 15 mmHg, and thus complete standstill of the circulation must therefore reduce capillary pressure by about 7 mmHg, disturb the balance of hydrostatic and osmotic forces across capillaries, and lead to fluid entering the circulation from the interstitial spaces. Lesser degrees of failure of the heart as a pump would lead to proportionately smaller falls of mean capillary pressure, but the effect would be of the same general kind, i.e. expansion of plasma volume. The mystery of heart failure is the continued accumulation of fluid in the plasma and interstitial space, leading to an increase in mean circulatory pressure and interstitial pressure. Oedema appears when interstitial pressure exceeds atmospheric pressure.

It is clear that the excess fluid filling the interstitial spaces in heart failure is due to active retention of sodium and water by the kidney. Up to a point this mechanism is valuable, because it allows the mean pressure filling the circulation to be increased, and for venous return to be enhanced. The increased filling of the heart stretches the heart muscle, and leads, according to Starling's Law, to an increase in output. This will obviously tend to compensate in some degree for any primary failure of the heart to pump blood adequately. However, there are three ways at least in which the sodium and water retention are disadvantageous to the body. Firstly, once cardiac filling pressure exceeds a certain point (the 'flat' portion of the Starling curve relating cardiac output to input pressure), there is no further increase in cardiac output, and if the heart is seriously overstretched it is possible that output may even start to fall (e.g. because of incompetence of the tricuspid valves). Secondly, excessive accumulation of fluid in the lungs can eventually prevent gaseous exchange. Thirdly, sustained overstretching of the heart appears to promote compensatory myocardial hypertrophy as well as permanent dilatation. Muscular hypertrophy obviously improves cardiac performance, but it may entail less efficient transfer of metabolites from cell to capillary, and of nutrients and oxygen from capillary to myocardial cell. This is especially liable to occur if there is occlusion or stenosis of the main coronary arteries. Also, according to the law of Laplace, as the diameter of the ventricle increases, the tension which the ventricular muscle has to develop to produce the same intraventricular pressure increases. A situation can be reached in which further increase in fibre length produces no further haemodynamic advantage, and the energy released by myocardial contraction falls.

As far as is known at present, there is no serious metabolic defect in the myocardium during cardiac failure. There appears to be no shortage of high energy phosphate materials, and the failing myocardium has a similar oxidation-reduction potential to a normal myocardium. There is some evidence for depletion of myocardial catecholamines. This may represent a basic fault, but may also simply reflect a chronic increase in sympathetic nervous activity.

Possible mechanisms of renal sodium and water retention
in heart failure
It is obvious that some message passes from heart to kidney, containing the instructions to retain sodium and water. It is well known that heart failure may be improved in two ways: either by improving myocardial performance, or by giving some drug which induces the kidneys to unload sodium and water. Experimental studies indicate that the following mechanisms could be responsible for sodium and water retention in heart failure:

A reduction of renal perfusion pressure. If no other influences are at work, a simple reduction in renal perfusion pressure results in a proportional falling off in sodium and water excretion. In established heart failure the systemic arterial pressure is not substantially different from that observed before the onset of heart failure. However, it could be argued that this mechanism played a part in the development of heart failure, but that it was shut off when the systemic arterial pressure returned to its accustomed level.

Renal vasoconstriction due to sympathetic nervous stimulation or to circulating catecholamines. A fall of systemic arterial pressure results in renal vasoconstriction and in adrenal catecholamine release by the reflex action of the systemic arterial baroreceptors (p. 42). There is much evidence that sympathetic vasoconstrictor activity is increased in heart failure, especially during the stage at which fluid is accumulating. The nature of the continuing stimulus to sympathetic vasoconstrictor activity once systemic arterial pressure has been restored to normal is not clear. However, the observations of slightly reduced glomerular filtration rate and considerably reduced renal plasma flow are fully compatible with nervous vasoconstriction. Increased sympathetic nervous activity in other areas is suggested by much evidence that neurogenic venoconstrictor tone is increased, and also by the effects of blockade of cardiac β-adrenergic receptors with drugs. Such drugs may precipitate or augment heart failure.

Renal sodium retention due to aldosterone. When renal perfusion pressure falls, it is well known that the enzyme renin is released into the blood-stream (p. 44). This in turn liberates angiotensin, which as well as being a powerful vasoconstrictor, is also a trophic hormone promoting the release of aldosterone from the adrenal cortex. Renin release can also be provoked by neurogenic renal vasoconstriction, even though arterial perfusion pressure does not fall. Thus there are good theoretical grounds for supposing that renin and hence aldosterone secretion might be increased in heart failure. Although the concentrations of renin and aldosterone in the blood probably rise during the phase at which fluid is accumulating in heart failure, there is fairly general agreement that the concentrations of both substances are usually normal in established chronic heart failure. However, this still leaves unexplained why renin and aldosterone secretion are not reduced, as they would be in any state of sodium and water overload not due to heart failure. Thus it seems reasonable to conclude that the renin/angiotensin/aldosterone system is at least permitting, if not actively encouraging, the retention of sodium in heart failure.

Vasopressin release. Similar considerations apply to vasopressin, whose secretion rate probably increases during the development of heart failure, even though in established cases the secretion rate returns towards normal.

It should be noted that all these mechanisms except the first involve the participation of the central nervous system. Although aldosterone secretion may increase when renal perfusion pressure falls (without central nervous participation), it is known that renal perfusion pressure is characteristically normal in established heart failure: therefore any apparently inappropriate increase in secretion rate could well be explained by renal vasoconstriction brought about by increased activity of the sympathoadrenal system.

Thus the message from heart to kidneys probably passes through the central nervous system, though it is not yet known which receptors are involved. Traditionally the 'volume' receptors of the circulation are the stretch receptors of the great veins and atria. Yet in heart failure these organs are demonstrably overstretched, and in acute experiments overstretching of the volume receptors is a stimulus for increased excretion rather than retention of fluid. Such a mechanism has been invoked to explain the diuresis characteristically associated with prolonged attacks of paroxysmal tachycardia. Attempts have been made to involve the volume receptors in the pathogenesis of heart failure by supposing that they respond only to a pulsatile stimulus, and that in heart failure the chronic overstretching of the great veins and atria reduces the pulsatile stimulation of the receptors. An alternative and perhaps more plausible explanation places the maintenance of an adequate systemic arterial pressure as the prime function of the heart, and suggests that any failure of the heart to sustain an adequate arterial pressure brings into action the many mechanisms under central nervous control which can increase cardiac output. By this hypothesis heart failure represents an attempt by the body to sustain arterial pressure by means which, though effective, eventually prove disadvantageous. An attractive feature of this hypothesis is that it explains why hypoxaemia, hypercapnia, anaemia, thyrotoxicosis, and arterio-venous fistula (all of which increase the demands of the tissues for the available blood, and lower peripheral systemic resistance) should provoke the same clinical syndrome as primary failure of the heart to pump blood.

Pulmonary oedema (*'left ventricular failure'*)
Pathological retention of sodium and water in the body can eventually lead to pulmonary oedema for purely hydrostatic reasons (when pulmonary capillary pressure exceeds plasma colloid osmotic pressure, and when the capacity of the pulmonary lymphatics is exceeded). However, pulmonary oedema, especially its acute form, which typically occurs during sleep, also has an important sympathetic reflex component. Characteristically in pulmonary oedema the blood pressure and heart rate are increased above normal, and there is sweating and pupillary dilatation. The condition is usually immediately responsive to very small amounts of sympathetic ganglionic blocking drugs. It is even possible in the experimental animal to produce acute pulmonary oedema without any pre-existing retention of sodium and water (e.g. by the injection of protein solutions into the cerebral ventricles). Acute pulmonary oedema may occasionally be precipitated in man by subarachnoid haemorrhage. However, in most cases there is a pre-existing expansion of the extracellular fluid, and the sympathetic reflex

3*

component is superimposed upon this and triggers off an attack, probably partly by peripheral venous constriction shifting blood into the thorax. The nature of the stimulus to the sympatho-adrenal system has not yet been discovered.

Constrictive pericarditis

Constrictive pericarditis causes many of the features of heart failure. In this condition the heart is encased in a rigid tube which limits its diastolic volume. Thus although the heart itself may be normal, increased filling pressure increases cardiac output very little. The heart fails because it cannot fill and not because it cannot empty. A similar situation may occur in some forms of cardiomyopathy in which there is myocardial fibrosis, and in constrictive endocarditis such as that due to endomyocardial fibrosis. By interfering with cardiac filling these produce an identical clinical picture, which is characterized by the signs of congestive cardiac failure usually unaccompanied by pulmonary congestion or orthopnoea.

CENTRAL CIRCULATORY OBSTRUCTION

One of the important syndromes of heart disease is that due to obstruction of the circulation at some point at which the whole, or most of the cardiac output must pass. The symptoms depend on the severity of obstruction, and tend to be similar whatever the site of obstruction. The cardiac output tends to be reduced, and cannot increase normally on exercise. There is usually a small pulse, low blood pressure, cold extremities and peripheral cyanosis in any severe obstruction. Evidence of a high cardiac output virtually rules out severe obstruction.

Left-sided central circulatory obstruction

When central circulatory obstruction is on the left side of the heart, it may cause congestion and oedema of the lungs, which alter pulmonary mechanics and gas exchange, and characteristically cause dyspnoea (p. 59).

Aortic stenosis. Resistance to left ventricular outflow by valve stenosis is countered by concentric myocardial hypertrophy; the distensibility of the ventricle is reduced as a result and increased force of atrial contraction becomes of importance in ventricular filling. Resting cardiac output is maintained at normal levels until left ventricular failure supervenes, at which time mean left atrial and right heart pressures rise, and there may be pulmonary oedema. In some forms of subvalvular stenosis the outflow of blood from the heart is not restricted throughout the whole period of systole, and the obstruction results from muscular hypertrophy of the ventricular outflow tract. Such a lesion may be part of an obstructive cardiomyopathy affecting the right and left ventricles, either singly or together. In this situation a high intraventricular pressure is developed during isometric systole, and when the pulmonary or aortic valves open there is an initial rapid ejection of blood which becomes interrupted by the hypertrophic septal segment of the outflow tract during the period of isotonic contraction. In severe aortic stenosis stroke volume fails to increase with exercise and the associated vaso-dilation may produce syncope or compromise the coronary circulation.

Mitral stenosis. Enhanced contraction of the hypertrophic left atrium becomes of major importance in maintaining ventricular filling, and the onset of atrial fibrillation often marks the onset of rapid clinical deterioration. As mitral obstruction becomes more severe the left atrial pressure rises, and enough pulmonary arterial hypertension develops to maintain the pulmonary arterio-venous difference, until the left atrial pressure reaches about 25 mmHg. There is then usually a disproportionate rise in pulmonary artery pressure, which may reach systemic levels. This is probably due to intimal thickening and muscular hypertrophy of the pulmonary arterioles, which shield the pulmonary capillary bed from excessive arterial pressure. However, this response is often disproportionate to needs, and imposes a strain on the right ventricle, and eventually congestive heart failure occurs. Pulmonary oedema occurs characteristically in the early stage of the condition. It makes the lungs stiffer and is probably the most important cause of shortness of breath.

Coarctation of the aorta (see also p. 89). Although the high proximal aortic pressure may overload the heart and cause cardiac failure, coarctation is often symptomless until cerebral haemorrhage or aortic rupture occur. The normal cerebral blood flow in coarctation cannot be taken to represent abnormal cerebral vasoconstriction, because it can be fully explained by cerebral autoregulation (p. 51). Thus the elevation of proximal aortic pressure could be the simple mechanical result of a mismatch between cardiac contractile force and proximal large vessel resistance. However, the proximal hypertension could have a renal origin (p. 68).

Right-sided central circulatory obstruction
Pulmonary stenosis and *pulmonary vascular obstruction*, by reducing blood flow to parts of the lungs, cause impaired gas exchange and

hyperventilation (p. 119). The enormous capacity of the right ventricle for hypertrophy often allows the maintenance of a normal resting cardiac output despite a many-fold increase in resistance either at the pulmonary valve or in the pulmonary vascular bed.

VALVULAR INCOMPETENCE

With incompetence of the aortic and pulmonary valves the degree of backflow depends not only on the valve itself but also on the mean diastolic pressure in the great vessel concerned. Because pulmonary diastolic pressure is generally low, pulmonary incompetence is usually unimportant. However, aortic incompetence is more serious, and may in itself be enough to cause heart failure. Mitral incompetence throws an extra load on both left ventricle and atrium, and is a common cause of heart failure and pulmonary oedema. Tricuspid incompetence is rare in the absence of heart failure. Tricuspid incompetence seems often to be a functional defect resulting from overstretching of the heart in several conditions which have in common an increased right ventricular pressure. When tricuspid incompetence is gross the systemic veins and the liver show exaggerated systemic pulsation (p. 90).

CARDIOVASCULAR SHUNTS

If there is an abnormal communication between two parts of the circulation, blood flows through the defect at a rate depending on the pressure difference across the shunt and the size of the defect. If the shunt is from the high pressure left side of the heart to the low pressure right side, the situation is physiologically similar to that found in valvular incompetence, in that part of the cardiac output passes through part of the heart twice and the work of the heart must increase if the systemic flow is to be maintained. Shunts may occur between any chambers of the heart or great vessels that are anatomically related to one another, but are commonly due to congenital defects in the atrial or ventricular septum or patency of the ductus arteriosus. The effect of a left to right shunt on the heart varies with the level of the shunt, as may be seen from Table 3.

Apart from the special case of pulmonary arteriovenous fistula a right to left shunt only occurs if there is an increase in the pressure on the right side of the heart, owing to some obstruction in the right heart itself or in the pulmonary circulation distal to the communication. Thus in persistent ductus arteriosus the blood only enters the aorta from the pulmonary artery if there is increased pulmonary vascular resistance. At the other end of the scale is atrial septal defect across

TABLE 3. Left to right shunts

Level of shunt	Ventricle doing increased work	Chambers through which flow is normal
Aorto-pulmonary	Left	Right atrium and ventricle
Interventricular	Left and right	Right atrium
Interatrial	Right	Left ventricle
Arteriovenous	Left and right	None

which the flow may be from right to left from any of the following causes: increased pulmonary vascular resistance, right ventricular failure, pulmonary stenosis, tricuspid stenosis or tricuspid atresia. The commonest example of a right to left shunt is Fallot's tetralogy in which the aorta arises from both the left and right ventricles, and there is pulmonary stenosis. The resistance to right ventricular outflow causes mixed venous blood to be ejected into the aorta.

The characteristic effect of a right to left shunt is arterial unsaturation. Cyanosis at rest is not obvious until the proportion of shunted blood in the peripheral arteries is over 30 per cent.

Under certain circumstances the shunt may not involve the whole aortic flow. Thus in persistent ductus arteriosus with reversed shunt only the lower half of the body (and sometimes the left arm as well) may be cyanosed, since the admixture of venous blood takes place distal to the origins of the innominate and left carotid arteries.

Pulmonary vascular hypertension

In the presence of large left-to-right shunts the pulmonary artery pressure is high although the pulmonary vascular resistance remains low. In some children there appears to be persistence of the foetal type of muscular arterioles in the lungs. In adult life patients with large left-to-right shunts develop atheromatous changes in the intima of the pulmonary arteries, and eventually there is progressive pulmonary hypertension and cardiac failure.

SYNCOPE: TRANSIENT CIRCULATORY ARREST

In a simple fainting attack there is a sudden fall in peripheral resistance, in filling pressure and in cardiac output. This causes faintness or loss of consciousness owing to insufficient cerebral blood flow. The sudden fall in peripheral resistance is caused mainly by relaxation of the vascular bed of skeletal muscle, which produces a big increase in muscle blood flow. There is now much evidence that the muscle vasodilatation is mediated by increased activity of cholinergic sympathetic nerves. The afferent limb of the reflex is not known.

Fainting attacks almost always occur in people who are standing still, and when they fall to the ground recovery starts, because the venous return and cardiac output tend to return to normal. The patient usually has premonitory symptoms of nausea, sweating and dizziness; and recovery is never immediate, taking several minutes to be complete.

Syncope due to failure to maintain an adequate cardiac output occurs on effort when there is severe obstruction to the circulation; for example, in aortic or pulmonary stenosis, and in pulmonary hypertension. The cardiac output cannot increase sufficiently to maintain an adequate cerebral circulation and at the same time supply the metabolic needs of the exercising muscles. Recovery occurs when the cerebral circulation is restored as the needs of the muscles decrease.

Fainting attacks due to disturbance in cardiac rhythm may result from extreme bradycardia, cardiac standstill or from extreme tachycardia. At the higher rates occurring with abnormal rhythms, the cardiac output begins to fall off because the heart cannot fill sufficiently during diastole, nor is there enough time for adequate coronary filling.

If the heart stops, unconsciousness follows in about 15 sec and irreversible cerebral changes occur within 4 min. Ventricular fibrillation is as harmful as cardiac arrest, for the output becomes negligible. Repeated (Stokes–Adams) attacks of cardiac syncope occur most commonly in patients with heart block who often have pulse rates of 28–36/min; this bradycardia is not the cause of their syncopal attacks, which are due to cardiac standstill or fibrillation. Syncope occurs without warning about 15 sec after the heart stops. If the heart starts beating again, there is a violent flush as fully oxygenated blood from the lungs flows into the vasodilated circulation. Recovery after cardiac standstill is immediate and complete provided that permanent cerebral damage has not occurred. The sudden onset and rapid recovery help to distinguish a Stokes–Adams attack from a simple faint and the history of flushing is also helpful. When the heart rate is extremely fast (over 250/min) any effort readily causes syncope, and although the cardiac output may be sufficient to maintain the cerebral circulation with the patient lying still, it cannot support the least exertion.

POSTURAL HYPOTENSION

Neurological disease processes interfering with circulatory reflexes adjusting peripheral vascular resistance, venomotor tone, and myocardial contraction during postural change can produce postural hypotension (e.g. diabetes mellitus, syringomyelia and tabes dorsalis). In other cases the filling of the circulation is inadequate (e.g. in the chronic sodium and water depletion of severe adrenocorticoid deficiency). In patients with neurological disorders the heart rate does not increase normally despite the profound fall of blood pressure on standing. The Valsalva manouevre (p. 72) provokes no change in heart rate and no overshoot of blood pressure on release of expiratory effort. In the few cases which have been studied at necropsy, spinal cord damage has been demonstrated, and the defect is presumably due to damage to efferent sympathetic fibres. The topographical pattern of damage shows itself clinically by patchy loss of sweating, especially in the trunk and legs.

PERPHERAL ISCHAEMIA

Atheroma affecting the major limb vessels results in a gradual reduction of the maximum attainable blood flow. The severity of the resulting disability depends on the extent to which a collateral arterial supply develops. During exercise the inflow of blood to the limb is limited and there is a drop in arterial pressure distal to the obstruction. Intermittent claudication represents ischaemic pain arising in muscles distal to the obstruction. Eventually occlusion of major vessels may lead to tissue death in the distal parts of the limb. Atheromatous plaques in major arteries may also be responsible for the formation of platelet thrombi and consequent embolism in the digits giving rise to one form of Raynaud's phenomenon (see below). Sudden occlusion of major limb arteries allows less time for the development of collateral circulation and resulting tissue death is more likely to occur.

Raynaud's phenomenon. This is a condition affecting the fingers, and less commonly, the toes. The skin shows paroxysmal colour changes and pallor followed by cyanosis and then redness, accompanied by severe pain. These changes are usually provoked by cold. In Raynaud's 'disease' the primary lesion involves digital arteries, rendering them unduly susceptible to normal constrictor stimuli, and leads eventually to organic narrowing, and atrophic changes in the tissues of the digits. The cause of the condition is not known, but in some cases it forms part of the clinical syndrome of a 'collagen' disease, especially scleroderma, systemic lupus erythematosus and rheumatoid arthritis.

DISORDERS OF THE VEINS

Obstruction. At most sites in the body there are several veins with free intercommunications draining the tissues. This protects against the development of a high venous pressure and consequent oedema following obstruction of just one vein. Furthermore, moderate elevation of venous and capillary pressures do not cause oedema because the normally negative interstitial pressure provides a safety factor. Oedema cannot appear until interstitial pressure has risen from its mean normal value (-7 mmHg) to atmospheric pressure. Although complete obstruction of a single vein thus produces no appreciable effects on a tissue, complete and sudden obstruction of all veins draining a tissue causes tissue death, accompanied by engorgement and haemorrhage. Severe but incomplete obstruction causes oedema.

Valvular incompetence. The valves are not essential for venous return, which can still occur passively (p. 46); but if valves are incompetent the massaging effect of the muscles elevates venous pressure distal to the valves and in the capillary bed. During exercise the venous pressure is higher in the leg than in normal subjects. Persistent elevation of venous pressure results in dilatation of veins and oedema, and has a bad effect on tissue nutrition. Although varicose veins often appear in association with raised venous pressure (either general, as in cardiac failure, or local, as in pregnancy) they occasionally occur without apparent cause. In these patients the vein wall is often defective in elastic tissue.

Loss of venous tone. The capacity of the veins is potentially very great, and their calibre is normally reduced by tonic contraction of muscle in their walls. Failure of this tone in enough veins below heart level causes pooling of the blood with failure of venous return and cardiac output. The role of this mechanism in syncope and other conditions of circulatory failure is not fully known, but it is probably the main reason for the postural hypotension following sympathectomy or the use of sympathetic-blocking drugs.

MYOCARDIAL ISCHAEMIA

Anginal pain occurs when the heart muscle is short of oxygen. Anything which interferes with the supply of oxygen to the heart muscle can provoke anginal pain. The usual cause is degenerative change in the coronary vessels, but anoxia or anaemia, by reducing the amount of oxygen carried in the coronary blood, can provoke anginal pain which may disappear when the oxygen content of the coronary blood is restored to normal. Both aortic stenosis and incompetence can interfere with the flow of blood to the coronary vessels, and syphilitic aortitis may involve the mouths of the coronary arteries and mechanically reduce the coronary flow. Any condition which increases the metabolic needs of the heart muscle will tend to provoke angina. Exercise and emotion are by far the most important precipitating factors, but thyrotoxicosis and hypertension also tend to make angina worse. Emotion may precipitate angina by increasing the cardiac output, by producing tachycardia, by raising the blood pressure and by increasing skin and muscle blood flow. The tendency for angina to be worse after a heavy meal is due to the fact that the circulatory needs of the stomach and intestines have also to be met. Nitrites are thought to relieve angina by lowering arterial pressure and hence reducing the work of the heart, but they also directly reduce the resistance offered by the larger coronary arteries.

ARTERIAL HYPERTENSION

Increased activity of the sympatho-adrenal system can raise the blood pressure acutely, as in emotion or exercise. Either cardiac output or peripheral resistance, or both, may increase. Other factors can acutely raise blood pressure (e.g. compression of venous reservoirs by contracting muscle, and increased levels of circulating angiotensin).

Chronic elevation of systemic arterial pressure is a feature of several distinct diseases, but in none is it fully understood. *Phaeochromocytoma* (p. 546) is perhaps the least enigmatic because the hypertension is probably caused by an excessive secretion of noradrenaline by the adrenal tumour. The increased secretion of both noradrenaline and adrenaline results in an increased rate of excretion of these amines in the urine, which can be shown by chemical or biological assay. The attacks of pallor, hypertension and (usually) reflex bradycardia seen when catecholamine release is intermittent may be reproduced by infusing noradrenaline intravenously. While surgical removal of the tumour is commonly followed by a fall in pressure, some degree of hypertension may persist or recur. These clinical failures illustrate a principle common to many hypertensive states: pathological elevation of arterial pressure from whatever cause may eventually induce a self-perpetuating hypertension that is uninfluenced by removal of the factor that initiated the rise in pressure.

In *coarctation of the aorta* the vascular obstruction is usually severe enough to limit the escape of blood to the periphery, so leading to a rise both in systolic and diastolic pressures proximally in the aorta. Beyond the coarcted segment the systolic pressure is reduced, but the diastolic is often above normal. Mean pressure may be high or normal, but is always lower than mean brachial artery pressure. From the failure of the central hypertension to evoke compensatory splanchnic vasodilatation it may be inferred that the carotid sinus regulating mechanism is probably reset at a higher than normal blood pressure, as in most other forms of chronic hypertension. The cause of the raised blood pressure is not known, but it seems reasonable that it may have features in common with the hypertension of renal artery stenosis (below). The hypertension is usually relieved but not always abolished by surgical correction of the anomaly.

The adrenal cortex plays some part in the maintenance of blood pressure, not only by the influence of its mineralocorticoids on salt and water balance, but also because glucocorticoids seem to be required for the maintenance of normal blood pressure. There is at present some dispute about the effects of adrenal cortical hormones on vascular reactivity to nervous and chemical influences. The hypertension of *Cushing's syndrome* is probably due to the oversecretion of cortisol, and the consistently raised systemic arterial pressure seen in primary hyperaldosteronism (p. 533) is probably due to an excess secretion of salt-retaining adrenal cortical steroids, notably aldosterone. The hypertension of *pre-eclamptic toxaemia* may also involve endocrine changes; though in neither disease has the cause of the disturbance been fully elucidated.

Renal hypertension remains enigmatic. A raised arterial pressure is common in acute and chronic glomerulonephritis, often found in chronic pyelonephritis and renal artery stenosis, and is occasionally seen in congenital, allergic, toxic, neoplastic and degenerative lesions of the kidney. The mechanism of the hypertension has not been ascertained with certainty. The available clinical and pathological data suggest that a reduction in the blood supply to the kidney is an important factor. This has led to intensive investigation of experimental hypertension in laboratory animals, from which it may be concluded, briefly, that the acutely ischaemic kidney liberates a specific secretion (renin) which interacts with a constituent of the blood to produce a vasoconstrictor substance (angiotensin). The latter is thought to be responsible for the generalized arteriolar narrowing that produces the initial rise in blood pressure. The extent to which this morbid sequence contributes to the hypertension of kidney disease in man remains conjectural (see p. 179) and attempts to demonstrate pressor substances in the blood in experimental renal hypertension in animals have only been successful in the very early stages. However, angiotensin can exert indirect and slowly developing pressor action when present in concentrations which are not enough to raise blood pressure acutely. It seems likely, therefore, that the renin–angiotensin system will prove to play an important part in the pathogenesis of chronic renal hypertension.

In most patients with hypertension no cause, renal or otherwise, can be found, and such patients are therefore described as having *essential hypertension*.

The malignant phase of hypertension. High arterial pressure of any origin may pass into a malignant phase characterized by papilloedema and focal necrotic lesions of small arteries. This syndrome is at present widely believed to be qualitatively different from 'benign' hypertension, although in some cases it may apparently be produced by an excessively high blood pressure alone. It has recently been observed that patients with malignant hypertension almost always secrete an excess of aldosterone, though they do not thereby become oedematous. We do not yet know whether this is functionally important; but it helps to explain the low plasma potassium concentrations sometimes seen in these cases. The aldosterone hypersecretion is probably brought about by the increased plasma concentrations of renin (see above) which are usually present.

Possible mechanisms of 'essential' hypertension
Theoretically only 5 haemodynamic changes can produce an abnormally high arterial pressure: (1) a rise in cardiac output, (2) an expansion in blood volume, (3) a reduction in vascular capacity, (4) an increase in blood viscosity, or (5) generalized constriction of the systemic arterioles. Sufficient evidence has accumulated to exclude the first four of these, and there are good grounds for attributing hypertension to an increase in the peripheral resistance, although there is some recent evidence that cardiac output may be increased in the early stages of the condition. It has generally been assumed that the arterioles throughout the whole systemic vasculature participate equally in the constriction, so that the distribution of blood throughout the body is not altered, although there is some evidence that the vessels of the upper limbs may not be involved early in the disease. The lability of the arterial pressure in many patients exculpates organic vascular narrowing as a major factor. On the other hand, if neurogenic vasomotor activity is arrested in an accessible tissue such as the forearm, there is only a normal (not an exaggerated) increase in blood flow.

Attempts to find alternative explanations for the increased peripheral resistance have led to the suggestion that there may be a specific functional increase in the constrictor responsiveness of the arteriolar sphincters as a result, possibly, of sensitization by some unknown humoral factor. The vascular smooth muscle, by this hypothesis, is unduly susceptible to normal constrictor stimuli.

An interesting suggestion has recently been made about the part that autoregulation (p. 49) may play in hypertension. If, for example, the kidneys retained sodium and water, there would be an expansion of plasma volume and an increase in cardiac output. However, if over long periods the tissues could adjust their vascular resistance to keep blood flow constant, then peripheral resistance and hence systemic arterial pressure should eventually rise. This type of slowly developing hypertension has been seen with prolonged use of sodium-retaining drugs in man. Its converse may be the slowly developing fall of blood pressure with prolonged diuretic treatment, and also with β-blocking drugs which reduce cardiac rate and contractile force.

The appearance of sustained high blood pressure signifies that the sino-aortic baroreceptors have been overruled, for if they were normally sensitive they would have brought the blood pressure down. There is direct animal evidence, and overwhelming indirect clinical evidence, that the sensitivity of the baroreceptors becomes reset, within weeks or months, to any level of systemic arterial pressure, whether high or low. Once this resetting has taken place, the baroreceptors, through their reflex connections with the sympathetic nervous system, will tend actively to resist departures from the new pressure level. Not only does this happen in 'essential' hypertension, but also in other forms, including renal hypertension. In all these cases, therefore, the central nervous system plays an active part in maintaining the high pressure. In experimental renal hypertension, the resetting is clearly an effect and not a cause of hypertension, for it lags behind the rise of pressure. An interesting paradox of experimental physiology is the recent confirmation of old observations that the blood pressure of a pithed animal falls to the same level whether the animal was previously hypertensive or not. There is clearly a link between the kidney and the nervous system in respect of blood pressure control, but it still awaits discovery.

Principles of Observations, Tests and Measurements

THE CHARACTER OF THE PERIPHERAL PULSE, AND ARTERIAL BLOOD PRESSURE

The rate of rise of the pulse wave is influenced by the rate at which blood is entering the aorta from the heart and by the compliance of the arterial tree. In aortic valve stenosis ejection is slowed. The pulse pressure (the volume of the pulse) depends chiefly upon the volume of blood ejected by the left ventricle into the aorta and to a lesser extent upon the force of this ejection and the rigidity of the arterial walls. If the cardiac output is low the pulse is 'small'. If the output is high the pulse is 'full' and may be abnormally prominent in the large arteries in the neck. The height of the diastolic pressure (the 'tension' of the pulse) is an indication of the peripheral resistance. Anything that allows the blood to run off from the arterial system too rapidly during diastole causes a low diastolic pressure and a 'water-hammer' pulse. Examples are onward run off, as in the vasodilatation of hyperthyroidism and anaemia, and backward run off, as in aortic incompetence.

Pulsus paradoxus

If the systemic arterial pressure and fullness of the pulse diminish appreciably during inspiration (pulsus paradoxus) it is likely either that the heart muscle itself or the pericardium is abnormally rigid, or that the pericardium is tightly stretched by fluid within it. In severe cases the systemic arterial pulse may disappear altogether during a deep inspiration. The phenomenon is clearly mechanical in origin, because it disappears immediately the pericardial pressure has been reduced in cardiac tamponade. The conventional explanation of the phenomenon is that the tug of the diaphragm on a rigid or tight pericardium during inspiration reduces the filling of the right side of the heart. However, this explanation fits neither with animal experiments nor with certain clinical observations. It seems more likely that when there is a limit to the total of right heart volume + left heart volume, any increase in right heart volume, such as occurs normally during inspiration because of augmented venous return, can only occur at the expense of filling of the left side of the heart. The cardiac septum is deflected, the filling of left atrium and ventricle is impaired, and left ventricular stroke output falls. If right atrial inflow of blood is kept constant, experimentally, then pulsus paradoxus cannot be produced by increasing intra-pericardial pressure.

VENOUS PRESSURE

The normal venous pulse consists of positive *a*, *c* and *v* waves, with *x* and *y* troughs (see Fig. 4). All venous pulses must be timed against carotid pulsation or the first heart sound and their identification needs practice. The *a* wave is due to atrial contraction and is absent in atrial fibrillation. It is presystolic in timing and increases on inspiration. It may be visible in normal subjects, but is seldom more than 3 cm above

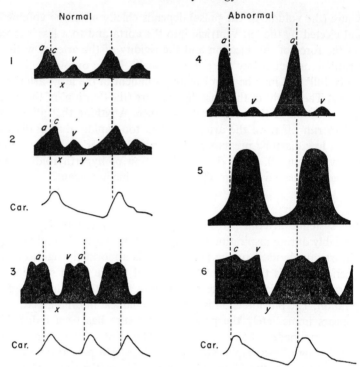

FIGURE 4. *Normal and abnormal forms of the jugular venous pulse.*

Normal

    1. Normal dominant *a* wave.

    2. Normal dominant *c* wave.

    3. Sinus tachycardia: summation of *v* and *a* waves.

Abnormal

    4. Giant *a* wave (see text).

    5. Ventricular pulse of tricuspid incompetence.

    6. Exaggerated *y* descent of constrictive pericarditis.

Car.

    Carotid pulse corresponding in time to the jugular pulse tracings above—
the broken line indicating the timing of the palpable beat.

    (Modified after Short, D. S., *Postgrad. Med. J.*, **33**, 389, 1957.)

the clavicle with the patient lying at 45°. The *a* wave is increased in
conditions in which the right atrium or right ventricle is beating against
a raised resistance. The best examples are seen in pulmonary stenosis
and pulmonary hypertension when the ventricular septum is intact,
and in tricuspid stenosis. In the presence of ventricular septal defect the
right ventricular pressure does not exceed that in the left ventricle and

the right atrial pressure wave is less marked. The *c* wave is unimportant: it was originally though to be due to displacement of the jugular vein by the carotid arterial pulse, but as it also occurs in the left atrium this explanation is incorrect.

The *x* descent after the *a* and *c* waves results from atrial relaxation plus the pull of the contracting ventricle, which tends to enlarge the atrium. It is followed by the *v* wave, which is caused by atrial filling during ventricular systole. The *v* wave is augmented by ventricular regurgitation in tricuspid incompetence and is then better called a positive systolic wave. The peak of the wave occurs at the time that the tricuspid valve opens, and it is followed by the *y* descent, which represents ventricular filling. In tricuspid stenosis the rate of fall of venous pressure during the *y* descent is slow while in tricuspid incompetence and constrictive pericarditis it is rapid.

The nature of the cardiac rhythm may also be determined by observing the venous pulse in the neck. In atrial fibrillation the *a* waves are absent. The appearance of 'cannon' waves indicates that the right atrium is contracting at a time when the tricuspid valve is closed. This occurs at irregular intervals in complete heart block where the atria and ventricles contract at different rates, and may also occur in nodal rhythm. In atrial flutter, waves due to atrial contraction are occasionally seen. Their frequency depends on the atrial rate which is usually 250–350/min.

The 'central' venous pressure

The mean jugular venous pressure is raised in all varieties of congestive heart failure (p. 55) and also in conditions of gross fluid overload (e.g. in oliguric renal failure) even though the heart is normal. If pressure is very high the venous pulse may be difficult to see, the head of the column of blood reaching above the ears. Ideally central venous pressure should be measured directly by means of a thin catheter passed into the superior vena cava. Clinically internal jugular pulsation is looked for first with the patient sitting upright, then at 45° to the horizontal, then supine. An empty external jugular vein which can be made to fill by pressure at the base of the neck is a reliable indication that mean central venous pressure is no higher than the point of pressure. A full external jugular vein may reflect a high pressure in the superior vena cava, but can also be produced by local compression. It is then necessary to rely on the observation of pulsation in the internal jugular vein to estimate central venous pressure.

Normally inspiration sucks blood into the chest and lowers pressure in the superior vena cava (it may be useful to ask a patient to breathe in sharply to demonstrate the upper level of filling of the neck veins in cases in which central venous pressure is excessively high). In some cases of cardiac tamponade and constrictive pericarditis cardiac filling may be impaired by inspiration (p. 60) so that the central venous pressure may rise paradoxically.

Central venous pressure is the cardinal measurement for distinguishing between circulatory failure and low blood pressure due to failure of the heart (venous pressure high) and that due to blood or plasma loss, or to dilation of veins (venous pressure low).

THE CARDIAC IMPULSE

Palpation of the cardiac impulse is valuable in deciding whether either ventricle is beating abnormally or against an excessive load. In the presence of ventricular hypertrophy the apex beat is sustained. Normally the apex beat is completed within the first half of systole, well before the second heart sound. The apex beat may be heaving as well as sustained when the left ventricle is dilated as well as hypertrophic. If both atrium and ventricle on one side are dilated, the site of the apex beat cannot be used to determine which ventricle is involved. Occasionally a double apex beat is palpable, and corresponds to the sound of forceful atrial contraction (4th heart sound, giving a presystolic triple rhythm).

Mechanical recording of the apex beat can give more exact information about the physical characteristics of the apical impulse.

ABNORMAL HEART SOUNDS

As a result of recent work physiological explanations can be advanced for most of the abnormal heart sounds heard in various conditions. Some extra sounds may occur in normal subjects, while others always indicate disease. Taking the cardiac cycle in sequence, the first abnormal sound is a presystolic or atrial sound, which gives rise to presystolic triple rhythm. This sound is always abnormal and is associated with forceful atrial contraction. It may be due to right atrial contraction in pulmonary stenosis, pulmonary hypertension or cor pulmonale; in left ventricular failure it is associated with left atrial contraction. The sound is probably due to blood entering the ventricle, because it occurs immediately after atrial contraction is finished.

Splitting of the first heart sound into its two components of tricuspid and mitral valve closure is commonly heard in health, but is widened when either bundle branch is blocked. The loudness of the first heart sound depends on the position of the atrioventricular valves when ventricular systole starts. In health, ventricular filling is complete before the end of diastole and the atrio-ventricular valves tend to close, so that ventricular contraction normally occurs when the valves are almost shut. In mitral or tricuspid stenosis, ventricular filling is prolonged and systole starts when the valve is still wide open. Its sudden closure increases the loudness of the first heart sound. The pliability of the valve also plays a part, because the first heart sound is not loud in patients with a heavily calcified valve. The timing of atrial contraction also influences the loudness of the first heart sound.

Systolic clicks occur during the ejection phase of ventricular contraction. They may originate in the pulmonary artery or aorta and are thought to be due to sudden changes in tension in the walls of the vessel concerned. They may occur in healthy hearts, but are loudest in mild pulmonary and aortic stenosis and pulmonary hypertension. The great vessel from which the click originates is usually dilated.

The normal splitting of the second heart sound and its variation with respiration have already been described (p. 41). The timing of either component may be delayed if ventricular contraction is prolonged. Thus in right bundle branch block, when right ventricular contraction is delayed, the second sound is widely split, but the width of the split still increases on inspiration. In atrial septal defect, the second heart sound is widely split and the width of the split is characteristically uninfluenced by respiration. The probable explanation for this is that inspiration produces such a small percentage increase in the large right ventricular stroke volume that pulmonary valve closure is not further delayed. If left ventricular contraction is prolonged in left bundle branch block or aortic stenosis the aortic valve closes after the pulmonary, and the normal relationship between the two components of the second sound is reversed. As a result expiration, by shortening right ventricular contraction, widens the gap between the two sounds. This phenomenon is referred to as reversed or paradoxical splitting of the second sound. Pulmonary valve closure may be inaudible in severe pulmonary stenosis, when the pulmonary blood flow is small. The second heart sound is then single. In less severe pulmonary stenosis pulmonary valve closure is delayed, but is often audible though faint. If the right and left ventricles are in free communication and have equal pressures as in Fallot's tetralogy and Eisenmenger's complex, the second heart sound is usually single.

Ventricular filling starts soon after the second heart sound and if there is mitral or tricuspid stenosis, the sudden opening of the atrio-ventricular valve often results in a loud, high-pitched sound known as an opening snap. It is caused by movement of the aortic cusp of the mitral valve. The opening snap is a distinctive feature of rheumatic mitral stenosis, and if the left atrial pressure is high the mitral valve will open soon after aortic valve closure, so that the opening snap will be early. If the valve is calcified and immobile the opening snap may be absent. The third heart sound occurs during the period of rapid ventricular filling, early in diastole. It is heard in normal children, but in adults is evidence of abnormal filling of either ventricle. It is also heard in conditions in which a large amount of blood enters the ventricle rapidly, as in mitral incompetence, ventricular septal defect, and patent ductus arteriosus. If the ventricle itself is abnormal, a third sound may occur with a normal flow as in left ventricular failure, constrictive pericarditis or cardiomyopathy ('constrictive myocarditis'). This sound gives rise to diastolic triple rhythm and with rapid heart rates, when diastole is short, the third sound may coincide with an atrial sound and produce a 'summation gallop'.

HEART MURMURS

Heart murmurs are due to the turbulent flow of blood through normal or abnormal valves or intra-cardiac defects. An increased flow through a normal valve may produce a murmur, the best example being the pulmonary systolic murmur of atrial septal defect. In this condition the right ventricular stroke volume at rest may be twice the normal maximum on severe exercise, and this large flow is thought to be the cause of the murmur. Systolic murmurs are of two types: those due to systolic ejection, which start after the first sound and finish before the second; and pansystolic murmurs which fill the whole of systole. These latter occur in mitral and tricuspid incompetence and ventricular septal defect, and fill systole because the pressure gradient, causing the flow responsible for the murmur, continues throughout systole. However, in some forms of mitral incompetence (e.g. ruptured chordae tendinae and cardiomyopathy) the murmur occurs in the second half of systole only. Ejection murmurs, often called 'diamond-shaped' because of their phonocardiographic appearance, are due to flow through the aortic or pulmonary orifices, and denote either increased flow through normal orifices or normal flow through stenotic orifices.

Diastolic murmurs also are of two types. Those due to incompetent flow from the aorta or pulmonary artery into the ventricle start immediately after the second sound and are high pitched. Diastolic murmurs due to impeded flow from an atrium into a ventricle do not start until isometric relaxation of the ventricle is complete, about 0·1 sec. after the second sound. These murmurs are low-pitched and their duration and intensity are related to the degree of stenosis and to the flow through the orifice. A similar murmur may occur with an increased flow through a normal valve, in patients with left to right shunts. The accentuation of the late diastolic (presystolic) murmur in mitral stenosis is due to atrial systole and is therefore absent in atrial fibrillation.

Continuous murmurs occur when there is a pressure gradient and flow between two parts of the heart throughout the cardiac cycle. The commonest example is patent ductus arteriosus, where the pressure in the aorta is higher than in the pulmonary artery. If there is no pressure gradient, because of pulmonary hypertension, the murmur is not continuous.

Inspiration, by increasing the venous return to the right heart, increases the right ventricular output, so that it makes right heart sounds and murmurs louder. Expiration squeezes blood out of the lungs and encourages flow into the left heart and consequently left-sided sounds and murmurs are louder on expiration.

EXERCISE RESPONSES

Cardiac function is most readily tested by exercising the patient. It is important either to observe the patient during exercise, or better to measure the ventilation, oxygen uptake and pulse rate during steady exercise either during a step test or on a treadmill or bicycle ergometer. In general, steady sustained exercise is limited by the maximum oxygen uptake. This is governed by different factors in different diseases (p. 112), but in heart disease it depends on the maximum cardiac output and the maximum extraction of oxygen from the blood in the tissues. By the Fick principle (p. 82):

$$\begin{array}{c} \text{Maximum oxygen uptake} = \\ \text{(in ml/min)} \\ \text{Max. cardiac output} \times \text{Max. O}_2 \text{ extraction} \\ \text{(in l/min)} \qquad\qquad \text{(in ml/l)} \end{array}$$

The maximum oxygen extraction depends on the level of haemoglobin in the blood and is normally about 140 ml/l. This value is relatively fixed, so that the maximum oxygen uptake in heart disease reflects the maximum cardiac output.

There is evidence in healthy subjects that the heart rate and oxygen consumption increase proportionately with increasing grades of steady exercise, and that the maximum oxygen uptake is reached with a pulse rate of about 195/min. The maximum oxygen consumption can be predicted by extrapolation from oxygen consumption at submaximal levels of exercise (e.g. at a pulse rate of 140/min), although not, of course, in atrial fibrillation. The cardiac output response varies with posture. In upright subjects stroke volume increases considerably during transition from rest to exercise, while in the supine position stroke volume is larger at rest and so does not increase as much when exercise begins.

VALSALVA'S MANOEUVRE

The measurement of the effect of Valsalva's manoeuvre on the arterial blood pressure has been used as a test of ventricular function. In the test, the patient blows up a column of mercury to 40 mmHg and maintains this pressure for 10 sec. The changes in systemic pressure which occur in normal subjects are shown in Fig. 5. The arterial pressure rises with the blow, as the increase in intrathoracic pressure is transmitted to the blood in the great vessels. The principal effect of the rise in intrathoracic pressure is to cut off the venous return to the right

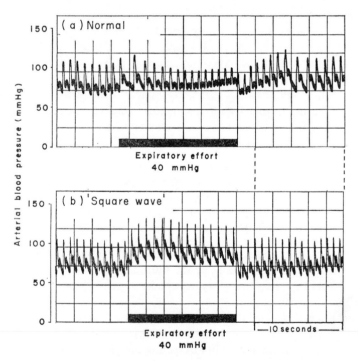

FIGURE 5. *Valsalva's manoeuvre* (see text).

atrium. As a result, filling of the heart is reduced and the arterial pressure falls as the central reservoir of blood in the heart and lungs is gradually emptied. The fall in arterial pulse pressure and mean pressure, acting through the baroreceptor reflexes, results in a rise in peripheral resistance, and towards the end of the period of strain there is often a slight tachycardia and rise in the mean arterial pressure. When pressure is released, the filling of the heart is suddenly restored and the cardiac output increases. At this stage there is still peripheral vasoconstriction and the increased flow into a constricted arterial bed produces a rise in arterial pressure above the resting level, which is usually referred to as 'overshoot'. This rise in pressure in turn stimulates the baroreceptors and produces cardiac slowing and the pressure returns to normal. Bradycardia after Valsalva's manoeuvre is the best clinical sign of a normal response.

In a typical abnormal response, shown in Fig.5(b), the arterial pressure does not fall when the venous return to the right atrium is arrested. This may be either because there is left ventricular failure, with excessively high filling pressure initially, or because there is an increased amount of blood in the central reservoir of the heart and lungs, or because of a combination of both factors. As the arterial pressure does not fall, there are no changes in rate or pressure during and after the period of strain. The abnormal response may be recognized clinically by the absence of bradycardia after the pressure is released. This abnormal response to Valsalva's manoeuvre has been called a 'failure' response, but it is better to call it a 'square-wave' response, because it occurs in patients with large left to right shunts with no evidence of heart failure. ('Square-wave' refers to the shape of the systemic arterial pressure tracing before, during and after the manoeuvre.)

When the autonomic nervous system is disabled (e.g. by diabetes, tabes dorsalis, or adrenergic neurone blocking drugs) no overshoot or bradycardia occur after release of expiratory effort. The arterial pressure gradually regains its previous level.

ELECTROCARDIOGRAPHY

Excitation of cardiac muscle is associated with a reversal of the electrical potential between the inside and outside of the membrane of the individual fibres. The spread of the excitation process through the heart causes a changing current field which can be recorded at the surface of the body. This account will be restricted to listing certain mainly empirical correlations which have become sufficiently well established for the electrocardiogram to give physiological information:

1. *The site of the pacemaker or the nature of the cardiac rhythm*
If the excitation process does not arise in the sino-atrial node the
P wave becomes abnormal in shape or position or disappears. The
disorder of rhythm and the site of the new pacemaker can be accurately
determined from the ECG.

2. *Disorder of conduction of the excitation process*
Blockage or delay of the spread of the excitation process at any site
can be accurately diagnosed.

3. *The size of the muscle mass in individual chambers of the heart*
Knowledge of the relative contributions of each of the chambers to
the various deflections as recorded at various sites on the surface of the
body has enabled considerable accuracy to be attained in judging the
relative muscular bulk of the individual chambers. This is particularly
true of the assessment of the size of the right and left ventricles from
the ECG recorded from the precordium. Since a sustained increase of
muscular work performed by any heart chamber ultimately produces
hypertrophy, the ECG can give valuable information about the work
each heart chamber has been performing, even though at the time of
the recording the work is diminished (e.g. after myocardial infarction).

4. *The state of viability or metabolism of the cardiac muscle*
Experience has shown that the state of the myocardium as a whole
and also the presence and site of localized disease or death of the
muscle can be diagnosed from the ECG. Thus death of a portion of the
muscle due to obstruction of the artery supplying it can be diagnosed
and localized with considerable precision. Experience has also shown
that electrolyte disturbances and the action of certain drugs cause
characteristic changes in the ECG which may be diagnostically helpful,
as in potassium depletion and intoxication, digitalis intoxication, and
hypothyroidism.

5. *Other information*
The ECG will show the electrical axis of the heart and indicate rotation
or displacement. It is also helpful in the diagnosis of pericarditis and
pericardial effusion.

RADIOLOGY
The information obtained from radiography of the heart tends to be
anatomical in nature and in general relates to the size and position of
different chambers of the heart and the great vessels. The assessment of

atrial size can best be made by X-ray and, while it is not always possible to distinguish the left ventricle from the right, radiology often gives information about ventricular size. The position and size of the great vessels may be of considerable importance in congenital heart disease, and radiology is particularly helpful in such conditions as coarctation of the aorta, patent ductus arteriosus, Fallot's tetralogy and transposition of the great vessels. The radiological examination of the lungs may give some indication of left atrial pressure. In pulmonary congestion, due to any cause, the presence of Kerley's horizontal interlobular lines at the bases of the lungs indicates that the left atrial pressure is raised.

A refinement of the technique is to inject radioactive agglutinated albumin intravenously. A scan with the subject seated will then accurately delineate the upper level of distribution and hence the mean left atrial pressure.

The amount of blood in the lungs can also be assessed radiologically and a distinction can be made between the oligaemic lungs of pulmonary stenosis and the pulmonary plethora in patients with a left to right shunt.

The principal use of fluoroscopy is in the detection of valve calcification, which may be of importance in determining the site of a lesion, and occasionally in distinguishing aortic stenosis from mitral incompetence. Fluoroscopy is also helpful in assessing pulsation in various parts of the heart and great vessels, and can give useful information about the volume of blood passing through a particular chamber.

ANGIOCARDIOGRAPHY

The anlysis of serial or cinematograph X-rays of radio-opaque dye passing through the heart and great vessels is an important method of outlining the anatomy, and is particularly valuable in the localization of shunts.

OXIMETRY

An ear oximeter is designed to measure the arterial oxygen saturation from the output of a photoelectric device recording the light transmitted through the warmed ear. It is thus a measure of the 'blueness' of the patient. Oximetry is particularly useful in detecting the changes in arterial oxygen saturation such as may occur when a patient exercises. The absolute level of saturation is difficult to measure accurately by oximetry. The clinical recognition of cyanosis is difficult until the arterial oxygen saturation falls below 75 per cent. It is important in

congenital heart disease to know whether the arterial saturation falls
with exercise, and this may be difficult to determine without oximetry.
The distinction between cyanosis due to a shunt and cyanosis due to
lung disease may be difficult to make on clinical grounds. The recording
of the change in arterial saturation by oximetry while the patient breathes
oxygen is an important means of determining the cause of the cyanosis.
In patients with lung disease, cyanosis is due to failure of the blood to
become fully saturated with oxygen during its passage through the lungs.
This deficiency is rapidly corrected by breathing 100 per cent oxygen
and the saturation rises at the rate of 15 per cent per minute or more.
The cyanosis of a shunt results from mixing of venous blood with fully
saturated blood coming from the lungs. In this case, when the patient
breathes 100 per cent oxygen, the saturation rises slowly because of
increased transport of oxygen in solution in the pulmonary blood.
The rate of rise is seldom more than 8 per cent per minute and depends on
the relative amounts of the pulmonary and shunt flows. This subject is
further discussed on p. 122.

Another use of oximetry is in the detection of atrial septal defect.
In patients with small- or medium-sized atrial septal defects, the left to
right shunt can be reversed by Valsalva's manoeuvre. This shunt reversal
produces a temporary drop in arterial oxygen saturation about 3 sec
after the end of the period of strain. The drop in saturation, which is
usually about 3 per cent, can be detected by oximetry. With large atrial
septal defects, the response to Valsalva's manoeuvre is square wave in
type and shunt reversal does not take place.

CARDIAC CATHETERIZATION, AND MEASUREMENT OF CARDIAC OUTPUT BY THE FICK PRINCIPLE

Cardiac catheterization sets out to measure the pressure and blood
flow in all the accessible chambers of the heart. Intracardiac pressures
are measured with an electromanometer connected to the catheter and
blood flows are estimated using the Fick principle, which involves the
analysis of the oxygen content of blood samples taken from different
parts of the circulation and measurement of the oxygen uptake in the
lungs.

By the Fick principle:

$$\frac{\text{Cardiac output}}{\text{(in l/min)}} = \frac{\text{Oxygen consumption (in ml/min)}}{\text{Arteriovenous oxygen content difference (in ml/l)}}$$

Oxygen is convenient for this purpose, but the Fick principle is, of
course, equally applicable to any substance taken up or removed by

the lung. The same principle is used to measure the blood flow of individual organs, in which case the flow is usually expressed as the 'clearance' of some substance (p. 180).

The determination of the cardiac output in the absence of a shunt entails the collection of blood from a systemic artery and mixed venous blood, usually from the pulmonary artery. These samples are taken during the collection of expired air for the measurement of oxygen uptake and the method is accurate only if the patient is in a 'steady state'. In patients with shunts, the Fick principle can be applied to measure both the pulmonary and systemic flows. In measuring the pulmonary flow, samples of pulmonary arterial and venous blood are required. A pulmonary venous sample cannot always be obtained and an oxygen content of 97 per cent must then be assumed. In measuring the systemic flow in the presence of a shunt, systemic arterial and mixed systemic venous samples are required. The systemic venous sample is obtained from a site where the blood is not mixed with blood shunted from the left side of the heart.

The measurement of *intra-cardiac pressures* is important in the diagnosis of pulmonary stenosis and pulmonary hypertension. In pulmonary stenosis there is higher systolic pressure in the right ventricle than in the pulmonary artery; and in pulmonary hypertension both pressures are increased. In assessing the severity of either condition, it is important to consider the pulmonary blood flow. The relationship between pressure and flow is normally expressed as *resistance:*

$$\text{Resistance (in mmHg/l./min)} = \frac{\text{Mean pressure difference (in mmHg)}}{\text{Blood flow (in l./min)}}$$

In this general formula, the mean pressure difference may be between any two points in the circulation. For example, in calculating the pulmonary vascular resistance, the mean pressure difference between the pulmonary artery and the left atrium is used; and for the systemic resistance, the mean right atrial pressure is subtracted from the mean systemic arterial pressure. The normal pulmonary vascular resistance is 1·5 mmHg/l./min and the normal systemic resistance about 10 times greater. The pulmonary artery pressure may be raised because of increased blood flow without any rise in resistance.

One of the most important diagnostic aspects of right heart catheterization in congenital heart disease is that the catheter may be passed into the left heart through a defect. The pressure tracing and oxygen content of the blood sampled are important means of identifying the chamber entered. In rheumatic heart disease right heart catheterization is more concerned with the assessment of the severity of the lesion than with the anatomical diagnosis. In mitral stenosis, the severity of the obstruction at the mitral valve can be assessed from the height to which the left atrial pressure is raised at rest and during exercise, and from the degree to which the cardiac output is reduced. The pressure in the left atrium can be measured indirectly by impacting the catheter in a distal branch of the pulmonary artery. This 'wedge' pressure has been shown to reflect the left atrial pressure in patients with mitral stenosis.

Direct measurement of the pressure gradient across the mitral valve can be obtained by remote puncture of the inter-atrial septum, and introduction of a catheter from the right into the left atrium.

Patients with mitral stenosis sometimes develop pulmonary vaso-constriction which causes further impedance to the circulation. Resistance from this cause can be calculated from the pressure gradient between the main pulmonary artery and the wedge pressure.

Severity of left ventricular and aortic lesions is assessed by left heart catheterization. An arterial catheter is advanced upstream into the left ventricle. Angiography can also be performed in the same way.

DYE DILUTION STUDIES, AND THE MEASUREMENT OF CARDIAC OUTPUT BY THE STEWART–HAMILTON METHOD

Dye dilution techniques may be used either for the measurement of the cardiac output or for the detection of shunts in congenital heart disease. The cardiac output can be calculated from a record of the concentration of injected dye passing a given point in the systemic circulation (Fig. 6). The technique used is to inject a known quantity of dye into a vein and record the change in colour due to the passage of dyed blood, either at the ear or in a systemic artery, with a photo-eléctric device.

The formula used for the calculation of cardiac output by the dye method is:

$$\text{Cardiac output (in l./min)} = \frac{60.I}{C.T}$$

where I is the amount of dye injected in mg, C is the mean concentration of dye during the first circulation in mg/l. and T is the time taken for the first circulation in seconds. The principal difficulty with the method is that blood containing dye starts to recirculate before the first systemic circulation is complete. As a result, the time taken for the first circulation has to be obtained by extrapolating the exponential decrease in dye concentration which occurs before recirculation starts. When dye

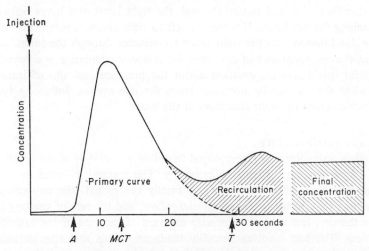

FIGURE 6. *Normal Indicator or 'Dye' Curve.*

The continuous curve shows the concentration of an indicator substance in the blood of a systemic artery following its injection into an arm vein at the time indicated. A is the time of first appearance of the dye at the sampling site. The dark shaded area is the 'primary' curve, i.e. the curve that would be obtained were there no recirculation. Its end, T, has to be drawn by eye, and its position judged by the early part of the descending primary curve. If concentration is on a logarithmic scale the early descending limb is straight. The area under the curve represents the sum of the concentrations at unit intervals of time (CT). Mean circulation time (MCT) is the time taken for half the dye to travel from the site of injection to the sampling site.

Cardiac output can be derived by dividing the quantity of dye injected by the area CT. Since the dimensions of the area CT are concentration (i.e. mass per unit volume) × time, the dimensions of mass (of dye) divided by CT become volume per unit time, which is the cardiac output. The *central blood volume*, i.e. that between the injection and sampling sites, can be calculated by multiplying the cardiac output by the mean circulation time (MCT). The *total blood volume* can be calculated by dividing the mass of dye injected by the final concentration attained after recirculation mixing is complete. If the dye is confined to the plasma, the volume must be divided by the haematocrit.

On-line computing systems have been developed by means of which these calculations can be carried out automatically.

dilution techniques are used for the detection of shunts during cardiac catheterization, the information obtained is qualitative. Dye can be injected into any chamber into which the catheter is passed. The time taken for the injected dye to appear in the systemic circulation will depend on the lesion. If the dye is injected into a chamber in the right heart from which blood is shunted to the left, the dye will appear earlier than if it had passed through the right heart and lungs before reaching the left heart. If there is a left to right shunt, a proportion of the dye injected into the right heart recirculates through the lungs, so that the disappearance of dye from the systemic circulation is delayed. Useful qualitative information about the presence and site of intra-cardiac shunts can be obtained from the dye curves, following dye injections into different chambers of the heart.

PLETHYSMOGRAPHY

Plethysmography may be employed to obtain an estimate of the volume of blood flowing through an extremity. The method is based on the principle that when the veins are briefly obstructed, the congestive swelling that occurs is due to arterial inflow, and the rate of swelling is for the first few seconds a precise measure of the rate of the arterial inflow. The test involves specially made apparatus and considerable technical experience, and has little place in routine clinical work, except possibly in the diagnosis of arteriovenous fistula of the extremity. In this condition considerable increase in flow occurs even when the lesion is small.

Practical Assessment

CARDIAC OUTPUT AND CIRCULATORY FILLING

Clinical observations: central venous pulse and mean pressure; peripheral arterial pulse; heart rate; cardiac impulse; sphygmomanometry; peripheral oedema; skin temperature; Valsalva's manoeuvre (p. 78).

Routine methods: central venous pressure and systemic arterial pressure by catheters; blood and plasma volume; radiology of heart and pulmonary vasculature; cardiac apex recording; circulation time; cardiac output (Fick and dye dilution methods) (p. 82).

Special tests: haemodynamic studies during exercise.

PERIPHERAL CIRCULATION

Clinical observations: Skin colour and temperature; dependent rubor; oedema; venous distension; peripheral arterial pulses (at rest and during exercise); arterial bruits; collateral vessels; speed of reactive hyperaemia flush after release of compression.

Routine methods: arteriography; venography; lymphangiography; skin temperature; loss of sweating (evidence of local sympathetic defect); effects on skin temperature of sympathetic blockade.

Special tests: venous occlusion plethysmography; rate of clearance of locally injected radioactive materials.

CENTRAL CIRCULATORY OBSTRUCTION

In general patients with central circulatory obstruction at any point show evidence of reduced systemic cardiac output (see above). The effects of circulatory obstruction depend on its site (see Table 4 overleaf).

VALVULAR INCOMPETENCE

Incompetence of any of the four cardiac valves is in the first instance usually compensated for by adjustments in the capacity of the chambers (or vessels) on both sides of the affected orifice. The stroke volume (and hence the work) of the related ventricle is increased, while on the other side of the affected valve there is a corresponding increase in the size or capacity of the related atrium or vessel. Thus the features that may be expected to result from regurgitation are summarized in Table 5.

SEPTAL DEFECTS WITH LEFT TO RIGHT SHUNT

In general, of course, such defects cannot produce cyanosis. They increase the work of the heart in proportion to the quantity of blood shunted. It is convenient to tabulate the features of the three commonest examples of pure left to right shunts (Table 6).

SEPTAL DEFECTS WITH RIGHT TO LEFT SHUNT

Irrespective of the level of the defect several features are commonly present. There is central cyanosis, roughly proportional to the volume of venous blood shunted into the systemic arterial system. The cyanosis increases on exercise, which by raising venous inflow and pressure in the right side of the heart increases the volume of blood shunted. Polycythaemia and clubbing usually occur eventually. In the special case of pulmonary-aortic communication, patent ductus arteriosus with right to left ('reversed') shunt, there may be cyanosis of the legs, without cyanosis of the arms or face.

There are usually signs either of pulmonary stenosis or pulmonary vascular bed obstruction (see over), with evidence of right ventricular hypertrophy except in the special case of tricuspid atresia in which the

TABLE 4. Types of central circulatory obstruction

	Tricuspid stenosis	Pulmonary stenosis (with intact ventricular septum)	Pulmonary vascular obstruction or hypertension
Clinical observations			
Peripheral pulse	Small	Small	Small
Venous pulse in neck	Dominant 'a' wave; slow 'y' descent	Prominent 'a' wave (if obstruction severe)	Prominent 'a' wave
Heart sounds	Loud tricuspid 1st sound (opening snap rare)	Reduced and delayed pulmonary 2nd sound	Loud pulmonary 2nd sound
Murmurs	Diastolic (increasing with inspiration)	Pulmonary systolic ejection murmur and thrill; ejection click (if stenosis mild)	Short pulmonary systolic ejection murmur and click
Routine methods			
ECG	'P pulmonale' (unless there is atrial fibrillation)	Right ventricular hypertrophy; 'P pulmonale' (unless there is atrial fibrillation)	Right ventricular hypertrophy; 'P pulmonale' (if no mitral lesion)
X-ray and fluoroscopy	Right atrial enlargement	Right ventricular enlargement; post-stenotic dilatation of pulmonary artery (if obstruction not infundibular); reduced lung vascularity (except when stenosis mild)	Dilatation of main pulmonary arteries with scanty peripheral branches and comparatively translucent lung fields
Special techniques			
Cardiac catheterization and other techniques	Diastolic pressure gradient between right atrium and right ventricle	Systolic pressure gradient between right ventricle and pulmonary artery (site of obstruction shown by withdrawal pressure trace and angiography).	Direct measurement of pulmonary vascular resistance (from flow and pressure) at catheterization

TABLE 4—*continued*

Mitral stenosis	Aortic stenosis (*valvular*)	Coarctation of aorta
Small	Slow upstroke (plateau)	Normal or increased in arms; small in legs (and delayed); palpable collaterals
		Marked arterial pulsation
Loud palpable 1st sound; opening snap (unless valve too rigid)	Reversed splitting of 2nd sound (if stenosis severe)	
Delayed diastolic murmur (length indicating severity); presystolic accentuation (if rhythm is sinus)	Systolic ejection murmur (and thrill); systolic ejection click (if stenosis mild)	Systolic ejection murmur (due to coarctation or collateral flow), continuing through 2nd sound
Right ventricular hypertrophy (only if pulmonary vascular resistance raised); 'P mitrale' (except in atrial fibrillation)	Left ventricular hypertrophy	Left ventricular hypertrophy
Left atrial enlargement; pulmonary congestion with Kerley's lines at lung bases; right ventricular enlargement (only if pulmonary vascular resistance raised); calcification of mitral valve	Left ventricular enlargement; post-stenotic dilatation of ascending aorta; calcification of aortic valve	Left ventricular enlargement; site of coarctation often visible on straight X-ray; rib notching after puberty
Measurement of indirect (wedge) pressure or of direct left atrial pressure; calculation of valve size from pressure and cardiac output measurements.	Direct arterial pressure tracing; systolic pressure gradient between left ventricle and aorta, if directly measured by left heart puncture or catheterization	Pressure gradient across coarctation; aortography, retrograde or direct

TABLE 5 Valvular incompetence

	Tricuspid incompetence	Pulmonary incompetence	Mitral incompetence	Aortic incompetence
Clinical observations				
Peripheral pulse			Normal; rarely collapsing	Water-hammer pulse; high pulse pressure
Venous pulse in neck	Raised pressure; giant systolic wave with rapid 'y' descent			Prominent carotid pulsation in neck
Heart sounds			Normal 1st sound; 3rd heart sound (occasional opening snap)	
Murmurs	Pansystolic (increasing in inspiration)	Immediate early diastolic (increasing in inspiration)	Pansystolic apical; short mid-diastolic (usually)	Immediate early basal diastolic
Other features	Common in severe heart failure; rare with normal rhythm; pulsating liver	Rare, except with pulmonary hypertension	Sustained left ventricular impulse	Sustained left ventricular impulse; skin warm; capillary pulsation
Routine methods				
ECG	Right ventricular hypertrophy	Right ventricular hypertrophy	Left ventricular hypertrophy; 'P mitrale'	Great left ventricular hypertrophy
X-ray and screening	Right atrial and right ventricular enlargement	Right ventricular enlargement; dilatation of main pulmonary artery	Left atrial and left ventricular enlargement; calcification of valve	Left ventricular enlargement; dilatation and increased pulsation of ascending aorta; calcification of valve
Special techniques				
Cardiac catheterization; other techniques	Right atrial pressure changes	Large pulse pressure in pulmonary artery at catheterization	Indirect left atrial pressure with rapid 'y' descent after high 'v' peak; left heart catheterization; angiography	Direct intra-arterial pressure tracing, rapid upstroke; left heart catheterization; angiography

TABLE 6 Left to right shunts

	Inter-atrial shunt	Inter-ventricular shunt	Aorto-pulmonary shunt (patent ductus)
Clinical observations			
Peripheral pulse			Water-hammer pulse; large pulse pressure (if shunt large)
Heart	Fixed splitting of 2nd sound (i.e. no variation with respiration)	2nd sound closely split, or single; 3rd heart sound (or short mitral diastolic flow murmur)	Hyperdynamic left ventricular impulse; reversed splitting of 2nd sound (occasionally only)
Murmurs	Pulmonary systolic ejection murmur (and thrill); tricuspid diastolic flow murmur in inspiration	Pansystolic murmur and thrill to left of sternum; short mitral diastolic flow murmur (or 3rd heart sound)	Continuous murmur increasing on expiration and accentuated at 2nd sound; short mitral diastolic flow murmur
Routine methods			
ECG	Incomplete right bundle branch pattern-RSR in VI	Right and left ventricular hypertrophy (mainly left)	Left ventricular hypertrophy
X-ray and screening	Enlargement of right atrium, right ventricle and pulmonary artery; 'hilar dance'; pulmonary plethora	Right and left ventricular enlargement; normal or small right atrium; pulmonary plethora	Left ventricular enlargement; dilatation of pulmonary artery; normal or small right atrium and right ventricle
Special techniques			
Cardiac cather-ization and other techniques	Jump in O_2 content of blood between venae cavae and right atrium; passage of catheter into left atrium; dye dilution methods to show left to right shunt; effect of Valsalva on arterial O_2 saturation	Jump in O_2 content of blood between right atrium and right ventricle; dye dilution methods to show left to right shunt; passage of catheter into left ventricle	Jump in O_2 content of blood between right ventricle and pulmonary artery; dye dilution methods to show left to right shunt; passage of catheter through ductus

left ventricle is dominant. It is difficult to identify the level of the shunt by clinical or routine methods. Cardiac catheterization is generally necessary. Dye dilution studies, with injections into different sites, may also help to localize the level of the shunt.

References

McDowall R.J.S. (1956) *Control of the Circulation of the Blood.* London, Dawson.
Hamilton W.F. (ed.) (1962–6). The Circulation. *Handbook of Physiology*, Section 2. Washington D.C., Amer. Physiol. Soc.
Guyton A.C. (1964) *Circulatory Physiology: cardiac output and its regulation.* Philadelphia, Saunders.
Brecher G.A. (1956) *Venous Return.* New York, Grune & Stratton.
Shepherd J.T. (1963) *Physiology of the Circulation in Human Limbs in Health and Disease.*
Guyton A.C. (1961) Physiologic regulation of arterial pressure. *Amer. J. Cardiol.* **8,** 401–407.
Lassen N.A. (1959) Cerebral blood flow and oxygen consumption in man. *Physiol. Rev.* **39,** 183–238.
Harris P. & Heath D. (1962) *The Human Pulmonary Circulation.* Edinburgh, Livingstone.
Hertzman A.B. (1959) Vasomotor regulation of cutaneous circulation. *Physiol. Rev.* **39,** 280–306.
Heymans C. & Neil E. (1958) *Reflexogenic Areas of the Cardiovascular System.* London, Churchill.
Goldman M.J. (1964). *Principles of Clinical Electrocardiography* 5th edn. Los Altos, Lange.
Friedberg C.K. (1966) *Diseases of the Heart,* 3rd edn. Philadelphia, Saunders.
Wood P. (1956) *Diseases of the Heart and Circulation,* 2nd edn. London, Eyre & Spottiswoode.
Allen E.V., Barker N.W. & Hines E.A., Jr. (1962) *Peripheral Vascular Disease,* 3rd edn. Philadelphia, Saunders.
Pickering G.W. (1955) *High Blood Pressure.* London, Churchill.
Braunwald E. (ed.) (1966) Symposium on beta adrenergic receptor blockade. *Amer. J. Cardiol.* **18,** 303–487.

3

Respiration

Normal Function

INTRODUCTION

Respiratory physiology deals with the processes concerned in the uptake of O_2 and the elimination of CO_2 from the lungs, and with certain aspects of the regulation of hydrogen ion concentration. The processes involved in gaseous exchange can conveniently be considered under four headings:

1. Ventilation: the mass movement of air in and out of the lungs.
2. Gas transfer: the exchanges of O_2 and CO_2 between the alveolar air and pulmonary capillary blood.
3. Pulmonary blood flow: this process is more conveniently considered as part of circulatory physiology (p. 51).
4. Blood gas transport.

Not only does this classification simplify the presentation of the subject but it is a convenient logical system of approach to clinical problems.

VENTILATION

Pulmonary ventilation is produced by the rhythmic contraction of the inspiratory muscles which cause expansion of the thorax and lungs. This rhythmic contraction is initiated in the brain stem. In ventilating the lungs the inspiratory muscles must overcome the elastic resistance of the tissues and the resistance of the airways to the flow of air through them. The volume of ventilation in any given period of time is adjusted in response to changes in the partial pressure of the gases in the blood, which themselves depend upon the ratio of ventilation to the metabolic activity of the tissues. The control is thus by a servo or 'feed-back' mechanism.

TOTAL, ALVEOLAR AND DEAD-SPACE VENTILATION

A normal subject at rest with a respiratory rate of 15 breaths/min and a tidal volume of 500 ml has a total pulmonary ventilation of 7·5 l./min (i.e. 7·5 l. inspired and 7·5 l. expired). However, about 140 ml of each breath are required to flush the conducting airways or anatomical dead-space, so that the ventilation of the alveoli is only about 5·5 l./min. If the depth of breathing is reduced, the dead-space ventilation becomes proportionately greater so that, in theory, if the tidal volume were to be less than the volume of the dead-space there would be no alveolar ventilation however great the total ventilation.

In recumbent normal subjects at rest the inspired air is almost perfectly distributed throughout the lungs and meets the blood in optimal proportions. However, if there are parts of the lung which have no blood flow or a reduced blood flow, the air going to those parts of the lung performs little or no exchange of O_2 or CO_2. This portion of the inspired air is therefore like the air in the conducting passages and can be regarded as dead-space ventilation. The anatomical dead-space plus the volume of this dead-space-like air (which is sometimes called 'alveolar' dead-space to distinguish it from the anatomical or airway dead-space) are usually referred to as the physiological dead-space. In the erect subject at rest there is an increased physiological dead-space because there is little blood flow, and therefore little gas exchange, in the apices of the upper lobes.

THE LUNG VOLUMES

It is customary for most accounts of respiratory physiology to begin with a diagram illustrating the terms used to describe the various subdivisions of the volume of the lungs. They are widely measured largely because overinflation of the lungs was for a long time considered to be the important functional disturbance in emphysema. Such emphasis is not really warranted because the changes in the lung volumes in disease are usually secondary to other abnormalities which can be studied with more profit.

The vital capacity is the volume of air expelled by a maximum voluntary expiration after a maximum voluntary inspiration; the residual volume is the volume of air left in the lungs after a maximum expiration; and the functional residual capacity is the volume of air in the lungs at the end of expiration when, during quiet breathing, no respiratory muscles are contracting. The total lung capacity, the volume of air in the lungs at maximum inspiration, is the sum of the vital capacity and residual volume.

THE RESPIRATORY MUSCLES AND THE MECHANICS
OF BREATHING

THE RESPIRATORY MUSCLES

During quiet breathing in normal subjects inspiration is produced by the action of the diaphragm and intercostal muscles; expiration is produced by the elastic recoil of the lungs. The diaphragm increases the volume of the thorax partly by its descent and partly by raising and everting the costal margin. If the diaphragm is depressed and flat, both of these actions become less efficient, its descent is restricted and the base of the thorax, instead of being expanded, may be contracted. Accessory muscles such as the sternomastoids, which are normally employed only during deep breathing, are then used even at rest. Their action is probably less efficient than the diaphragm and they tend to expand mainly the upper thorax where the pulmonary blood flow and gaseous exchange are less.

In patients who have obstructed breathing, and in normal subjects during deep or forced breathing, expiration may be assisted by the abdominal muscles. These muscles play little, if any, part in normal breathing although they are, of course, employed in coughing and straining.

THE MECHANICS OF BREATHING

The mechanical properties of the respiratory muscles and the ribs are important in governing the change of shape of the thorax—and therefore of the lungs—during breathing. In recent years much attention has also been devoted to the physical ('visco-elastic') properties of the lungs themselves.

The 'elasticity' of the lungs governs the amount of air that can be taken in by a given muscular effort. The calibre of the airways governs the resistance to airflow and therefore the rate at which air flows in for a given muscular effort.

The elastic properties of the lungs

In the preceding paragraph the word elasticity has been placed in inverted commas because the common use of the term to describe 'stretchiness' does not accord with that of physics. Elasticity strictly means the property of a substance or structure of returning to its original shape and dimensions after a deforming force has been removed. The quantitative expression of the relation between the magnitude of deformity and force is the modulus of elasticity. Several terms have been used to describe the elastic properties of the lungs, the most popular being 'compliance' (p. 137), which describes the increase in lung volume per unit increase in distending pressure (ml or 1. per cm H_2O). Compliance is therefore akin to a modulus of elasticity in that it relates strain (the increase in volume) to stress (the change in pressure). It is not, however, a true modulus because it does not take account of size. The 'elasticity' of the lungs can also be looked at from the reverse standpoint as the pressure required to distend them by a given volume. This is usually called the 'elastance' (cm H_2O per 1.).

The elastic properties of the lungs are not just functions of the elastic tissue proper but also of the structural pattern of the lung. Furthermore, many other structures within the thorax exert elastic forces, and the surface tension of the liquid lining the alveoli provides about half the elastic recoil.

Surface tension

The small size of the alveoli minimizes the distance O_2 and Co_2 have to diffuse and also maximizes the area of alveolar surface. But the alveoli have a liquid lining and the pressure generated by surface tension becomes progressively greater the smaller the volume or radius of the alveoli—from Laplace's law applied to a spherical bubble:

$$\text{Pressure} = 2\frac{\text{Tension}}{\text{Radius}}.$$

If the lining liquid had a surface tension like that of water either the alveoli would have to be bigger than they are or the intrathoracic pressure (intrapleural pressure) would have to be several times more sub-atmospheric ('negative') to hold them open.

The surface tension of the liquid lining the alveoli is also important for the stability of the alveoli. Consider two bubbles of the same surface tension but different size. The equation given above shows that the smaller one would exert a greater pressure on the gas within it so that, if they were in communication, the smaller one would empty into the larger. If they are both to stay open the smaller one must have a smaller surface tension. It has been shown that the surface tension of the liquid lining the lung depends on the area over which it is spread. This layer is composed of a lipoprotein which is synthesized by the alveolar cells.

Loss of this normal 'surfactant' property of the lung lining is now recognized in a number of conditions such as the respiratory distress syndrome of the newborn (hyaline membrane disease) and the 'post-perfusion lung' syndrome; but whether such changes are the cause or the result of the conditions is not yet known. The loss of surfactant causes a stiffness or loss of compliance and a tendency to atelectesis even when the main airways are patent.

The viscous or resistive properties of the lungs and airways

The initiation and maintenance of airflow through the airways from the mouth to the alveoli or vice versa requires a pressure difference between the mouth and the alveoli. The narrower the airways, the greater their resistance to airflow and the greater must be the pressure difference. If the flow of the air were entirely streamlined (laminar) the resistance would be constant and the pressure difference would be proportional to the rate of flow. However, at various sites in the respiratory tract, particularly in the larynx and large upper airways the flow of air is turbulent. When airflow is turbulent, an increase in the rate of airflow demands a disproportionate increase in the pressure difference. For this reason it is difficult to give a single value for airflow resistance. Furthermore, when air flows in or out of the lungs the shape of the thorax changes and, apart from the elastic forces already mentioned, this involves resistance from tissues sliding over each other and from the displacement of blood and tissue fluids. These viscous resistances add to the flow resistance of the airways to form a resistance which depends upon the *rate* of change of shape and volume and is usually called non-elastic resistance to distinguish it from elastance which depends simply upon the *magnitude* of the change of shape or volume. The measurement of the elastic and non-elastic properties of the lungs is discussed on page 137.

The mechanics of expiration

In ordinary breathing expiration is produced by the recoil of the stretched elastic tissue of the lungs. The recoil pressure forces the air up the respiratory passages and maintains the pressure inside them above the surrounding intra-pleural pressure. The elastic recoil pressure of the lungs is much greater than is required for quiet expiration in normal subjects and the inspiratory muscles 'pay off' by gradual relaxation. During the deep breathing of muscular exercise the greater distension of the lungs provides greater recoil pressure and the inspiratory muscles 'pay off' more rapidly. If the elastic recoil pressure of the lungs is partially lost or if the airflow resistance of the respiratory passages is increased, the passive mechanism of expiration becomes less effective. There are two possible compensations for this. The first is the use of expiratory muscles and the second is further distension of the lungs so as to increase recoil pressure. In fact, the second reaction is the usual one and helps to explain the increase in lung volume seen in conditions such as asthma and emphysema. The use of expiratory muscles is of limited value because not only do they increase the pressure in the terminal airspaces, but they raise the pressure surrounding the airways. If they contract too forcibly, they cause narrowing of the airways, which increases flow resistance and limits the rate of flow. This limitation may be so severe that 'air-trapping' occurs. The narrowing of the airways by forced expiration, while unhelpful to pulmonary ventilation, is valuable in coughing because the *linear velocity* of the airflow through these narrowed airways is greatly increased even though the *rate of volume flow* is reduced. During a vigorous cough all the intrathoracic airways are compressed and the velocity of airflow in the trachea of a normal subject may reach Mach 1 (600 m.p.h.).

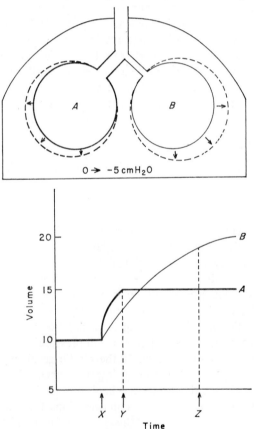

The mechanical properties of the lungs and the distribution
of ventilation (Fig. 7)

If the elastance of a part of the lungs is high (i.e. its compliance is low) the volume of air that enters or leaves it for a given pressure difference is reduced, however long the pressure difference operates. If the non-elastic resistance is high, the rate at which air enters the part of the lung is reduced. Thus a part of the lung with a low compliance and a high non-elastic resistance requires a greater pressure difference or a longer time to undergo the same proportionate ventilation as one with a high compliance and a low non-elastic resistance. At a high rate of breathing the part with the low resistance therefore receives a greater ventilation than the part with high resistance. The distribution of the inspired air in the lungs is the same at all rates of breathing only if the resistance and compliance of all parts of the lungs are equally matched.

THE WORK OF BREATHING

The *mechanical* work of breathing can be estimated by measuring the pressures developed and the volumes of air displaced. The work performed on the lungs can be derived from records of the intra-pleural

FIGURE 7. *The mechanical properties of the lungs and the distribution of ventilation.*

A and B are two 'lung units' (which could be alveoli, lobules or lobes) having the same resting volume (say, 10 mm^3). They are enclosed in the thorax. A is less distensible (less compliant) than B so that, when the pressure round them (intrathoracic or intrapleural pressure) is lowered from 0 to -5 cm H_2O, A only enlarges to 15 mm^3 whereas B enlarges to 20 mm^3. In addition, the airway leading to A is wide and of low resistance to airflow, whereas the airway to B is of high resistance. The effect of this difference in resistance is shown in the tracing of change in volume against time (lower figure). If the surrounding pressure is suddenly lowered at time X, air enters A rapidly and B slowly. If the inspiration stopped at time Y, A would be more ventilated than B, but if the rate of breathing were slower so that inspiration lasted till time Z, B would be more ventilated than A.

Air will flow into A or B until the pressure in A and B is the same as that at the mouth. At time Y airflow into A stops because the pressure in A has become the same as the pressure at the mouth. Air continues to flow into B between times Y and Z because the pressure in B is still lower than mouth pressure. If, at time Y, the intra-thoracic pressure were raised (i.e. returned towards O), there would be an interval before the pressure rose sufficiently to stop air flow into B, although A would start to empty immediately. During this period air would flow from A not only to the mouth but also into B. This phenomenon is called 'paradoxical respiration' or *pendelluft* (swinging air). (Reproduced from the *Postgraduate Medical Journal*, **34**, 30, 1958.)

or intra-oesophageal pressure, but the work on the thoracic cage is technically difficult to measure. The total mechanical work of breathing in normal subjects is about 0·6 kilopond metres per minute, of which at least two-thirds is expended on the lungs. In patients with chronic lung or heart disease the mechanical work of breathing may be increased five or tenfold.

The *metabolic cost* of breathing can be assessed by estimating the O_2 consumption of the respiratory muscles; this amounts to 1–3 per cent of the total O_2 intake at rest (i.e. about 0·5 ml O_2 per l. ventilation, or 4 ml O_2 per min). At higher levels of ventilation the O_2 consumption of the respiratory muscles increases disproportionately, but in normal subjects it only represents a small portion of the total O_2 intake even at the highest levels of pulmonary ventilation reached during strenuous physical exertion. In patients with disease of the heart or lungs the O_2 consumption of the respiratory muscles during exercise may reach very high levels. As the maximum rate of O_2 intake is also limited in these patients, the O_2 consumption of the respiratory muscles may severely restrict the amount of O_2 available to the rest of the body.

The mechanics of breathing and the respiratory rate (frequency)

If the compliance of the lungs is reduced, the work and force required for a normal sized breath are increased. It therefore becomes more economical to breathe shallowly and more frequently. However, the smaller the tidal volume, the larger must be the total pulmonary ventilation to flush the dead-space and maintain alveolar ventilation. The consequence is that, for any given combination of dead-space volume, compliance and non-elastic resistance, there is an optimal combination of rate and depth for each level of alveolar ventilation. The frequency of breathing of normal subjects is close to the optimum and, although the mechanism is not understood, the rapid breathing seen in conditions of reduced compliance approximates to an optimum.

THE CONTROL OF VENTILATION

The rhythm of breathing is generated and its rate and depth determined in the pons and medulla. It is customary to attribute this control to a 'respiratory centre' although the concept of a localized centre is inadequate on both structural and functional grounds. The rhythm of breathing is probably entirely generated in the brainstem and does not depend on any vagal feedback from the lungs. The volume of breathing, the pulmonary ventilation, is chiefly regulated by the chemical state of the blood, particularly its CO_2 tension (PCO_2), as sensed by medullary chemoreceptors. In the conscious subject, however, and particularly during exercise, the chemical drive is probably supplemented by other factors including conditioning and proprioceptive reflexes. The rhythm, depth and frequency of breathing having been decided by the 'respiratory centres', the execution of the necessary muscular actions is probably mediated by neural mechanisms analogous to those subserving voluntary movement. In normal subjects breathing air at sea-level the pulmonary ventilation is adjusted to keep the arterial PCO_2 at 40 mmHg (± 4). There are no cells in the brain which adjust the ventilation in response to changes in the O_2 tension of the blood. However, there are chemoreceptors in the aortic and carotid bodies which respond to anoxia and stimulate the breathing. In normal subject exposed to anoxia (e.g. at high altitude) this stimulation lowers the arterial PCO_2. The medullary chemoreceptors appear then to have their sensitivity to the PCO_2 adjusted to this new lower level and over a short term will resist any tendency for the PCO_2 to rise. In patients with respiratory paralysis who are chronically overventilated by a mechanical respirator a similar situation develops. They also become accustomed to a low PCO_2 and are distressed if the artificial respiration is reduced and their PCO_2 rises, even though the level to which it rises is still below the normal level of 40 mmHg. On the other hand, in patients with chronic lung disease whose ventilation may be partly maintained by reflex anoxic stimulation via the aortic and carotid chemoreceptors, the administration of O_2 may cause a severe reduction in pulmonary ventilation and the PCO_2 may rise to narcotic levels without increasing the ventilation. When normal subjects return to sea-level conditions, and when patients with lung disease improve sufficiently, there is usually a return to the normal sensitivity to PCO_2. It is not yet certain whether in normal subjects at sea-level there is a reflex anoxic stimulation of ventilation, but it is certainly small compared with that provided by the arterial PCO_2.

GAS TRANSFER

The exchange of O_2 and CO_2 between the alveolar air and pulmonary capillary blood depends on three processes: first, the correct distribution of ventilation and blood flow; secondly, diffusion through the alveolar air, the various membranes and liquid layers; thirdly, chemical reactions within the red cells.

Distribution

The distribution of ventilation and blood flow within the lungs can be studied and discussed in several ways. One approach is the anatomical in which the regional distribution in terms, say, of the lobes is examined. A second is by examination of the homogeneity of distribution in terms of the alveoli; that is to say, the extent to which all alveoli receive inspired air or pulmonary blood flow in proportion to their size. A third approach is to consider the ventilation and pulmonary blood flow in relation to each other, ignoring in what part of the lungs or in which alveoli the air and the blood meet.

Although these approaches are obviously related to each other in theory, in practice each of them has demanded the use of different techniques of considerable difficulty and the information so far obtained is not easily collated.

In most studies the distribution of the inspired air to the alveoli has been regarded as a dilution or mixing process taking as the criteria of perfect distribution that each alveolus shall receive air of the same composition at the same time and in an amount proportional to its volume. These criteria demand perfection in both temporal and spatial distribution. Most of the information available deals with the spatial distribution and shows that in normal subjects the spatial distribution is very good but not perfect. The *temporal* factor—i.e. the sequence in which alveoli are ventilated during a single inspiration—is very difficult to study quantitatively and we know little about it.

Studies of the anatomical distribution of air and blood show that the lower lobes receive more ventilation and blood flow per unit volume of lung than the upper lobes. The disparity in blood flow is greater than that in ventilation. These inequalities are greater in the erect than in the supine posture. Because of the effect of gravity, the ratio of ventilation to perfusion is always lower in the lower parts of the lung.

From the functional standpoint of maintaining the normal gaseous composition of the arterial blood, the distribution of ventilation relative to blood flow is more important than either the gross anatomical distribution or the perfection of the distribution of inspired air throughout the alveolar volume. By *reductio ad absurdum* it will be appreciated that if every alternate alveolus is ventilated but not perfused and every other one is perfused but not ventilated, then no gaseous exchange will occur although the techniques available for studying distribution from the other standpoints may suggest that distribution is perfect. In this situation the total pulmonary ventilation would behave as dead-space ventilation and the total pulmonary blood flow would behave as a right-to-left shunt. In fact, unless the proportion of ventilation to blood flow in all alveoli is similar, the arterial blood gas composition cannot be normal. Although overventilated alveoli will excrete more CO_2 and thus partially compensate for the CO_2 retention in the under-ventilated alveoli, they cannot compensate for inequality of O_2 uptake because overventilation produces little increase in the quantity of O_2 taken up by the blood (see p. 105). Increasing the total ventilation to increase the ventilation of the relatively underventilated alveoli may correct the oxygenation of the blood, but by causing further increase in the ventilation of the already overventilated alveoli it causes a reduction in the arterial CO_2 concentration.

Little is known about the adjustment of local ventilation-perfusion ratios within the lungs. If one lung is ventilated with a low O_2 or high CO_2 concentration the blood flow is redistributed to the other lung, and bronchial obstruction is usually followed by a reduction of pul-monary blood flow through the affected lobe. Similarly, reduction of the blood flow to a part of the lung is followed by a reduction in its ventilation, apparently produced by an increase in the airway resistance and a reduction in the compliance of the part. These are, however, relatively gross observations and the fine adjustment of ventilation and blood flow at alveolar level is as yet little understood.

When distribution is very imperfect the definition or measurement of 'the' alveolar air composition becomes very difficult (p. 129).

DIFFUSION

Ventilation moves the gases in bulk up and down the airways but their movement in the depths of the lungs is by molecular diffusion. Oxygen and CO_2 diffuse at almost equal rates in the gas phase. The gases also diffuse through the aqueous layers and membranes between the alveolar air and the interior of the red cells but, because of its greater solubility, CO_2 diffuses through these media much more readily than O_2. Indeed, one of the historical debates of physiology was whether the volume of O_2 uptake could be accounted for by diffusion alone or whether some 'secretion' or active transport was required. We now know that diffusion alone adequately accounts for movement from alveolus to red cell and, furthermore, that there is little O_2 pressure gradient between the alveolar air and the red cell even during stresses such as exercise or disease.

CHEMICAL REACTIONS IN THE RED CELL

Although movement of O_2 and of Hb within the red cell and changes in shape of the Hb molecule and the formation of intermediate compounds (Hb_2O_2, Hb_2O_4, Hb_2O_6, etc.) must eventually be taken into account, it is convenient to consider only the chemical reaction of O_2 with Hb_4 to form Hb_4O_8. (This polymeric representation is not given elsewhere in this chapter, it being sufficient to distinguish between Hb and HbO_2). Accepting this simplification: the volume of O_2 that can be taken up by the red cells per unit time is the product of the rate of this chemical reaction and the volume of Hb present in the pulmonary capillaries.

No analogous simplification is possible or justifiable in the case of CO_2. The key chemical reaction is the dehydration of H_2CO_3 to form CO_2 and H_2O. This reaction is catalyzed by carbonic anhydrase in the red cells. But there are a number of other processes to be considered, particularly the diffusion of HCO_3^- ions from the plasma into the red cells and the other reactions dealt with in the next section. It is doubtful if chemical reaction rates ever limit CO_2 exchange in the lungs sufficiently to cause a capillary–alveolar PCO_2 difference except when carbonic anhydrase is artificially inhibited.

BLOOD GAS TRANSPORT

The main facts about blood gas transport from the standpoint of pulmonary physiology have been established for so long and are so well known that a reiteration is unnecessary. There are, however, certain aspects which are insufficiently appreciated clinically and which will be discussed.

Oxygen
The relationship between the partial pressure of O_2 (PO_2) and the volume of O_2 carried in the blood is given by the dissociation curve. Usually the curve is plotted with percentage saturation along the ordinate. In Fig. 8 the actual O_2 content is plotted as well as the percentage saturation because this mode of presentation stresses the differences between the curves of O_2 and CO_2. Anaemia lowers the O_2 curve as plotted from the left-hand ordinate, and polycythaemia raises it.

Clinically the 's' shape of the curve is important in several ways. Firstly, a considerable reduction in the PO_2 below the normal arterial value does not significantly reduce the oxygenation of the arterial blood. Hence a reduction of arterial saturation below 90 per cent does not occur until arterial PO_2 has fallen to 60 mmHg. Secondly, the change in shape below 60 mmHg means that any further reduction in PO_2 causes a disproportionately severe desaturation. Thirdly, this change in slope means that overventilation of parts of the lung cannot compensate for underventilation of other parts of the lung because further increase in Po_2 above the normal arterial value causes a negligible increase in the volume of O_2 taken up.

The shape of the O_2 dissociation curve is affected by a number of physiological variables, the most important of which are raised Pco_2,

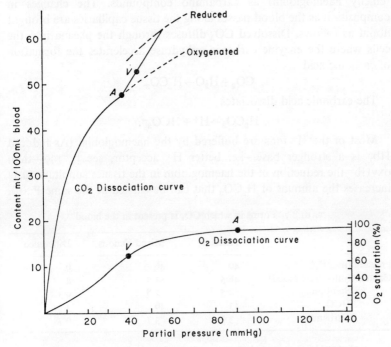

FIGURE 8. *The carbon dioxide and oxygen dissociation curves of blood.*

These curves were obtained by equilibrating blood with CO_2 or O_2 at various partial pressures and measuring the quantity of the gas contained by the blood. *V* and *A* represent the usual findings in mixed venous (*V*) and arterial (*A*) blood in a resting normal subject. The O_2 dissociation curve as plotted on the left hand ordinate (i.e. ml/100 ml) is that of blood with a normal haemoglobin concentration. The right-hand scale (per cent saturation) is independent of variations in haemoglobin concentration.

The CO_2 dissociation curve is that of blood with normal bicarbonate and haemoglobin concentration. Reduction of haemoglobin allows more CO_2 to be carried at any given partial pressure. Therefore, the simultaneous addition of CO_2 to, and the removal of O_2 from, blood in the tissues produces the solid line *A-V*. The importance of the steeper slope of the CO_2 curve and the 'S' shape of the O_2 curve are described in the text.

(Modified from Riley, R. L., and Cournand, A., *J. appl. Physiol.*, **1**, 825, 1949.)

increased (H^+) and raised temperature, all of which shift the curve to the right and therefore facilitate the removal of O_2 in the tissues.

Carbon dioxide

Carbon dioxide is carried in the blood in three main forms (Table 7): in simple solution, as bicarbonate, and combined with protein (chiefly haemoglobin) as carbamino compounds. The changes in composition as the blood passes along the tissue capillaries are brought about as follows. Dissolved CO_2 diffuses through the plasma into the cells where the enzyme carbonic anhydrase accelerates the formation of carbonic acid

$$CO_2 + H_2O \rightarrow H_2CO_3.$$

The carbonic acid dissociates

$$H_2CO_3 \rightarrow H^+ + HCO_3^-.$$

Most of the H^+ ions are buffered by the haemoglobin. (As reduced Hb^- is a stronger base—i.e. better H^+ acceptor, see p. 199—than oxyHb^- the reduction of the haemoglobin in the tissues simultaneously increases the amount of H_2CO_3 that can be carried at the same P_{CO_2}).

TABLE 7. Forms in which CO_2 is present in the blood

	Arterial	Mixed Venous	Difference
Pressure (mm Hg).. ..	40	46	6
Content (ml/100 ml blood)	48·5	52·5	4
Solution	2·5	2·8	0·3
HCO_3^-	43	46	3
Carbamino ..	3·0	3·7	0·7

Most of the HCO_3^- ions diffuse out into the plasma, and Cl^- ions enter the cell to restore equilibrium. Reduced haemoglobin has a greater capacity for forming a carbamino compound than oxy-haemoglobin so the removal of O_2 enables more CO_2 to be carried in this form. In the pulmonary capillaries all these processes are reversed.

The importance of the red cells in CO_2 transport should be noted. Although most of the CO_2 is carried in the plasma as HCO_3^-, the red cells are important in four ways:

1. The hydration of CO_2 to form carbonic acid can only occur at sufficient speed in the red cells, there being no carbonic anhydrase in the plasma.

2. The reactions described by the above equations can only proceed fully to the right (converting CO_2 into HCO_3^-) if H^+ ions are removed.

Similarly, the reactions can only proceed to the left if H^+ ions are donated. Haemoglobin is the buffer which accepts and donates H^+ ions.

3. Changes in the degree of oxygenation of the haemoglobin alter its affinity for H^+ ions in such a way as to facilitate CO_2 uptake when O_2 is removed and vice versa.

4. The greater the reduction of the haemoglobin in the tissues, the greater is its capacity for forming carbamino-haemoglobin.

The second and third points noted above, coupled with the exchange of HCO_3^- and Cl^- mentioned earlier, account for the difference between 'true' plasma and 'separated' plasma. Thus, if whole blood is exposed to a high CO_2 tension these factors enable the plasma to take up more CO_2 than it does if the cells and plasma were previously separated at a low CO_2 tension and the plasma then exposed to the high CO_2 tension by itself (see also p. 216 and Fig. 27).

Table 7 gives typical values for arterial and mixed venous blood at rest; that is, at CO_2 tensions of 40 and 46 mmHg respectively. The relationship between total CO_2 content and tension is expressed in the CO_2 dissociation curve (Fig. 8). The main curve is that of normal oxygenated or arterial blood. The upper dotted segment is that of completely reduced blood. The curve crossing from the oxygenated to the reduced segments is the one obtained if an equivalent amount of O_2 is removed from the blood as CO_2 is added. It is therefore called the 'physiological' dissociation curve.

Fig. 8 shows the two very important differences between the dissociation curves of O_2 and CO_2. First, the CO_2 curve is much steeper, implying that much larger volume changes occur for the same change in partial pressure. Secondly, the slope of the curve above and below the arterial values for CO_2 is such that overventilation of parts of the lungs (producing a low PCO_2) can remove CO_2 to compensate for underventilation of other parts of the lungs. Such compensation for local variations in ventilation cannot occur for O_2.

Table 8 shows that the bulk of the CO_2 in the blood is in the form of HCO_3^-. Any alteration in the HCO_3^- concentration due to non-respiratory changes therefore alters the CO_2 dissociation curve. The concentration of HCO_3^- is increased in metabolic alkalosis and reduced in metabolic acidosis (Chapter 5). Metabolic alkalosis therefore 'raises' the CO_2 dissociation curve and metabolic acidosis 'lowers' it.

Body gas stores

The body of a normal man (excluding the gases in the lungs) contains 'stores' of 1 l. O_2 and 17 l. of CO_2. Practically all the O_2 is in the blood, whereas the bulk of the CO_2 is in the tissue fluids as bicarbonate. (There are even larger amounts of CO_2 in bone, but little of it is exchangeable.) These differences in storage capacity and distribution are of considerable clinical importance. A change in the volume of ventilation or of the composition of the inspired air changes the O_2 stores to a new level within 2 min, whereas the CO_2 stores take more than 15 min to reach a new level. Also, addition or removal of O_2 produces a much greater change in the tension than is produced by the same change in volume of CO_2. A clinical example which illustrates the importance of these differences is provided by a patient who has underventilated while breathing O_2. If he is given air to breathe instead of O_2, the O_2 tension in the blood and tissues will fall rapidly. Increasing the ventilation to normal cannot completely counteract this fall because the high partial pressure of CO_2 in the mixed venous blood maintains the alveolar CO_2 tension high for several minutes, thus diluting the O_2 in the alveolar air. The maintenance of a normal alveolar O_2 concentration during this time requires considerable overventilation, often beyond the ventilatory capacity of such patients.

Respiratory exchange ratio

The respiratory exchange ratio is the ratio of the volume of CO_2 expired from the lungs to the volume of O_2 taken in (Vol. CO_2 exp. $\div$ Vol. O_2 insp.). In a steady state this ratio is the same as the metabolic respiratory quotient. If ventilation is changed some minutes elapse before the body gas stores adjust to the new steady state. During this unsteady state the respiratory exchange ratio does not reflect the metabolism of the tissues. The dissociation curves of CO_2 and O_2 (Fig. 8), as pointed out above, imply that the volume of CO_2 given off for a change in the gas tension of the alveolar air is much greater than the volume of O_2 exchanged for an equal change in tension. Changes in ventilation (which affect the alveolar tensions of O_2 and CO_2 almost equally, but in opposite directions) therefore cause an initially much greater change in CO_2 output than in O_2 uptake. An unsteady state with overventilation therefore causes a high respiratory exchange ratio, and an unsteady state with underventilation causes a low respiratory exchange ratio. Once the body gas stores have changed to their new level—i.e. once a new steady state is reached—the respiratory exchange ratio again equals the metabolic RQ.

In the preceding paragraph it has been shown that overventilation causes a high respiratory exchange ratio and underventilation causes a low one. This is true not only of the lungs as a whole in an unsteady state; it is also true of individual regions of the lungs (lobes, alveoli) in the steady state. Those with a high ventilation/perfusion ratio have a high respiratory exchange ratio; those with a low ventilation/perfusion ratio have a low one.

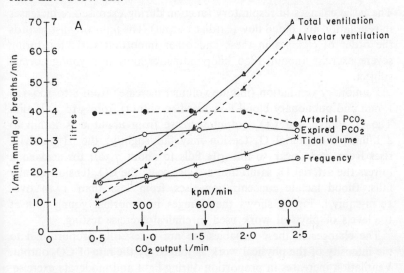

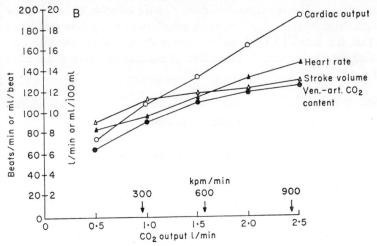

FIGURE 9. *The respiratory (A) and circulatory (B) changes during progressively increasing work.*

These are average values obtained in young men. 300 kpm is approximately equivalent to walking on the level, 600 kpm/min to bicycling and 900 to running.

RESPIRATORY AND CIRCULATORY CHANGES
IN EXERCISE

The basic changes in respiratory function during exercise are increases in ventilation and blood flow (cardiac output). The following list records the order of changes in these and other important variables during severe exercise (about 1800 kilopondmetres/min) in a young normal subject.

Pulmonary ventilation (minute volume) increases from 8 to 100–120 l./min and pulmonary blood flow (cardiac output) from 5 to 30 l./min. The O_2 intake and CO_2 output increase from about 0·25 l./min to 4 l./min; the arterial O_2 tension may fall slightly; the H^+ activity rises from 40 to near 50 nm (pH falls to about 7·30); the acidaemia lowers the arterial O_2 saturation 2–3 per cent; the CO_2 tension usually falls. Blood lactate concentration rises from less than 1 to over 10 m-equiv/l. Fig. 9 shows the changes in a normal young man at the levels of physical work used in clinical exercise testing.

The changes in these variables are not necessarily proportional to the intensity of the physical work as judged by the rate of CO_2 output. Ventilation increases in proportion during light and moderate exercise, but increases disproportionately during severe exercise, chiefly because of the development of acidaemia. A corollary of this excess ventilation is that the arterial CO_2 tension is lower during severe exercise than during moderate exercise. Limitation of exercise tolerance is discussed on p. 112.

Disordered Function

HYPOXIA AND DYSPNOEA

HYPOXIA

The physiology of hypoxia is so clearly related to the processes of pulmonary and circulatory physiology that a detailed account would be largely a reiteration of much that has already been said. This section therefore merely summarizes the main points.

The following list of causes of hypoxia is logically based upon the stages in the passage of O_2 from the environment to the tissue cells and therefore also helps to indicate the rational treatment.

1. Reduced O_2 tension in the inspired air.

2. Inadequate alveolar ventilation.
3. Impaired pulmonary O_2 uptake.
4. Venous-arterial shunts.
5. Insufficient functioning haemoglobin.
6. Inadequate blood flow through the tissues.
7. Poisoning of cellular enzymes.

Conditions in groups 1-4 cause 'hypoxic' hypoxia; that is to say, a reduction in the arterial Po_2. Conditions in group 5 cause 'anaemic' hypoxia; that is to say, a reduction in the amount of O_2 in the arterial blood but no reduction in the Po_2. Conditions in group 6 cause 'stagnant' hypoxia; that is to say, normal arterial O_2 values but excessive O_2 extraction from the blood leaving the tissues. Conditions in group 7 cause 'histotoxic' hypoxia and are associated with normal arterial O_2 values and diminished O_2 extraction from the blood.

Hypoxia and cyanosis
Conditions in groups 1 to 4 cause central cyanosis (p. 122) if sufficiently severe. Cyanosis does not occur in simple anaemia or carbon monoxide poisoning but does occur in methaemoglobinaemia and sulphaemoglobinaemia. Peripheral cyanosis may occur in group 6. Cyanosis does not occur in group 7.

Hypoxia, hypoxaemia and dyspnoea
Although the supply of oxygen available to the tissues is necessarily reduced in hypoxaemia, this reduction causes little damage until the arterial saturation falls to about 50 per cent and the arterial Po_2 falls to about 30 mmHg (Fig. 10). An arterial Po_2 of 20 mmHg seems to be intolerable. Lesser degrees of hypoxaemia cause increases in ventilation, blood flow, red cell formation and other changes but these are essentially adaptive responses.

Although acute hypoxia causes some disturbance of the breathing and often a slight degree of hyperpnoea it does not usually cause dyspnoea. Chronic hypoxia in the presence of normal ventilatory control causes hyperpnoea and undue breathlessness on exertion.

Suspicion of hypoxia must depend not upon respiratory but on neurological disturbance. The neurological manifestations of hypoxia are protean, varying from impairment of the highest cerebral functions in mild chronic hypoxia to convulsions and irreversible cerebral damage in a few minutes of acute severe hypoxia.

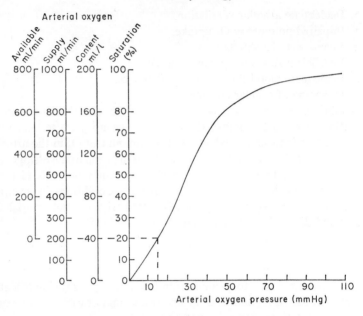

FIGURE 10. *The O₂ dissociation curve and O₂ supply.*

The inner ('saturation') vertical scale is the usual one which expresses (content÷capacity) × 100. The next scale ('content') gives the O_2 content per l. of blood assuming a normal Hb concentration (15 g/100 ml, 150 g/l.) and O_2 combining power (1·3 ml O_2/gHb). The next scale ('supply') gives the systemic O_2 flow per min assuming a cardiac output of 5 l./min. The outer scale ('available') allows for the fact that many vital tissues cannot extract the last 20 per cent of O_2 from Hb because they cannot tolerate a capillary PO_2 below about 15 mmHg. Therefore 40 ml/l. or 200 ml/min of O_2 are 'unavailable'. As the O_2 requirement of a resting subject is about 200 ml/min, an O_2 saturation of 40 per cent providing an O_2 supply of 400 ml/min is about the tolerable lower limit in uncomplicated hypoxaemia. Evidence of disordered function in the brain, liver and other vital organs appears at saturations below 50 per cent, but may appear at higher levels if there is anaemia or if the circulation is impaired.

LIMITATION OF EXERCISE TOLERANCE

In all exercise lasting more than a minute or so the rate of work is limited by the capacity to exchange and transport O_2 and CO_2. The effects of a limited capacity in each of the links in the chain of respiratory and circulatory systems connecting the tissues with the air will be considered individually.

Ventilation

Inability to increase ventilation in proportion to CO_2 output and O_2 intake should cause the alveolar and arterial P_{CO_2} to rise and the alveolar and arterial P_{O_2} to fall. Usually dyspnoea caused by the ventilatory stimulus of rising P_{CO_2} causes the subject to stop before significant hypoxaemia develops.

Pulmonary oxygen transfer

Inability to increase the capacity of the lungs to transfer O_2 in proportion to an increasing O_2 uptake causes an increased alveolar–arterial P_{O_2} difference. The fall in arterial P_{O_2} brings into play two adaptive responses: first, an increase in ventilation which, by increasing alveolar P_{O_2}, decreases the hypoxaemia; secondly, an increased cardiac output. This compensates for the lessened arterial oxygen content by increasing the total arterial flow.

Cardiac output

Inability to increase cardiac output in proportion to CO_2 output or O_2 intake causes a wide veno-arterial difference for CO_2 and oxygen, and a fall in the tissue P_{O_2}. This may cause an increase in anaerobic metabolism (see below).

Anaemia

The effect of anaemia is similar, with respect to O_2, to a reduction in cardiac output in that the flow of O_2 to the tissues is reduced. The important difference, however, is that in anaemia the cardiac output is often increased thereby compensating for the reduced content per unit volume of blood by an increased total volume flow.

Peripheral oxygen transfer

Inability of the muscles and their vascular bed to increase their capacity to transfer O_2 in proportion to an increasing O_2 usage causes an increased P_{O_2} difference between the blood and the tissues and may cause an increase in anaerobic metabolism. The difference between this form of limitation and a reduction in cardiac output is that the arterio-venous O_2 difference is not increased.

Metabolism

If the processes discussed above are unable to increase the supply of O_2 to the exercising muscles in proportion to the energy consumption, excessive anaerobic metabolism may occur causing the addition of lactic acid to the tissue fluid. This lactic acid displaces CO_2 from HCO_3^-. As anaerobic metabolism is relatively inefficient, the total CO_2 evolved through this mechanism is about four times that released by aerobic metabolism for the same work. This excess of CO_2 increases the load on all the above mechanisms and the rise in blood H^+ activity causes an excessive increase of ventilation so that the arterial P_{CO_2} falls.

What actually stops you?

Excessive demands on local muscle groups may cause local symptoms, and disease may signify the limit of tolerance by symptoms of local significance such as angina pectoris, intermittent claudication or wheezing. But in many diseased states including unfitness, heart disease, lung disease, anaemia the message is provided by breathlessness. The above considerations have shown how often limitation at some other site in the chain of respiratory and circulatory processes throws a strain on the breathing either by causing an increased CO_2 load or by increasing the ventilatory drive in other ways.

DYSPNOEA

Before defining dyspnoea it is as well to consider three situations. First, a normal subject performing strenuous exercise is conscious of his breathing and knows that it is increased, but recognizes that it is appropriate to his activity and is not distressed by the act of breathing. Second, a subject with anaemia, metabolic acidosis or a low cardiac output finds that his breathing is inappropriate to his activity on mild exercise or even at rest, but is not distressed by the act of breathing. Third, a subject with abnormal chest or lungs may be distressed by the act of breathing. Some definitions of dyspnoea include any condition of increased respiratory effort, whether or not it is accompanied by distress in the act, and even allow the term to be applied to unconscious subjects. Narrower definitions restrict dyspnoea to distress in the act, the third situation above, and prefer 'hyperpnoea' to describe the first two situations. In the absence of general agreement, and in view of the fact that beyond a certain point hyperpnoea causes distress in the act, the wider definition must be recognized.

If this starting-point is adopted the mechanism of dyspnoea can be approached in three stages. First, anything increasing ventilation is an indirect cause of dyspnoea, the factors responsible for the hyperpnoea of exercise being particularly important. Second, diseases which cause distress in the act at low levels of ventilation are associated with changes in the mechanical state of the lungs or chest. Third, the sensation itself probably arises in the nervous control of the respiratory muscles or in the chest wall. The sensation appears to arise from an imbalance or 'inappropriateness' between the volume demanded and the forces required to meet this demand. Inappropriateness may result from an excessive demand or from deranged mechanics or from a combination of the two.

Orthopnoea is probably due to an increase of pulmonary blood volume causing a reduction in compliance, but other factors such as disturbed ventilation/perfusion relationships and the mechanical advantage of the respiratory muscles may be important.

Cheyne-Stokes breathing is due to a hunting behaviour of the respiratory control. The possibility of hunting is intrinsic to any system in which the sensing element (in this case the medullary chemoreceptors) is separated from the effector element (the lungs) so that there may be a time lag between the two (between the medullary Pco_2 and the alveolar Pco_2). Hunting normally does not occur because this lag is small, because the respiratory demand is not sufficiently sensitive to CO_2 and because the volume of gas in the lungs damps the change in alveolar gas composition when ventilation changes. In Cheyne-Stokes breathing the most important causal factor appears to be an excessive ventilatory response to CO_2 which overcomes the smoothing properties of the system. The excessive ventilatory response is due to damage to supra-medullary nervous pathways which normally inhibit either the respiratory centres or the motor pathways to the respiratory muscles. A prolonged lung-to-brain circulation time may also be important.

REDUCED VENTILATORY CAPACITY

The ventilatory capacity may be reduced first by conditions which obstruct the airways; secondly, by conditions which hinder the expansion of the lungs or thoracic cage and, thirdly, by weakness of the respiratory act.

Airways obstruction

Obstruction of the upper extrathoracic airways, particularly in the larynx, affects inspiration more than expiration; obstruction of the intrathoracic airways affects expiration more than inspiration. Narrowing of the intrathoracic airways may result from processes in their walls such as increased bronchial muscle tone, swelling of the bronchial mucosa or the presence of secretions; it may also be due to loss of support because of destruction of the lung so allowing the airways to be narrowed by high external pressure in expiration.

Non-obstructive defects

Restrictive defects. This term is used to describe limitation of expansion of the lungs due to pulmonary causes such as fibrosis or congestion or to extrapulmonary causes such as pleural effusion, pneumothorax, or kyphoscoliosis.

Hypodynamic. This term is used to describe weakness of the respiratory muscles, disease of the central or nervous peripheral system or of the muscles themselves. This group is often included under the general heading 'restrictive' but it is as well to separate them because there is no real restriction to the expansion of the lungs.

INADEQUATE VENTILATION: HYPOXAEMIA
WITH HYPERCAPNIA

If ventilation is inadequate for the metabolic requirements of the body, whether at rest or exercise, the alveolar P_{CO_2} rises and P_{O_2} falls. The arterial P_{CO_2} also rises and the arterial P_{O_2} falls but because of the shape of the O_2 dissociation curve the O_2 saturation does not fall until the degree of underventilation is considerable. The alveolar and arterial P_{O_2} can fall by half (from about 100 mmHg to about 50 mmHg) before hypoxaemia becomes manifest as cyanosis (p. 122).

Inadequate ventilation may be due either to a reduced ventilatory capacity or a reduced central ventilatory drive. Although the first is much commoner it is important to remember that the degree of ventilatory incapacity at which underventilation appears varies very much between patients. Many develop inadequate ventilation with hypercapnia when, as judged by assessment of their ventilatory capacity, they could maintain normal alveolar gases. In these patients it appears that there is also some defect of central respiratory drive. In a small group of patients, inadequate ventilation occurs in the presence of a normal ventilatory capacity (p. 121).

Although the term 'ventilatory failure' can be used to describe the state of respiratory function when arterial P_{CO_2} is increased we must recognize that in many conditions the inadequate gas exchange is largely due to a disturbance of ventilation : perfusion relationships. In parts of the lung with a reduced blood-flow, ventilation accomplishes little removal of CO_2 or uptake of O_2. This is commonly called the 'dead space-like effect' of unequal ventilation : perfusion relationships.

Although in theory hypercapnia could be caused solely by an extreme imbalance between ventilation and perfusion, in practice it occurs only if ventilatory capacity is limited because total ventilation can usually be increased sufficiently to maintain an alveolar ventilation despite the increased physiological dead space.

DEFECTIVE GAS TRANSFER: HYPOXAEMIA WITHOUT HYPERCAPNIA

The exchange of O_2 and CO_2 between the alveolar air and the pulmonary capillary blood may be unduly hindered first, when the membrane is thickened or reduced in area. The uptake of O_2 is more severely affected than the elimination of CO_2 because, being less soluble, O_2 diffuses much less readily. Secondly, exchange may be hindered if the volume of the capillary bed is too small to permit the diffusion of gases through the red cells and the various chemical reactions in the red cells to reach equilibrium in the time available. Oxygen is again at a disadvantage compared with CO_2 because it accomplishes these processes more slowly. The term 'alveolar-capillary block' is often applied to defective O_2 transfer because there appears to be a 'block' or increased pressure drop in O_2 between the alveolar air and the pulmonary capillary—and hence systemic arterial—blood. But in fact the disturbance of ventilation : perfusion relationships is more important in causing defective transfer than any diffuse affection of the alveolar-capillary membrane. In parts of the lung with reduced ventilation, the blood-flow accomplishes little O_2 uptake or CO_2 removal. This blood has a big 'shunt-like' effect on the arterial oxygenation but, although in principle it should cause hypercapnia, in practice it has little effect. One reason is that the Pco_2 of the 'shunted' blood is little greater than that of the arterial blood (Fig. 8); the other is that the slight hypercapnia which might result is readily abolished by a very slight increase in ventilation.

BLOOD GAS TRANSPORT

In anaemia or in the presence of abnormal compounds of haemoglobin the volume of O_2 that can be taken up by the blood in the lungs is reduced but the Po_2 of the arterial blood is normal. As there is no impairment of CO_2 transport or exchange, the arterial Pco_2 and CO_2 content, and therefore ventilation, are usually normal. In severe or chronic situations, however, ventilation may be increased by hypoxic stimulation of the sino-aortic chemoreceptors with consequent lowering of the arterial Pco_2.

Changes in CO_2 transport affect ventilation by altering the arterial P_{CO_2} or H^+ concentration (Chapter 5). Thus in metabolic acidosis the increased (H^+) stimulates ventilation and reduces the arterial P_{CO_2}. For reasons as yet incompletely known the converse is not always true in metabolic alkalosis when the P_{CO_2} is often normal and not, as would be expected, raised (p. 211).

DISORDERED FUNCTION IN SPECIFIC DISEASES

Nearly all diseases which affect respiration disturb all aspects of lung function. There are no patterns of disordered function which are pathognomonic of individual diseases. In this chapter a few common conditions have been chosen to illustrate the inter-relationships of the various functional changes that can occur. The functional changes in other conditions can usually be deduced from a knowledge of their pathology.

Paralysis of the respiratory muscles
Partial paralysis reduces the ventilatory capacity but causes no disturbance at rest. Extensive paralysis causes ventilatory failure with elevation of the arterial P_{CO_2} and reduction of the P_{O_2}. Arterial unsaturation only occurs if the ventilatory failure is severe. Selective failure of individual muscles groups, or coughing too feeble to clear accumulated secretions often leads to atelectasis of parts of the lungs, causing a reduced P_{O_2} and (if sufficiently severe) arterial desaturation, by a 'shunt-like' effect.

Pneumothorax
The introduction of air into the pleural space, by allowing the thoracic cage to expand and causing the lungs to shrink, raises the intrathoracic pressure. No serious disturbance results from these changes unless—say as a result of a valvular opening—the intrathoracic pressure rises above atmospheric pressure. The effect of a severe reduction of lung volume or of a rise of intrathoracic pressure above atmospheric is to occlude intrathoracic airways during expiration causing air trapping. The maintenance of ventilation then requires a forceful contraction of the inspiratory muscles to overcome the elastic forces of the distended thoracic cage. In a severe case there may be areas of atelectasis in the underlying lung causing a reduction in arterial P_{O_2}, but the effect is seldom sufficient to reduce the saturation significantly because blood-flow in the affected lung is reduced. Only in very severe cases is there ventilatory failure with raised P_{CO_2}.

Lung cysts

Cysts in the lung substance produce virtually the same functional effects as a pneumothorax. Only those with a valvular bronchial communication produce an important disturbance of function. Cysts with free ventilation just increase the dead-space.

Pneumonia, congestion, fibrosis (fibrosing alveolitis)

These all cause a restrictive reduction in ventilatory capacity and defective gas transfer. The compliance is reduced; there is hypoxaemia without hypercapnia—the P_{CO_2}, in fact, is often low because either hypoxaemia or abnormal stimuli from the lungs or circulation (or both) cause the ventilation to increase.

Pulmonary arterial obstruction

Cessation of blood flow through a part of the lung causes its ventilation to become 'dead-space'. This effect is much less than would be predicted because there is a rapid increase in the elastance and resistance of the part which has the effect of reducing its ventilation. A characteristic feature of this and other forms of pulmonary vascular disease is alveolar overventilation causing a low arterial P_{CO_2}. The mechanism is uncertain.

Asthma (variable obstruction of airways)

There is narrowing of the airways by contraction of the bronchial muscles, by swelling of the lining of their walls and by increased mucus secretion. The resistance to airflow (non-elastic resistance) is increased particularly during expiration. The inspiratory muscles contract forcibly to stretch the lungs and hold the airways open. The work of breathing is greatly increased, but as the non-elastic rather than the elastic work is chiefly responsible, the optimum rate is not much increased. As the disorder is ventilatory there is usually equal difficulty with O_2 uptake and CO_2 excretion and equal liability to a raised arterial P_{CO_2} and reduced P_{O_2}. If, however, the airway obstruction is very unequal in different parts of the lungs there may be a 'shunt' effect producing a disproportionate reduction in P_{O_2}. The presence of atelectatic areas intensifies this 'shunt' effect.

Chronic lung disease with airways obstruction
(chronic bronchitis and emphysema)

Chronic bronchitis is characterized by excessive mucous secretion in the bronchial tree. Emphysema implies an abnormal enlargement of the air spaces distal to the terminal non-respiratory bronchiole, accompanied by destructive changes in their walls. A feature common to patients with these conditions is some degree of 'fixed' airways obstruction in that, although it varies, some degree of obstruction is always present. Although most patients have features of both conditions it is possible to recognize extremes of 'pure' bronchitis and 'pure' emphysema. It must be stressed that the disordered pulmonary function in these patients cannot be simply attributed to bronchitis or emphysema; these just happen to be the terms most commonly applied to these patients. Typically patients with bronchitis develop underventilation with hypercapnia more readily than the reduction of their ventilatory capacity would suggest; they are also more prone to develop cardiac enlargement and oedema. The gas exchanging surface as assessed by the CO transfer factor (p. 134) is fairly well maintained. Nevertheless, at rest, they do have an increased alveolar–arterial Po_2 difference which is due to a large volume of poorly-ventilated but well-perfused lung. When the total ventilation is increased on exercise the ventilation of the poorly-ventilated regions is also increased and the alveolar-arterial-Po_2 difference falls.

Typically, patients with emphysema do not underventilate but remain severely dyspnoeic and maintain normal alveolar gas concentrations until their ventilatory capacity is severely reduced. They are not so prone to cardiac enlargement and oedema. Their gas exchanging surface as assessed by the CO transfer factor is reduced. On exercise they develop an increased alveolar–arterial Po_2 difference and hypoxaemia.

'*Cor pulmonale*'. Heart failure may occur acutely or terminally in any respiratory condition in which there is severe hypoxia, but chronic venous engorgement and oedema usually occur only when there is CO_2 retention. Although this fluid retention is usually attributed to failure of the right ventricle caused by pulmonary hypertension, the explanation is not entirely satisfactory because many such patients have a normal cardiac output and it increases normally on exercise.

CO_2 *narcosis*. Patients with any chronic lung disease who are persistently hypoxic have part of their stimulus to breathe supplied by the arterial hypoxia. If hypoxia is relieved by the administration of excessive O_2, ventilation may fall acutely, causing severe CO_2 retention and acidosis, the effects of which are largely on the nervous system causing unconsciousness, muscular twitching and raised intracranial pressure. Drugs which depress the respiratory centres may produce a similar effect.

'Primary' alveolar hypoventilation

This term has been applied to a group of patients who can breathe normally but do not. The characteristic finding is a raised Pco_2 in a patient who has a relatively normal ventilatory capacity. Other common features include: arterial unsaturation, polycythaemia, obesity, oedema, somnolence and neurological damage. The resemblance to Dickens' fat boy has led to the popular synonym of 'Pickwickian' syndrome, but the term is misleading because obesity is not an essential feature.

In fact, it is unlikely that these patients are a homogeneous group. Hypoventilation may be produced by damage at various levels in the brainstem and the other features are very variable.

Principles of Clinical Observations Tests and Measurements

THE EVALUATION OF EXERCISE TOLERANCE
BY QUESTIONING

Exercise on the level has to be vigorous to stress the respiration or circulation. A normal man has an aerobic capacity considerably greater than is required for running or bicycling (Fig. 9, p. 109) and he can lose three-fifths of his capacity before walking becomes difficult to sustain. So, when trying to assess exercise tolerance, it is usual to supplement enquiry about exercise on the level with questions about hills and stairs. Most people climb stairs at a rate which requires the performance of physical work which is greater than their steady state aerobic working capacity, that is, at a rate they cannot sustain for more than a minute or so. And yet it is possible to exercise for half a minute or so without making any demand on the respiration or circulation. This is why we think nothing of climbing one or two floors but will usually wait for the lift if we should want to go up three or more. It also means that the answer to the common type of question 'How many stairs can you climb without getting unduly short of breath' must lie somewhere between 30 and 120 stairs or 2–6 domestic flights. In answering this question, patients base their estimate not on their steady state aerobic working capacity but on the distress they experience in repaying the oxygen debt and CO_2 accumulation during the unsteady state. The more severe the limitation of exercise tolerance, the more it becomes a matter of 'unsteady state' and the less reliable are changes in the patient's exercise tolerance as judged by questioning in indicating the true state of cardiorespiratory capacity. If important decisions of prognosis or treatment are at stake it is always preferable to supplement an assessment by questioning with an objective evaluation by studying the patient's performance during exercise. The measurements made need not be complex; measurement of the subject's true working capacity on a treadmill or ergometer together with such simple measurements as the ventilation, pulse rate and gas exchange will often be adequate.

PHYSICAL SIGNS OF AIRWAYS OBSTRUCTION
The forced expired time
The best physical sign of diffuse intrathoracic airways obstruction is a prolongation of the time taken to deliver the vital capacity (p. 123 and Fig. 11). In a normal subject this is accomplished in 3–4 seconds. Prolongation beyond 6 seconds means that the ratio of FEV_1 : VC is less than 60 per cent.

Over-inflation of the chest
The physiological response to airways obstruction is to inflate the lungs so as to hold the airways open and provide elastic recoil. This causes an increase in the areas of resonance on percussion. If the process goes on over a few years the thoracic cage itself becomes deformed: the anterior–posterior diameter of the chest is increased; the sternum becomes elevated so that the suprasternal portion of the trachea is shortened; the diaphragm is flattened and the heart becomes lower and more medial in position. The movements of the chest are also distorted: the expansion ('bucket handle' movement) of the upper ribs is lost, and replaced by exaggeration of the upward lift ('pump handle' movement). The depression of the diaphragm causes it to lose its mechanical advantage on the costal margin. The normal diaphragm lifts the costal margin and gives little downward pull on the mediastinum; the depressed diaphragm pulls the costal margin inwards and pulls the mediastinum downwards; this can be felt as a descent of the thyroid cartilage during inspiration.

Wheezes and squeaks (*rhonchi*)
Musical sounds are produced by fluttering of airways on the point of closure. Their pitch depends on the linear velocity of airflow rather than on the dimension of the airway in which they arise. Their loudness is no guide to severity; severe airways narrowing may be silent because the rate of airflow is insufficient to generate a sound.

CYANOSIS
Cyanosis is a blue colour of the skin or mucous membranes usually due to the presence of an excessive amount of reduced haemoglobin (or of methaemoglobin or sulphaemoglobin) in the small blood vessels

of the tissues. It is widely taught that there must be 5 g of reduced Hb per 100 ml blood before cyanosis occurs. This figure is a very rough approximation whose chief merit is to stress that cyanosis cannot occur in the presence of severe anaemia. Clinically cyanosis can most conveniently be subdivided into central, in which the arterial blood is unsaturated, and peripheral, in which the arterial blood is normally saturated but the extraction of O_2 from the blood in the tissues is excessive. The distinction is best made by examining the mucous membranes inside the mouth where blood flow is always good. If these are blue the cyanosis is of central type. Central cyanosis is an unreliable sign even under the best conditions of illumination. It can only be reliably detected if the saturation is below 75 per cent, and conversely it may be present (due to other causes such as pigmentation or thickness of the tissues) when the saturation is over 95 per cent.

Doubts about the presence or absence of cyanosis due to pulmonary disease can usually be resolved by the administration of O_2 (p. 126). If a patient who has indefinite cyanosis thought to be due to pulmonary disease does not become pink on breathing O_2, then the 'blue colour' is not due to arterial unsaturation of pulmonary cause.

THE VITAL CAPACITY

Interpretation of changes in the VC requires an understanding of the factors which limit the depth of voluntary inspiration and of those which limit the depth of voluntary expiration.

Maximum inspiration: the total lung capacity at full inspiration is, of course, governed to a considerable extent by the volume of the thorax and therefore by body size. In normal subjects there is a good correlation with height. Deformities or loss of mobility of the bony cage reduce this volume. Weakness of the inspiratory muscles, and decreased compliance (whether due to loss of functioning lung tissue or to increased stiffness of the lungs), also reduce the volume that can be inspired (Fig. 11).

Maximum expiration: the residual volume of air in the lungs at full expiration is also partly dependent on the size and integrity of the thoracic cage and the power of the respiratory muscles, but to a smaller extent than the total lung capacity. The physiological event which limits expiration is closure of the intrathoracic airways. The patency of these airways depends on a number of factors: the elastic tension in the lungs tending to hold them open, the strength of their walls and the presence or absence of processes such as oedema or muscular spasm tending to narrow them. In a normal subject expiration ceases when the elastic

5*

tension of the shrinking lung falls to a low level and the intrathoracic pressure rises sufficiently to collapse the small airways which are without cartilaginous support. Loss of elasticity, such as occurs in emphysema, causes the volume at which this closure occurs to be increased. In bronchitis, however, and particularly in asthma, the airways also tend to close prematurely because of the disease processes in their walls.

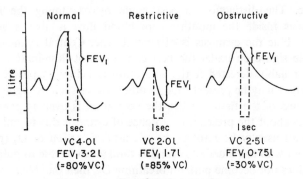

FIGURE II. *Forced expiratory spirograms.*

The three records are taken from spirometer tracings. Inspiration is up and expiration down, and the records read from left to right. After a deep inspiration the subjects breathed out as rapidly and forcibly as they could. The total volume expired is the (Forced) Vital Capacity (VC) and the volume expired in the first second is the Forced Expired Volume in one second (FEV_1). The 'restrictive' record was obtained from a patient with kypho-scliosis; the 'obstructive' record from a patient with emphysema. Although the vital capacity is more severely reduced in the patient with kypho-scoliosis than in the patient with emphysema, the proportion of the vital capacity expired in the first second is normal.

The complexity of factors affecting the vital capacity make it almost valueless in the diagnosis of specific diseases and of limited use in distinguishing between different disease processes. Moreover, the range of normal values, even when allowance is made for age, sex and size (Table 8, p. 144), is large and limits its value as a general 'screening' test or as a standard of comparison between patients. However, in the individual subject the VC is sufficiently reproducible to make it a useful measurement in assessing the progress of a large number of conditions.

Airways obstruction slows the delivery of the VC so that the FEV_1 : VC ratio is reduced (Fig. 11). Non-obstruction reduction of ventilatory capacity reduces the VC but does not slow its delivery so that the FEV_1 : VC ratio is normal (see below).

THE FORCED EXPIRED VOLUME

In normal subjects and in patients whose airways are healthy the closure of the airways which limits the end of voluntary expiration occurs almost simultaneously throughout the lungs. As a result 75 per cent of the VC is expelled smoothly and rapidly in 1 second and the remaining 20 per cent only takes a further 2 or 3 sec. However, in conditions causing diffuse airways obstruction (asthma, bronchitis, emphysema) the inequality of the disease process in different airways causes them to close irregularly and progressively as expiration proceeds. The result is that in a severe case, less than 40 per cent of the vital capacity is expelled in the first second and the remainder takes much longer. In fact, airflow continues for as long as the patient can wait before asphyxia forces him to take another breath.

A number of methods of quantitatively expressing the rate of delivery of the forced vital capacity have been used. The most popular is to measure the volume expired in the first second (FEV_1) with a spirometer and kymograph. This should normally be over 75 per cent of the vital capacity (Fig. 11). The FEV_1 is reduced by all conditions, obstructive and non-obstructive, which reduce the VC but the FEV_1 : VC ratio is reduced only by airways obstruction. FEV_1 is a much more sensitive index of the severity of airways obstruction than the vital capacity, but unfortunately it does not distinguish between the different causes. Thus a patient in an attack of asthma whose lungs between attacks are normal may have the same reduction in FEV_1 as a patient with emphysema who has no 'bronchospasm'. The effect on the FEV_1 of bronchodilator drugs helps in distinguishing between the mechanisms of airway obstruction, but measurement of non-elastic resistance, when the narrowing effect of the high intrathoracic pressure used to produce a FEV_1 is absent, may be required (p. 139).

'Peak' Expiratory Flow

The Wright peak flow meter measures the volume expired in the first tenth of a second of a forced expiration and gives a reading in l.min. Like the FEV_1 this is reduced in all conditions reducing the ventilatory capacity—both obstructive and non-obstructive.

Maximum Breathing Capacity

The maximum breathing capacity (MBC), better called the maximum voluntary ventilation (MVV), is measured by asking the patient to breathe as rapidly and as deeply as he can for about 15 sec. The volume breathed is either collected in a bag or recorded with a spirometer, and the result expressed as l./min. The MBC is little used now because it is no more informative than the FEV_1 and is much more difficult for the subject to perform.

Attempts to extrapolate from such measurements as the VC, FEV_1 or MBC to the ventilation which the subject can sustain during exercise are very approximate. During exhausting exercise a normal subject only achieves a ventilation equal to half his MVV. It is not uncommon on the other hand for a patient with severe airways obstruction to attain a ventilation during exercise which is greater than his MVV.

ARTERIAL OXYGEN SATURATION AND PRESSURE

The arterial O_2 saturation is the percentage saturation of Hb with O_2 ($100 \times$ content $\div$ capacity). It is measured volumetrically or spectrophotometrically on blood drawn from an artery. It can also be measured in the heated ('arterialized') pinna of the ear by oximetry, which is a form of spectrophotometry.

The systemic arterial blood is normally 95–98 per cent saturated with oxygen. Reduction of the saturation is an overall measure of the severity of respiratory disease but it is not a discriminating measurement in that the saturation is reduced by underventilation, defective gas transfer and anatomical right–left shunts. These causes can be distinguished from each other by measurement of the arterial Pco_2 and by observation of the effects of breathing oxygen. If the cause of a reduction in saturation is underventilation the arterial Pco_2 is raised. If it is due to an anatomical right–left shunt, breathing oxygen will produce little increase. Breathing oxygen raises the saturation to 100 per cent both in underventilation and in defective gas transfer because raising the Po_2 in the alveolar air of even very poorly ventilated parts of the lung raises the saturation of the blood to 100 per cent however much blood flows past—that is, however low the ventilation : perfusion ratio. Parts of the lung in which the alveolar–capillary membrane is so thick or ventilation is so low that oxygenation of the blood cannot be achieved by breathing 100 per cent oxygen are functionally indistinguishable from anatomical shunts with respect to both O_2 and CO_2 exchange.

The development of the polarographic electrode has enabled the evaluation of O_2 uptake by the lungs to be studied more accurately but the principles are the same. Breathing 100 per cent oxygen raises the alveolar Po_2 to about 650 mmHg. The small normal anatomical right-to-left shunt through such vessels as the Thebesian veins reduces the arterial Po_2 to about 600 mmHg. The Po_2 only falls below this level if there is anatomical right-to-left shunt or if there are regions of completely unventilated lung.

The sensitivity of arterial Po₂ and saturation to the inspired oxygen in defects of gas transfer is so great that 25–30 per cent O₂ causes a considerable increase in arterial Po₂ (fig. 12).

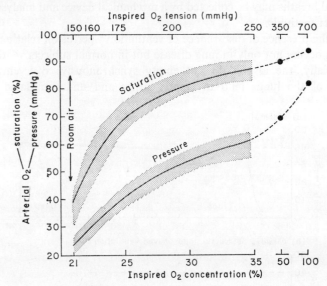

FIGURE 12. *The effect of increasing inspired O₂ concentration on arterial oxygenation in lung disease.*

These curves are derived from studies of patients with severe generalized lung disease causing underventilation, very uneven ventilation/blood-flow relationships and loss of diffusing capacity. Despite these defects, an increase in the inspired O₂ tension of 28 mmHg (4 per cent O₂) caused an increase of 17 mmHg in the arterial Po₂. As the arterial blood was on the steep part of the O₂ dissociation curve, this increase in tension was sufficient to increase O₂ saturation by 30 per cent. (*Lancet*, 1960, ii, 10.)

MEASUREMENT OF ALVEOLAR GAS PRESSURES

The classical (Haldane–Priestley) method of obtaining alveolar air is by forcibly and rapidly expiring down a long tube and analysing the last gas to be expelled. In a trained normal subject the alveolar air obtained by this method is of relatively constant composition and has O₂ and CO₂ tensions close to those of arterial blood (Fig. 13a 'H–P'). An untrained subject may hold his breath or overbreathe just before the forced expiration. This produces an 'unsteady state' in which the alveolar air and arterial blood differ from the 'steady state' values. A way of overcoming this (which is very satisfactory in normal subjects breathing spontaneously) is to analyse the last gas expelled during each expiration while the subject is breathing naturally. This is called 'end-tidal' sampling (Fig. 13a 'E-T'). This gas may be analysed breath-by-breath with a rapid gas analyser or a small proportion of each of several breaths may be collected by a mechanical device and analysed by simpler methods.

In the presence of disturbance of ventilation : perfusion relationships which occurs not only in lung disease but in normal subjects ventilated artificially, the alveoli do not empty synchronously; overventilated areas of the lungs tend to empty earlier and underventilated ones

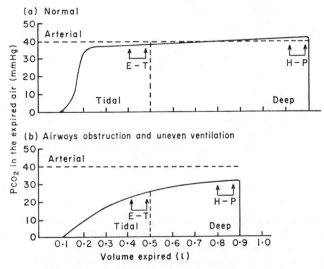

FIGURE 13. *The* CO_2 *concentration in the expired air during a single expiration.*

These records show the instantaneous CO_2 tension of the air coming out of the mouth during a resting (tidal) expiration and during a forced rapid deep expiration. There is no CO_2 in the first air to be expelled and then a steep S-shaped curve as the anatomical dead-space is flushed. Following this in the normal subject there is a slightly sloping plateau with a Pco_2 close to arterial Pco_2 so that either an end-tidal (E-T) or a Haldane–Priestley (H–P) sample provides a good estimate of the Pco_2 both of homogeneous alveolar air and of arterial blood. In the lower trace there is no plateau; the record continues to rise fairly steeply as long as the expiration continues. Homogeneous alveolar air therefore cannot be obtained either by an end-tidal or a Haldane–Priestley sample, nor can the arterial Pco_2 be estimated by these methods.

In both normal and abnormal subjects, slowing of the rate of the expiration would cause the slope to become steeper because the mixed venous blood is continuously adding CO_2 to a diminishing volume of air in the lungs.

empty later. The tracing of CO_2 tension during expiration is therefore much more sloping than in the normal subject (Fig. 13b). Therefore neither the Haldane–Priestley (H–P) nor end–tidal (E–T) samples correspond to 'true' alveolar air.

When ventilation : blood flow relationships are abnormal it becomes very difficult to define 'true' alveolar air, let alone to determine its composition. Theoretically, if the volume and composition of the gas in all the alveoli could be determined a 'true' mean value for alveolar composition could be calculated. However, this cannot be done, and, moreover, it might give an erroneous idea of the *effective* alveolar composition—i.e. the composition of the air in the alveoli which are in contact with blood flow—because many of the alveoli contributing to this 'true' value may be so poorly supplied with blood that their contribution to gaseous exchange is negligible.

'Ideal' alveolar air (Fig. 14)
The concept of ideal alveolar air represents an attempt to overcome these difficulties. It makes use of two facts. (1) The respiratory exchange ratio (p. 108) of any average value for alveolar air must be the same as that of the body as a whole (i.e. the metabolic respiratory quotient). Unless this is so, the values obtained will not represent a steady state. (2) The differing dissociation curves for O_2 and CO_2 mean that there is only one value of alveolar air which would, if present in all alveoli, cause the volumes of gaseous exchange appropriate to the respiratory quotient.

In practice this 'ideal' value cannot be determined exactly because too much accurate information about ventilation, blood flow and metabolism is required, but an 'effective' value very close to it is obtained by assuming that the arterial CO_2 tension and the alveolar CO_2 tension are equal. CO_2 diffuses so readily through biological media that at any site along the alveolar membrane the P_{CO_2} of the air on one side and the blood leaving a pulmonary capillary on the other side are the same. Hence, the P_{CO_2} of the arterial blood is the mean P_{CO_2} in those alveoli from which the 'average' blood has come. Obviously this estimate of alveolar P_{CO_2} is weighted by the over-perfused alveoli in the same way that estimates based on expired air would be weighted by the over-ventilated alveoli. However, at rest the arterial and mixed venous P_{CO_2} only differ by about 6 mmHg whereas alveolar and inspired air differ by about 40 mmHg. Hence the presence of venous or 'shunted' blood (i.e that from overperfused underventilated alveoli) affects estimates of alveolar P_{CO_2} based on the arterial blood to a smaller extent than the presence of 'dead-space' air (i.e. that from overventilated underperfused alveoli) affects any estimate based on expired air.

If the arterial Pco_2 is known and is taken to equal the 'effective' alveolar Pco_2, then the 'effective' alveolar Po_2 can be calculated (p. 133, p. 137).

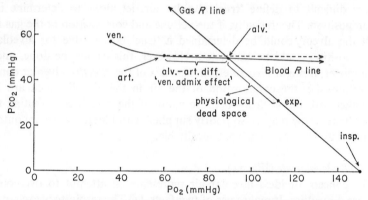

FIGURE 14. *The 'ideal' alveolar air analysis illustrated with the $CO_2 : O_2$ diagram using data obtained on a patient with underventilation and disturbance of ventilation : blood flow relationship.*

Inspired air (insp.) at sea level has a Po_2 of 150 mmHg and a Pco_2 of O. All possible expired and alveolar combinations of Po_2 and Pco_2 which have a respiratory exchange ratio (R) equal to that of the body's R.Q. must lie on the Gas R line. Similarly, all combinations of Po_2 and Pco_2 in blood which satisfy the body R.Q. must lie on a line (the blood R line) which starts from the mixed venous point (ven.); this line is not straight because the O_2 and CO_2 curves are not straight but it is both nearly straight and flat at Po_2's above 60 because the upper part of the O_2 dissociation curve is flat.

In practice, three points are known: the inspired (insp), the mixed expired (exp.) and the arterial (art.). The problem is to find the ideal alveolar point (alv.'), the physiological dead space and venous admixture. There are 4 steps. Step 1 says that the gas R line extrapolated from insp through exp must pass through alv'. Step 2 says that the difference between the Pco_2 of arterial blood and alveolar air (the vertical interval alv.'−art.) is very small (the blood R line is nearly flat) so that a horizontal (dashed) line from art passes close to the alv' which is thus fixed by the intersection of this line with the gas R line. The horizontal difference (alv'−art) is the alveolar to arterial Po_2 difference. Step 3 says that the ratio of dead space ventilation to total ventilation is the distance (alv'−exp) divided by (alv'−insp). Step 4 says that the venous admixture component is the difference in O_2 content of the blood between alv' and art divided by the difference in O_2 content between alv' and ven (the mixed venous point). This fourth step strictly requires that the mixed venous point and the slope of the O_2 dissociation curve be known; in practice both can be estimated with sufficient accuracy for clinical purposes. (From West, slightly modified.)

Physiological dead-space and venous admixture

If all the alveoli were to receive air and blood in the same proportion (e.g. all receive 80 units of air to 100 of blood, or 60 units of air to 100 of blood), the alveolar air expelled from all alveoli would have the same composition and the blood leaving all the pulmonary capillaries would have the same composition. Alveoli which have a higher ventilation in relation to blood flow than the average contribute air with a lower CO_2 concentration and higher O_2 concentration. This air therefore resembles dead-space air (i.e. air with no CO_2 and 21 per cent O_2). The blood in the capillaries leaving alveoli which have a lower ventilation in relation to blood flow than the average has a higher CO_2 tension and a lower O_2 tension and therefore resembles mixed venous blood. The problem is to decide what is the true or average alveolar composition. As discussed the best practical approach is to assume that the arterial CO_2 tension is equal to the 'effective' alveolar CO_2 tension. If this assumption is made, then the overventilated alveoli can be quantified as the increase in physiological dead-space they cause. The under-ventilated alveoli cause an increase in the Po_2 difference between the 'effective' alveolar air and the systemic arterial blood. This can be quantified as an apparent right-to-left shunt or 'venous admixture effect'. This is the basis of the 'ideal' alveolar air analysis which gives the most complete assessment of the distribution of ventilation in relation to pulmonary blood flow at present available.

Rebreathing methods

As has been shown above, when pulmonary function is disturbed, the determination of effective alveolar gas composition requires the measurement of arterial blood CO_2 tension. The techniques involved are difficult. It has, however, recently been appreciated (or rather re-appreciated) that, at rest, mixed venous Pco_2 is only 6 mmHg more than arterial, with a variation of only a few mmHg even when the cardiac output changes considerably. Mixed venous CO_2 tension can be relatively simply determined in the following way. A small bag containing CO_2 at a tension estimated to be a few mmHg higher than mixed venous Pco_2 is rebreathed. The gas in the bag mixes with that in the lungs (which has a Pco_2 lower than mixed venous blood) and the resultant mixture then has a Pco_2 close to that of mixed venous blood. The mixed venous blood then gives off or takes up CO_2 from the lungs until their tensions are equal. Blood then passes through the lungs without changing its Pco_2, and the CO_2 tension of the gas passing backwards and forwards between the lungs and the bag does not change. This equilibrium is recognized by recording the P_{CO_2} at the mouth with a rapid CO_2 analyser which shows a 'plateau' of unchanging CO_2 concentration (lower record, Fig. 15). The P_{CO_2} recorded during this equilibrium is that of the mixed venous blood. About 20 seconds are available for the attainment and recognition of this equilibrium before blood which has left the lungs unable to give off CO_2 comes back again from the tissues with its P_{CO_2} increased. It is possible to determine mixed venous P_{CO_2} (and thus to estimate arterial P_{CO_2}) using this principle without a rapid CO_2 analyser by getting the subject to 'prepare' the initial CO_2 mixture in the bag by rebreathing O_2. Such is the storage capacity of the body for CO_2 that, once having reached mixed venous P_{CO_2}, the P_{CO_2} in the bag, lungs and blood only rises slowly (upper record, Fig. 15). At any time between 75 and 120 seconds after beginning to rebreathe O_2, the P_{CO_2} in the bag is close to the true mixed venous value and is therefore suitable for use as the starting gas in the rebreathing

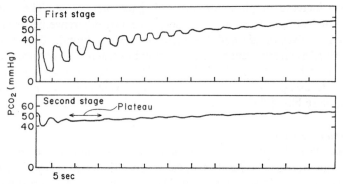

FIGURE 15. *The two-stage method for estimating mixed venous CO_2 tension.*
This is the record of P_{CO_2} at the mouth of a subject rebreathing from a bag initially containing 100 per cent O_2, its volume being less than twice the subject's tidal volume. During the early part of the first stage the P_{CO_2} rises quickly until the mixed venous P_{CO_2} is reached. The rate of rise then slackens to about 1 mmHg every 10 sec as CO_2 is stored in the body. This rise is allowed to continue until the bag is 'prepared' for the second stage, that is, until the the P_{CO_2} is a few mmHg above mixed venous. This first stage in practice usually requires about $1\frac{1}{2}$ min and is followed by a rest of about 3 min during which the subject breathes normally to allow the blood P_{CO_2} to return to normal. During the second stage the subject rebreathes from the bag that he had 'prepared' in the first stage. The CO_2 in the bag, lungs and mixed venous (pulmonary arterial) blood come into equilibrium which is shown as the plateau. The gas in the bag at any time within 20 to 40 sec after the start of the second stage has a P_{CO_2} within 1–2 mm of that of the mixed venous blood.

technique proper. It has also been shown that rebreathing a CO_2 mixture so prepared for 20–40 seconds brings the Pco_2 in the bag sufficiently close to that of mixed venous blood for most clinical purposes (lower record, Fig. 15).

THE INTERPRETATION OF ARTERIAL Pco_2

In interpreting measurements of arterial Pco_2 three equations must be borne in mind.

1. *The alveolar ventilation equation.* This relates CO_2 production (which is dependent on metabolic rate), alveolar ventilation (the effective volume of breathing) and arterial Pco_2.

$$\text{Arterial } Pco_2 = \frac{CO_2 \text{ production}}{\text{Alveolar ventilation}} \times 0\cdot86$$

0·86 is an average value at sea level for a factor depending chiefly upon barometric pressure.

This equation can be paraphrased:

$$\text{Arterial } Pco_2 \propto \frac{\text{Metabolic rate}}{\text{Effective volume of breathing}}$$

Thus, at any given metabolic rate, an inadequate ventilation causes an increased Pco_2.

2. *The alveolar air equation.* This equation depends upon the fact that the sum of the partial pressures of O_2, CO_2, N_2 and H_2O in the alveolar air equals barometric pressure. Nitrogen and H_2O are not exchanged in the lungs, so if the relative volumes of O_2 and CO_2 exchanged (i.e the respiratory exchange ratio or RQ) are known the alveolar Po_2 can be calculated from the arterial Pco_2.

$$\text{Alveolar } Po_2 = \text{Inspired } Po_2 - \frac{\text{Arterial } Pco_2}{\text{RQ}}$$

(This is a shortened version of the full equation which is used when the RQ is far from 1·0 or when greater accuracy is required.)

Thus, for any given inspired Po_2, an increase in arterial Pco_2 is associated with a fall in alveolar Po_2.

3. *The acid : base equation.* The derivation of this equation, of which the following are two versions, is given in chapter 5.

$$\text{Arterial H}^+ \text{ activity} = 24 \; \frac{\text{Arterial Pco}_2 \text{ (mmHg)}}{\text{Arterial plasma [HCO}_3^-\text{] (m-equiv/l.)}}$$
(nm)

$$\text{Arterial pH} = 6{\cdot}1 + \log \frac{\text{Arterial plasma [HCO}_3^-\text{] (m-equiv/l.)}}{0{\cdot}03 \; \text{Arterial Pco}_2 \text{ (mmHg)}}$$

These equations show that the changes in blood H$^+$ activity or pH depend upon both the Pco$_2$ and the HCO$_3^-$ concentration.

THE TRANSFER FACTOR (DIFFUSING CAPACITY)

For many years it was thought that the most important process concerned in the exchange of gases between the alveolar air and the pulmonary capillary blood was diffusion and that loss or damage to the alveolar-capillary membrane by disease would impair diffusion. Much effort was therefore devoted to the measurement of the 'diffusing capacity' of the lungs. Latterly, however, it has emerged that these measurements are more dependent on ventilation : blood flow relationships and chemical reactions than on diffusion and that the less specific term 'Transfer Factor' would be preferable.

The transfer factor for any gas X is calculated from the following equation:

$$\text{Transfer factor} = \frac{\text{Vol. of X taken up}}{\text{Alv. press. of X} - \text{Mean capill. press. of X}}$$
(ml/min/mmHg)

Three measurements are therefore required:
1. The volume of X taken up by the pulmonary capillary blood (ml/min).
2. The partial pressure (tension) of X in the alveolar air (mmHg).
3. The mean partial pressure of X in the pulmonary capillary blood (mmHg).

The volume of a gas that will diffuse from the alveolar air to the red cells in the pulmonary capillaries each minute depends upon many factors: the difference between the partial pressure of the gas in the alveolar air and the interior of the red cell; the solubility of the gas in aqueous solutions; its molecular weight; the area and thickness of the following barriers: the alveolar fluid, the alveolar membrane, the capillary membrane, the plasma, the red cell membrane, and the interior of the red cell; and on the volume of red cells in the pulmonary capillaries and the speed of certain physico-chemical processes in the red cells.

In respect of movement of O_2 and CO_2 across the alveolar-capillary membrane and the other liquid barriers, the much greater solubility of CO_2 outweighs all other factors. For many years, however, there was uncertainty about the ability of the lung to take up oxygen by diffusion in health and/or in disease and much effort was expended in attempts to estimate the diffusing capacity of the lungs for O_2. The major difficulty lies in the estimation of the mean partial pressure of O_2 in the pulmonary capillary blood because the Po_2 changes as Hb takes up the O_2.

The transfer factor for carbon monoxide
Although CO is not a physiological gas, its rate of diffusion throughout the physiological media resembles that of O_2 and the measurements of the transfer factor for CO can give information bearing upon O_2 transfer. The advantage of CO is that it largely removes the difficulty of estimating the mean pulmonary capillary tension for the following reason: the affinity of haemoglobin for CO is so great that, for all tolerable concentrations, the CO is so completely taken up by the Hb that the partial pressure in the capillary blood is zero. Only the first and second measurements listed above therefore need be made.

Several methods for the estimation of the CO transfer factor have been introduced. They fall into two main groups: the *steady state* methods in which the uptake of CO and the alveolar tension are measured over a period of several minutes; and the *single breath* methods in which the rate of uptake and alveolar tension are calculated from the change in composition of a gas mixture containing CO which is inspired, held in the lungs for about 10 seconds and then expired.

All these methods use low concentrations of CO ($<$0·3 per cent) in the inspired air. The chief differences between them lie in the estimation of alveolar CO tension. As discussed on page 129, the determination of the composition of alveolar air is not easy when pulmonary function is abnormal. Few methods of estimating transfer factor are entirely satisfactory in this respect because disturbance of ventilation/blood flow relationships cause reductions in the values obtained with them.

Partition of the diffusion pathway into the membrane and intracapillary components. O_2 and CO compete for haemoglobin but do not affect each other's diffusion through the alveolar-capillary membrane. Therefore, by measuring the CO transfer factor at different alveolar O_2 tensions, it can be broken down into a component dependent on diffusion through the membrane and a component dependent on events within the red cell. In normal subjects rather less than half the resistance to CO uptake lies in the membrane. This approach has also permitted estimation of the volume of blood in the pulmonary capillaries exposed to the alveolar air at any instant. In a normal subject, this volume is about 80 ml.

The concept of diffusing capacity is valuable and the transfer factor measurement can provide a quantitative description of the ability of a subject's lungs to transfer O_2 from the air to the blood. Its use to examine the area and permeability of the alveolar-capillary membrane in disease has, however, been disappointing for two reasons. First, it has proved difficult to devise a practicable method which is not affected by ventilation/perfusion inequality. Secondly, changes in the pulmonary blood volume and flow obscure the effect of disease of the membrane. With none of the methods in general use is it possible to maintain that a low value means that the alveolar-capillary membrane is shrunken or thickened. Indeed, it is doubtful if reduction of the diffusing capacity of the alveolar-capillary membrane is ever an important cause of defective O_2 transfer. It is certainly very much less important than inequality of ventilation : blood flow ratios.

METHODS OF ASSESSING THE EVENNESS OF DISTRIBUTION OF THE INSPIRED AIR

Methods of studying the distribution of the inspired air all measure the effects on the expired air composition of a sudden change in the composition of the inspired air.

The single breath nitrogen test

In this test a breath of oxygen is taken. The concentration of nitrogen throughout the next expiration is recorded. Were the breath of oxygen to be uniformly distributed throughout the lungs the nitrogen concentration in the succeeding expiration should be uniform. In fact overventilated parts of the lungs tend to empty first and underventilated parts to empty last so that the nitrogen concentration tends to rise throughout the course of a single expiration. If the rate of this rise is increased it implies that the preceding breath of oxygen was distributed less evenly than normal.

Nitrogen emptying rate. If the inspired gas is changed from air to 100 per cent O_2, nearly all of the N_2 in the lungs should be washed out in 7 minutes of quiet breathing. A nitrogen concentration in the alveolar air in excess of 2·5 per cent at this time indicates maldistribution.

Mixing efficiency. If a foreign gas such as helium is added to the inspired air in a closed spirometer circuit (i.e. one in which the same air, minus CO_2, is rebreathed by the subject) it is possible to calculate how many breaths should be required to attain 90 per cent (or some other proportion) of complete mixing between the spirometer gas and the lung gas. If the number of breaths actually required is measured, it can be related to the predicted number and expressed as a 'percentage efficiency'.

'Poorly' or 'slowly' ventilated space. A breath by breath record of the change in composition of the expired air is taken during the manoeuvres described above and plotted against time or number of breaths on semilogarithmic paper. It is usually found that the points form a curve with a single inflexion. This curve can thus be analysed as though it were derived from two separate processes, one representing mixing in a volume of the lung which is well or rapidly ventilated and the other representing mixing in a volume which is poorly or slowly ventilated. In the presence of maldistribution the volume of the poorly or slowly ventilated space is increased.

The above techniques only study the distribution of the inspired air in relation to the lung air. They give no information about the distribution of the inspired air in relation to the blood flow in the lungs.

THE MECHANICAL PROPERTIES OF THE LUNGS:
COMPLIANCE AND NON-ELASTIC RESISTANCE

The estimation of the compliance and non-elastic resistance of the lungs requires measurement of the transpulmonary pressure, that is, the pressure difference between the alveoli and the surface of the lungs; and also between the alveoli and the mouth. The pressure at the surface of the lungs—i.e. outside the lungs but inside the thoracic cage—is called the intrathoracic pressure and is usually measured in the oesophagus. The alveolar pressure is equal to mouth pressure when there is no airflow.

The intrathoracic pressure at rest, with no airflow and the respiratory muscles inactive, is normally about 5 cm H_2O below atmospheric (-5 cm H_2O) (Fig. 16, point A). This pressure is due to the elastic tension or relaxation pressure of the lungs pulling inward on the thoracic cage. [If the thoracic cage were removed at this volume and air prevented from leaving the mouth, the recoil or relaxation of the lungs would cause the pressure in the air spaces to rise to $+5$ cm H_2O.] If the subject breathes in very slowly, so that the rate of airflow is negligibly small, the intrathoracic pressure falls, producing the record

AOB in Fig. 16. The volume inspired (500 ml) divided by the change in oesophageal pressure (-5 to $-7\cdot5 = 2\cdot5$ cm H_2O) gives the compliance of the lungs (200 ml/cm H_2O in the example) and the reciprocal is the elastance (5 cm H_2O/l. in the example). If the subject breathes in at a normal speed the oesophageal pressure produces the record AIB. The difference between *I* and *O* is due to the non-elastic resistance offered by the airways to the flow of air and to the viscous resistances of the lung tissues. If a simultaneous record of the rate of airflow is taken, an instantaneous value for $I-O$ divided by the simultaneous rate of airflow is a measure of the non-elastic resistance. A normal expiration produces the record *BEA*, the horizontal distance $E-O$ divided by the rate of airflow again being a measure of non-elastic resistance.

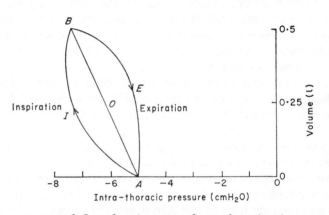

FIGURE 16. *Intra-thoracic pressure changes during breathing.*

A record of the relation between lung volume (ordinate) and intra-thoracic (pleural or oesophageal) pressure (abscissa). *AIB:* the changes in volume and pressure during a normal inspiration; *BEA:* the changes in volume and pressure during a normal expiration; *AOB:* the changes during a very slow inspiration when the effects of airflow are negligible.

In practice, the subject breathes normally while simultaneous records of oesophageal pressure, the rate of airflow and/or the tidal volume are obtained. A 'loop' such as *AIBE* is then constructed (it can be obtained electrically from the other records) and the diagonal joining the points of no flow (i.e. the line *AOB*) is used to calculate the compliance, and the non-elastic resistance is obtained as described above. Reduction of compliance causes the diagonal to be flatter; increased non-elastic resistance causes the loop to be fatter. Unfortunately, although the points *A* and *B* represent no flow through the mouth, in subjects whose lungs are not mechanically uniform there may still be regional differences of pressure causing air to flow within the lungs (p. 99 and Fig. 7). These pressure differences are reflected in the oesophageal pressure causing it to be lower (i.e. 'more negative') than it would be if there were complete cessation of airflow within the lungs. The compliance as calculated by the diagonal *AOB* is then lower than the true or 'static' compliance of such subjects. The difference between the apparent or 'dynamic' compliance and the true or 'static' compliance is an index of the degree of non-uniformity of the mechanical properties of the lungs. The effect of the non-uniformity on the measurement of non-elastic resistance (as described above) is to cause it to be overestimated.

As previously pointed out (p. 96), the compliance depends upon other factors besides the amount, arrangement and integrity of the elastic tissue proper, particularly surface tension. Moreover, it does not take account of lung size; thus reduction of the amount of functioning lung tissue reduces the compliance although the elastic properties of the functioning lung tissue have not changed. A reduced compliance may be due to any of four factors: stiffer lung tissue; higher surface tension of the alveolar lining fluid; reduction of the functioning lung volume; or damage to the normal architecture.

Measurements of compliance have considerably increased under standing of pulmonary physiology in general. They are, however, of limited value in the assessment of individual patients partly because of the difficulty of interpreting changes and partly because the normal range is so wide.

An apparently satisfactory measure of *non-elastic resistance* of the lungs and airways would be the pressure difference between the mouth and the alveoli per unit rate of airflow (cm H_2O/l./sec). However, as pointed out earlier (p. 97), the presence of turbulent airflow prevents the pressure difference from being simply proportional to the rate of airflow. Techniques for separately estimating the laminar and turbulent components of the total flow resistance have been used but the results are of doubtful validity. Moreover, the usual methods measure other sources of resistance besides that due to the air passages; for example, the sliding of tissues over each other and the viscous resistance of the tissue fluids. At present, therefore, the most popular term is 'non-elastic resistance' and it is usually expressed as the pressure difference between the mouth and the alveoli at a given rate of airflow (e.g. 1·5 cm H_2O at 0·5 l./sec, or 3·5 cm H_2O at 1 l./sec). Alternatively the relationship between pressure and rate of flow can be shown graphically. The non-elastic resistance, like compliance, partly depends on lung size; if the amount of functioning lung is reduced the rate of airflow per unit pressure difference is reduced because there are fewer passages for the air to flow through.

In spite of all these difficulties and uncertainties the measurement of non-elastic resistance promises to be of more clinical value than compliance because the normal range is smaller in relation to the changes in disease, and because the resistance of the airways is much the most important of all the factors affecting the non-elastic resistance.

Sufficient information about the severity of airway obstruction can usually be obtained from analysis of spirographic tracings of a single forced expiration (p. 124). Unfortunately, these simpler measurements do not discriminate between increased resistance due to swelling, or spasm of the wall of the airway (such as occurs in asthma) and increased resistance due to closure of the airways by external pressure (such as occurs in emphysema).

The *work of breathing* can be calculated from graphs such as Fig. 16 in which pressure and volume-change are plotted against each other because areas on such graphs have the dimension of work; that is, pressure × change in volume.

The methods described above, based on the measurement of intra-thoracic pressure, only estimate the compliance and non-elastic resistance, and work due to structures within the thorax. The thoracic cage also has elastic and non-elastic properties but they cannot easily be studied by available techniques.

Whole body plethysmography

A more convenient technique than the registration of oesophageal pressure for the measurement of non-elastic resistance is obtained by a subtle application of Boyle's Law while the whole body is in a plethysmograph. This method has the additional advantage of measuring the lung volume simultaneously so that the variation of non-elastic resistance with lung volume can be allowed for. The body plethysmograph cannot however be used for the measurement of lung compliance.

ASSESSMENT OF REGIONAL LUNG FUNCTION

Fluoroscopy. On fluoroscopy the intensity of 'lighting-up' of the lungs, the movement of the ribs, the mediastinum and the diaphragm indicate the proportion of ventilation received by individual lobes. Lags in the movement of the diaphragm and the mediastinum indicate unequal obstruction of the airways. A forced voluntary inspiration and expiration magnify regional differences of pressure in the lungs and therefore magnify these regional changes in movement.

Broncho-spirometry and bronchial catheterization. In these procedures the air from the different lungs or lobes is separately analysed and, by using such devices as the inspiration of foreign gases and the measurement of the regional respiratory exchange ratio, the regional ventilation and blood flow can be assessed.

Radio-isotope techniques. After administration of an isotopically labelled gas to a subject, the concentration can be followed in regions or 'cores' of lung by external counting. This elegant approach permits the assessment of regional ventilation and blood flow. A good example is provided by the use of ^{133}Xenon, an insoluble gas, to study either ventilation or blood flow. If ^{133}Xe is inspired it is not taken up by the blood and its local concentration in the underlying lung is therefore dependent on regional volume and ventilation. If ^{133}Xe is injected intravenously it comes out of solution completely on passage through the lungs, and its local concentration in the underlying lung is therefore dependent on regional blood flow.

A less subtle but more widely available technique is to scan the radioactivity in the lungs after intravenous injection of macro-aggregates of ^{131}I- or ^{99m}Tc-labelled albumin. These impact in the precapillary pulmonary blood vessels producing regional radioactivity proportional to the local blood flow.

Practical Assessment

VENTILATORY CAPACITY
Clinical observations
Exercise tolerance and severity of dyspnoea as assessed by questioning; supplemented by observation at rest and when exercising (climbing stairs) as fast as possible.

Note frequency, depth, movements of the chest (p. 122), action of accessory muscles, wheezing, ability to talk or count between breaths.

Differentiate reduced ventilatory capacity from: overventilation, fatigue, angina or other chest pain, poor morale.

Signs of airways obstruction (p. 122): forced expired time; over-inflation; wheezes.

Signs of conditions likely to hinder expansion, e.g. basal congestion, air or fluid in pleura, obesity, deformed thorax.

Signs of muscular weakness.

Routine methods
Peak flow (p. 125): reduced in obstructive and non-obstructive defects.
   Spirometry (p. 123): FEV_1: VC ratio reduced in airways obstruction.
   Effect of bronchodilators.
Ventilatory response to exercise.

Special techniques
   Compliance by oesophageal pressure (p. 137).
   Resistance by oesophageal pressure (p. 139) or plethysmography (p. 140).
   Distribution of inspired gas (p. 136). Lung volumes.
   Arterial P_{CO_2} on exercise.

GAS TRANSFER
Clinical observations
If impaired: overbreathing and cyanosis; usually inconspicuous at rest but may be provoked by exercise. Cyanosis abolished, ventilation reduced and exercise tolerance improved by O_2.

Routine methods
CO transfer factor (diffusing capacity) (p. 134).
Ventilatory response to exercise.
Arterial saturation on exercise.
Restrictive ventilatory defect usually present in conditions causing impairment.

Special techniques
Arterial P_{O_2} and P_{CO_2}; physiological dead space; alveolar-arterial P_{O_2} difference and venous admixture particularly on exercise. Effects of O_2.

HYPERCAPNIA
Clinical observations
Many signs may be present; none is pathognomonic, all may be absent: mental confusion proceeding to coma, tremor, vasodilation, tachycardia, raised blood pressure, sweating, papilloedema. Absence of cyanosis does not exclude.

Routine methods

Pco_2 by rebreathing (p. 131) or interpolation method (Astrup; p. 215).
In chronic hypercapnia, plasma [HCO_3^-] secondarily increased.

Special techniques

Arterial Pco_2 and pH (p. 213-5).

HYPOXAEMIA

Clinical observations

'Central' cyanosis, i.e. of mucous membranes where blood flow good.
If caused by arterial hypoxaemia due to respiratory failure, the central
cyanosis is abolished by breathing O_2. Persistence of cyanosis on O_2
signifies anatomical R–L shunt or abnormal pigment (p. 122).

Routine methods

Arterial saturation.
Pco_2 indicates relative importance of underventilation and defective
gas transfer.

Special techniques

Arterial Po_2: partition of cause of desaturation by measuring Pco_2 and
by breathing O_2 (p. 126).

REGIONAL LUNG FUNCTION

Assessment must always include, and is helped by, assessment of total
lung function.

Clinical observations

Physical and radiographic signs of local aeration.

Routine methods

Fluoroscopy (p. 140).

Special techniques

Bronchospirometry or bronchial catheterization (p. 141).
Radioactive gas isotopes or macroaggregates (p. 141).

TABLE 8. Respiratory function tests: normal values and changes in disease

A range is given where one is well established; a single value indicates either that the range is not well established or that it varies considerably with such factors as age or body size. Reference must then be made to one of the works listed in the bibliography. There are several hundred measurements which may in some circumstances be used to evaluate pulmonary function. Only those are given which are of established value in general use or which appear likely to become so.

Measurement	Usual units	Normal value	Comments	Changes in disease
Vital Capacity (VC)	litres (BTPS—i.e. Body Temperature and Pressure, Saturated with water vapour)	[Height (in.)×0·12]−[Age×0·03]−2·4 l. Women 20% less.	Wide variation between individuals even when standardized for age, sex and size. More value in following changes in a given individual.	Reduced in large number of conditions affecting neuro-muscular system, thoracic cage, lungs, airways, pulmonary circulation.
Forced (Fast) Vital Capacity (FVC)	litres (BTPS—see above)	Equal to VC.	The volume obtained for the VC when the measurement is made on a forced expiration.	In diffuse airways obstruction the FVC may be less than the VC.
Residual Volume (RV)	litres (BTPS—see above)	20% TLC at age 20 40% TLC at age 60 (TLC=Total lung capacity, i.e. VC+resid. vol.).		Increased in all conditions causing diffuse airway obstruction (e.g. asthma, emphysema). May exceed 70% TLC.
Forced Expired Volume in 1 second (FEV₁)	litres (BTPS—see above)	>75% FVC	Reduction of VC from any cause reduces FEV₁, but ratio FEV₁ : VC only reduced in diffuse obstruction.	Decreased if airways obstructed. <1·5 l. (50% VC), moderate reduction; <0·8 l. (30% VC), severe reduction.

Maximum Breathing Capacity (MBC) (Max. Voluntary Ventilation)	l./min (BTPS—see above)	Man age 20 > 150 age 60 > 100 Woman age 20 > 100 age 60 > 70	May be performed at a set rate of breathing but usually subject allowed to choose his own.	Reduced in all conditions which interfere with mechanics of breathing. Particularly marked in diffuse-airways obstruction. Under 40 l./min, moderate reduction; under 25 l./min, severe reduction.
Pulmonary Compliance	l./cm H_2O	0·120–0·250	$\text{Compliance} = \dfrac{1}{\text{Elastance}}$ Values depend to considerable extent on technique.	Compliance reduced (elastance increased) in many conditions, particularly diffuse infiltrations and vascular congestion. Findings in emphysema vary with technique but 'true' compliance probably increased.
Pulmonary Elastance	cm H_2O/l.	4–8		
Pulmonary Non-Elastic Resistance	cm H_2O/l./sec.	1·0–3·0	Pressure/Flow relationships can only be described by this simple approximation at low flow rates	Moderately increased in bronchitis and emphysema (4–10), more marked when oedematous (10–20). Greatest increase in severe asthma (> 20).
Physiological Dead-Space	ml	100–170 ml (Approx. = body weight in lb)	Not normally greater than anatomical dead-space and less than 35% of tidal vol. Increases on exercise but less than tidal vol. so that the ratio falls below 20%	Increased in all conditions with maldistribution of ventilation/blood flow.

TABLE 8 (*continued*)

Measurement	Usual units	Normal value	Comments	Changes in disease
Pulmonary Nitrogen Emptying Rate	$\%N_2$	$<2\cdot5\%$	$\% N_2$ in alveolar air after 7 minutes breathing $100\% O_2$.	Increased in all conditions with maldistribution of inspired air.
Arterial Carbon Dioxide Pressure (Pa_{CO_2})	mmHg.	36–44	See also Table 9, p. 218. Falls in heavy exercise	Increased (respiratory acidosis) when alveolar ventilation inadequate. >60, moderate; >80, severe. Reduced (respiratory alkalosis) in hyperventilation and metabolic acidosis.
Arterial Plasma CO_2 Content	m-mole/l.	21–29	Bicarbonate conc. (m-eq./l.) $1\cdot1$–$1\cdot5$ less. Corresponding venous values approx. 2 more. See also Table 9, p. 218.	Increased in metabolic alkalosis and compensated respiratory acidosis. Reduced in metabolic acidosis and compensated respiratory alkalosis.
Arterial H^+ Concentration	nm pH	36–44 } 7·36–7·44}	See also Table 9, p. 218. Falls in severe exercise	(H^+) increased (pH reduced) in acidaemia. (H^+) reduced (pH increased) in alkalaemia. See Chap. 5.

Arterial Oxygen Saturation	%	93–98% Normally (even at low altitude) varies slightly with alveolar ventilation, respiratory quotient and barometric pressure.	Does not fall on exercise	Both reduced in 'hypoxic' hypoxia (p. 111). Commonest cause of reduction is defect of O_2 transfer due to ventilation: perfusion inequality. Reductions due to true shunts distinguished by effects of O_2 (p. 126).
Arterial Oxygen Pressure (Pao_2)	mmHg	80–110 Varies considerably with alveolar ventilation, respiratory quotient and barometric pressure	More sensitive to minor abnormality than saturation. Should be interpreted in relation to alveolar Po_2 (see below).	
Alveolar-arterial Po_2 Difference (A–a gradient)	mmHg	<15	Most of the difference is normally due to inequality of ventilation/blood flow ratios (i.e. the 'physiological shunt'—see below). Increases slightly on exercise.	Increased if O_2 transfer defective or R–L shunt (see above)
Venous admixture effect	% of cardiac output	<5%	Normally due to 'shunt-like effect' of uneven ventilation : perfusion ratios (p. 102) and very small amount of true shunt (Thebesian veins, etc.). Falls on exercise	Derived from, and same significance as, alveolar-arterial Po_2 difference
Transfer Factor for CO (CO Diffusing capacity)	ml/min/mmHg	Rest : 15–25 Exercise : 30–50	Varies with method and physique	Reduced if alveolar-capillary gas transfer defective from any cause.

6

References

FENN W.O. & RAHN H. (ed.) (1965). Respiration. *Handbook of Physiology.* Section 3. Vols. I & II. Washington D.C., Amer. Physiol. Soc.

COMROE J.H. (1965) *Physiology of Respiration.* London, Lloyd-Luke.

DEJOURS P. (1966) *Respiration.* Trans. by L.E. Farhi. Oxford University Press.

COTES J.E. (1965) *Lung Function: Assessment and Application in Medicine.* Oxford, Blackwell Scientific Publications.

BATES D.V. & CHRISTIE R.V. (1964) *Respiratory Function in Disease.* Philadelphia, Saunders.

WEST J.B. (1965) *Ventilation/Blood Flow and Gas Exchange.* Oxford, Blackwell Scientific Publications.

CAMPBELL E.J.M. (1966) Exercise Tolerance *Sci. Basis. Med. Ann. Rev.* 128–144.

HOWELL J.B.L. & CAMPBELL E.J.M. (ed.) (1965) *Breathlessness.* Oxford, Blackwell Scientific Publications.

CAMPBELL E.J.M. (1965) Respiratory Failure. *Brit. Med. J.* **i,** 1451–1460.

FORGACS P. (1969) Lung Sounds. *Brit. J. Dis. Chest,* **63,** 1–12.

4

The Kidney

Normal function

ANATOMY

Each kidney contains $1-1\frac{1}{4}$ million nephrons. Each nephron is composed of a glomerulus, proximal tubule, loop of Henle, distal tubule and collecting duct, the nephron being invested by highly specialized blood vessels.

Vascular anatomy. The renal arteries, which are often multiple, enter the kidney at the hilum, and divide into branches which pass dorsal and ventral to the pelvis, forming interlobar arteries passing between the pyramids. At the corticomedullary junction the interlobar arteries form the arcuate arteries, running over the bases of the pyramids. From the arcuate arteries the interlobular arteries turn off at right angles and run towards the cortex. There are short arterioles, the afferent arterioles, running off from the interlobular arteries to the glomeruli. The interlobular arteries run at right angles from the parent arcuate arteries, and the afferent arterioles at right angles from the interlobular arteries. This arrangement is of particular importance for the 'plasma skimming theory' (see p. 152). The afferent arterioles split up into the glomerular capillary network, which drains into the efferent arterioles.

Juxta-glomerular apparatus. As the afferent arteriole approaches the glomerulus it comes into contact with the distal tubule. At this point the distal tubule cells are columnar and close packed and are termed the 'macula densa'. The afferent arteriolar wall at this site is also modified, the media and adventitia containing large epithelioid granular cells forming a perivascular cuff, the 'polkissen' or juxta-glomerular apparatus. These cells are thought to be the site of renin secretion (see p. 165).

Efferent arterioles. The efferent arterioles split up to form the peritubular capillary complex, which drains in the cortex into cortical venules. These join interlobular veins, which combine to form arcuate veins running in a similar position to the arcuate arteries. The arcuate veins form arches over the bases of the pyramids and join to form the renal veins.

Blood supply of the medulla. The anatomy of the blood vessels supplying the medulla is quite distinct from that of the cortex. Blood entering the juxtamedullary glomeruli leaves through wide bore efferent arterioles, which send off a few branches to a peritubulary capillary network. The efferent arterioles then branch repeatedly, the branches descending parallel to Henle's loops into the pyramids; they are termed 'vasa recta'. They branch into a capillary network in part, and then bend with the loop of Henle into the ascending vasa recta, joining interlobular veins close to their junction with the arcuate veins. The structure of the vasa recta is closely applied to both Henle's loops and the collecting ducts which pass through the medulla.

Glomerulus. The glomerulus is an invagination of a capillary tuft into the proximal tubule. Bowman's space is on the outer side of the glomerulus and is continuous with the lumen of the proximal tubule. The glomerular surface is covered with epithelial cells; these have discrete and separate foot processes or podocytes resting on the surface of the capillary basement membrane. In proteinuric states these become fused.

The basement membrane is continuous with the basement membranes of the tubules. The basement membrane supports the endothelium of 20–40 capillary loops which are divided into 4–8 or more lobules. The endothelium is flat. The area occupied by the capillaries is 5000 to 15,000 cm²/100 g of kidney. The glomerular capillaries behave as if they are penetrated by pores 75–100 Å in diameter and there are narrow slit-like pores about 100 Å in diameter passing between the foot processes of the epithelial cells; the endothelial cells are likewise perforated by many holes about 800 Å in diameter. In the basement membrane, however, there are three layers, a central osmophilic layer and two outer non-osmophilic layers. There are no pores visible in the basement membrane on electron microscopy but it may be a semi-permeable gel.

Proximal tubule. The proximal tubule is a coiled tube connecting Bowman's capsule with the loop of Henle; the proximal tubules are in the cortex and outer layers of the medulla. Histologically they are cuboidal cells with a 'brush border' projecting into the lumen. The basement membrane is a highly infolded and convoluted structure, interdigitating with that of other proximal tubular cells and of the peri-tubular capillaries. The cytoplasm is granular.

The loop of Henle. In 1 loop of Henle out of 7 the long hairpin bend reaches down into a papilla, some reaching as far as the papillary tip. The nephrons with glomeruli in the outer two-thirds of the renal cortex have short loops of Henle, many of which are restricted to the cortex. The long loops of Henle originate from the juxtamedullary glomeruli which lie in the inner third of the cortex, closest to the medulla. The site and number of these long loops and their investing vasa recta is important in the counter current theory of urinary concentration (p. 160).

The loop of Henle consists of a short descending thick limb continuous with the proximal tubule, long descending and ascending thin limbs and a thick ascending part joining the distal convoluted tubule. The thin segment has flattened epithelial cells, whereas the thick segment consists of cuboidal cells. It is these cuboidal cells which may have a sodium pump located inside them with the ability to pump sodium out of the tubular lumen and into the interstitium (see p. 161).

Distal tubule. The distal tubule extends from the thick section of the loop of Henle to the collecting duct, coiling round in the neighbourhood of the parent glomerulus. The cells are cuboidal with columnar cells at the macula densa—the area where the afferent arteriole comes into contact with the distal tubule. The columnar cells of the macula densa are closely packed.

Collecting tubule. The distal tubular cells, when they approach the collecting tubule, are dark granular cells, gradually being replaced by the clear cuboidal cells of the collecting tubules. Two or more distal tubules fuse to form collecting tubules, which pass through the outer and inner cortex into the medulla. Here they fuse to form papillary ducts in the calyces.

RENAL BLOOD FLOW

The renal blood flow (RBF) in man is 1·0–1·2 l./min, one quarter to one fifth of the cardiac output. About 90 per cent of the renal blood flow is distributed to the cortex, the medulla receiving 8–10 per cent and the papilla 1–2 per cent. The relatively low blood flow of the medulla is important in the process of urine concentration (see p. 162). Nevertheless the medulla receives a blood flow per unit tissue weight 15 times that of resting muscle, half that of the brain, and one third that of the resting myocardium.

Control of renal blood flow

In the intact animal, and to a less extent in the isolated perfused kidney, as the blood pressure is increased above 90 mm Hg the RBF remains constant: this phenomenon is known as 'autoregulation'. It is also found that glomerular filtration rate (see p. 153) and the filtration fraction (see p. 154) also remain constant in spite of wide variations of blood pressure, suggesting that the changes in resistance in response to alteration in blood pressure are in the preglomerular arterioles. The hypotheses which have been advanced to explain the autoregulation of renal blood flow are (1) plasma skimming or the theory of cell separation; (2) theory of intrarenal pressure; (3) myogenic-renin theory.

Plasma skimming. This theory suggests that when the blood pressure increases the renal blood flow remains constant due to an increase in the viscosity of the blood. When blood flows down interlobular arteries the plasma is distributed peripherally, with an axial stream of red cells. The afferent arterioles are so positioned as to skim off the plasma, leaving behind blood of increasing haematocrit value. If perfusion pressure is higher, the greater is the plasma skimming and so the haematocrit increases distally even more. When the haematocrit reaches 80 per cent small increases in haematocrit cause very great increases in viscosity, so that most of the energy of a higher blood pressure is expended in overcoming the increased viscosity and thus there is little increase in RBF. This attractive theory is not borne out by the experimental evidence, for in the isolated kidney perfused by fresh cell-free plasma autoregulation of renal blood flow is maintained.

Intra-renal pressure theory. If there is an increase in arterial pressure it may be presumed that there will be an increase in interstitial fluid pressure which will compress the peritubular capillaries and veins. This results in an increased resistance to renal blood flow which is thus held constant in spite of increases in blood pressure. Micropuncture experiments with direct measurements of intra-renal pressures do not support this theory.

Myogenic-renin theory. It is known that prior treatment of an animal with drugs which paralyze smooth muscle (such as papaverine, cyanide or procaine) abolishes autoregulation of RBF. In addition there is a delay in autoregulation compatible with the known relative slowness of response of smooth muscle. This theory has been further developed to emphasize the role that renin might play in triggering the contraction of the smooth muscle. There is some evidence that an autoregulatory mechanism operates as a result of the higher sodium content in distal tubular fluid which would result from a transient increase in RBF and raised filtered load of sodium. This high sodium content of fluid in the distal tubule at the macula densa might stimulate the secretion of renin from the juxta-glomerular apparatus. The renin so liberated then acts on the smooth muscle of the afferent arteriolar wall causing constriction. This theory has considerable evidence to commend it but is somewhat difficult to reconcile with other evidence linking renin secretion to sodium balance (p. 13).

Other factors affecting renal blood flow. The sympathetic nerve supply to the kidneys comes from the fourth dorsal to fourth lumbar segments. In the normal animal there is no sympathetic tone because renal denervation does not increase RBF. Asphyxia decreases RBF, probably by stimulating sympathetic activity. Adrenaline and noradrenaline reduce RBF. RBF is lowered in hypopituitarism and hypoadrenocorticism, being partially or completely restored to normal by adequate hydrocortisone replacement therapy. In hypovolaemia, due to severe haemorrhage or salt depletion, with a profound fall in blood pressure the RBF is greatly reduced. Similarly in cardiac failure the RBF may be reduced to less than one tenth the normal value.

Increases in RBF are associated with pyrexia, pregnancy, polycythaemia and the administration of aminophylline and hydrallazine.

GLOMERULAR FILTRATION RATE

About 120 ml of plasma are filtered each minute through the walls of glomerular capillaries into Bowman's space. The filtrate is virtually protein-free, the glomerular capillary wall preventing passage of the plasma proteins but permitting the filtration of crystalloids. This type of filtration in which colloids such as proteins are retained while crystalloids pass through the filter is known as 'ultrafiltration'. The driving force for this ultrafiltration is provided by the hydrostatic pressure in the glomerular capillaries and ultimately by the heart. If the blood pressure falls below 60 mmHg the hydrostatic pressure is insufficient to overcome the combined plasma oncotic pressure and the hydrostatic pressure in Bowman's space, and so filtration ceases. There is considerable evidence that filtration occurs through pores in the glomeruli. Estimation of pore size has been carried out by observation on the ability of haemoglobin to pass from plasma to urine causing haemoglobinuria, the haemoglobin molecule being roughly pill shaped and 54 Å in diameter. On the other hand serum albumin with a molecule which is ellipsoid, 150 Å in its long diameter, is only filtered in very small quantities. The amount of sieving of haemoglobin is in agreement with a pore diameter of at least 75 Å; studies with dextrans of graded molecular size indicate a pore size of about 100 Å. The difference between these results is possibly due to the lack of charge on dextran particles, whereas protein molecules are charged and suffer from electrostatic hindrances to filtration. Calculations indicate that the pore areas occupy about 5 per cent of the glomerular capillary surface areas, a proportion over 50 times greater than the ratio of pore to capillary areas in muscle.

The volume of plasma filtered through the glomeruli in 1 minute is termed the glomerular filtration rate (GFR). The normal GFR in man is about 125 ml/min for 1·73 m^2 of body surface.

Control of GFR

The GFR is related to the glomerular capillary blood pressure, itself controlled by the relative tone of the afferent and efferent arterioles and by the systemic arterial pressure. Thus afferent arteriolar constriction reduces mean glomerular pressure and so GFR falls; afferent arteriolar dilation leads to an increase in glomerular capillary pressure and a rise in GFR results. Efferent arteriolar constriction leads to a rise in glomerular capillary pressure and in GFR; dilation of the efferent arteriole leads to a fall in GFR. The renal blood flow changes remarkably little despite wide fluctuations in systemic blood pressure, and autoregulation of the GFR and filtration fraction (see below) likewise minimizes the effects of variations in the blood pressure. GFR is increased by hypertonic saline, aminophylline and mannitol infusion, and in the hypertensive subject by injection of angiotensin. In normal man angiotensin causes a fall in GFR.

Filtration fraction

The filtration fraction is the ratio of plasma filtered at the glomeruli/minute to the total renal plasma flow/minute, i.e. GFR/RPF where RPF = renal plasma flow. It represents approximately the proportion of plasma passing through the glomeruli which is actually filtered off, the approximation being due to a small percentage of the renal plasma flow never traversing glomeruli (i.e. in supplying the pelvic renal tissues, papillary tip, fat and capsule). The normal filtration fraction is 15–20 per cent in man. It rises in congestive heart failure because of a relatively greater fall in RPF than in GFR. In severe haemorrhagic shock when there is a profound fall in blood pressure the GFR and RPF both fall, but the GFR is reduced more than the RPF so that the FF falls. This has been interpreted as due to an intense vasoconstriction of the afferent arteriole in an ischaemic kidney. In the renal hyperaemia caused by fever, the RPF is increased relatively more than GFR, so that FF falls.

TUBULAR FUNCTION

The function of the renal tubules is predominantly reabsorption of and secretion into the glomerular filtrate in accordance with the need for homeostasis of the body fluids. It is convenient to consider the tubular functions as predominantly proximal and predominantly distal, although in health many processes take place in both proximal and distal tubular sites.

The proximal tubule

Eighty per cent of the glomerular filtrate is reabsorbed in the proximal tubule. Proximal tubular functions include reabsorption of glucose, amino-acids, phosphate, bicarbonate, sodium, potassium, calcium and water and, as has been recently shown, acidification of tubular fluid and secretion of ammonia.

Glucose reabsorption. The urine of normal man contains virtually no glucose, because glucose is actively reabsorbed from the proximal tubular lumen. If the plasma glucose concentration is increased, plasma glucose will be filtered at an increased rate, so that there will be an increased filtered load to be reabsorbed in the proximal tubule. Ultimately, a point is reached at which the active absorption mechanism can no longer reabsorb any further glucose, presumably because of saturation of the carrier. Further elevation of the plasma glucose level leads to spill over of glucose in the urine—'glycosuria'. This is shown in Fig. 17. The level of tubular reabsorption at which no further tubular glucose reabsorption can occur is known as the T_m glucose, or tubular maximal reabsorption of glucose. The term T_m can be applied to many other substances handled by the tubules either secreted (e.g. PAH) or reabsorbed (e.g. phosphate) (see overleaf).

Amino acids. Small quantities of amino acids are found in the urine, but most of the plasma amino acids are reabsorbed proximally. Amino-acid reabsorption is complex, and probably involves two transport systems, one group-selective, and the other uniquely selective for each amino acid. Thus three group selective systems control the absorption of (1) cystine, lysine, arginine and ornithine; (2) glutamic and aspartic acids,

6*

threonine and most other amino-acids; (3) proline, hydroxyproline and glycine.

The amino acids within each group compete with each other for absorption and several of the amino acids (e.g. lysine and glycine) have a measurable T_m for reabsorption.

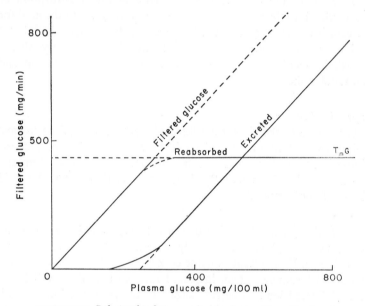

FIGURE 17. *Relationship between plasma glucose filtered load and tubular reabsorption of glucose.*

Phosphate. The tubular reabsorption of phosphate is a complex phenomenon influenced by several factors including the filtered load of phosphate, parathyroid hormone, the dietary intake of phosphate, hydrocortisone and metabolic acidosis. Tubular reabsorption of phosphate is a proximal tubular function with a T_m which is lower than that for glucose, so that at normal plasma levels of phosphate the filtered load of phosphate exceeds the T_m. A moderate decrease in plasma concentration may so reduce the filtered load (i.e. the amount filtered per unit time) as to cause it to be below the T_m; the filtered load is then entirely absorbed and the urine is phosphate-free. Phosphate apparently competes with glucose for reabsorption by the proximal tubule cell, and administration of phlorizin causes decreased glucose reabsorption and increased phosphate reabsorption. Similarly, infusion of alanine and acetoacetate significantly reduce phosphate reabsorption, presumably by competition for energy available for reabsorption in the tubular cells.

Phosphate reabsorption is reduced by the administration of parathyroid hormone. In the absence of parathyroid hormone phosphate reabsorption increases and the T_m phosphate increases.

Vitamin D administration depresses phosphate T_m, but this effect may be mediated indirectly through the parathyroid glands (p. 314). Hydrocortisone administration reduces phosphate T_m and consequently increases urinary phosphate excretion.

High dietary phosphate intakes reduce phosphate T_m. This is of importance in measurement of phosphate T_m clinically (see principles of tests, p. 185).

Urate. Urate is absorbed from the proximal tubular lumen and there is some evidence that proximal tubular reabsorption of urate is complete, leading to a urate-free fluid, and that the urate found in the urine is entirely derived from urate secreted in the distal tubule. When lithium urate is infused intravenously into normal man the plasma level increases and there is a simultaneous increase in tubular reabsorption of urate and of urate excretion in the urine. At very high levels of plasma urate (15 mg/100 ml—far higher than is found in the normal subject) a T_m for urate can be demonstrated, the curve showing marked splay (p. 185). The splay indicates, in one view, that there is heterogeneity of the tubular population in the tubular ability to reabsorb urate. Because some tubules reabsorb urate very inefficiently, urate may be excreted in the urine at the low levels of plasma urate found in the normal individual. However, this explanation is incompatible with a complete proximal tubular reabsorption of urate.

Urate excretion is enhanced by large dosage of salicylates and probenecid. These are known as 'uricosuric' drugs. In small doses they have a paradoxical effect, reducing urate excretion. This might be interpreted as suggesting that small doses of uricosuric drugs inhibit the secretory mechanism of urate in the distal tubules whereas large doses inhibit both proximal reabsorptive and distal secretory sites. Lactate infusion reduces urate excretion, possibly by inhibition of the postulated tubular urate secretion.

Sodium, chloride and water reabsorption

The reabsorption of sodium, chloride and water are closely linked in the proximal tubule. About 80 per cent of the filtered load of water, sodium and chloride is reabsorbed there.

Sodium reabsorption. By means of micropuncture studies in which minute pipettes and electrodes are inserted into the proximal tubules of the living kidney, it has been established that sodium can be reabsorbed against a concentration gradient. It has also been shown that the tubular lumen is at a potential of 20 mV negative to the peritubular fluid. Sodium ions are thus reabsorbed against an electrochemical gradient, and the absorptive process must be an active one for which energy is needed. This is corroborated by the finding that at least 80 per cent of the oxygen consumption of the kidney is attributable to sodium re-absorption. It has been calculated that 13 per cent of the oxygen consumption of resting man is devoted to the reabsorption of sodium in the renal tubules.

The mechanism by which sodium is transported out of the tubular lumen is uncertain; it is postulated that a carrier mechanism, energized partly but not completely by high-energy phosphate bonds, is involved. This carrier mechanism is referred to as the 'sodium pump' and is referred to in more detail elsewhere (p. 4).

Chloride transport. Chloride ion can be absorbed passively along an electrochemical gradient. However there is some recent evidence to suggest that chloride ion can be actively reabsorbed, and that it does not function merely as a passive partner to the sodium ion.

Water reabsorption. Eighty per cent of the filtered water is reabsorbed in the proximal tubule, this process being passive. Micropuncture studies have shown that the fluid in the proximal tubule remains isotonic to plasma, i.e. it is isosmotic. Water reabsorption is a result of the osmotic forces set up by the passage of sodium and chloride ions out of the tubular lumen, water accompanying the ions so that no osmotic gradient is set up. Micropuncture studies have demonstrated that the proximal tubule is freely permeable to water in both directions, into and out of the tubular lumen.

The final concentrations of sodium, chloride and water appearing in the urine are determined by the distal tubule. The latter acts as a fine adjustment to the metabolic needs of the body, the proximal tubule acting as a coarse adjustment. This has been referred to as 'obligatory reabsorption' by the proximal tubule and as 'facultative reabsorption' by the distal tubule.

Potassium reabsorption
Eighty per cent of the filtered load of potassium is reabsorbed in the proximal tubule, so that the concentration of potassium in the tubular

fluid as it leaves the proximal tubule is identical with that in the glomerular filtrate. The electrochemical gradient opposes potassium reabsorption from the proximal tubule so that the reabsorptive process must be active. Micropuncture studies in dogs have shown that proximal reabsorption of potassium is unaffected by changes in GFR or inhibition of sodium reabsorption or hydrogen ion secretion. This suggests that, as with sodium, chloride and water reabsorption, the distal tubule is responsible for the fine control of the amount of potassium excreted in the urine.

Bicarbonate

The proximal tubular cells synthesize carbonic acid from CO_2 (Fig. 18). The carbonic acid dissociates and the HCO_3^- ions, together with reabsorbed Na^+ ions, are transferred to the peritubular fluid and thence to the blood. H^+ ions are passed into the tubular fluid where most of them combine with HCO_3^- to form carbonic acid. The P_{CO_2} of the tubular fluid therefore rises and the CO_2 diffuses back into the cells and blood.

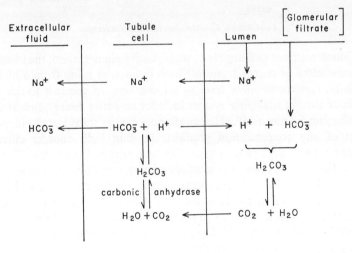

FIGURE 18. *Handling of bicarbonate and sodium by the proximal renal tubules.*

The net effect of this particular mechanism in a normal subject is a reabsorption of 20–28 mEq of Na^+ per litre of glomerular filtrate, an apparent reabsorption of 20–28 mEq/l of HCO_3^- and little net effect on H^+ concentration.

COUNTER CURRENT SYSTEM OF
URINE CONCENTRATION

The urine concentrating mechanism is a joint function of the loop of
Henle and distal tubules. The principles of counter current exchangers
are familiar to heat engineers, in machines in which hot exhaust gas is
conducted past the cold incoming gas so warming the latter and conserving heat (Fig. 19). This method of counter current *exchange* is
found in many situations in biology, a typical example being the
arrangement of the circulation to conserve heat in the legs of wading
birds.

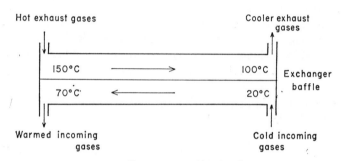

FIGURE 19. *Counter current heat exchanger.*

Counter current exchange is a purely passive phenomenon, the transfer
of substances or energy from one limb to another being from a higher
activity, concentration or level to a lower one. In contrast to this the
counter current *multiplier* system includes an active energy consuming
mechanism by means of which substances can be transported independent of any concentration gradient. In man both counter current
exchanger and multiplier systems can take part in the process of concentration of the urine, the multiplier being important in establishing
the initial medullary hypertonicity both in the interstitium and in the
intraluminal fluid in the long loops of Henle. A counter current exchanger system is thought to be present in the vasa recta of the medulla
where it maintains interstitial hypertonicity. It is probable that the long
loops of Henle themselves do the actual work of urine concentration by
sodium and water transport, although a minority view invests the vasa
recta with this ability. In this chapter the majority view is presented.

Figure 20 represents the loop of Henle, descending limb above,
ascending limb below. In (a) the fluid from the proximal tubule is not
being concentrated, so that fluid enters and leaves the system without
change in its concentration of 280 m-osmole per kg. In (b) the multiplier

is activated so that the maximum gradient between lower and upper limbs of 50 m-osmole can be achieved by pumping sodium in or water out; thus the osmolality in the upper limb reaches 305 m-osmole/kg, and in the lower limb 255 m-osmole/kg. In (c) more fluid has entered and pushed previously concentrated fluid further on so that at the right

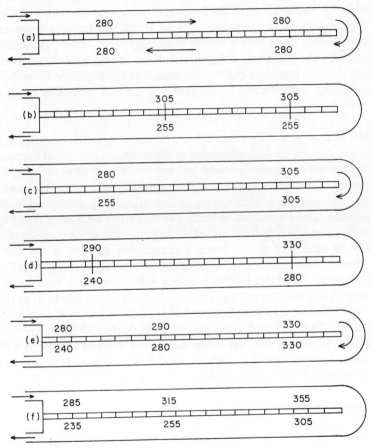

FIGURE 20. *Counter current multiplier system* (after R.W. Berliner).

hand of the loop its concentration is 305 m-osmole/kg. The sodium pump again sets up a concentration gradient, and (d) shows the results, an osmolality of 330 being achieved. In (e) further fluid has entered and the 330 m-osmole fluid has been pushed round the tip, and by (f) it is again subjected to the sodium pump gradient so that the osmolality reaches

355. The multiplication of the osmolality can go in man until the urine reaches an osmolality of 1400 m-osmole/kg. It will be noticed that the fluid coming out of the distal end of Henle's loop is hypotonic to plasma; this fluid then traverses the hypertonic medulla when it passes through the collecting tubules, being once again concentrated to the concentration of the fluid at the tip of the loop of Henle. It has been shown by micropuncture techniques and tissue slice analysis, including cryoscopy, that the tips of the loops of Henle, the vascular loops and the collecting ducts have a similar osmolality. This osmolality is maintained by the peculiarly sluggish circulation of the medulla, whereby high osmotic pressures can be maintained at the papillary tip without their being washed away by the blood in the vast medullary capillary network.

Rôle of urea in urine concentration. The major osmotically-active substances causing the high osmolality of the urine and interstitial tissues of the papillary tip in man are urea and sodium. The effect of reducing the amount of available urea can be observed by putting normal men on a low protein intake. This results in less urea being excreted and the maximal urine concentration being less than when on a normal or high protein diet. Part, but not all, of the reduction in urine concentration may be attributed to the lower concentration of urea in the urine, indicating that urea may play an active rôle in maintaining medullary hyperosmolality. Urea itself is a unique substance. It can pass through many tissues as if the cell walls were completely permeable to it, so that in these tissues, for example the red blood cells, it can exert no osmotic pressure. There are at least two exceptions to this in which the movement of urea is slower, the first being the central nervous system and the second being the renal medulla, so that in both tissues urea can exert an appreciable osmotic pressure.

DISTAL TUBULE
Urinary dilution
The formation of a dilute urine is predominantly a distal tubular function. Sodium is actively reabsorbed from the distal tubular fluid, but unlike the process of sodium reabsorption in the proximal tubules, this is not an isosmotic process. When dilute urine is formed the reabsorbed sodium takes with it a lesser amount of water due to the impermeability of the distal tubule to water in the absence of circulating vasopressin. The excess of water remaining is known as 'free water' (p. 186).

The distal ion-exchange mechanism

The final regulation of the sodium, potassium and hydrion concentration in the urine takes place in the distal tubule, and there is good evidence for a final ion exchange in the collecting tubules themselves (Fig. 21). However, as in the case of sodium and potassium, most filtered bicarbonate is reabsorbed in the proximal tubules, leaving final adjustment of acid-base balance to distal tubule mechanisms. Bicarbonate reabsorption probably depends on the secretion of hydrogen ions by tubular cells. There is a powerful 'sodium pump' in the collecting tubules which is probably activated by aldosterone, so that sodium is pumped from the tubular fluid into the tubular cells and so into the peritubular capillaries. In exchange for sodium either hydrogen ion, potassium ion, or both, are pumped out of the cell. The exchange is so effective that in health on a sodium-free diet the urine is virtually sodium free.

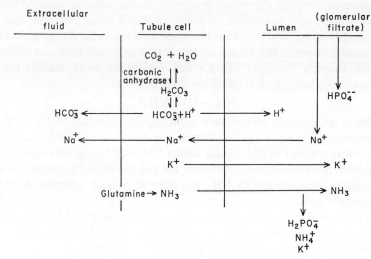

FIGURE 21. *Ion exchanges in the distal renal tubules.*

The ability of the hydrion pump to deliver hydrion to tubular fluid is such that hydrion gradients of urine to plasma as high as 1000:1 are produced when acid urine is formed. Potassium is secreted distally by the ion-exchange mechanism, and this may, under certain circumstances, lead to excessive potassium loss in the urine if hydrion excretion is impaired.

Bicarbonate is absorbed at this distal site so that the urine is bicarbonate-free if its pH is below 6·0. Bicarbonate reabsorption is itself dependent on changes in arterial P_{CO_2}, potassium content of cells, chloride depletion and corticosteroids. In normal man bicarbonate is completely reabsorbed if plasma bicarbonate is below 28 m-mole/l. If arterial P_{CO_2} is raised, intracellular carbonic acid formation is enhanced; this tends to increase bicarbonate reabsorption.

Acidification of the urine

Reabsorption of bicarbonate with a fall in urinary pH due to hydrion secretion into the tubular lumen occurs by both proximal and distal mechanisms already considered. The important mechanisms of excretion of acid are as ammonium and buffered hydrogen ion (titratable acidity).

Ammonia excretion. Ammonia can be detected in increasing amounts in the terminal part of the proximal tubule, but most of the ammonia formation is carried out in the distal tubule and collecting ducts. Ammonia is formed in the kidney mainly from the amide nitrogen of glutamine although the amino groups of glycine, alanine, aspartic acid and leucine also contribute. Urinary ammonia excretion is inversely related to urinary pH, so that the more acid the urine the greater the ammonia content. The reason for this is that ammonia itself can diffuse back through the lipid tubular cell membrane more readily than ammonium ion, which is relatively lipid insoluble.

$$NH_3 + H^+ \rightleftharpoons NH_4^+$$

This is an example of *non-ionic diffusion*, an important factor in the excretion of many drugs. Hydrogen ion secreted by tubular cells is therefore trapped in the tubular lumen by combination with ammonia to form ammonium ion. The lower the pH the more hydrogen ion is available to combine with NH_3 and prevent its back diffusion. So the ammonia excretion increases as pH of urine falls. Ammonia excretion increases in the presence of acidosis, the mechanism by which this occurs being unknown. Ammonium ion saves cation such as Na^+, K^+ and Ca^{++} from being excreted with obligatorily excreted anions.

Titratable acidity. Hydrion can be excreted in combination with the urinary buffers phosphate, creatinine and organic acids. The extent of this hydrion excretion can be estimated by titrating acid urine with alkali up to a pH of 7·4 (i.e. the pH of plasma), and the amount of alkali required is referred to as 'titratable acidity' (TA).

Total hydrogen ion excretion can therefore be expressed as urinary ammonia excretion (in m-mole/l.) plus titratable acid minus bicarbonate excretion (m-equiv/l.) thus:

$$H^+ = (NH_4^+ + TA - HCO_3^-)$$

In normal man the urinary pH can vary from 4·6 to 8·2. It is important to note that at a pH of 4·6 the concentration of free H^+ ion is only 0·025 m-equiv/l. titratable acidity is normally about 50 m-equiv/day, but in systemic acidosis with increased buffer excretion it may exceed 400 m-equiv/day.

Potassium and chloride handling in the distal tubule
Potassium is secreted in the distal tubule and the collecting duct, most of the proximal tubular potassium having been absorbed before the fluid enters the distal tubule. Ammonia and hydrion are secreted at the site of potassium secretion, sodium being reabsorbed at this site. This site is referred to above as the distal ion exchange site (p. 163). Potassium is excreted in increased amounts by oral loading with salts, the administration of alkalinizing substances such as citrates, or by administration of salts of non-reabsorbable anions (e.g. ferrocyanide or sulphate).

Chloride ion is actively reabsorbed in the distal tubule, according to micropuncture studies which show that the electrical gradient present is adequate to account for the passive absorption of chloride against the chemical gradient observed when the urine contains a chloride concentration of less than 1 m-equiv/l.

Calcium excretion
The calcium content of normal urine is related to sodium content, for reasons at present unknown. Calcium excretion during a calcium infusion is found to vary inversely with the level of circulating parathyroid hormone. Calcium and magnesium clearances both increase fourfold within 5 hr after parathyroidectomy. Generally, calcium and phosphate excretion parallel each other. Calcium is excreted in various forms: 30 per cent is excreted as citrate, but much citrate is reabsorbed in the proximal tubular site for citrate reabsorption. Some calcium is excreted as free ionized calcium, the principal site of reabsorption being in the distal tubule overlapping the sodium reabsorptive site there.

RENIN AND BLOOD PRESSURE
Renin is an enzyme produced in the juxta glomerular apparatus which acts on a plasma protein, an α-globulin, to produce a decapeptide, angiotensin I; the latter is converted to an octapeptide, angiotensin II, which has pressor activity. In addition to its direct pressor effect, angiotensin II stimulates the production of aldosterone from the adrenal glands (see p. 526). The possible roles of renin in the regulation of blood pressure and sodium balance are considered on pp. 68 and 13.

ERYTHROPOIETIN (see also p. 223)

The kidney is one of the sources of a humoral agent, erythropoietin, which increases the rate of red cell production in the marrow and the rate of release of red cells from both marrow and spleen. Erythropoietin migrates electrophoretically as an α-globulin. Its presence in the kidney can be demonstrated by the amelioration of the anaemia in dialyzed nephrectomized dogs by the injection of kidney extracts. Anaemia in renal disease is discussed below in the section on abnormal renal function (p. 171).

OSMOTIC DIURESIS

Osmotic diuresis occurs when the plasma contains large quantities of osmotically active substances, e.g. mannitol, glucose, urea, in such quantity that the maximal reabsorptive capacity of the tubules is considerably exceeded by the quantity of solute present. In osmotic diuresis the urine volume increases until it may reach one third of the filtration rate. Because the distal tubule is capable of reabsorbing not more than 10-20 per cent of the filtered fluid, it is presumed that in osmotic diuresis there is incomplete proximal tubular reabsorption of water and solute. In osmotic diuresis the urine is consequently approximately isosmotic with plasma or not far from this. The sodium content depends on the agent producing the diuresis, but may be as high as 40-50 m-equiv/l., with a urinary pH of between 6 and 7. It is likely that this is due to the tubular fluid streaming past the tubule cells so fast that the reabsorptive and secretory tubular processes cannot reach completion and the fluid appears as partially processed glomerular filtrate.

Disordered function

RENAL FAILURE

Both homeostatic and excretory functions of the kidneys are impaired in renal failure. In some conditions a localized portion of the tubules is involved—e.g. proximal tubule in Fanconi syndrome or distal tubule in pyelonephritis, while the remaining parts of the tubules and the glomeruli are healthy; this leads to selective impairment of specific renal functions. In other cases all the glomeruli may be totally destroyed, so that all the excretory and homeostatic functions of the kidney are completely absent.

ACUTE RENAL FAILURE

In acute renal failure there is usually—but not constantly—a profound reduction in the urine volume below the minimum necessary for the excretion of the normal metabolic load. (This minimum volume has been calculated to be 700 ml per day, but this is dependent on the dietary load, and on the ability of the kidney to produce a concentrated urine (p. 9).) In acute renal failure the osmotic work that can be carried out by the kidneys is impaired, so that the minimum volume required to excrete the normal solute load in health is much smaller than the minimum volume necessary to excrete the same load in the diseased kidney. The majority of patients with acute renal failure in the initial stages of their illness excrete a daily urine volume of less than 400 ml per day; this is known as 'oliguria'. These small urinary volumes are unable to cope with the osmotic load to be excreted. Later in the disease the urine volumes may be over 1500 ml/day but the renal damage is such that the kidneys are still unable to excrete the metabolic solute load. Occasionally, as in acute interstitial nephritis, the urine volume is never reduced but renal function is so impaired that excretion of metabolic products is inadequate. The urine in acute renal failure has an osmolality (see p. 31) which is close to that of plasma, an illustration of the inability of the kidneys to concentrate the urine in spite of the severe oliguria present. Urine urea concentration falls below 1 g/100 ml compared to the normal 2–4 g/100 ml. Urinary cation composition may be inappropriate in some cases of acute renal failure, in which the inability of the distal renal tubules to function normally is demonstrated by the sodium concentration in the urine sometimes approaching that of plasma and being frequently over 70 m-equiv/l. RBF is reduced to half or one third normal. There is some evidence that some glomerular filtration may occur, but that the filtrate is rapidly reabsorbed by the tubules or leaks back into the peritubular capillaries through the damaged tubular cells or between them. In acute tubular necrosis the low urine volumes usually found are the result of the cessation of glomerular filtration, rather than of tubular disruption *per se*. An exception to the rule of the urine being isosmolar to plasma in acute renal failure is provided by acute glomerulonephritis, in the early stage of which a more concentrated urine may be found. Pre-renal uraemia, discussed below (p. 172) is, however, the most frequent cause of a high urine osmolality in the presence of severe oliguria; in this condition the tubular cells are therefore capable of performing osmotic work.

Metabolic effects
Water balance. In a normal afebrile man whose kidneys have been removed, the water requirements are about 500 ml/day in temperate climates. Although 1000 ml of water/day are lost in the expired air and

by insensible sweating, the metabolically produced water from carbohydrate and fat oxidation, together with water from cell breakdown, liberate approximately 500 ml of water in the body (p. 6). Hence the net water requirement is only 500 ml/day. In acute renal failure the urine volume (usually below 400 ml/day) has to be taken into account. A daily water intake of 500 ml plus the urine volume/day is required to keep the patient in water balance. Fever increases water loss.

Nitrogenous products accumulate in the body in acute renal failure. Urea accumulates as a result of the breakdown of protein. The rate of protein catabolism varies from 20 g to 150 g per day depending partly on the diet and partly on 'hypercatabolism' due to trauma, sepsis, fever or the involuting uterus. 40 g of protein yields 13·7 g of urea. This accumulates in the total body water of 50 l. and causes a blood urea rise of 27·5 mg/100 ml of blood every day. Similarly, phosphate and potassium are liberated from broken down cells and gradually accumulate in the ECF. Hyperkalaemia may prove fatal if severe enough to stop the heart.

Acid base balance. The catabolism of protein yields hydrogen ion in quantities of about 50 m-equiv/day on a normal diet, and about 20 m-equiv/day on very severely protein restricted diets. In the absence of renal function, or with depression of renal function the hydrogen ion produced cannot be excreted in the urine and accumulates in the blood causing a metabolic acidosis (p. 210). The over-breathing associated with severe metabolic acidosis is a common feature of advanced renal failure.

Anaemia. In acute renal failure a normochromic anaemia develops rapidly. There is inhibition of ^{59}Fe uptake, the half life of injected ^{59}Fe being tripled in the nephrectomized dog maintained on peritoneal dialysis. Examination of the bone marrow shows depression of erythropoiesis but the speed of development of anaemia is suggestive of a haemolytic process. This has been demonstrated experimentally in animals.

Calcium, magnesium and phosphate metabolism. Plasma calcium levels fall in acute renal failure and cannot be elevated to normal levels by repeated injections of calcium gluconate, nor by parenteral administration of parathyroid hormone. The fall in plasma calcium levels is usually associated with a rise in plasma phosphate levels and a metabolic acidosis. When the serum calcium has fallen to 6–7 mg/100 ml correction of the acidosis may result in tetany due to a low ionized calcium level (see p. 330). Plasma magnesium levels increase in renal failure and may result in central nervous system depression, with drowsiness and eventual coma.

Diuretic phase. Recovery from acute renal failure is accompanied by an increase in urine volume to between 1 and 2 l./day in the majority of cases and occasionally up to 5 l. a day in those patients given too much water in the oliguric phase. The urine is hypotonic or isotonic to plasma, and has a high sodium concentration. The renal tubules are unable to respond to vasopressin (see p. 158) so that the urine volume remains high; the tubules are also unable to respond to aldosterone, and cannot conserve sodium. The urine composition is similar to that found in osmotic diuresis, with a high sodium and chloride content and an osmolality approaching that of plasma. The sodium loss may be so profound as to lead to a fall in whole body sodium with a contraction of ECF volume and intravascular volume, leading to hypotension and even to peripheral circulatory failure.

CHRONIC RENAL FAILURE

In chronic renal failure there is a reduction in number of the functioning glomeruli. The extent of the reduction is variable, but there are few manifestations of chronic renal failure until more than 75 per cent of the total nephron population is destroyed. When only 2 per cent of nephrons survive life can only be maintained if the solute load requiring excretion is reduced. Nocturia is an early sign of renal failure, due initially to a loss of the normal diurnal rhythm in which the urine volume falls at night. It is often accompanied or followed by polyuria. This increase in the urine volume due to a loss in the urine concentrating ability may be due to either:

(1) loss in functioning nephrons so that the few remaining nephrons are undergoing osmotic diuresis and thus are unable to produce a urine osmolality higher than that of plasma (see below); or

(2) a change in cortical and medullary blood supply may occur due to structural changes in advanced chronic renal failure, or fibrosis in the kidney may prevent the normal passage of urea and sodium into the papillae of the kidney so that no counter current multiplier system can be established.

At the commencement of chronic renal failure, the urine may be hypertonic to plasma although less concentrated than in health, but as the disease progresses the urine approaches the osmolality of plasma. Ability to secrete dilute urine is retained after the ability to concentrate the urine has been lost.

The '*intact nephron hypothesis*' suggests that in renal failure the residual nephrons behave as if they were working normally but under an excess load; only those nephrons which are normal in both glomerular and tubular structure can function, the others being functionless. There is considerable evidence to support the hypothesis in man and the experimental animal suffering from diffuse renal disease. Thus the GFR is reduced in chronic renal failure, say to 10 ml/min and T_mPAH is correspondingly reduced, so that the ratio GFR/T_mPAH is constant and the same as in health. Similarly, GFR/T^cH_2O ratio is constant and identical with that in health (p. 187). These ratios indicate that the ratio of functioning glomeruli and functioning proximal and distal tubules remain constant in disease as in health, and it is therefore probable that all functioning glomeruli are connected to functioning proximal and functioning distal tubules.

Sodium excretion. If only a small percentage of glomeruli are functioning, and as in chronic renal failure the same amount of urea, for example, is excreted per day as in health, then the load of urea and other solutes per functional nephron will be very high. This will in effect cause each nephron to excrete a relatively high percentage of its filtered solute load —about 10 per cent of filtered sodium, for example, compared with the normal of less than 1 per cent. There is an osmotic diuresis in the remaining nephrons, the rate of passage of fluid along the tubular being too great to allow tubular secretion and reabsorption to proceed to completion. This gives rise to an obligatory sodium 'leak' for, unlike the normal, many patients with chronic renal failure are unable to produce a virtually sodium-free urine in response to a very low sodium intake in the diet; the urine contains a minimal loss of about 50–80 m-equiv of sodium/day in many cases of advanced renal failure given a 10 m-equiv/day intake. In some specific types of renal disease— medullary cystic disease and pyelonephritis—the sodium loss may be very large—over 200 m-equiv/day. This is known as 'salt losing nephritis'. In this condition and in specific tubular lesions, such as are found in renal tubular acidosis and Fanconi syndrome, it is apparent that the specific tubular function concerned is impaired to a greater degree than the reduction of GFR. This is evidence against the 'intact nephron hypothesis' being universally applicable in renal failure.

In addition to an obligatory sodium leak in advanced renal failure there is a maximum sodium excretion, limited by the reduced filtered load of sodium. If more sodium is ingested than can be excreted the sodium will be retained in the body, expanding ECF and plasma volume, and causing oedema and hypertension.

Water requirements are similarly fixed in chronic renal failure. Inability to concentrate the urine makes a water intake of 1·5–2 l. necessary in most patients to excrete the solute load. If too much water fluid is drunk there will be fluid retention with increasing hypotonicity of the body fluids, a condition of 'water intoxication'.

Potassium excretion. Potassium retention is rarely a problem until renal failure is far advanced because, firstly, considerable amounts of potassium can be excreted via the gastro-intestinal tract, and secondly, overall potassium secretion occurs in renal failure so that potassium clearance is 2 or more times larger than inulin clearance (p. 181).

Ultimately, dietary intake and catabolic production of potassium exceed renal and gastrointestinal capabilities to excrete potassium and a state of hyperkalaemia results. This is associated with high peaked T waves in the ECG and ultimately venticular standstill develops at levels of serum potassium of 7·5 to 9 m-equiv. Occasional patients have a spontaneous obligatory potassium loss but this is uncommon.

H+ excretion. In renal disease H^+ excretion is impaired, due to a decrease in both ammonia formation and in titratable acidity (TA). TA is reduced because of the reduced filtered load of phosphate and creatinine. The H^+ which is formed but not excreted is in part buffered by the bone salts and this may be a factor in the genesis of azotaemic renal osteodystrophy (p. 324).

Anaemia is common in chronic renal failure and is usual in patients with blood levels of more than 200 mg/100 ml. It is due to a combination of reduced red cell production from the bone marrow and, in severe anaemia, to a decreased red cell life span. The cause of the decreased red-cell production from the marrow may be due to metabolic factors, e.g. nitrogenous products of protein metabolism inhibiting the marrow, or due to lack of erythropoietin. The reduction of red cell life span is related to the level of urea rather than to the amount of functioning renal tissue.

URAEMIA

The pathogenesis of individual symptoms in the clinical picture of acute and chronic renal failure is only partially understood.

Gastro-intestinal disturbances have been attributed to the production of increased amounts of ammonia in the gastro-intestinal tract by bacterial urease acting on high concentrations of urea. Evidence in favour of this hypothesis consists of the demonstration of increased gastric ammonia secretion plus the absence of gastro-intestinal symptoms at low levels of blood urea in spite of severe renal failure.

Central nervous symptoms. Central nervous depression with somnolence has been found in association with high levels of plasma magnesium—as high as 6·4 m-equiv/l. in one case. Convulsions and twitching are sometimes due to tetany caused by a low plasma ionized calcium concentration. Tetanic fits are particularly frequent after correction of the metabolic acidosis by intravenous sodium bicarbonate, so that the ionized calcium level falls to low levels and tetany results.

The causes of pericarditis and skin itching in uraemia are unknown.

Extra-renal uraemia
Renal failure is sometimes due to factors other than renal disease, this being referred to as 'extra-renal uraemia'. The causes of extra-renal uraemia can be divided into two classes—pre-renal and post-renal.

Pre-renal uraemia. This is due to a failure of adequate filtration in the glomeruli, caused by either an inadequate blood pressure or an inadequate number of perfused nephrons, although the kidney tissues are initially healthy. Failure of glomerular filtration occurs at mean arterial pressures less than 60 mmHg, such as may occur after severe haemorrhage or extracellular fluid depletion (p. 16), or severe impairment of cardiac function. However, renal vasoconstriction may also reduce glomerular filtration rate even though the arterial perfusion pressure is maintained. The urine that is formed is of higher osmolality than that found in true renal uraemia, because there is commonly an increased output of vasopressin caused by hypovolaemia.

Post-renal uraemia results from obstruction of the urinary pathways, which may be unilateral if the contralateral kidney is absent or diseased. More frequently there is obstruction to both kidneys. Obstruction may be partial, with slowly progressive damage to renal function, causing a general decrease in GFR and RBF and specifically damaging distal tubular functions of urine concentration, acidification and sodium conservation, and so causing acquired diabetes insipidus with renal tubular acidosis. Release of the obstruction occasionally is associated with massive polyuria—12 l. in 24 hr—the urine containing high concentrations of sodium and chloride ions. The mechanism of this is unknown, but it is likely to be due to proximal tubular abnormalities in water and sodium reabsorption.

TUBULAR DEFECTS

Renal tubular defects can be classified in a number of ways. The simplest is to consider separately for the proximal tubule the *selective* disorders of function, most of which are inherited as recessive characters (p. 573) and the *non-selective* group of disorders, in which proximal tubular cells may be damaged by inherited disorders such as those in which cystine, copper or galactose are present in excess, or by acquired disorders such as heavy metal poisoning, vitamin D deficiency, hyperparathyroidism, and myelomatosis. In the first group, selective disorders of reabsorption have been recognized for glucose, phosphate, and for three groups of amino-acids (cystine and others, threonine and others, and proline and glycine). There are also still more selective disorders of amino-acid reabsorption, affecting one amino-acid only (e.g. 'pure' cystinuria, alaninuria). In the non-selective disorders, glucose, phosphate, many amino-acids, and uric acid are not reabsorbed normally in the proximal tubule.

There are also disorders of distal tubular function, which may be partially or wholly selective. Disorders have been recognized in which there is failure of hydrogen ion secretion, failure to conserve water, and failure to conserve sodium. Failure to conserve potassium is probably always secondary to mineralocorticoid excess (p. 522).

Various combinations of disorders also occur. There are combined selective disorders (e.g. for glucose and phosphate reabsorption in the same individual). Combined proximal and distal tubular defects may also occur, for example in cystinosis (see below).

PROXIMAL TUBULAR DEFECTS
Selective
Glucose reabsorption (renal glycosuria). T_m glucose varies from nephron to nephron in renal glycosuria. Some of the nephrons have such a low T_mG that the filtered load of glucose exceeds T_mG and therefore the urine contains glucose when blood sugar concentrations are normal. Tubular functions other than T_mG are normal in renal glycosuria. The evidence about nephron heterogeneity is given below.

Phosphate reabsorption. Phosphate reabsorption is decreased so that there is an excess urinary excretion of phosphate and a lowered plasma phosphate. This defect is associated with rickets and osteomalacia, which is very resistant to treatment with Vitamin D (p. 322).

Cystine reabsorption. The condition of cystinuria, in which cystine stones are formed, usually signifies a metabolic block in the reabsorption of 4 amino acids which share a common transport system: cystine, lysine, arginine and ornithine. Since the solubility of cystine in urine is so much less than that of the other amino-acids, especially when the urine is acid, the stones formed in this condition consist of cystine. It is interesting that a similar metabolic block can be demonstrated in the intestinal absorption of these amino-acids.

Some reabsorption of each amino-acid still takes place by means of the individually specific transport systems. 'Pure' renal cystinuria, without the presence of lysine, arginine or ornithine in excess, has recently been recognized. This is likewise an incomplete defect, because some cystine reabsorption can still occur by the group-specific transport system.

Hartnup disease. In Hartnup disease, those amino-acids other than the cystine group (see above) and proline and glycine (see below) appear in excess in the urine because of a selective failure of proximal tubular reabsorption. The amino-acids affected are threonine, serine, asparagine, glutamine, valine, methionine, isoleucine, leucine, tyrosine, phenylalanine, and tryptophane. As in the case of cystine and the related amino-acids mentioned above, all these other acids presumably share a common reabsorptive mechanism, the defect of which is also demonstrable in the intestine. However, in the case of Hartnup disease, the failure of intestinal absorption of at least one substance (tryptophane) leads additionally to a skin rash resembling pellagra.

Proline and glycine reabsorption. A defect in the metabolism of proline, resulting in hyperprolinaemia, can lead not only to failure of proline reabsorption in the proximal tubule, but also to an inhibition of glycine reabsorption since these 2 amino-acids probably also share a common proximal tubular reabsorptive mechanism.

Non-selective proximal tubular defects
Damage by cystine deposition. Cystinosis (Lignac-de Toni-Fanconi syndrome) is a condition in which cystine is deposited in the tissues. There

are non-specific defects of proximal tubular function with 10 or more amino-acids appearing in the urine, cystine not being prominent among them. There is also renal glycosuria and phosphaturia with osteomalacia, and the plasma uric acid concentration is low because of failure of tubular reabsorption of urate.

Damage by tubular copper deposition. In Wilson's disease there is defective reabsorption of many amino-acids, threonine and cystine being particularly prominent. It has been suggested that the aminoaciduria is the result of the presence in the proximal tubular fluid of specific oligopeptides. These compete with the amino-acids for reabsorption proximally. Glycosuria is present with a substantially reduced T_m glucose. The ability to excrete hydrogen ion is impaired, as in renal tubular acidosis (p. 176). Uric acid reabsorption is also impaired, and phosphate reabsorption impairment results in hypophosphataemia. This occasionally may be responsible for osteomalacia.

Damage by galactose. In galactosaemia there is an inherited defect in galactose metabolism, as a result of which galactose is present in excess in blood and urine and there is a non-selective aminoaciduria and proteinuria due to renal damage, probably caused by galactose-1-phosphate. The abnormal amino-acid excretion is related closely to the presence of galactose in the urine, disappearing gradually on a galactose-free diet, which renders the urine galactose-free.

Damage by heavy metals. Poisoning with cadmium, lead, uranium, and mercury causes a generalized aminoaciduria and glycosuria due to inhibition of proximal tubular reabsorption.

Vitamin D deficiency, hyperparathyroidism and myelomatosis can also cause multiple defects of proximal tubular reabsorption, particularly of amino-acids, presumably by their general metabolic effects. In addition, parathyroid hormones and vitamin D have specific effects on the renal handling of calcium and phosphate which will be mentioned more fully later (p. 317).

DISTAL TUBULAR DEFECTS
Water: nephrogenic diabetes insipidus
Ability to produce a concentrated urine is impaired in the inherited sex-linked disease, nephrogenic diabetes insipidus, in which male children are usually affected, and in which the nephron is insensitive to vasopressin. Nephrogenic diabetes insipidus is also found as an

acquired lesion in Fanconi syndrome, renal tubular acidosis, hydronephrosis, pyelonephritis, hypokalaemia, hypercalcaemia, amyloid disease and polyarteritis. In these conditions there is both structural and functional damage to the distal and collecting tubules. A form of acquired nephrogenic diabetes insipidus may be induced by drinking 10 or 11 l. of water a day, the defect in urine concentration persisting after water ingestion has ceased. In sickle cell disease there is a defect in urinary concentration, due to sickling which occurs due to the low oxygen tension of the medullary blood and this causes interference with medullary blood flow.

Hydrogen ion
The ability to produce an acid urine is impaired in renal tubular acidosis, which may be a rare familial disease, or more commonly an acquired disease due to hydronephrosis, pyelonephritis, hypokalaemia or hypercalcaemia. The damage to the distal acidification site may be associated with damage to other functions, such as those responsible for sodium conservation, potassium secretion and urinary concentration. In renal tubular acidosis there may be a moderate or severe metabolic acidosis which differs from that found in generalized advanced renal disease. In the latter both plasma bicarbonate and the plasma chloride levels are low, there being an increase in plasma sulphate, phosphate, organic acids, and a high blood urea. In renal tubular acidosis, the ability to secrete hydrogen ion against a gradient of up to 1000:1 is impaired. The urine secreted has an inappropriately high pH (in the region of 7) and contains much bicarbonate. Bicarbonate reabsorption is dependent on H^+ secretion, and if bicarbonate is not adequately reabsorbed chloride ion is available in the renal tubules as the anion to accompany sodium reabsorption. This increased chloride reabsorption leads to a high plasma chloride. The plasma bicarbonate level is depressed due to the increased loss of the bicarbonate filtered load. In contrast to generalized renal failure, in RTA the plasma chloride is elevated and the plasma bicarbonate depressed with a normal blood urea and normal phosphate and urate levels, until late in the course of the disease. The cause of the nephrocalcinosis and renal stone formation is not certain. It may be due to secondary hyperparathyroidism.

DIURETICS (see also p. 187)
Diuretic drugs cause sodium loss: for example, ethacrynic acid and frusemide act on the ascending loop of Henle inhibiting sodium transport out of the lumen. Ethacrynic acid and frusemide also may

inhibit proximal sodium reabsorption. Thiazide diuretics inhibit both proximal and distal sodium reabsorption partly by inhibiting the action of renal carbonic anhydrase (CA) but have no inhibitory effects on extra-renal CA. The mechanism of action of the non-thiazide diuretics, such as frusemide or mercurials is ill-understood but is thought to be the binding of S-H groups in the sodium carrier preventing normal sodium transport. It is known that the presence of adequate plasma chloride levels is necessary for the diuretic action of mercurial diuretics, but the evidence is in favour of a primary effect on sodium transport, not on chloride transport. Carbonic anhydrase inhibitors, such as acetazoleamide, act by preventing the secretion of hydrogen ion from the tubular cells into the lumen, so that bicarbonate reabsorption is reduced and alkaline urine with a high bicarbonate and sodium content is formed. The increased sodium excretion is due to the lack of HCO_3^- ion reabsorption in the proximal tubules.

Diuretics, potassium and distal tubular ion exchange. Diuretics which inhibit sodium reabsorption proximal to the site of Na/K exchange produce, inevitably, changes in the rate of potassium excretion. For example an increased delivery of sodium to the distal tubule increases potassium excretion by this mechanism alone. Other factors such as the inhibitory action of organic mercurials on potassium excretion may modify this. (See also p. 187.)

COMBINED DEFECTS OF PROXIMAL
AND DISTAL TUBULE
In some diseases both proximal and distal tubular functions are impaired. Thus in cystinosis (p. 174) there is impairment not only of proximal tubular function, resulting in glycosuria, aminoaciduria, hypophosphataemia, and hypouricaemia, but also of the distal tubular functions of acidification and urine concentration. This leads to the excretion of a urine with an inappropriately high pH in spite of the presence of a severe systemic acidosis (the functional abnormality of renal tubular acidosis) and a polyuria due to inability to form a concentrated urine. Cystinosis may be associated with similar defects affecting proximal and distal tubules.

PROTEINURIA
Protein may appear in the urine associated with glomerular or tubular disease.

Glomerular proteinuria. There is normally very little protein in the glomerular filtrate in man, and much of this small amount is reabsorbed in the proximal tubule. In renal disease proteinuria is a common finding, most frequently due to 'leaky' glomeruli permitting the filtration of increased amounts of protein, above the upper limit of the normal of 150 mg/day. Detailed investigation of urinary protein excretion suggests that the sizes of abnormal pores vary (p. 189).

Tubular proteinuria. In some diseases of the tubules, such as Fanconi syndrome, and, classically, cadmium poisoning, the glomeruli are normal but the urine contains a particular protein pattern quite distinct from that found in glomerular disease. In tubular disease α_2- and β-globulins are prominent, and albumin is very low. This pattern is known as 'tubular proteinuria'. The disorder represents a failure of the normal proximal tubular function of reabsorption of low molecular weight proteins, such as the 'light' κ and λ chains of immunoglobulins (Bence Jones' proteins). The presence of albumin excess always signifies glomerular damage.

GROSS PROTEINURIA: NEPHROTIC SYNDROME

When protein excretion reaches high levels of 5 g or more/day, the loss of serum proteins may be so great that the anabolic activity of the liver in making albumin is unable to keep pace with the increased synthesis required. The serum albumin level has usually to fall below 3·0 g/ 100 ml (normal 3·5–5·0 g/100 ml) before oedema appears. The increase in ECF volume and oedema are due to the lower plasma oncotic pressure being insufficient to attract tissue fluid back into the venous end of the capillaries in the normal manner (p. 5). At the same time as the serum albumin falls, the plasma cholesterol level rises due to the hepatic production of cholesterol being linked to that of albumin. The syndrome of massive proteinuria (usually 5 g or more/day), serum albumin below 3·0 g/100 ml, peripheral oedema and (often) a raised serum cholesterol level is known as the 'nephrotic syndrome'. In the nephrotic syndrome although the ECF volume is expanded, the lower plasma oncotic pressure results in a fall in the intravascular volume, which may be the stimulus to increased aldosterone production (p. 13). The hypovolaemia of the nephrotic syndrome may lead to a fall in RBF and GFR and the development of renal failure which may be fatal.

URETEROSIGMOIDOSTOMY

Patients who have the ureters implanted into the sigmoid develop a curious metabolic syndrome if they do not empty the urine out of the rectum at frequent intervals. This consists of a hypokalaemic, hyper-chloraemic metabolic acidosis; it is due to the action of the sigmoid in secreting potassium and HCO_3^- into the urine pooled in the large bowel, and reabsorbing H^+ and chloride from the urine. The same phenomenon happens if a normal person is given a litre of saline into the sigmoid.

HYPERTENSION AND THE KIDNEY

In essential hypertension the earliest sign of abnormal renal function is a fall in T_mPAH and RBF, but with a GFR which is initially maintained at normal levels, giving rise to a raised FF. There is a decrease in the ratio of RBF to T_mPAH. The renal function changes are probably due to efferent arteriolar constriction. There is an increase in RBF and a small fall in GFR in hypertensive patients given spinal anaesthesia up to T5 dermatome, suggesting that some of the increased renal vascular resistance is nerve dependent. In essential hypertension there is an abnormal response to an intravenous loading with isotonic saline, with a more rapid excretion of sodium than is found in normotensive persons given a similar loading. Similarly, a water load is abnormally handled in essential hypertension, with a delay in the excretion of water. Some studies suggest an impairment of urinary concentrating ability, and in malignant hypertension $T_m^c H_2 O$ (p. 186) seems to be constantly reduced.

In benign hypertension renal failure is the cause of death in 8 per cent of patients, whereas 50 per cent of patients with malignant hypertension die of renal failure.

In hypertension due to unilateral renal disease caused by renal artery stenosis or pyelonephritis, there are differences in function between the two kidneys. The affected kidney has a lower GFR than the contra-lateral side, with lower RBF and a lower T_mPAH. The filtered load of sodium on the affected side is reduced, so that the reabsorption of sodium proceeds further to completion. Similarly, there is a smaller volume of filtered water, and because proximal sodium reabsorption is isosmotic there is a reduced urine volume from the affected kidney. These findings are the basis of the 'divided renal function' test of Howard (see p. 193).

THE KIDNEY AND PREGNANCY
Normal pregnancy

In normal pregnancy there is an increase of GFR by up to 50 per cent from the second month to the thirty-eighth week, the RBF increasing by up to 25 per cent in the middle trimester and falling to normal values in

7

the last trimester. FF is elevated throughout pregnancy. It is possible that the hypervolaemia of pregnancy is responsible for some of these increases. Serum uric acid levels fall below the normal levels in pregnancy due to an increase in uric acid clearance. Glycosuria is common in pregnancy, and is due to an increase in the filtered load of glucose so that T_mG is exceeded. Sodium retention is found up to the thirty-eighth week of pregnancy and may be due to the effect of oestrogens, hydrocortisone and aldosterone. There is no significant difference between the normal and the pregnant woman in the excretion of a hypertonic sodium load.

Pre-eclamptic toxaemia is associated with a fall in GFR, RBF and FF. Uric acid clearance is reduced, leading to a rise in serum uric acid levels. The cause of the decrease in uric acid clearance is thought to be related to the elevated plasma lactate levels associated with toxaemia, for high plasma lactate levels have been shown to depress uric acid clearance. Sodium excretion is impaired in pre-eclamptic toxaemia; there is a delay in the excretion of an intravenous hypertonic sodium chloride load in pre-eclampsia when compared with the normal pregnant woman.

Principles of tests and measurements

RENAL CLEARANCE

The concept of clearance can be applied to any organ. The clearance of a substance is the volume of plasma completely cleared of that substance each minute by passage through the organ. In practice the blood flowing through an organ may not have the substance under consideration completely removed from the blood, so that some of the substance is still present in the venous blood coming from the organ. Hence the clearance of a substance is defined as the volume of plasma containing the amount of that substance removed by the organ in 1 minute. Taking the kidney as the example of the particular organ, this can be expressed mathematically as follows:

$$C_A = \frac{U_A V}{P_A}$$

where C_A is clearance of substance A in ml/min.

U_A = Urine concentration of A.

V = Urine volume ml/min.

P_A = Plasma concentration of A.

GLOMERULAR FILTRATION RATE

If substance A is filtered by the glomeruli but is neither secreted nor reabsorbed by the kidneys, then the amount of A appearing in the bladder urine each minute will be identical with the amount of A being filtered in the glomeruli. In these circumstances, the renal clearance of A is termed the 'glomerular filtration rate'. The glomerular filtration rate (GFR) in a normal adult male is about 125 ml/min/1·73 sq. m. of body surface. Substances which are predominantly reabsorbed in the renal tubules, such as urea and sodium, have a lower renal clearance than the GFR. Substances which are predominantly secreted, such as para-aminohippurate (PAH) have a renal clearance greater than the GFR. Unfortunately, many substances are both secreted and re-absorbed in the tubules, so that the value of a renal clearance above or below GFR indicates that secretion or reabsorption predominates, but does not exclude that both reabsorption and secretion are simultaneously taking place.

Ideal properties for substance used for GFR measurement. A substance suitable for the measurement of GFR must be small enough to filter freely through the glomerular capillary walls, it must not be handled by the tubules in any way, and, as a corollary, its renal clearance must be independent of the plasma concentration. In general substances which do not penetrate cell membranes (and so also may be used to measure the ECF volume) often satisfy these criteria. The concentration in plasma water must be determined, and for substances such as inulin, creatinine, thiosulphate, hypaque, and polyfructosan S, which are not bound to protein, this is the same as the concentration in whole plasma, but with cyanocobalamin only the concentration of its non-protein bound moiety must be used. Endogenous creatinine is widely used in clinical medicine for assessment of the GFR; being present in normal plasma endogenous creatinine requires no infusion. However, in infancy and in patients with congestive heart failure endogenous creatinine is pre-dominantly reabsorbed by the tubules. In advanced renal failure and in the nephrotic syndrome creatinine is predominantly secreted by the tubules. Further, there are technical difficulties in plasma creatinine measurement.

UREA CLEARANCE

The urea clearance in health is about 60 per cent of the GFR providing the urine volume is at least 2 ml/min (p. 162 where dependence of urea clearance on urine flow is described). When the GFR falls below 10 ml/min, urea clearance approaches GFR.

BLOOD UREA

Measurement of the blood urea is one of the most frequently carried out measurements in the assessment of renal function. It is important that the factors affecting blood urea level are understood before interpreting the measuring of individual blood urea levels in patients. Blood urea levels depend on:

Renal function. On a normal diet the blood urea level does not rise above the upper limit of normal (40 mg/100 ml) until the GFR has fallen to about 30 ml/min. This is shown in Fig. 22. When GFR is 5 ml/min blood urea levels of 200–250 mg/100 ml can be expected, and at a GFR of 2 ml/min a blood urea of 400–500 mg/100 ml is found.

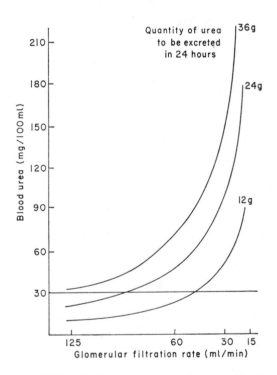

FIGURE 22. *Relationships between urea load, glomerular filtration rate and blood urea.*

Note that with a low urea load the glomerular filtration rate must be halved before the blood urea concentration rises above the normal range. (Modified from Gamble, 1954.)

Dietary intake. If a high protein diet is taken the blood urea will be higher for any given value of GFR than if a low protein intake is taken. An extreme example of the application of this principle is seen in the patient on taking 18 g protein per day with a GFR of 3 ml/min, in whom the blood urea is 50 mg/100 ml. The dependence of blood urea on GFR and dietary intake of protein is also shown in Fig. 22. The reason for this dependence of blood urea on protein intake is that urea is the principal nitrogenous breakdown product of protein metabolism; the greater the load of urea to be excreted the higher will be the blood level assuming that excretion is impaired as indicated by a low GFR.

SERUM CREATININE

Levels are normally below 2·0 mg/100 ml and, like the blood urea, they rise above normal only after the GFR has fallen to 30 ml/min or less. An important principle to bear in mind is that the serum creatinine level is independent of the amount of dietary protein, and behaves quite differently from the blood urea in this respect.

PAH AND RENAL PLASMA FLOW

P-aminohippurate (PAH) is removed by a combined process of tubular secretion and glomerular filtration. If one assumes that all the PAH is removed from the blood in passing through the kidney, then the renal clearance of PAH will be equal to the renal plasma flow.

It is more accurate to avoid the assumption that PAH extraction is complete by measuring PAH extraction by the kidneys. This necessitates catheterizing the renal veins and determining the percentage extraction of PAH from the blood stream in passing through the kidneys. Thus

$$\text{true renal plasma flow (RPF)} = \text{Clearance of PAH } \frac{A}{(A-V)}$$

where A = arterial concentration of PAH
V = renal venous PAH concentration.

It is impracticable to catheterize the renal veins for the routine clinical estimation of RPF, so that the PAH clearance measured without renal venous samples is used. This is the effective renal plasma flow (ERPF) to distinguish it from the true RPF determined by renal vein catheterization.

It has been estimated that at low plasma levels 92 per cent of the PAH is extracted in a single passage through the kidneys, and that the extraction is virtually 100 per cent complete for blood which passes through the peritubular capillaries. The unextracted 8 per cent is thought to be largely accounted for by blood passing through non-excretory tissues, such as renal capsule, renal pelvis and peri-renal fat. Thus ERPF, in terms of renal function, is more meaningful than RPF.

Diodrast or hippuran labelled with ^{131}I is easy to estimate accurately and, being handled by the kidney in the same way as PAH, can be used for measuring ERPF.

T_mPAH AND T_mG

There is a maximal and reproducible limit to the rate of secretion of PAH by the renal tubule. This is known as T_mPAH and is an index of the number of functioning proximal tubules or 'proximal tubular mass'. Similarly there is a maximal limit to the rate of reabsorption of glucose by the proximal tubule. This is known as T_mG and likewise is a measure of the amount of functioning proximal tubular tissue.

To measure T_mPAH it is necessary to increase plasma PAH levels to 15–30 mg/100 ml so as to provide adequate amounts of PAH to saturate the sites of tubular secretion. T_mPAH is calculated by measuring T_{PAH} over a series of increasing plasma concentration of PAH, using the expression

$$T_{PAH} = UV - P.C_{in}$$

where   T = tubular secretion of PAH
         UV = PAH excreted/min
         $P.C_{in}$ = filtered load of PAH, derived from
         P = plasma concentration of PAH
         C_{in} = inulin clearance.

When T_{PAH} reaches a constant value this is taken as T_mPAH.

T_mG

If an increasing plasma glucose level is produced by an intravenous infusion of glucose, then the maximal rate of tubular reabsorption of glucose can be determined. The principles involved in calculating T_mG offer a great deal of insight into the mechanisms of renal glycosuria. Tubular reabsorption (T_G) is calculated from the formula $T_G = P.C_{in} - UV$, i.e. tubular reabsorption of glucose is equal to the filtered load minus the amount of glucose excreted/min. The latter can only be measured if glycosuria is present. In Fig. 17 (p. 156) it will be seen that no filtered glucose should be excreted until T_mG is exceeded. Theoretically the graph of reabsorbed glucose should have a sharp bend at B when the T_mG is exceeded. In practice it is found that no such sharp bend occurs, but that glucose starts to appear in the urine at point A and that instead of the reabsorption curve proceeding from A through B to C it is found to have a gentle curve direct from A to C. This is referred to as 'splay' of the filtration curve.

Origin of splay in glucose titration curve. There are two explanations of the origin of splay in glucose titration curves. The first is that there is nephron heterogeneity, some of the glomeruli produce a lower volume of filtrate than normal, but have proximal tubules which can reabsorb glucose normally. In these nephrons the plasma glucose level will have to be higher before the reabsorption capacity of the tubules is exceeded and glycosuria appears. In other glomeruli normal filtration may occur in combination with relatively deficient proximal tubular reabsorptive capacity. In these nephrons glucose will spill over into the urine at lower plasma glucose levels. The nephrons are heterogeneous and demonstrate 'glomerulo-tubular imbalance', i.e. not all the glomeruli and tubules are functionally matched. This explanation seems applicable to many cases of renal glycosuria where there is an increased splay on measuring T_mG.

The second explanation is dynamic and assumes that reabsorption of glucose is mediated by a carrier substance which requires an appreciable quantity of glucose in the tubular lumen before the carrier is saturated. Inevitably some glucose will therefore spill over into the urine before the carrier is totally saturated with glucose.

The evidence at the moment is in favour of the nephron heterogeneity or glomerular tubular imbalance theory, largely because of the correlation between the splay of T_mG in dogs and the actual measurements of glomerular and proximal tubular size.

Phenolsulphonephthalein (PSP; phenol red)

PSP is a dye which is 80 per cent bound in plasma albumin. It is secreted by the proximal tubules as well as by glomerular filtration and has a T_m value. Injection of phenol red with measurement of its rate of excretion is an empirical test of renal function introduced in 1910. The dye is easy to estimate colorimetrically but the test does not measure any specific renal function.

Phosphate

There is a T_m for inorganic phosphate reabsorption (T_mPO_4) but this differs qualitatively from that for glucose in two important ways:
1. T_mPO_4 is small enough to permit part of the filtered load of phosphate to be excreted at normal plasma levels of phosphate.
2. T_mPO_4 is influenced by many factors including dietary intake of phosphate, parathyroid activity, hydrocortisone and vitamin D. If

the glucose reabsorptive mechanism is saturated by infusing glucose intravenously, T_mPO_4 falls; the reverse occurs on giving phlorizin, suggesting that the phosphate and glucose reabsorptive mechanisms share a common step. In clinical medicine it is unusual to measure T_mPO_4: more frequently tubular reabsorption of phosphate (TRP) is measured, and expressed as a percentage of the filtered load. TRP is depressed by increased parathyroid hormone secretion, vitamin D and a high phosphate diet. TRP is increased in hypoparathyroidism.

Free water clearance

The process of urinary dilution can be examined mathematically. To do so we have to assume that urine, which is hypotonic to plasma, is composed of two parts: the first part being the urine which would be produced with the same osmolality as plasma; this is expressed by the *osmolal clearance*:

$$C_{osm} = \frac{U_{osm}V}{P_{osm}} \qquad (1)$$

where U_{osm} = urine osmolality
V = urine volume (ml/min)
C_{osm} = osmolal clearance (ml/min)
P = plasma osmolality.

The second part is the water which would have to be added to urine which was isotonic with plasma to bring the concentration down to the observed osmolality of the urine. This is known as 'free water' and if expressed as ml/min is known as 'free water clearance'. Expressed mathematically:

$$V = C_{H_2O} + C_{osm} \qquad (2)$$

where V = urine volume per minute
C_{osm} = osmolal clearance
C_{H_2O} = free water clearance.

By combination and rearrangement of (1) and (2)

$$C_{H_2O} = V\frac{(1 - U_{osm})}{P_{osm}} \qquad (3)$$

Thus it will be seen from (3) that if the urine is hypotonic to plasma, then C_{H_2O} will have a positive value; if the urine is hypertonic to plasma then C_{H_2O} is negative. It is then usually referred to as T^cH_2O or tubular reabsorption of free water. Under the conditions of *maximal* free water reabsorption during an osmotic diuresis with mannitol and under maximal exogenous vasopressin stimulation, free water reabsorption reaches a maximal value; this is known as $T_m{}^cH_2O$ or tubular maximum reabsorption of free water. Its value in normal man is 5·2 ml/min/100 ml of GFR. Like all tubular functions it is related to the GFR in health. If urine concentration is achieved in the absence of osmotic diuresis the term T^cH_2O is used to indicate negative free water clearance. T^cH_2O rarely exceeds 1 ml/min, whereas C_{H_2O} may readily reach values of 15 ml/min. Therefore ADH acts to prevent the loss of large volumes of water as hypotonic urine (i.e. diabetes insipidus) rather than to make the urine particularly hypertonic for extreme water conservation. Man is not an efficient desert animal.

T^cH_2O and C_{H_2O}. In practice both T^cH_2O and C_{H_2O} are rarely estimated other than in research projects. The use of these factors in determining the probable sites of action can be understood if the following principles are accepted:

1. Diuretics which act only on the proximal tubule do not reduce T^cH_2O or C_{H_2O}. Acetazoleamide falls into this category of diuretics.

2. Diuretics which act on the ascending loop of Henle and limit sodium reabsorption there reduce both T^cH_2O and C_{H_2O}. They do this by reducing the entry of sodium into the medullary interstitium, so preventing a maximal value for T^cH_2O being achieved under the influence of ADH. They also prevent sodium being removed from the tubular fluid under conditions of water diuresis and so reduce the value of C_{H_2O}. Ethacrynic acid and mercurials are in this group of diuretics.

3. Diuretics which act on the distal and collecting tubule by inhibiting or reducing sodium transport, reduce the value of C_{H_2O} but have no effect on T^cH_2O. Chlorothiazide falls into this group of diuretics.

CONCENTRATION TEST

The principle of the urinary concentration test is to stimulate adequate endogenous ADH production so that the urine becomes concentrated. Obviously maximal urinary concentration to 1400 m-osmole/kg is not necessary because this would entail prolonged water deprivation. Usually an empirical 12–14 hr of fluid deprivation overnight is adequate, the inconvenience or discomfort being minimal and a urine osmolality of 700 m-osmole/kg being achieved by the normal person.

DILUTION TESTS

Dilution tests are less frequently carried out. Their interpretation is difficult because ability to produce a dilute urine (i.e. hypotonic to plasma) is retained in advanced renal disease. The majority of patients

7*

with a GFR of 5 ml/min can readily excrete 2500 ml of water/day, although the response to a water load is delayed. Inability to excrete a water load by producing a dilute urine hypotonic to plasma is also present in cirrhosis of the liver, some cases of congestive heart failure and hypoadrenocorticism (p. 538).

URINE/PLASMA OSMOLALITY RATIO

This is a test used in the differential diagnosis of oliguria. In pre-renal uraemia reduction in extracellular fluid volume causes ADH release; tubules not completely refractory to ADH concentrate urine to a urine/plasma osmolality ratio of 4:1. In acute tubular necrosis, the tubules cannot concentrate urine as well and so urine/plasma osmolality ratio falls to 1·1:1.

PROTEINURIA

The normal urine protein loss is up to 150 mg/day. In the nephrotic syndrome (p. 178) the urinary protein loss is usually at least 5 g/day although it may occur with a daily loss as low as 3·5 g/day. This protein loss is sufficient to cause a fall in serum albumin levels below 3·0 g/ 100 ml due to the inability of the liver to synthesize enough albumin to account for the albumin loss in the urine plus the loss in normal protein catabolism. The maximum urine protein loss recorded is over 50 g/day but 10–14 g/day is more frequently met with in nephrotic syndrome. If the serum albumin level is raised by infusion of albumin, the clearance of albumin either remaining constant or increasing as the GFR increases with correction of the hypovolaemia, then protein loss in the urine will increase proportionately so that after a day or two all the albumin infused is excreted. The plasma albumin level once again falls back to its previous level. Unfortunately, one of the most remarkable principles of protein homeostasis is rarely appreciated—that albumin anabolism can increase many times in the face of a continued urinary loss in nephrotic syndrome. An example is the patient with a serum albumin of 0·9 g/ 100 ml who excretes 37 g of albumin/day in his urine. To maintain a serum albumin level of 0·9 g/100 ml the liver must synthesize 37 g of albumin/day above and beyond the normal daily albumin catabolism. Normal daily albumin catabolism in health is 10–12 g, the half life of human albumin being 14 days. In hypoalbuminaemic states albumin catabolism is reduced, but at a conservative estimate albumin formation can be 4 times normal in nephrotic syndrome.

Protein clearances

If the protein content of the urine in different types of renal disease is analysed, it is found to consist of various types of proteins. In membranous glomerulonephritis, the glomerular pore size is large so that the larger molecules can readily escape from the capillaries into Bowman's space and so into the urine. In proliferative glomerulonephritis on the other hand, the glomerular pore size is smaller, so that the large molecules cannot get through the pores into Bowman's space and so do not pass into the urine.

The amount of any individual protein appearing in the urine is dependent not only on glomerular permeability (or pore size) but also on the plasma concentration, shape and charge of the protein (p. 178).

Differential protein clearances. It is convenient to compare the clearances of proteins of different sizes to estimate the pore size distribution, and so arrive at a tentative diagnosis of the type of glomerular disease. This is done by comparing the protein clearances of several proteins by an immunological technique, and using as a reference protein transferrin (siderophilin). The estimation is described as 'differential protein clearance'. Transferrin makes particularly sharp precipitin lines with its antisera, and being only slightly larger than albumin is convenient to take as the standard of 100 per cent. Thus if there is a clearance of β lipoprotein only a fifth of that transferrin, the differential β lipoprotein clearance is 20 per cent.

Selectivity of protein excretion. If the differential protein clearances are plotted against the molecular weight of the proteins (see Fig. 23) then for an individual disease the variation in protein clearances according to protein size can be seen. The differential clearance of the larger proteins can be compared to those of the smaller proteins. If the differential protein clearance is plotted the angle θ gives an indication of the degree to which larger proteins are actively excluded from the urine by the glomerular capillary wall. This is known as selectivity. If none of the larger proteins are present θ is a very small angle (θ'' in Fig. 23), and the proteinuria is described as 'highly selective'. If the larger proteins are able to get through the glomerular capillary wall, the proteinuria is described as 'non-selective' and θ is large (θ' Fig. 23).

In membranous glomerulonephritis, proteinuria is non-selective; in proliferative glomerulonephritis it is selective. In the small amount of protein found in normal man non-selectivity is present.

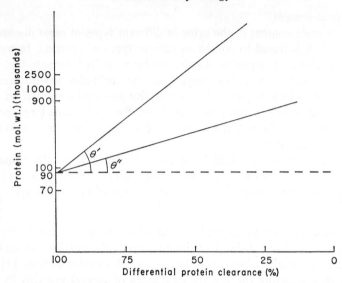

FIGURE 23. *Differential protein clearance related to protein molecular weight.*

Bence Jones protein. Bence Jones proteins are found in plasma and urine in myelomatosis but also occur in small amounts in 'tubular proteinuria' (p. 178). They are interesting in that their structure is made up of the light chains or 'L' part of the normal gamma globulin molecule (γ-globulin is made up light L and heavy H chains with a sulph-hydryl linkage) (p. 273). Bence Jones proteins have a characteristic thermo-coagulabity, precipitating between 45° C and 55° C and redissolving at 95° C. If albuminuria is also present the urine has to be filtered at 100° C to demonstrate the presence of Bence Jones protein and albuminuria together.

AMINO-ACIDURIA
There are normally small amounts of many amino-acids in the urine, but any abnormal increase usually signifies either a selective or non-selective failure of renal proximal tubular reabsorption, or alternatively, a generalized metabolic defect of amino-acid metabolism. A number of examples of renal amino-aciduria have been discussed on p. 173; so-called 'overflow' amino-aciduria occurs in conditions in which one or many amino-acids are present in increased concentrations in the blood (e.g. acute liver cell failure) (p. 444), phenylketonuria (p. 590) and maple-syrup urine disease (failure to metabolize branched-chain amino-acids).

In any case of amino-aciduria, an approximate quantification of each acid present can be obtained by chromatography, which is usually diagnostic of the cause of the defect.

INTRAVENOUS PYELOGRAPHY

This is a valuable test carried out by intravenous administration of organic iodine contrast media such as hypaque (sodium diatrizoate) or sodium acetrizoate. The compounds are excreted both by glomerular filtration and tubular secretion; they are radio-opaque. Dense radio-opaque shadows of the calyces and pelvis are found on X-ray if GFR and tubular secretion of dye are adequate and also if concentrated urine is being formed. This is due to the radio-opacity of a solution being related to the concentration of iodine present, i.e. the number of atoms of iodine per ml of urine. In the first 3–5 min of an IVP, renal parenchyma is opacified due to the presence of intratubular iodide (nephrogram phase). If the water reabsorption is greater in one kidney than in its fellow (as in renal artery stenosis) the kidney may appear more radio-opaque in spite of a lower GFR and lower tubular secretion of the contrast medium. If the blood urea is above 70 mg/100 ml poor shadows are formed due to low renal clearance of contrast medium. To improve the quality of an IVP in renal failure, the amount of organic iodine filtered and secreted can be increased by raising plasma concentration. This technique involves giving a double dose of contrast medium intravenously as a drip—the drip infusion pyelogram (DIP).

RADIOACTIVE RENOGRAM

The radioactive renogram is simple in principle. Radioactive hippuran, labelled with ^{125}I or ^{131}I, is injected intravenously. The hippuran is secreted by the proximal renal tubules and the γ-rays emitted can be detected by collimated counters placed over the renal angles. Several different patterns of radioactivity can be seen if the radioactivity is counted and automatically transcribed onto moving graph paper.

Normal pattern (Fig. 24 (1)). The first part of the graph (a) is a steep climb related to the blood flow to the kidney. Then comes a reduced slope (b) indicating the passage of hippuran into the tubules, and loss of some into the urine; finally there is a downward slope as radioactivity diminishes due to its being carried away in the urine. The two kidneys give symmetrical patterns.

Renal disease (Fig. 24 (2)). Severe generalized renal disease modifies the renogram. RBF is reduced so that the height of the initial part of the graph (a) is low. Because of reduced proximal tubular mass (b) is also small. Finally little radioactive hippuran is secreted into the urine so that there is no fall-off in (c).

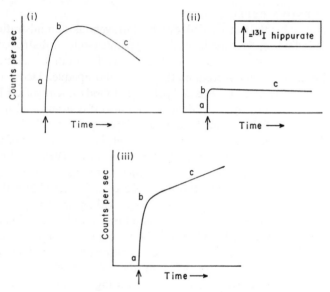

FIGURE 24. *The radioactive renogram.*
(i) Normal.
(ii) Over a non-functioning kidney.
(iii) Over an obstructed kidney.

Obstruction to the urinary pathways (Fig. 24 (3)). In obstructive uropathy of recent onset RBF may be only slightly reduced, so that (a) is not obviously different from normal. The functioning proximal tubular mass (b) is appreciably smaller than normal, but the characteristic abnormality is the rise in (c) instead of the decrease in urine concentration, due to radioactive hippuran entering the urine in the pelvis, the radioactivity accumulating there in the presence of renal tract obstruction.

SCINTILLOGRAM
If chlormerhydrin ^{197}Hg is injected the renal tubules take up the organic mercurial diuretic which emits γ-rays. The diuretic persists for several days in the kidney and it has been shown that there is a good correlation between the intensity of γ-irradiation from the mercurial diuretic and the RPF. Essentially the scintillogram is an autoradiograph and its

principal use is in the diagnosis of abnormal shapes of kidney due to tumours, cysts, infarcts. It has also been used to locate the kidney for biopsy.

ACIDIFICATION TESTS

The principle of acidification tests is the administration of acid load. Usually, ammonium chloride is given. The ammonium moiety is metabolized to urea, giving rise to I hydrogen ion per molecule of ammonium chloride.

$$NH_4Cl = NH_4^+ + Cl^-$$
$$2NH_4^+ + CO_2 \rightarrow CO(NH_2)_2 + H_2O + 2H^+$$

The increased plasma (H^+) concentration reduces plasma HCO_3^- concentration $H^+ + HCO_3^- \rightleftharpoons H_2CO_3 \rightleftharpoons H_2O + CO_2$. The CO_2 is excreted by the lungs. The filtered load of HCO_3^- is reduced and despite buffering and a lowered P_{CO_2}, the (H^+) of the body fluids is increased, causing an increase in tubular H^+ secretion. The H^+ (I) combines with filtered HCO_3^- in the tubule (2) provides H^+ for NH_4^+ production and TA, and (3) causes increased urine H^+ concentration (fall in pH). If the ammonium chloride stimulus is adequate the minimum urine pH produced in health is 4·6 to 5·3. In RTA the minimum urine pH is > 5·3 and usually > 6·0. The distal H^+ secretion mechanism is impaired in this disease.

SPLIT RENAL FUNCTION TESTS

In normal health there is little difference in the amount and composition of the urine being formed by each kidney, but in renal artery stenosis or pyelonephritis affecting I kidney, urinary volume may be decreased to less than 50 per cent of that excreted on the normal side. Similarly, the urinary sodium concentration may be decreased by 15 per cent or more on the diseased side. This is because the lower filtered load of sodium is readily absorbed proximally. On the other hand, creatinine concentration and PAH concentration are increased due to very efficient water reabsorption caused by a lower filtered load of water. To determine the function of each kidney separately, ureteric catheterization has to be carried out with catheters that collect all the urine from each kidney. Infusions of urea and sodium chloride are sometimes used to increase the filtered load of solute and water bilaterally and so to demonstrate more clearly the difference between the two sides.

SODIUM CONSERVATION UNDER MINERALOCORTICOID STIMULATION

Sodium conservation ability is tested in two ways; the first is by giving 20 m-equiv sodium diet and estimating the sodium loss in the urine/24 hr.

After 5 days a normal person has reached a urinary sodium excretion of 20 m-equiv/day. Retention is probably mediated through aldosterone secretion. The second method is to give intravenous aldosterone (10 mg intravenously) and the urine/sodium content falls after 2 hr. Care should be taken to avoid errors caused by normal diurnal variations in sodium output; Na excretion reaches a peak in the forenoon. In salt loss due to poor sodium conservation, urine/sodium excretion exceeds the dietary intake even after 5 days.

Practical Assessment

CLINICAL OBSERVATIONS
Acute renal failure
Duration of oliguria and size of fluid losses when related to salt and water intake indicate fluid balance. Hypertension, oedema, heart failure suggest a fluid excess; hypotension and signs of sodium depletion suggest a fluid deficit. Urine volume low initially (less than 400 ml/24 hr means that a normal solute load cannot be excreted) and it rises with recovery; the osmolarity approximates to that of plasma (and urine SG approaches 1010). Concentrated urine suggests pre-renal uraemia and the need for fluid repletion; dilute urine suggests a renal lesion and the need for regulating the fluid intake. Casts, blood and protein in the urine indicate renal damage.

Chronic renal failure
Duration indicated by the history, presence of anaemia and the duration of nocturia. Symptoms include polyuria, thirst, abnormal diurnal rhythm of urine flow (failure to concentrate); nausea (acidaemia, gastritis); convulsions (hypertensive encephalopathy, water intoxication, hypocalcaemia); air-hunger (acidaemia); cramps (sodium depletion); tetany (hypocalcaemia); pruritus (raised blood urea); bone pain and tenderness (secondary hyperparathyroidism). A bleeding tendency is common. Sodium homeostasis is poor so predisposing to either hypertension and heart failure (sodium excess) or hypotension (sodium depletion).

The nephrotic syndrome
Peripheral oedema, ascites, pleural effusion indicate hypoproteinaemia and massive proteinuria. Degree of frothing of the urine and turbidity with sulphosalicylic acid gives a rough guide to the degree of proteinuria.

ROUTINE METHODS

The urinary deposit in timed urine specimens indicates pyelonephritis if the leucocyte excretion exceeds 200,000/hr. Granular casts (debris of tubular cells) indicate glomerular disease; doubly refractile casts, which contain lipoprotein, are associated with massive proteinuria. Some hyaline casts are normal. In haematuria, erythrocyte casts point to a renal lesion.

The blood urea concentration is normally 15–40 mg/100 ml when the protein intake is 80–100 g/day. Above 60 mg/100 ml means that the glomerular filtration rate is probably less than 30 ml/min. When protein is severely restricted (e.g. to 20 g/day) the blood urea concentration may be hardly elevated despite very low glomerular filtration rate; the plasma creatinine concentration is then a more useful index of renal function.

Plasma sodium concentration is either high or low depending on the water and sodium balance.

Plasma potassium concentration is high in advanced renal failure; above 8 m-equiv/l. cardiac arrest may occur.

Plasma chloride concentration is low with severe vomiting. If high it suggests renal tubular acidosis. The acidosis of chronic renal failure is not associated with hyperchloraemia unless the diet is low in protein.

Plasma bicarbonate concentration low (metabolic acidosis). Low bicarbonate without azotaemia and a urine pH of over 6 suggest renal tubular acidosis.

Plasma calcium and phosphate concentration. The plasma calcium concentration tends to be low, especially when plasma phosphate concentration is high. A normal or high calcium concentration suggests hyperparathyroidism. Correction of acidosis lowers ionized calcium and so predisposes to tetany.

Plasma albumin and cholesterol concentrations are usually inversely related in the nephrotic syndrome but cholesterol may be normal in the nephrotic syndrome of systemic lupus erythematosus (SLE) or acute nephritis.

Plasma globulin concentration is high in SLE and some patients with amyloidosis.

Proteinuria may be normal in the upright position when the liver rotates and compresses the inferior vena cava (benign orthostatic proteinuria). Otherwise it indicates renal disease or infection of the urinary outflow tract. If all components of the plasma proteins are present it suggests tubular disease; and, if low molecular weight globulins (Bence Jones protein) are present it suggests a dysproteinaemia, such as myelomatosis. Daily protein excretion indicates progress in nephrotic syndrome.

Concentration test. After 15 hr fluid deprivation the urine osmolality usually exceeds 700 m-osmole/kg (approximately equivalent to SG 1025). In renal disease it approaches the osmolality of plasma water (SG 1010), progressively more so as renal function deteriorates. Powers of concentration are specifically impaired in potassium depletion, hypercalcaemia and pyelonephritis.

Injection of supramaximal doses of vasopressin does not concentrate the urine in severe glomerular disease and nephrogenic diabetes insipidus, whether congenital or acquired. Compulsive water drinking impairs the response to vasopressin but the response to dehydration is usually normal; the reverse is true in pituitary diabetes insipidus.

Intravenous (or excretory) pyelography (IVP) defines anatomical boundaries and indicates function semi-quantitatively. The rate of appearance of the radio-opaque material is directly proportional to renal function; the rate of disappearance depends on the patency of the outflow tract. Unilateral renal ischaemia is indicated by a small kidney which concentrates slowly and does not flush easily when a diuresis is induced. Unless a large dose of radio-opaque material is given, an IVP is usually only successful if the blood urea concentration is below 100 mg/100 ml.

[131]*I-hippuran renogram* gives similar functional information as an IVP but it is more accurate and the rate of appearance is measured continuously.

SPECIAL TECHNIQUES

Inulin, creatinine, cyanocobalamin, ^{125}I-hypaque clearances measure the glomerular filtrate rate. PAH, diodrast, ^{131}I-hippuran measure effective renal plasma flow. T_mPAH, T_mG measure the functional tubular mass. These methods are research tools. In renal disease the criteria for relating clearances to components of renal function may not remain valid, e.g. the extraction ratio for PAH often falls. Endogenous creatinine clearance and urea clearance overestimate and underestimate GFR respectively but are most useful for clinical assessment, especially when considering changes with time.

Urine acidification (p. 193).

Other tubular tests (p. 184).

References

BERLINER R.W. (1963). Outline of Renal Physiology. In *Disease of the Kidney*. (Ed. M.B. Strauss & L.G. Welt.) London: Churchill.

BERLYNE G.M. (1966). *A course in Renal Diseases*. Oxford: Blackwell.

PITTS R.F. (1963). *Physiology of the Kidney and Body Fluids*. Chicago: Year Book Publishers Inc.

SMITH H.W. (1956). *Principles of Renal Physiology*. New York: Oxford University Press.

Hydrogen Ion (Acid:Base) Regulation

Normal function

INTRODUCTION: DIFFICULTIES IN TERMINOLOGY

Water partially dissociates to form H^+ and OH^- ions:

$$H_2O \rightleftharpoons H^+ + OH^- \tag{1}$$

In pure water and in neutral solutions the concentration of each is equal to 10^{-7} Eq/l. at 20° C and about $10^{-6.8}$ at body temperature. Their product is a constant (the ionic product of water, 10^{-14} at 20° C) even in solutions containing other ionic material. Therefore the concentration of one ion automatically fixes the concentration of the other.

pH. pH was originally introduced as a mathematical convenience in dealing with the very wide range of H^+ concentrations $[H^+]$ met in chemistry. As conceived, pH would be the negative logarithm to the base 10 of $[H^+]$. Thus pH 7 would represent $[H^+] = 10^{-7}$ Eq/l. or, in the usual units of chemical pathology, 0·0001 m-equiv/l. Unfortunately neither pH nor $[H^+]$ as defined in this way can readily be measured (p. 213). pH as measured in practice approximates to the H^+ *activity* rather than the H^+ *concentration*. The activity of a solute is an expression not of how many particles there are but of how many there seem to be and is commonly indicated by round brackets: (H^+). This is equal to $[H^+]$ multiplied by an activity coefficient which is 1 only at infinite dilution. As most of the quantitative relationships to be quoted are based on pH measurements, (H^+) rather than $[H^+]$ will be used in this chapter. This distinction is biologically important in that it is the activity rather than the concentration of a substance which matters (c.f. Ca^{++}, p. 311). Unfortunately most techniques used in chemical pathology, such as flame photometry, measure concentration. One further point: pH and (H^+) are related to a molal (mass/mass) rather than a molar (mass/volume) scale so that (H^+) should be quoted, for example, in nanoEquivalents/kg (n-equiv/kg) of solvent, or as nano-molality (nm) (nano is 10^{-9}).

Acids and bases. An acid is a substance which increases (H^+) (lowers pH); a base is a substance which decreases (H^+) (raises pH). A buffer is a system of an acid and base in which the acid is only partly dissociated. The degree of this dissociation varies in such a way as to oppose any change in (H^+). There is no difficulty about these general statements, but in the more detailed use of the terms there are important differences between orthodox chemical and physiological usage. Although it must be admitted that acid-base physiology is a difficult subject, the terminology and approach used by many clinicians and physiologists make it more difficult. The orthodox chemical usage will therefore be described first. Fortunately the contradictions in nomenclature can usually be avoided. Where they cannot be avoided the chemical system is used.

In the most widely used chemical terminology (that of Bronsted) the term 'acid' is used to describe hydrogen ion (proton) donors:

$$HX \rightleftharpoons H^+ + X \qquad (2)$$
Acid

'Base' is used to describe hydrogen ion (proton) acceptors:

$$X + H^+ \rightleftharpoons HX \qquad (3)$$
Base

In fact, free protons as such are very rare in these solutions, most being associated with water molecules to form hydronium ions, H_3O^+. As these react by virtue of the extra proton, no serious inaccuracy results from considering the processes in terms of H^+ alone.

Substances which neither donate nor accept H^+ ions are neither acids nor bases. Acids and bases are not the same as anions and cations. An acid, for example, may be electrically neutral, an anion, or a cation:

e.g. $$HCl \rightleftharpoons H^+ + Cl^- \qquad (4)$$
Electrically
neutral

$$H_2PO_4^- \rightleftharpoons H^+ + HPO_4^{--} \qquad (5)$$
Anion

$$NH_4^+ \rightleftharpoons H^+ + NH_3 \qquad (6)$$
Cation

Whether a substance behaves as an acid or a base is not necessarily a fixed characteristic. Substances having two or more modes of dissociation may be acids or bases depending on the (H^+) of the solution. For instance, HCO_3^- (a base at physiological (H^+)) is an acid at low (H^+): $HCO_3^- \rightarrow H^+ + CO_3^{--}$; and $H_2PO_4^-$ (an acid at physiological (H^+)) is a base at high (H^+): $H_2PO_4^- + H^+ \rightarrow H_3PO_4$.

Some physiologists and clinicians call a substance an acid if it tends to cause an increase of $[H^+]$ by virtue of certain physiological reactions. Similarly a substance which tends to cause a fall in $[H^+]$ is referred to as a base. The contradiction between the two systems is well exemplified by hydrochloric acid and carbonic acid.

$$HCl \rightleftharpoons H^+ + Cl^- \tag{7}$$

$$H_2CO_3 \rightleftharpoons H^+ + HCO_3^- \tag{8}$$

Chemists restrict the use of the term acid to HCl and H_2CO_3, whereas physiologists and clinicians frequently call Cl^- and HCO_3^- acids. Hydrochloric acid is a strong acid (i.e. fully dissociated) and the difference is not likely to cause confusion, but carbonic acid is a weak acid (i.e. only partly dissociated). So, in equation (8) above, HCO_3^- is a base in chemical usage:

$$HCO_3^- + H^+ \rightleftharpoons H_2CO_3$$

Substances, such as the sodium ion, which are often called bases, are in chemical usage neither acids nor bases because they can neither donate nor accept H^+ ions.

The following further definitions of physiological usage are included to help in following the literature, but will not be used in this book.

The term 'fixed acid' is usually used to refer to the anion formed by the dissociation of a strong acid. Sometimes it is used only to refer to those radicals (e.g. Cl^-, SO_4^{--}), which cannot be formed or destroyed in the body. 'Organic acids' are those radicals (lactate, citrate, aceto-acetate) which are formed and destroyed by metabolic processes. 'Buffer acids' are those radicals (HCO_3^-, Protein$^-$) which are derived from weak acids whose degree of dissociation varies with $[H^+]$. 'Fixed base' is used to describe the quantity of those radicals (Na^+, K^+, Ca^{++}, Mg^{++}) which is 'covered by' (i.e. equivalent in amount to) the 'fixed acids'. 'Buffer base' is used to describe the quantity of the same radicals which is 'covered by' 'buffer acids'.

PHYSIOLOGICAL ACTIVITY OF HYDROGEN IONS

Extracellular fluid. The normal (H^+) of arterial blood is about 0·00004 m-molal (pH 7·4). As the decimal places are unwieldy it is convenient to multiply by a million to yield 40 n-molal (nm). The normal range is about 36–44 nm (which happens to be 7·44–7·36 pH units—the similarity of these numbers is a logarithmic accident—see Fig. 25). The (H^+) of the interstitial fluid is probably 3–25 nm higher than in the arterial blood, depending on the local balance between metabolism and blood flow. The range of extracellular (H^+) compatible with life is about 20 to 160 nm (pH 7·7–6·8). These figures show that the 'reaction of the blood' need not be as constant as is often implied.

Intracellular fluid. Estimates of intracellular (H^+) vary from 50 to 1000 nm (pH 7·3–6·0). Even if an average figure were more accurately known it is doubtful what it could mean because regional variation within individual cells must be very great.

REGULATION OF (H^+)

There is no one receptor or centre which is specifically sensitive to (H^+) and which integrates all aspects of its regulation. Nevertheless, the mechanisms which resist change in (H^+) are efficient and well co-ordinated. They are 3 in number:
  1. Buffer systems within the body.
  2. The renal regulation of H^+ excretion.
  3. The respiratory regulation of CO_2 excretion.

THE BUFFERING ACTION OF BODY FLUIDS

The first line of defence against a change in (H^+) is provided by the buffer systems of the body fluids. If a strong acid or alkali is added to the extracellular fluid, 30–50 per cent is buffered by systems immediately available in the extracellular fluid (notably bicarbonate–carbonic acid) and the remainder is either buffered in the cells and bone or by the release of buffers from these. This buffering is so effective that the addition of 1 m-equiv of strong acid per l. of body fluid only increases (H^+) by about 5 nm. That is, all but 5 of every million H^+ ions added are buffered. The sites of these buffers govern their availability and the magnitude and rate of the resultant change in (H^+). The buffers of blood and extracellular fluid are immediately available; those of intracellular fluid are less so but still operative in a few minutes; the immense buffer capacity of bone requires hours or days to become effective. These differences are partly due to blood flow and also to the rates of exchange with interstitial fluid.

BICARBONATE, CARBONIC ACID, DISSOLVED CO_2
AND HYDROGEN ION CONCENTRATIONS

Bicarbonate and carbonic acid are quantitatively the most important buffer system in the extracellular fluid.

$$HCO_3^- + H^+ \rightleftharpoons H_2CO_3 \qquad (9)$$

Addition of H^+ ions causes the equilibrium to move from left to right and removal causes it to move from right to left. Chemically this is not a very good buffer system because carbonic acid is quite a strong acid. Its unique physiological virtue lies in the fact that H_2CO_3 is in equilibrium with the dissolved CO_2 of the body fluids:

$$H_2CO_3 \rightleftharpoons CO_2 + H_2O \qquad (10)$$

Hence, by varying the volume of CO_2 excreted from the lungs, the equilibrium in equations (9) and (10) can be adjusted to resist changes in (H^+) (see also p. 205).

The equilibrium conditions for equation 9 can be expressed in the following version of the law of mass action*:

$$(H^+) = K' \frac{[H_2CO_3]}{[HCO_3^-]} \qquad (11)$$

Carbonic acid forms a small virtually constant portion (about one molecule per 1000) of the CO_2 in solution (equation 10), so equation 11 can be rewritten:

$$(H^+) = K' \frac{[CO_2]k}{[HCO_3^-]} \qquad (12)$$

where k is the equilibrium constant of the reaction of CO_2 with water to form H_2CO_3. Usually k is incorporated in K' and Hasselbalch's version of the equation is used:

$$pH = pK' + \log \frac{[HCO_3^-]}{[CO_2]} \qquad (13)$$

---

* The Henderson–Hasselbalch equation is derived from the equilibrium constant (K) of the reaction as follows:

$$(H^+) = K' \times \frac{[H_2CO_3]}{[HCO_3^-]}$$

Taking logarithms, and changing the sign of all terms:

$$-\log (H^+) = -\log K' - \log \frac{[H_2CO_3]}{[HCO_3^-]}$$

which can be rewritten:

$$pH = pK' + \log \frac{[HCO_3^-]}{[H_2CO_3]}$$

If $[HCO_3^-]$ and $[CO_2]$ are expressed as molar and (H^+) as nm, K' for plasma is about 800. Using the same units for $[HCO_3^-]$ and $[CO_2]$, pK' is about 6·1.

As the concentration of dissolved CO_2 is proportional to the partial pressure of CO_2 ($[CO_2]$ mM = 0·03 Pco_2 in mmHg), the equations can be further rewritten:

$$(H^+) = 24 \frac{Pco_2}{[HCO_3^-]} \tag{14}$$

$$pH = 6·1 + \log \frac{[HCO_3^-]}{0·03\, Pco_2} \tag{15}$$

These equations enable the third variable to be calculated if the other two are known. There are many nomograms and other graphical ways (Fig. 25) for solving the equations. Although satisfactory for most clinical purposes, such calculations of the third variable from knowledge of the other two are not entirely accurate, chiefly because the 'constants' K' and pK' vary slightly with temperature, (H^+) and other factors.

OTHER BUFFERS: HAEMOGLOBIN

The acid formed in the largest quantity in the body is, of course, carbonic acid itself which is formed from the CO_2 produced in the tissues. The most important buffer for dealing with carbonic acid is haemoglobin:

$$H^+ + Hb^- \rightleftharpoons HHb \tag{16}$$

This reaction minimizes the rise in blood (H^+) associated with the transport of CO_2 from the tissues to the lungs. Haemoglobin is of particular importance in this respect because its buffering power varies with oxygenation and reduction. Reduced Hb^- is a stronger base (i.e. will bind more H^+ ions) than oxy-Hb^- so that the removal of O_2 from the blood in the capillaries of the tissues simultaneously and inevitably provides a buffer for much of the H_2CO_3 added to it.

Haemoglobin is able, of course, not only to buffer carbonic acid but also all acids, and in the blood (as opposed to the interstitial fluid) the concentration of haemoglobin makes it quantitatively as important a buffer as carbonic acid–bicarbonate. The plasma proteins also act as buffers but their capacity in m-equiv/g is only one-third that of haemoglobin. As the haemoglobin concentration is normally twice that of the plasma proteins, haemoglobin is normally six times as important as the plasma proteins in the total buffer capacity of the blood.

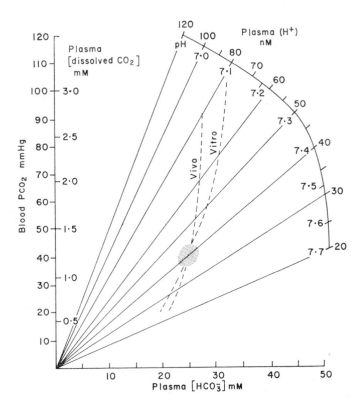

FIGURE 25. *The* P_{CO_2} : $[HCO_3^-]$ *diagram.*

This is a graphical representation of equations 14 and 15 in which the acid : base ratio of the CO_2 : HCO_3^- system is used to indicate (H^+) and pH. The central shaded ellipse represents the normal range found in arterial blood in resting subjects. The 'vitro' curve shows the changes in (H^+) and $[HCO_3^-]$ when the P_{CO_2} of blood with a normal Hb concentration is changed *in vitro*; the 'vivo' curve shows the changes in the arterial blood when the P_{CO_2} of the body is changed acutely (over a few minutes or hours). The *in vivo* curve is steeper and the change in (H^+) greater because the buffering effect of Hb, instead of being concentrated in the blood, is shared throughout the extra-cellular fluid. In this diagram, as in others, such as the Astrup-Siggaard-Andersen log P_{CO_2} : pH diagram and the Davenport $[HCO_3^-]$: pH diagram, changes in position of the buffer or dissociation curve are produced by non-respiratory changes in $[HCO_3^-]$ while changes in slope of the curve are due to changes in the concentration of the blood buffers, particularly Hb.

HYDROGEN ION BALANCE AND THE KIDNEY

Hydrogen and hydroxyl ions are taken in with the diet and are also produced by many metabolic processes. Normally there is an excess absorption and production of H^+ ions amounting to about 50 m-equiv or more daily. Most of these H^+ ions are derived from sulphuric and phosphoric acids formed by the breakdown of protein and other complex substances. The concentration in the body is maintained constant by the excretion of an equal amount in the urine. The two most important mechanisms by which the kidney tubules accomplish this are: (1) by adding H^+ to buffers such as the HPO_4^{--} in the glomerular filtrate, to form $H_2PO_4^-$, and (2) by forming ammonia NH_3, which carries H^+ out as ammonium NH_4^+.

An alkaline diet tends to cause a decrease of (H^+) in the body fluids. In such circumstances the kidney reduces ammonia formation, excretes more HPO_4^{--} and less $H_2PO_4^-$, and may also excrete HCO_3^-.

HYDROGEN ION BALANCE AND THE LUNGS

CO_2 and water are the end products of many metabolic processes. The CO_2 is formed in solution and some of it combines with H_2O to form carbonic acid which in turn partly dissociates

$$CO_2 + H_2O \rightleftharpoons H_2CO_3 \rightleftharpoons H^+ + HCO_3^- \qquad (17)$$

CO_2 is excreted in the lungs and the reactions move from right to left so that the H^+ ions formed in the tissues disappear. The concentration of CO_2 in the blood leaving the lungs depends upon the partial pressure of CO_2 in the alveolar air. A change in the alveolar P_{CO_2} therefore alters the equilibria in equation (17). A rise in alveolar P_{CO_2} shifts the reactions to the right, thereby increasing (H^+).

It will be appreciated, therefore, that, although H^+ ions are not excreted through the lungs, any alteration in the balance of CO_2 production and elimination alters the (H^+) of the body fluids by altering the P_{CO_2}. The relation between CO_2 production, the volume of the breathing and P_{CO_2} is a simple one, as will be appreciated from the following derivation.

The amount of CO_2 excreted by the lungs each minute equals the amount of CO_2 in each litre of alveolar air multiplied by the number of litres of alveolar air expired. This can be restated as follows: the volume of CO_2 expired equals the alveolar concentration of CO_2 times the alveolar ventilation:

Vol. CO_2 excreted = Alv. CO_2 concentration × Alv. ventilation.

The alveolar CO_2 concentration has the same partial pressure as the arterial blood, and in a steady state the CO_2 excreted by the lungs must equal the amount produced by the tissues; so: Vol. CO_2 produced is proportional to Arterial P_{CO_2} × Alv. ventilation or:

$$\text{Arterial } P_{CO_2} = \frac{\text{Vol. } CO_2 \text{ produced}}{\text{Alveolar ventilation}} \times \text{Barometric press.} \quad (18)$$

It follows, therefore, that any disturbance of the balance between CO_2 production and alveolar ventilation causes a change in P_{CO_2} and therefore in (H^+), not only in the arterial blood but throughout the body fluids. The size of the potential changes involved is very great. A normal subject at rest excretes 15,000 m-equiv (330 l.) of CO_2 through the lungs each day. This contrasts with the 50 m-equiv of H^+ excreted by the kidneys normally, and the 600 m-equiv they can excrete when functioning maximally. An illustration of this contrast is that suppression of urinary formation of H^+ for 30 minutes causes no detectable change in the (H^+) of the extracellular fluid. Suppression of respiratory CO_2 excretion for 30 minutes would cause the (H^+) to exceed 100 nm (pH below 7).

Disordered function

ACIDOSIS AND ALKALOSIS: DIFFICULTIES IN TERMINOLOGY

Much of the difficulty in following accounts of acid : base disturbances hinges on differences in usage. The chief of these is the ambiguity of the meaning of the terms acidosis and alkalosis. Sometimes they are used in a chemical sense; sometimes in a physiological one. Thus, some people imply that 'an acidosis is an increased blood (H^+)' that is, the disturbance in the chemical composition is the acidosis. Others imply that 'an acidosis is a disturbance of function causing an accumulation of H^+ ions'; i.e. the disturbance of function rather than a change in chemical composition is the acidosis. Although logically undesirable the distinction would not matter very much if the change in function always caused the change in composition; but this is not so. Because of compensatory or opposing disturbances the (H^+) may be normal or low. The physiological usage is to be preferred and in this account the terms acidosis and alkalosis will be used to imply abnormal processess or conditions which would cause a deviation of (H$^+$) if there were no secondary changes. When describing abnormalities of chemical composition it is preferable to specify the variable in question and to say whether it is increased or decreased. But it is sometimes convenient to use the following terms: *acidaemia* and *alkalaemia* mean a high and low blood (H$^+$); *hypercapnia* and *hypocapnia* mean a high and low blood Pco_2. *Hyperbasaemia* and *hypobasaemia* have been suggested as terms to describe an increased or decreased non-respiratory variable (see p. 216).

The (H$^+$) in the intracellular fluid is different from that in the extracellular fluid and may vary independently in disease. The terms intracellular and extracellular acidosis or alkalosis should therefore be used to make it clear which fluid compartment is under discussion. If the site is not specified then it is usual to imply that the extracellular fluid is being considered. This usage is observed throughout the following account and elsewhere in this book.

RESPIRATORY (GASEOUS) AND METABOLIC (NON-GASEOUS) ACIDOSIS AND ALKALOSIS

There are many ways in which (H$^+$) can be increased or decreased. Physiologically and clinically they are best separated into two groups.

1. Disturbances of respiration which affect H$^+$ through their effects on CO_2 and H_2CO_3.

2. All other disturbances.

Changes in the first group are usually called 'respiratory' acidosis or alkalosis, and those in the second are called 'metabolic'. These terms are not really satisfactory. For instance, an increase in (H$^+$) due to increased metabolic CO_2 production has to be called 'respiratory'. Also, renal causes of acidosis or alkalosis are not well termed 'metabolic'. More satisfactory terms are 'gaseous' for those due to changes in CO_2 concentration and 'non-gaseous' for the others. However, these terms have not gained acceptance so 'respiratory' and 'metabolic' will be preferred in the following account.

There are four types of disturbance: respiratory acidosis, metabolic acidosis, respiratory alkalosis and metabolic alkalosis. These rarely occur clinically in isolation; there is usually a secondary change tending to restore (H$^+$) to normal and often a complicating primary disorder which may tend to restore or aggravate a change in H$^+$. The main effects of the primary disorders of H$^+$, Pco_2 and HCO_3^- will now be described. It must be emphasized that this account will mention only simple features of the underlying physiology; a fuller description would require an extensive consideration of many other topics notably in respiratory and electrolyte physiology.

A. *Respiratory (gaseous) acidosis*

Respiratory acidosis is present whenever the ratio of CO_2 production to alveolar ventilation rises (see p. 206, equation 18) whether by a rise in CO_2 production or a fall in alveolar ventilation; it is characterized by hypercapnia, an increase in arterial P_{CO_2}. Primary respiratory acidosis is synonymous with ventilatory failure (p. 116). The primary change is a rise in P_{CO_2} (arrow 1, Fig. 26). The kidney compensates for the rise in (H^+) by excreting more H^+ ions and retaining bicarbonate (causing the secondary change illustrated by arrow 2 in Fig. 26). Thus the secondary response to a respiratory acidosis is an increase in $[HCO_3^-]$. Whether or not an acidaemia occurs depends on the rapidity

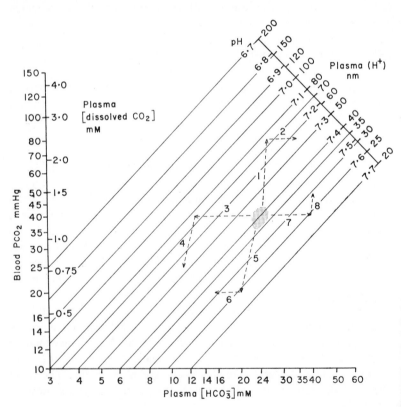

of development and severity of the acidosis. If P_{CO_2} is acutely increased to say 80 mmHg, some (about 1 in 20) of the CO_2 molecules remain in solution; the remainder are hydrated to form H_2CO_3 which then dissociates. Most of the HCO_3^- ions remain in the extracellular fluid; the H^+ ions are buffered mainly by Hb and partly by intracellular buffers. The changes in blood (H^+) and [HCO_3^-] (the '*in vivo* dissociation or titration curve of blood') are shown in Fig. 26. In acute respiratory acidosis the renal response even if immediate cannot compensate adequately. If ventilation ceased H^+ ions would accumulate in the body at a rate of about 10 m-equiv. per minute. This rate is over 20 times faster than the rate at which the kidney can excrete H^+ ions.

FIGURE 26. *The changes in pH, P_{CO_2} and bicarbonate in the four primary disturbances of hydrogen ion regulation.*

The axes are the same as Fig. 25, but they are plotted logarithmically, thus covering a greater range and increasing the discrimination at lower values of P_{CO_2} and [HCO_3^-].

$$CO_2 + H_2O \rightleftharpoons H_2CO_3 \rightleftharpoons H^+ + HCO_3^-$$

$$(H^+) = 24 \frac{P_{CO_2}}{[HCO_3^-]}$$

$$pH = 6 \cdot 1 + \log \frac{[HCO_3^-]}{0 \cdot 03 P_{CO_2}}$$

Respiratory acidosis. Pulmonary ventilation is reduced. Alveolar and arterial P_{CO_2}, and therefore [H_2CO_3], increase (arrow 1). (H^+) increases (pH falls). The kidney retains HCO_3^- and excretes H^+ and therefore tends to restore (H^+) towards normal (arrow 2).

Respiratory alkalosis. Pulmonary ventilation is increased (arrow 5). Alveolar and arterial P_{CO_2}, and therefore [H_2CO_3], fall. (H^+) decreases (pH rises). The kidney excretes more HCO_3^- and retains H^+ and therefore tends to restore (H^+) towards normal (arrow 6).

Metabolic acidosis. Addition or production of H^+ causes a rise in (H^+) (fall in pH). Buffering of the rise in (H^+) involves the combination of H^+ and HCO_3^- to form H_2CO_3, thus causing a reduction in [HCO_3^-] (arrow 3). As a result of this buffer action there should also be increases in [H_2CO_3], in the concentration of dissolved CO_2 and therefore in P_{CO_2}. Two things prevent this. Firstly, the excess CO_2 would be very easily excreted by the lungs to maintain P_{CO_2} constant. Secondly, the rise in (H^+) stimulates the breathing so much that, in fact, more CO_2 is washed out, causing P_{CO_2} and [H_2CO_3] to fall. The (H^+) is therefore returned towards normal (arrow 4).

Metabolic alkalosis. Loss or neutralization of H^+ ions causes a reduction in (H^+) (increase in pH). Buffering of the reduction in (H^+) is partly effected by dissociation of H_2CO_3 to H^+ and HCO_3^-, thus increasing [HCO_3^-] (arrow 7). This buffer action would tend to cause a fall in [H_2CO_3] and in P_{CO_2}. However, the fall in (H^+) depresses the breathing so that reduced amounts of CO_2 are excreted and P_{CO_2}, and [H_2CO_3], rise. The (H^+) is therefore restored towards normal (arrow 8). (*Lancet*, 1962, **ii**, 154, modified.)

Both the primary and secondary changes cause an increase in the plasma HCO_3^- concentration, but the increase in plasma CO_2 content produced by a primary respiratory acidosis is so small that it hardly exceeds analytical error.

B. *Metabolic (non-respiratory, non-gaseous) acidosis*

Metabolic acidosis is present if there is an accumulation of acid other than H_2CO_3 in the extracellular fluid, or a loss of base.

An increase of acid occurs: if an excess of H^+ ions is ingested (e.g. $NH_4Cl \rightarrow H^+ + Cl^- + NH_3$); if an excess of organic acids is produced (e.g. lactic acid or aceto-acetic acid); or if the kidney fails to excrete sufficient acid.

A decrease of base occurs if there is loss of alkaline alimentary secretions as by diarrhoea or biliary fistula.

The primary change in metabolic acidosis (arrow 3, Fig. 26) is a rise in (H^+) and a fall in $[HCO_3^-]$. The rise in (H^+) causes an increase in pulmonary ventilation and a reduction in PCO_2 so the direction of the secondary change is as indicated by arrow 4 in Fig. 26. The response to a metabolic acidosis therefore causes hypocapnia, and both cause a reduction in plasma HCO_3^- concentration.

Minor degrees of metabolic acidosis can be compensated by the respiratory response, but in severe metabolic acidosis an acidaemia occurs which can only be corrected by excretion of the acid, or (in the case of the organic acids such as lactic and aceto–acetic) by its degradation to CO_2 which can be excreted by the lungs. It is important to remember that, although buffering and hypocapnia can prevent acidaemia, the full restitution of normal acid : base composition requires the removal of the offending acid or addition of the missing base.

Unless there is a disorder of renal secretion of H^+, the urine in metabolic acidosis is always acid (the pH usually being less than 5·3).

C. *Respiratory (gaseous) alkalosis (hypocapnia; hypocarbia)*

Respiratory alkalosis occurs whenever alveolar PCO_2 is lowered by excessive ventilation. It occurs in artificial or voluntary overbreathing and during excessive stimulation of the breathing by a number of nervous and chemical disorders such as anoxia, various forms of cerebral disease, hepatic failure and salicylate poisoning. Respiratory alkalosis is also a feature of certain disorders of the pulmonary circulation, notably thrombo-embolic pulmonary hypertension.

The primary change is a reduction in PCO_2 (arrow 5, Fig. 26). The kidney reacts by excreting more HCO_3^- ions and reabsorbing more

H⁺ ions (thus excreting an alkaline urine) causing the secondary changes illustrated by arrow 6, Fig. 26. Thus the secondary response to a respiratory alkalosis is a decrease in $[HCO_3^-]$ and both cause a reduction in plasma HCO_3^- concentration. Another factor which opposes the change in (H⁺) during an acute respiratory alkalosis is an increase in the blood concentration of lactic and pyruvic acids; this is to be regarded as a complicating metabolic acidosis rather than as a compensatory response.

As in the case of respiratory acidosis, the presence or absence of an alkalaemia depends chiefly on the acuteness of the development of the alkalosis. If it develops rapidly the kidney is overwhelmed, but in a chronic state severe alkalaemia is unusual.

The urine is initially alkaline but usually becomes acid later (p. 205).

D. *Metabolic (non-respiratory, non-gaseous) alkalosis*

Metabolic alkalosis is a loss of acid other than H_2CO_3 from the extracellular fluid or an increase of base.

A loss of acid occurs during vomiting when there is loss of HCl, and a gain in base occurs when absorbable alkalis such as sodium bicarbonate are administered in excess. There are also several conditions associated with potassium depletion in which altered renal function causes a metabolic alkalosis because the kidney excretes too many H⁺ ions (see p. 14).

It is in the group of disorders causing metabolic alkalosis that the dissociation between extracellular and intracellular (H⁺) is best recognized. Potassium depletion commonly causes an extracellular alkalosis at the same time as an intracellular acidosis. This is believed to be caused by H⁺ ions taking the place of K⁺ inside the cells.

The primary change in metabolic alkalosis (arrow 7) is a fall in (H⁺) and rise in $[HCO_3^-]$. The secondary change should be a rise in P_{CO_2} (arrow 8), but this is often small and may not occur at all. The reason for this lack of respiratory response is not clear but may be connected with the divergence between the intracellular and extracellular change in (H⁺).

The lack of respiratory response leads to the development of an alkalaemia in many cases of primary metabolic alkalosis.

Both the primary and secondary changes cause an increase in plasma HCO_3^- concentration. The urine is alkaline at some stage in all those conditions due to abnormal loss of H⁺ or abnormal absorption of base, because the kidney responds by an increased excretion of basic ions (HPO_4^{--} and HCO_3^-) and an increased reabsorption of H⁺.

8

However, in the metabolic alkalosis of potassium depletion the urine is acid because the alkalosis is actually produced by an excessive renal excretion of H^+ ions. The urine is also paradoxically acid when metabolic alkalosis is associated with extreme sodium loss, as after prolonged vomiting.

MIXED DISTURBANCES
Mixed disturbances are very common and may have opposing or additive effects on blood (H^+).

Opposing disturbances
Respiratory alkalosis and metabolic acidosis. This combination occurs, for example, if renal failure is combined with heart failure and pulmonary congestion. It may also be common in uraemia when the ventilation may be stimulated by amines. A better example is salicylate poisoning in which an initial respiratory alkalosis due to the stimulation of the ventilation by the salicylate radical is complicated by a later lactic-acidosis.

Respiratory acidosis and metabolic alkalosis. This combination commonly occurs in patients with ventilatory failure and oedema ('cor pulmonale') who are overtreated with diuretics causing K^+ and/or Cl^- depletion. This combination is commonly associated with intracellular acidosis.

Additive disturbances
These set particularly sinister traps for the unwary partly because they usually occur in patients who are so ill in other ways that they are overlooked and partly because they have opposing effects on the plasma [HCO_3^-] which may thus not be very high or very low. This may mislead those who rely only on a measurement of venous [HCO_3^-] or alkali reserve as part of routine electrolyte examination in management.

Respiratory acidosis and metabolic acidosis. This combination is probably the final common pathway of respiratory and circulatory failure. The poor pulmonary circulation and underventilation cause CO_2 retention; the poor peripheral circulation causes stagnant hypoxia and lactic acidosis; and the poor renal circulation reduces the ability of the kidney to excrete H^+ ions.

Respiratory alkalosis and metabolic alkalosis. This combination occurs as a complication of respiratory failure in the presence of K$^+$ and/or Cl$^-$ depletion if, for example, excessive artificial ventilation is given.

DISTURBANCES OF INTRACELLULAR [H$^+$]

As indicated on page 201 little is known about intracellular (H$^+$) and it is doubtful to what extent values quoted for it are meaningful. Certain generalizations are, however, important. First, CO$_2$ appears to cross cell membrances so easily that respiratory (gaseous) disturbances tend to alter the intracellular (H$^+$) in the same direction as the extracellular. Secondly, this parallelism does not necessarily apply to metabolic (non-gaseous) disturbances. Thus in potassium depletion there may be a raised intracellular (H$^+$) associated with a low extracellular (H$^+$) (see above). The addition of strong acids or bases to the extracellular fluid may cause an acute paradoxical shift in the intracellular reaction. For example, the addition of HCl (as NH$_4$Cl) increases the extracellular (H$^+$) and stimulates the breathing thus lowering intracellular Pco$_2$ and [H$_2$CO$_3$]. As the added H$^+$ and Cl$^-$ ions do not enter the cells at once, the intracellular (H$^+$) may temporarily fall.

Studies of isolated muscle suggest that intracellular (H$^+$) may change less when extracellular (H$^+$) is raised (by manipulation of either Pco$_2$ or [HCO$_3$$^-$]) than when it is lowered.

Principles of tests and measurements

A full evaluation of the acid : base state requires knowledge of 2 of the 3 components of the acid : base equation so that the third can be calculated. Two of them (pH and Pco$_2$) are not often measured but are easy to understand; the third (HCO$_3$$^-$ or one of the related measurements discussed below) is commonly measured but is more difficult to understand.

It is important to realize that a description of the chemical composition of the blood, however complete, does not necessarily explain the mechanism causing any disturbance and also to realize that the same change in chemical composition can result from different disturbances.

pH or (H$^+$)

Although pH as originally conceived was the negative logarithm to base 10 of H$^+$ concentration, in fact pH as measured approximates more to the negative logarithm of the H$^+$ activity (p. 198). But even this definition cannot be rigorously observed and in practice an 'operational' scale of pH has been developed by assigning certain pH values to certain buffer solutions. pH measurement now consists of an electrometric comparison between the unknown solution (in this case blood) and one of the standard solutions. Modern millivoltmeters have made this process fairly easy, but difficulties remain. The present position is that changes in pH in a given solution can be measured very accurately

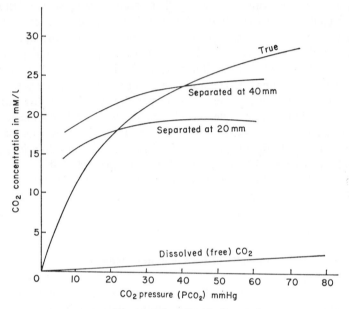

FIGURE 27. *Plasma carbon dioxide dissociation curves.*

These curves were obtained from blood with an initially low normal bicarbonate concentration.

True: This is the curve obtained when whole blood is equilibrated with a range of CO_2 tensions and the CO_2 content of the plasma determined. Its relatively steep slope depends upon the presence of haemoglobin (see text).

Separated: These are the curves obtained when the plasma is separated from the red cells before equilibration with a range of CO_2 tensions. The height of the curve depends upon the P_{CO_2} at the time of separation. The curves are relatively flat because of the absence of haemoglobin during equilibration.

Dissolved: This curve shows the amount of CO_2 in simple solution in the plasma at body temperature. Subtraction of this curve from any of the others at any given P_{CO_2} gives the *plasma bicarbonate* concentration in m-eqiv/l. The relation between bicarbonate concentration and P_{CO_2} is expressed in another form in Figs. 25 and 26.

($\pm$0·005 units in the physiological range); the absolute pH value in terms of the agreed scale can be less certainly determined; the interpretation of the 'absolute' pH value in terms of H^+ ionic activity is, in turn, less certain; finally, the relation between the H^+ ionic activity and the H^+ concentration of a solution is uncertain.

The respiratory variable: arterial P_{CO_2}
Arterial P_{CO_2} can be measured in one of 3 main ways: first 'directly' by a tonometric method in which a bubble of gas is brought into equilibrium with the blood. (This method is not used much in practice); secondly, by measuring the P_{CO_2} of alveolar air or by using rebreathing to estimate the P_{CO_2} of mixed venous blood from which at rest the arterial P_{CO_2} can be calculated with acceptable accuracy (p. 131); thirdly, by use of one of the following methods based upon pH measurement.

Blood P_{CO_2} measurement using a pH meter
The locked relationship between (H^+) (or pH), P_{CO_2} and [HCO_3^-] outlined on pages 202–3 means that P_{CO_2} can be calculated from pH measurements if [HCO_3^-] is known.

The 'indirect' method. Blood P_{CO_2} can be estimated by measuring pH and bicarbonate or CO_2 concentrations (see above) and calculating P_{CO_2} making use of the Henderson–Hasselbalch equation or one of its graphical forms.

The 'interpolation' (Astrup) method. The pH of the blood is measured and then the blood is equilibrated with 2 gases of known P_{CO_2} and the pH measured again after each equilibration. This procedure allows the standard bicarbonate concentration to be determined. The original P_{CO_2} can be calculated from the original pH. In practice these steps can be performed rapidly and semi-automatically.

The 'electrode' or 'titration' method. The pH electrode is covered with a membrane permeable to CO_2 but not to HCO_3^-. The thin space between the electrode and this membrane is occupied by a matrix such as cellophane holding a dilute bicarbonate solution. When the whole is placed in blood, the CO_2 diffuses through the membrane, forms H_2CO_3 and changes the pH of the solution to a value depending on the P_{CO_2} of the blood.

THE NON-RESPIRATORY (METABOLIC) VARIABLE:
BICARBONATE, ALKALI RESERVE, BASE EXCESS.
As a starting point, non-respiratory factors (including renal function) can be said to create an extracellular fluid with [HCO$_3^-$] of 25 m-mole/l. and respiratory function to create an extracellular fluid with a PCO_2 of about 40 mmHg having a concentration of dissolved CO_2 of 1·25 m-mole/l. so that the ratio of 20 : 1 produces a (H$^+$) of 40 nm or a pH of 7·4. So why not simply measure the [HCO$_3^-$]? Most people would say that this is the best thing to do but, unfortunately, the [HCO$_3^-$] is not entirely independent of changes in PCO_2. If PCO_2 is raised or lowered it is equivalent to the addition or removal of [HCO$_3^-$] and the H$^+$ ions liberated by the dissociation of [H$_2$CO$_3$] are buffered by protein, notably Hb;

$$H_2CO_3 + Hb^- \rightleftharpoons HHb + HCO_3^-$$

The effect of this is that the plasma [HCO$_3^-$] as eventually recorded by whatever analyser is used depends, first, on *in vivo* factors. It is necessary to consider the PCO_2 of the body as a whole and the PCO_2 of the particular sample of blood taken (which in turn depends upon the local blood flow and metabolism of the tissues and the presence or absence of any stagnation in the vessel from which the sample was taken). Secondly, recorded values reflect *in vitro* changes induced as a result of contact with air during sampling, storage, transport etc. Thus if blood is allowed to lose CO_2 so that, say, its PCO_2 falls to 20 mmHg and the plasma is then separated from the cells, re-equilibration of the plasma with a PCO_2 of 40 mm will not restore the [HCO$_3^-$] concentration to its original value (Fig. 27).

In vitro, the sum of [Hb$^-$] + [HCO$_3^-$] per unit volume of blood is unaffected by changes in PCO_2. The change in [HCO$_3^-$] due to a change in PCO_2 is accompanied by an equal and opposite change in [Hb$^-$] (ionized Hb). But this is not true *in vivo* because HCO$_3^-$ ions migrate to the interstitial fluid so that, per unit volume of blood, [Hb$^-$] + [HCO$_3^-$] falls. Hence a change in PCO_2 occurring *in vivo* may appear to produce a non-respiratory change when compared with what would happen to the same blood if its PCO_2 were changed *in vitro*.

Practical solutions

A number of approaches to these problems have been advocated and 3 are in common use.

1. Use arterial or arterialized blood and interpret the [HCO$_3^-$] in relation to the PCO_2.

2. Use venous or capillary blood and equilibrate it with a P_{CO_2} of 40 mmHg and enough oxygen to saturate the haemoglobin so that the respiratory variable is standardized. The $[HCO_3^-]$ of the plasma is then measured. This is the principle of the standard bicarbonate and the alkali reserve.

3. Use venous or capillary blood and titrate the blood to determine its base concentration either in absolute terms or by reference to a given value. The first of these is the principle underlying the buffer base measurement and the second underlies the base excess measurement. The easiest acid to titrate the blood with is carbonic acid; this is essentially what the Astrup technique uses when the relationship between change in P_{CO_2} and change in pH is measured and its slope indicates the base excess.

Choice of measurement.

For the evaluation of non-respiratory disturbances the best measurement is probably the first in which the $[HCO_3^-]$ is evaluated by making allowance for the P_{CO_2}. In other words, $[HCO_3^-]$ is compared with the value which is to be expected for the titration curve or dissociation curve of the body as a whole. Unfortunately, of course, much of clinical practice is based upon sampling venous blood and, for the chemical pathologist receiving blood whose state at the time of sampling and whose fate since sampling are unknown, the best solution may be the second or third. The argument continues about which is better but, provided the Hb concentration and the oxygen saturation of the blood are also recorded (even approximately) both views can be taken. Fortunately, over the ranges of concentration most often met in practice the *in vitro* and *in vivo* dissociation curves do not differ so much that important mistakes will be made.

Practical assessment

CLINICAL OBSERVATIONS
Four lines of evidence:
1. *Nature of underlying disease*
eg. Renal disease, diabetes mellitus likely to cause metabolic acidosis; chronic lung disease more likely to cause respiratory acidosis.

2. *Symptoms and signs of abnormal (H^+) or P_{CO_2}*
Of limited value, firstly because, with few exceptions, they are not discriminating; secondly because they are often dominated by the

manifestations of the underlying condition or associated electrolyte changes; thirdly, (H^+) may vary from 30–60 nm (pH 7·5–7·3) and Pco_2 from 30–60 mmHg without symptoms.

Increased (H^+): twitching, flapping tremor, confusion; proceeding if (H^+) over 80–100 nm (pH 7·1–7·0) to convulsions and coma.

Increased Pco_2: similar, plus tachycardia, hypertension, peripheral vasodilatation, sweating, papilloedema; coma (CO_2 narcosis) if Pco_2 over 100 mmHg

Decreased (H^+) or Pco_2: paraesthesia, tetany, convulsions.

TABLE 9. Normal values for arterial blood

Measurement	Definition	Unit	Normal range
Hydrogen ion activity		Eq/l nm	$36–44 \times 10^{-9}$ 36–44
pH	Neg. $\log_{10}$ H^+ activity		7·44–7·36
Plasma CO_2 content. (Plasma Tco_2)	Vol. CO_2 extractable at existing Pco_2	m-mole/l	21–29
Plasma Bicarbonate Concentration	At existing Pco_2	m-mole/l	20–28
Plasma Standard Bicarbonate concentration	At Pco_2=40 mmHg, and O_2 saturation 100% (True plasma: see Fig. 27)	m-mole/l	21–27
CO_2 Pressure (Pco_2)		mmHg	36–44
Base Excess	Base concentration as measured by titration to pH 7·4 at Pco_2 40	m-mole/l whole blood	$-3–+3$
Whole Blood Buffer (Buffer Base) Concentration	The sum of concentrations of the buffer anions of whole blood bicarbonate, plasma proteins, haemoglobin	m-mole	42–55

3. *Altered respiration*

Of most value in metabolic acidosis and respiratory alkalosis when ventilation is increased ('air hunger').

Of less value in metabolic alkalosis and respiratory acidosis because: firstly, normal breathing is so unobtrusive that reduction is difficult to detect; secondly, underventilation is uncommon in metabolic alkalosis (p. 211); thirdly, in respiratory acidosis the breathing is usually disturbed by deranged pulmonary function: total ventilation may be normal or increased but much of it is wasted on dead space so that alveolar ventilation is decreased (Chapter 3).

TABLE 9.—*continued*

Changes in Disease		Remarks
Increased	Decreased	
Acidaemia > 70 severe	Alkalaemia < 30 severe	
Alkalaemia > 7·55 severe	Acidaemia < 7·15 severe	
Primarily in metab. alkalosis > 36 severe. Secondarily in respirat. acidosis	Primarily in metab. acidosis < 12 severe. Secondarily in respirat. alkalosis	Venous blood taken without stagnation 1–2 m-mole/l. greater
Resp. Acidosis > 90 severe	Resp. Alkalosis < 20 severe	If lungs healthy, alveolar P_{CO_2} = arterial P_{CO_2} (p. 127). Rebreathing methods (p. 131) can be used for most clinical purposes
Metab. Alkalosis	Metab. Acidosis	Normal range and severity of disturbance depend on blood Hb. concentration and saturation. Negative values may be called 'base deficit'

4. *Urinary reaction*

Urine acid (pH less than 7·4, usually less than 6·0) in metabolic and respiratory acidosis.

Urine alkaline (pH greater than 7·4) in acute respiratory alkalosis but may be acid if chronic because urinary reaction then depends chiefly on the diet and metabolism. Urine may be alkaline in metabolic alkalosis but usually not, because inappropriately acid urine is the cause (e.g. in K^+ depletion, p. 14).

ROUTINE METHODS

Venous plasma $[HCO_3^-]$ or standard $[HCO_3^-]$.
Mixed venous P_{CO_2} by rebreathing method.
(H^+) by calculation from these.

Also: Plasma electrolytes for evidence of associated or causative conditions: $[K^+] + [Na^+] - [Cl^- + HCO_3^-]$ indicating presence or absence of abnormal ions.

SPECIAL TECHNIQUES

pH by glass electrode.
Astrup method with arterialized capillary blood gives P_{CO_2} pH, standard bicarbonate, base excess (p. 215).

Also; Blood for abnormal radicals: ketones; lactate, salicylate.
Tests for renal capacity to acidify urine.
Respiratory function tests.

Intracellular (H^+). There is as yet no easy way of estimating intracellular (H^+) but the use of organic amine buffers seems promising. The intracellular concentration of these and their degree of dissociation can be measured. The mean pH or (H^+) can then be calculated from the dissociation constant. This is, in principle, the same procedure as the estimation of (H^+) from knowledge of the total CO_2 content and the $[HCO_3^-]$. When applied to the whole body the directional changes are probably more informative than the actual values and then overwhelmingly represent the intracellular changes in muscle because the bulk of muscle is so great.

References

KAUFMAN H.E. & ROSEN S.W. (1965) Clinical Acid-base Regulation—the Bronsted Schema. *Surg. Gynec. Obstet.*, 103, 101–12.
DAVENPORT H.W. (1958) *The A.B.C. of Acid-Base Chemistry* (4th ed.) Chicago, University of Chicago Press.

WADDELL W.J. & BATES R.G. (1969) Intracellular pH. *Physiol. Rev.* 49, 285–329.
ATKINS E.L. (1969) Assessment of acid-base disorders. A practical approach and review. *Canad. med. Ass. J.* 100, 992–8.
SIGGAARD ANDERSON J. (1963) The acid-base status of the blood. *Scand. J. Clin. Lab. Invest.* 15, Suppl. 70.
Current Concepts of Acid-base Measurement. *Ann.N. Y. Acad. Sci.* 133, 1–274 (1966).

6

Formed Elements of Blood and Haemostasis

RED CELLS

Normal function

The function of the red cells is to provide an efficient exchange of gases between tissues and environment. Animals low in the phylogenetic scale have haemoglobin or other oxygen carrying compounds free in solution in the plasma. During evolutionary development, haemoglobin has become enclosed within cells and in this way more haemoglobin can be carried per unit volume of blood without a concomitant rise in blood viscosity.

RED CELL PRODUCTION

In common with most other tissues, there is a continual turnover of red cells and the rate of production is closely controlled. Red cells are produced outside the marrow sinusoids and they enter the circulation by diapedesis through the sinusoid walls. Maturation of red cells is thought to take place as follows. The existence of a multipotential stem cell has been postulated although this has never been satisfactorily defined microscopically; this stem cell divides and one of the cells remains in a primitive condition while the other develops into a proerythroblast. Iron enters the cell at this stage, which is followed by three mitotic divisions, when the normoblast stage is reached. No further division occurs, but maturation of the cells proceeds to the reticulocyte stage with formation of haemoglobin and loss of the nucleus.

The reticulocyte retains some ribosenucleic acid (RNA) which can be precipitated and stained as reticulin granules with cresyl blue. Development from primitive cell to the reticulocyte probably takes about 4 days. Approximately 50 per cent of the total body content of reticulocytes are present in the marrow at any given time. The remainder are present in the circulation, and take approximately 1–2 days to mature into adult cells.

The rate of red cell production is approximately 15–20 ml red cells each day (0·25 ml/kg body weight). This maintains the haematocrit at approximately 45 per cent. This value of the haematocrit represents the optimum for the efficient delivery of oxyhaemoglobin to the tissues. Lower values reduce oxygen delivery because of inadequate haemoglobin concentration, and higher values decrease blood flow because the blood becomes more viscous. The basic controlling factor in the rate of red cell production has not yet been identified, but there is considerable circumstantial evidence that production is dependent on tissue oxygen tension which regulates the secretion of erythropoietin. This hormone is probably formed in the juxtaglomerular cells of the kidney. Erythropoietin stimulates proerythroblast division and increases the rate of differentiation of the multipotential stem cell.

The long-recognized affect of cobalt on stimulating erythropoiesis is probably the result of stimulation of erythropoietin production. Large doses of testosterone also increase erythropoietin secretion. In addition, hormones from the gonads and thyroid have an indirect effect on red cell production by setting the level of tissue oxygen needs. Failure of secretion from these glands thus leads to a reduction in red cell mass.

Studies on the excretion of ^{15}N-labelled urobilinogen after feeding ^{15}N-glycine suggest that some 10–15 per cent of red cells produced by the marrow are destroyed *in situ* or are destroyed very shortly after reaching the circulation.

Red cell life span

The life span of red cells has been studied in man either by crosstransfusion experiments in which the survival of transfused cells has been followed by means of blood group antigens (Ashby technique), or by labelling a subject's own cells with radioactive isotopes. The evidence indicates that red cells are delivered to the circulation with a potential life span of approximately 120 days. However, there is also some random destruction of cells irrespective of age. The rate of random destruction is small, being of the order of 0·1 per cent of the total red cell mass per day, compared to 0·85 per cent destroyed on reaching the end of the life span. The normal adult destroys between 15 and 20 ml of red cells each day.

Red cells do not lyse in the circulation but are removed intact by the reticuloendothelial system. Phagocytosis may be due to structural or biochemical changes at the red cell surface. The most favoured hypothesis is that the red cell is delivered to the circulation with a fixed quantity of enzymes which are concerned with energy metabolism and that the concentration of one or more of these enzymes slowly falls so that after approximately 120 days the energy required to maintain the normal constitution of the red cell surface becomes insufficient. Several enzymes concerned with glucose metabolism have been found to decline during red cell ageing but as yet there is no evidence that energy production is critically reduced. The spleen is usually said to be the main site of normal red cell destruction but the evidence for this is meagre and it is possible that the bone marrow and liver are as important.

The rate of red cell destruction is predetermined by the biochemical constitution of the cell and therefore red cell volume is controlled by adjustments in the rate of production. The normal red cell volume is maintained at 30 ml/kg in men and 25 ml/kg in women, or approximately 2000 ml for a 70 kg man. The total blood volume is about 75 and 65 ml/kg in men and women respectively. It should be noted that the body haematocrit, that is, the ratio of red cell volume to total blood volume is not the same as the venous haematocrit but is lower by a factor of 0·91. This results from the fact that in the small vessels such as arterioles and capillaries the axial streaming of red cells results in a relatively great proportion of plasma to red cells compared to that found in the venous blood.

ENERGY SOURCES AND METABOLISM (Fig. 28)
The mature red cell requires energy for its continued survival in the circulation and this is obtained from the breakdown of glucose. Approximately 90 per cent of the metabolism proceeds along the non-oxidative Embden–Meyerhof pathway via phosphorylated glucose intermediates to pyruvic acid (p. 472) and energy is transferred through adenosine triphosphate (ATP) and nicotinamide adenine dinucleotide (NADH) (Fig. 28). The remaining 10 per cent of the glucose metabolism is oxidative and proceeds along the pentose phosphate pathway from the first intermediate (glucose-6-phosphate) of the non-oxidative pathway. The enzyme involved in this initial step is glucose-6-phosphate dehydrogenase. Pentose phosphates and CO_2 are produced and the former fed back into the Embden–Meyerhof pathway. The pentose mono-phosphate pathway produces the energy-rich compound, reduced nicotinamide adenine dinucleotide phosphate (NADPH). Energy is necessary for the maintenance of surface structure and cell shape, for lipid turnover and for the sodium and potassium pumps.

One of the functions of NADPH is to maintain the red cell content of reduced glutathione (GSH) which is a store of energy. The 3 compounds

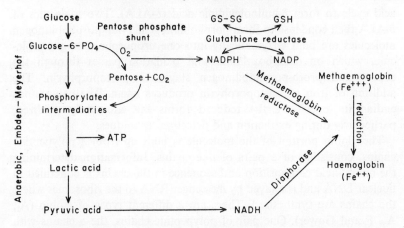

FIGURE 28. *Schematic diagram for the transfer of energy from glucose for the maintenance of haemoglobin and enzymes in the reduced state.*

NADH, NADPH and GSH all have a high reductive capacity and they play an essential role in the maintenance of haemoglobin in the reduced form assisting by in the enzymatic conversion of methaemoglobin (ferric ion) to haemoglobin (ferrous ion). Two enzymes have been isolated which carry out this conversion, methaemoglobin reductase (NADPH dependent) and diaphorase (NADH dependent). The NADPH-dependent pathway is probably the more important and hence the maintenance of the oxygen-carrying capacity of the red cell is dependent on the oxidative catabolism of glucose via the pentose phosphate pathway. Although this pathway represents only about 10 per cent of the total glucose metabolism under normal conditions, the entrance of oxidants such as drugs (page 234) into the red cell stimulates metabolism along this pathway and hence maintains a normal supply of NADPH.

HAEMOGLOBIN

The marrow produces approximately 7 g of haemoglobin each day. The haemoglobin molecule contains 4 haem molecules, each of which lies in surface indentations of one of the 4 polypeptide chains of globin. Synthesis of both haem and globin proceeds simultaneously in the RNA-rich normoblast. Haem is produced in mitochondria and the essential steps in its synthesis are as follows:

Haem synthesis starts with the condensation of 8 molecules of the amino-acid glycine and 8 of succinate obtained from the Krebs citric acid cycle to form δ-aminolevulinic acid (δ-ALA). Two molecules of δ-ALA then condense to form porphobilinogen. Four porphobilinogen molecules are built enzymatically into one uroporphobilinogen molecule, which on decarboxylation and oxidation passes through the copro- and proto-porphobilinogen stages to protoporphyrin. The addition of iron to protoporphyrin produces haem. The compounds ending in 'ogen' are the reduced forms but are easily oxidized, particularly during extraction and detection techniques.

The globin portion of the molecule is built up from 4 polypeptide chains, consisting of 2 pairs of like chains. Information determining the amino-acid composition and sequence in the chains is contained in nuclear DNA and is relayed by messenger RNA to the ribosomes where the chains are synthesized. There are 4 different types of globin (A_1, A_2, F and Gower). One pair of polypeptide chains, the α chains with 141 amino-acids, is common to all 4 globins, but the other pair of chains is different in each case. Thus haemoglobin A (97 per cent of the total Hb in an adult) consists of two α chains and two β chains (146 amino-acids), i.e. $\alpha_2\beta_2$. Haemoglobin A_2 (3 per cent of the total) has δ chains ($\alpha_2\delta_2$). Haemoglobin F has γ chains ($\alpha_2\gamma_2$). These β, γ and δ chains differ in their amino-acid sequences. Until 3 months of intrauterine life, the foetus contains haemoglobin Gower ($\alpha_2\epsilon_2$ and ϵ_4) which is then replaced by Hb F. At birth 70–90 per cent of the haemoglobin is F, but new cells produced after birth contain Hb A so that the percentage of F is reduced to 10 per cent or less by 4 months; small amounts (0·5–1 per cent) can be detected in some children up to 10 years. It is still debated whether very small amounts (less than 0·5 per cent) persist throughout adult life. The difficulty lies in the accurate determination of Hb F at this low concentration.

One gene locus (cistron) on the chromosomes is responsible for the production of one polypeptide chain. Thus each cell contains 2 cistrons for the α chains, 2 for the β chains and so on. Mutations may be present in either one or both cistrons, giving rise to the heterozygous or homozygous state. Cistrons for the polypeptide chains are present on autosomal chromosomes and inheritance is not sex-linked.

ACCESSORY FACTORS IN RED CELL PRODUCTION
The cobalamins (Vitamin B_{12}) and intrinsic factor
The cobalamins are composed of (1) a ring structure closely related to the porphyrin ring of haem in which a cobalt atom replaces iron, (2) a nucleotide moeity, (3) a CN group (cyanocobalamin) or other

groups such as OH, (hydroxycobalamin) attached to the cobalt atom. These are the stable but inactive forms of the vitamin and they must be converted to the active coenzyme forms (cobamides) which have a deoxyadenosyl group attached to the cobalt. All animal tissues require vitamin B_{12}. Recent evidence on its function suggests that it has isomerase activity, i.e. the transfer of H from one carbon atom to an adjacent carbon atom. It is also concerned in the synthesis of methionine, a pathway which involves folic acid. Vitamin B_{12} accepts a methyl group from 5-methyl-H_4-folate and transfers it to homocysteine to form methionine. Vitamin B_{12} is also concerned in the conversion of nucleotides to deoxynucleotides and hence in the production of DNA; this activity is linked with the observation that there is an altered DNA/RNA ratio in pernicious anaemia. Vitamin B_{12} is synthesized exclusively by micro-organisms and is only found in bacteria and animal tissues, usually combined with protein. The intake is variable, about 1–100 μg each day. The minimum daily requirement is of the order of 1·0 μg.

Intrinsic factor (IF) is probably a mucoprotein secreted by the peptic cells of the fundus and body of the stomach. It has not been isolated and its concentration in gastric juice can only be estimated in terms of its binding capacity for B_{12} (one unit of IF is defined as that which will bind 1 mμg of B_{12}). Only about 1000 units, which is only 1–2 per cent of the normal daily secretion are required for the absorption of B_{12}.

The function of intrinsic factor is to bind the B_{12} in the food. The intrinsic factor-B_{12} complex is then adsorbed onto specific sites on mucosal cells of the distal half of the ileum, the chief site of absorption. The method of transfer of B_{12} across the gut wall is not known. Absorption is slow as B_{12} does not appear in the plasma until 4 hours after oral intake and reaches a peak at 8–12 hr. Normal plasma levels of B_{12} vary between 100 and 900 $\mu\mu$g/ml and estimation of this level is considered to be an accurate guide to body stores. The total body content of B_{12} is approximately 4 mg; the liver stores 1 mg, which has a biological half-life of about 1 year. There is no metabolic breakdown of vitamin B_{12} and the main loss is through desquamation of gut endothelium; only traces of B_{12} are lost in the urine (0–270 $\mu\mu$g/day). Approximately 0·2–0·3 per cent of the total body B_{12} is lost each day. At this rate of loss, it takes 2–3 years for the B_{12} content to be reduced to 10 per cent of its original level, if intake is drastically reduced. Vitamin B_{12} is also secreted in the bile (3–7 μg each day) but all except 1 μg of this is reabsorbed.

Folate compounds

The term 'folate' refers to those compounds which are related to pteroylglutamic acid (folic acid). Pteroylglutamic acid consists of a pteridine group linked through *p*-aminobenzoic acid to glutamic acid. The active derivatives of pteroylglutamic acid are in the reduced form known as tetrahydrofolates, with 4 H atoms attached to the pteridine ring. The several active derivatives contain different single carbon units, the most important being formyl (—CHO), methyl (—CH$_3$) and methenyl (=CH—), and folates act as coenzymes by transferring these single carbon units in the synthesis of purines, pyrimidines and methionine, and in the degradation of histidine. Thus folate compounds assist in the insertion of a single carbon atom unit in the final stage of purine ring synthesis, bring about methylation of uracil to give thymine (5—CH$_3$ uracil) and methylate homocysteine to give methionine. Folate compounds are therefore concerned, like vitamin B$_{12}$, with both nucleic acid and methionine synthesis. It is these relationships which account for the fact that deficiency of either gives the same megaloblastic changes in the marrow.

Folates are synthesized by plants and certain micro-organisms. Those micro-organisms which synthesize folate are sensitive to sulphonamides which block folic acid synthesis by competitive inhibition with *p*-amino-benzoic acid. Vertebrates require preformed folates and hence are not affected by sulphonamides. The minimum daily requirement is 50–200 μg, and the average diet contains up to 2000 μg. Food folate is in conjugated form and only part of this is available for absorption. Folates are absorbed in the jejunum and transferred to the plasma where folate levels are 5–16 ng/ml and thence to the liver where storage occurs (total liver content is 4–6 mg; total body content, 6–10 mg).

The ultimate fate of folate compounds is not yet known in detail. The greatest loss results from metabolic destruction; approximately 5 μg/day is lost in the urine. Organisms in the large gut synthesize folates so that six times as much folate is excreted in the faeces as is ingested, but this source is not available to the body.

The main storage form of folates is tetrahydrofolate. Stores are not large in relation to turnover and 2 per cent of the total body folate may be lost each day. Depletion of body stores can thus occur in 3–4 months when intake is greatly reduced.

IRON METABOLISM

Iron is present in all tissues of the body. Every cell contains small quantities in the haem group of the respiratory enzymes. The highest concentration of iron is found in the red cells, containing approximately 2 g in a normal adult (1 ml of red cells contains approximately 1 mg Fe). A small amount (0·15 g) is present as myoglobin and the remainder is present as stores (approximately 1 g) in the liver, bone marrow and spleen.

Free Fe ions in solution are toxic as they cause denaturation of proteins and enzymes. Thus iron is only found in the body attached to proteins which are able to bind it without becoming denatured. Transport of iron in the plasma is by attachment to the protein transferrin. Iron is stored within the cells of the reticuloendothelial system either as ferritin, which is a combination of iron and the protein apoferritin, or as haemosiderin; the nature of the protein in this latter compound has not yet been defined. The cells involved in storage are the reticulum cells of the bone marrow and spleen, and the Kupfer cells of the liver. Haemosiderin appears as golden-brown granules in the reticulum cells of marrow aspirates but ferritin is water-soluble and is thus removed during the normal preparation of histological sections. Iron is released from both ferritin and haemosiderin in response to need. Iron is also present as ferritin in red cell precursors, prior to its incorporation into haem. It can be demonstrated there as blue-staining granules by the Prussian-blue reaction. Nucleated cells showing these granules are known as sideroblasts and non-nucleated cells as siderocytes.

There is a continuous turnover of iron in the body. The main metabolic pathway is derived from the destruction of red cells (approximately 20 ml/day) releasing 20 mg of iron, which is transported in the plasma from the cells of the reticuloendothelial system to the red cell precursors. A further 10 mg of iron passes through the plasma each day. This is the resultant of iron absorption, iron transport to and from stores, and metabolism of iron in myoglobin and the respiratory enzymes.

There is approximately 10–20 mg of protein-bound iron in an average daily diet. Approximately 10 per cent of this iron is absorbed by normal people, although there is considerable variation depending on the source of the iron. Organic iron is less well absorbed than inorganic, and iron in vegetables is less well absorbed than that from animals. Iron is split from protein in the stomach, converted to the ferrous form by reducing agents and absorbed by the duodenum and jejunum. Hydrochloric acid is not necessary for absorption. The body content of iron is regulated by control of absorption but the mechanisms involved are at present unknown. It has been suggested that the iron absorbed into the mucosal cells of the gut is bound to apoferritin; then, depending on the total body content, the iron is either transported into the plasma or remains in the cell to be lost by exfoliation. There is no specific excretory mechanism for iron but it is continuously lost from the body owing to desquamation of epithelium, endothelium, nails and hair. The amount lost in this way is approximately 1 mg/day. Loss through menstruation also amounts to an average of 1 mg/day, (approximately 30 ml of cells with each period). Pregnancy requires an extra 250 mg; the child requires 300 mg and a further 200 mg is lost at parturition, but approximately 250 mg is saved through 9 months of amenorrhea. Loss through lactation is also approximately 1 mg/day. Thus throughout the child bearing period, women lose about 2 mg/day, that is 1 mg more than men. As absorption of iron normally is only 1–2 mg/day it is not surprising that iron deficiency anaemia is so common in women in the child-bearing period.

The iron stores in the liver (approximately 100 mg) of the newborn are deposited in the last month of intrauterine life so that prematurity leads to reduced iron stores. Furthermore, both human and cow's milk are poor in iron. Thus iron deficiency anaemia is common in children aged 1–3 years.

BLOOD GROUPS

The biochemical nature and configuration of the red cell surface is not known but probably consists of polysaccharides, proteins and lipids. There is considerable variation between individuals in the nature of these biochemical compounds. This variation has come to light, not from a biochemical analysis of red cells, but from the fact that transfusion of cells with a particular biochemical substance to a person lacking that substance gives rise to antibody production. From an analysis of the specificity of these antibodies, variation is known to occur at 12 different locations on the cell surface, the biochemical configuration at each of the locations being controlled by 12 different sets of genes, each set of genes being present on a different chromosome. The 12 different blood group systems are thus manifestations of the variations in the genetic material. More than 50 substances at the red cell surface are known to vary, and each has given rise to difficulties in blood transfusion. It is fortunate that only 3 of the substances, A and B of the ABO system and D of the Rhesus system, commonly give rise to antibody production. The A and B substances, which are polysaccharides, are also present in food and bacteria and their absorption gives rise to anti-A or anti-B in those people who lack the antigen themselves. D substance (also known as the Rh substance) is not present in food or bacteria and hence anti-D is not found in Rh-negative people (those with 'd' substance), but over half the number of Rh-negative people transfused with 5 ml or more of Rh-positive blood will develop anti-D.

Abnormal function

The abnormalities found in the physiology of the red cell can be classified into 3 groups: (1) abnormalities of production and destruction, (2) abnormalities in haemoglobin structure, and (3) abnormalities in the energy-producing systems necessary for the maintenance of viability.

By convention, the term anaemia refers to a reduction of the haemoglobin concentration below the normal levels, and not to any changes in total red cell volume. Although there is usually a direct relationship between these two values, this is not always the case. For instance, owing to the increase in plasma volume often seen in pregnancy, it is possible for the haemoglobin concentration to be reduced while the red cell mass is raised above the usual values for the individual. No precise value for the normal level of haemoglobin can be given owing to the considerable variation found between healthy people; arbitrary lower limits must therefore be taken and values commonly used are given on page 267.

Anaemia is the result of an imbalance between the rate of red cell production and the rate of their disappearance from the circulation. Functional disorders of these two aspects will be examined separately.

RED CELL PRODUCTION:
HYPOPLASIA AND HYPERPLASIA
In hypoplasia of the bone marrow, the extent of the reduction of marrow activity may vary from only a small diminution to almost complete cessation of activity. When marrow hyperplasia is present both the number of differentiating cells per unit volume and the total volume of marrow tissue are increased. Marrow volume is normally about 10 per cent of that of the blood volume but an increase of up to 50 per cent can take place. However, marrow hyperplasia does not always result in a concomitant increase in the rate of supply of red cells into the circulation. In certain diseases (notably pernicious anaemia and thalassaemia) a large proportion of the red cells are defective and are either destroyed in the marrow, or, if they reach the circulation, do not survive for more than a few minutes. Thus, a

differentiation must be made between total erythropoiesis and *effective* erythropoiesis.

The immediate response of the marrow to anaemia is the release of red cell precursors, usually reticulocytes, but occasionally nucleated cells. Following this, the total rate of production increases and after long-standing stimulation can reach 60–160 ml/day, that is 4–8 times the normal rate. Thus a healthy marrow can compensate for a considerable shortening of red cell survival in the peripheral circulation. On the other hand, when the production of viable red cells is impaired by an abnormality such as folate or vitamin B_{12} deficiency or by the production of an abnormal haemoglobin, erythropoiesis is ineffective and there is destruction of red cells within the marrow. Despite a 4–8-fold increase in total marrow activity, effective production of viable cells delivered to the circulation may be only normal or perhaps twice normal.

RED CELL DESTRUCTION

Normally, red cells are destroyed after 120 days on reaching the end of their life-span. When abnormal destruction takes place the cells are usually destroyed at random irrespective of their age. Thus, if a sample of cells from a patient with haemolytic anaemia is labelled with radioactive chromium (^{51}Cr) and their survival followed, it is usually found that the survival curve is exponential, i.e., a constant percentage of those cells remaining in the circulation is removed each day. In certain diseases such as sickle cell disease or paroxysmal nocturnal haemoglobinuria, two populations of cells are found: a population which is destroyed quickly, and a population with a longer mean cell life. The average red cell life span may be reduced to 20–30 days in mild cases of haemolytic anaemia, whatever the cause i.e. about $\frac{1}{4}$ to $\frac{1}{6}$ normal. This is about the maximum that can be compensated for by an increase in the rate of production by the marrow; in severe cases of haemolytic anaemia the average life span may be only 5 days.

Apart from haemorrhage, red cells are usually removed from the circulation by phagocytosis and only occasionally by intravascular lysis. Phagocytosis in the spleen, liver and bone marrow can remove as much as 20 per cent of the total red cell mass each day, but the relative part played by each of these organs in various diseases is not well-defined. An indication of the site of destruction can be obtained by labelling the cells with ^{51}Cr and determining the site of ^{51}Cr accumulation by surface counting. ^{51}Cr is deposited mainly in the spleen in hereditary spherocytosis, elliptocytosis, in children with Hb–S disease and in certain acquired haemolytic anaemias. In adults with Hb–S disease liver accumulation of ^{51}Cr-labelled cells is found. In other patients with acquired haemolytic anaemia and some patients with non-spherocytic haemolytic anaemia, ^{51}Cr accumulates in both organs, but most patients with the non-spherocytic type and those with paroxysmal nocturnal haemoglobinuria show no accumulation in either organ. It is possible that the marrow plays a predominant role in the destruction of red cells in some of these latter diseases.

Intravascular lysis is not common, but is usually found after incompatible transfusions involving complement-binding antibodies (usually anti-A or anti-B), in paroxysmal nocturnal haemoglobinuria, and in the haemoglobinuria following exercise (march haemoglobinuria, where it may be due in part to damage to red cells in the soles of the feet). Intravascular lysis has also been produced by plastic heart valves, where it is due to mechanical damage. The role of antibodies in haemolytic anaemia is discussed on page 289.

Haemolytic disease of the newborn.
Approximately 1 in 20 of all Rh-negative mothers who give birth to an Rh-positive child subsequently produce anti-D. This is the result of a leakage of Rh-positive cells into the maternal circulation: this occurs to a small extent during the last trimester, but particularly during parturition when 0·2 ml or more of foetal cells may cross the placental barrier. The disease is thus not seen with the firstborn (unless the mother has been previously transfused with Rh-positive blood) but in subsequent pregnancies anti-D crosses the placenta and brings about destruction of the foetal cells, if these are Rh-positive. The passive injection of anti-D into the Rh-negative mother within 36 hours of giving birth to an Rh-positive child will prevent her from actively producing anti-D. The injected anti-D is metabolized by the time of the next pregnancy. The mechanism of this action is unknown; it has been suggested that the passively administered anti-D prevents the foetal cells reaching the antibody-producing organs.

Anti-A can also cause haemolytic disease of the newborn in a group O mother giving birth to group A infant. The disease is almost invariably mild.

ABNORMAL ENERGY METABOLISM
Glucose-6-phosphate dehydrogenase (G-6PD) deficiency
This is an inherited defect of intermediate dominance linked to the X chromosome. Males are hemizygous (X) Y (where (X) is the abnormal

chromosome) and have approximately 10 per cent of the normal level of G-6PD; most females are also heterozygous, (X)X, but because of the presence of 1 normal X chromosome, they usually only have a small reduction in G-6PD levels. Homozygous females (X) (X) are rare but have enzyme levels similar to males. The abnormality is widely distributed, the incidence varying from 60 per cent in Kurdish Jews to less than 1 per cent in Caucasians.

When G-6PD concentration is reduced to 10 per cent of the normal level the oxidative pentose phosphate pathway becomes defective, resulting in a lowered content of NADPH. As NADPH is the coenzyme for glutathione reductase, there is a consequent reduction in cell GSH. When NADPH and GSH are deficient the entrance of oxidizing compounds into the cell causes damage to proteins and consequent cell destruction. Thus haemoglobin is first oxidized to methaemoglobin, followed by oxidation of the globin portion of the molecule (especially the —SH, groups) with resultant precipitation of haemoglobin as Heinz bodies. Usually G-6PD deficiency is benign, the only abnormality being a 25 per cent reduction in the lifespan of the red cells, but there are over 40 drugs which are known to accentuate G-6PD deficiency. The most important are primaquine and quinine, some sulphonamides, the nitrofurans, aspirin and phenacetin. Certain bacteria and viruses (bacterial pneumonias, infectious hepatitis, viral respiratory infection and infectious mononucleosis) and the Fava bean also have the same action. Some of these agents may react with oxyhaemoglobin to form hydrogen peroxide which causes a rapid fall in the already depressed levels of NADPH and GSH. Red cells are destroyed and the haemoglobin concentration falls. The older red cells, already depleted of enzyme (p. 223), are mainly destroyed, so that after 7–10 days the haemoglobin level ceases to fall and partial recovery may occur despite continuation of the drug. The severity of the anaemia depends on the nature and concentration of the drug and on the extent of the pre-existing G-6PD deficiency.

An almost complete absence of G-6PD is responsible for some of the cases classified as congenital non-spherocytic haemolytic anaemia.

Methaemoglobin reductase and diaphorase deficiency are the cause of diseases grouped as *hereditary methaemoglobinaemia*; in these conditions the rate of conversion of methaemoglobin to reduced haemoglobin is inadequate (page 225). Methylene blue and ascorbic acid are both able to reduce methaemoglobin without the presence of the enzymes.

ABNORMAL HAEMOGLOBIN

Over 36 abnormal haemoglobins have now been described. These are the result of a mutation in a cistron leading to substitution of an amino-acid in either the α- or β-chains of haemoglobin. Abnormal haemoglobins can only be detected by changes in their electrophoretic properties. Thus only those mutations which change the surface charge of the molecule can be detected, and there may be many other mutations of which we are unaware because the substituted amino-acid does not affect total charge. In the heterozygous state all haemoglobin abnormalities are harmless, with the exception of haemoglobin S which may give rise to disease following extreme anoxia. In the homozygous state, Hb S gives the most severe disease and haemoglobins C and E (β-chain defect), and D (α-chain defect) give rise to only a moderate reduction in haemoglobin.

Haemoglobins and sickle-cell disease

An uncharged valine molecule is substituted for a negatively-charged glutamic acid in the β-chain. This single alteration causes Hb–S molecules to form polymers or 'tactoid' bodies when oxygen tension is reduced with a resultant change in shape of the red cell. In homozygous SS disease, polymer formation occurs at the oxygen tension of normal venous blood, whereas in the heterozygous SA disease polymer formation does not occur until the haemoglobin oxygen saturation falls below 40 per cent. The formation of haemoglobin polymers not only leads to sickling but also increases the ridigity of the red cell. The viscosity of whole blood therefore rises and it has been suggested that this change is the cause of the infarcts which characterize the disease. However, patients with Hb-SS disease are always anaemic and the viscosity of Hb-SS blood with a haematocrit of 25 per cent is the same as that of normal blood with a haematocrit of 45 per cent. It is perhaps more likely that the infarcts result from the blocking of small capillaries by rigid sickled cells which leads to a damming up of other cells behind them. Delay in passage through the capillaries must also play a part as sickling takes 2–3 min to appear *in vitro* on exposure to low oxygen tensions and passage through the capillaries is normally of the order of 5 sec. Prolonged stagnation of cells certainly occurs in the spleen; studies with ^{51}Cr-labelled cells have shown sequestration in that organ and splenic puncture has demonstrated that most red cells in the spleen are sickled, many of them irreversibly.

The red cells are destroyed by phagocytosis. In children this may occur in the spleen, but in adult life the spleen is usually destroyed by infarction, so that destruction is presumably either in the liver or bone marrow. The changes on the surface of the red cells which lead to phagocytosis are not known. A small proportion of cells have a decreased resistance to osmotic lysis and also to mechanical stress *in vitro*, but it is not known whether either of these mechanisms play a part *in vivo*.

The severity of the anaemia is approximately proportional to the amount of Hb-S present. Homozygous SS disease is the most severe, and the Hb-S content is 80–100 per cent, the remainder being Hb–F. The disease does not manifest itself in the immediate post-natal period because there is still a high concentration of Hb-F in the circulation. Hb-S is also seen in association with other abnormal haemoglobins which modify the severity of the anaemia. Thus, sickle-cell-thalassaemia, SF, has 67–82 per cent Hb-S and is less severe than SS disease; the SC combination produces only 50 per cent Hb-S and is milder still, although there is considerable overlap in extent of the anaemia in the different types. Sickle-cell trait (SA) does not give rise to anaemia unless there is a severe lowering of oxygen tension.

Haemoglobins C, D, and E
When these abnormalities are found in the homozygous state there is some shortening of the red cell life span. The haemoglobin concentration may also be reduced, but not below 10 g/100 ml. Target cells are a marked feature of the peripheral blood. The low red cell haemoglobin content results in flattening of the cells. Most examples of these abnormalities are found as a result of the routine screening of red cells for abnormal haemoglobins.

Abnormal haemoglobins with defective
oxygen-carrying capacity
A number of abnormal haemoglobins have been found in which the oxygen carrying capacity is impaired. The haemoglobins M are a group in which the oxidation product, methaemoglobin, is not easily reduced by the normal cell methaemoglobin reductase, thus causing cyanosis. Other haemoglobins have been described where there is an abnormally high or low affinity for oxygen. In the latter case, cyanosis also results (haemoglobin Kansas).

Unstable haemoglobins
A number of congenital nonspherocytic haemolytic anaemias of variable severity are due to the presence of abnormal haemoglobins

(haemoglobins Koln, St. Mary's, Seattle, Ube-1, Zurich and 'heat unstable haemoglobins') which are easily oxidized and denatured within the cells. The disease is present from the time of changeover from foetal to adult haemoglobin and the instability of the haemoglobin is manifested by the presence of Heinz bodies (page 250) and by the rapid appearance of methaemoglobin on *in vitro* incubation without glucose.

Thalassaemia
The basic lesion of thalassaemia is an inability to produce an adequate amount of either α- or β-chains for the formation of adult haemoglobin A, the diseases being known as α-chain and β-chain thalassaemia respectively. There is only a partial gene suppression so that some production of these chains continues; the genetic defect probably causes an alteration in messenger RNA and this results in the failure of chain production on the ribosomes.

The commonest form is β-chain thalassaemia, resulting in a deficiency of haemoglobin A $(\alpha_2\beta_2)$; the α-chains on their own are unstable and predispose to early destruction of the red cells. There is a compensatory increase in the other two haemoglobins, haemoglobin A_2 $(\alpha_2\delta_2)$ and haemoglobin F $(\alpha_2\gamma_2)$. In the homozygous state compensatory production of these haemoglobins is inadequate and the patients die in childhood. In the heterozygous state, sufficient β-chains are usually produced to maintain the haemoglobin concentration at 10 to 12 g/100 ml.

In α-chain thalassaemia there is an inability to form sufficient α-chains, which are common to the 3 types of haemoglobin A_1, A_2 and F. In the homozygous state, production of α-chains is reduced to such an extent that it is incompatible with life and the child is still-born. In the heterozygous state, the normal gene can bring about adequate production of α-chains and adults are healthy and usually haematologically normal.

Haemoglobin H disease is a variant of α-thalassaemia in which there are 2 abnormalities, 1 parent supplying the α-thalassaemia gene and the other an unknown silent gene which is undetectable on its own. There is a deficiency in the production of α-chains, resulting in a compensatory production of β- and γ-chains which combine to form tetramers. Thus in infancy, haemoglobin Bart's (γ_4) is formed and in adults haemoglobin H (β_4). These tetramer haemoglobins are unstable and are more easily oxidized to methaemoglobin than haemoglobin A. Inclusion bodies can thus be readily produced *in vitro*. Haemoglobin H binds oxygen tightly and is useless as an O_2 carrier. Patients with this disease have only a mild anaemia and the haemoglobin H content of the cells ranges from 1 to 40 per cent.

Where there is insufficient haemoglobin synthesis resulting from any of these genetic abnormalities, the red cells in the peripheral blood are abnormally thin. Their survival in the circulation is shortened and there is considerable amount of ineffective erythropoiesis in the marrow.

B_{12} DEFICIENCY

There are 3 main causes of deficiency. (1) *Inadequate diet.* This is rare, but may occur in strict vegetarians, and takes 10 to 20 years to develop. (2) *Diversion of* B_{12} *in the gut. Diphylobothrium latum* and intestinal bacteria utilize B_{12} and hence the presence of this tape worm or of a diverticulum or blind loop giving rise to sepsis in the ileum results in the diversion of B_{12} away from the intestinal mucosa. (3) *Failure of absorption mechanisms*, due either to failure to secrete intrinsic factor (pernicious anaemia, gastrectomy) or to functional failure of the gut wall, as in steatorrhoea.

Pernicious anaemia is the result of a failure of the gastric mucosa to secrete sufficient intrinsic factor for the absorption of B_{12}. Gastric atrophy is always found together with a failure to secrete hydrochloric acid so that failure to produce intrinsic factor is probably secondary to a general functional failure of the stomach. Evidence from family studies suggests that the disease is genetically determined and that there is a predisposition to a failure of intrinsic factor secretion which is probably inherited as dominant autosomal factor. There is only a gradual loss of ability to secrete intrinsic factor and as B_{12} absorption is not affected until intrinsic factor secretion is reduced below 1–2 per cent of the amount normally secreted, the disease only manifests itself in the later decades of life. After extensive gastrectomy it takes at least 5 years for the stores to become sufficiently depleted to lead to megaloblastic changes in the marrow. The body content of B_{12} must be reduced to 5–10 per cent of the normal amount before abnormalities appear.

B_{12} deficiency affects all tissues and histological abnormalities are found in endothelial and epithelial cells. Since marrow tissue probably has the highest turnover rate in the body, the disease is most manifest there. There is a failure in the development of red cell precursors accompanied by the characteristic histological changes of megalo-blastosis. Microspectrophotometry has shown that there is an increase in the RNA/DNA ratio and a delay in the disappearance of RNA from the cytoplasm. The rise in marrow erythrocyte/granulocyte ratio, faecal urobilinogen output and plasma iron turnover in pernicious anaemia indicates approximately a three-fold increase in total erythropoietic activity. However, studies on the survival of red cells in the peripheral circulation have shown that not only is the life span shortened but also that, despite the increased marrow activity, the rate of production of viable cells is only normal or less than normal, depending on the stage of the disease. Thus there is a considerable amount of ineffective erythropoiesis with destruction of red cells before they leave the marrow.

A haematological response to $1-3$ μg B_{12}/day is evidence of B_{12} deficiency. Megaloblastic changes of B_{12} deficiency respond temporarily to folic acid administration in doses of 5 mg/day, which is approximately 100 times the minimal daily requirement.

FOLATE DEFICIENCY

The clinical effects of folate deficiency are the result of a failure of the production of nucleic acid. This is chiefly manifested in haemopoietic tissue, but also results in dermatitis, and in gonadal failure, leading to azoospermia and amenorrhoea. Histological changes in the marrow are similar to those seen in B_{12} deficiency. The peripheral blood shows pancytopenia with macrocytes and hypersegmented neutrophils. If iron deficiency is also present, then the morphology of iron deficiency predominates and megaloblastic changes in the marrow may only appear after iron treatment.

The causes of folate deficiency fall into 3 main groups. (1) The diet may be low in folate compounds or there may be malabsorption due to disease of the gut, when folate deficiency is part of a general picture of malabsorption. (2) Deficiency occurs when the requirements for folate are increased and exceed that present in the diet. Approximately 25 per cent of pregnant women in Britain develop folate deficiency if cytological changes in the marrow are used for evaluation; the incidence is higher than this if serum and red cell folate levels are used as criteria for diagnosis. This is the result of increased requirements by the foetus. Megaloblastic anaemia in pregnancy is almost always due to folate deficiency, unless malabsorption is present, when B_{12} deficiency may also occur. The onset of lactation will precipitate deficiency if the dietary intake of folate is only just sufficient to meet daily requirements. Folate deficiency may develop as a result of increased marrow activity in chronic acquired haemolytic anaemia, hereditary spherocytosis and sickle-cell anaemia. It may also be the cause of the aplastic crises seen in these diseases. Finally, both hyperthyroidism and infection increase the demand for folates, which can result in megaloblastic changes in a person whose total body content of folate is already depleted. (3) Deficiency also results from interference with folate metabolism by drugs, such as the folic acid antagonists, (methotrexate, pyrimethamine), anticonvulsants (diphenylhydantoin, barbiturates and pyrimidone) and alcohol (which depresses formylase activity, an enzyme concerned with transfer of formyl groups from folic acid derivatives). Folate deficiency is seen in alcoholics both with and without cirrhosis.

IRON DEFICIENCY

Iron deficiency anaemia is probably one of the commonest diseases in the world; it has been estimated that there are approximately 100 million sufferers. It is usually the result either of poor diet, malabsorption, excessive loss of blood from the intestinal or genital tracts, or of such physiological events as growth and pregnancy. Because of the considerable iron stores, there may be a long delay between cause and effect as anaemia does not develop until iron stores are exhausted. If the loss of iron is 1 mg/day greater than intake, then it takes approximately 6 years before the haemoglobin concentration falls to half the normal value. When iron stores are almost depleted, the plasma iron begins to fall and in severe depletion falls below 20 μg/ml. The total iron binding capacity of the plasma is consistently increased (to 350–450 μg/100 ml). At this stage, the marrow is hyperplastic (erythroid/myeloid ratio 1 : 1) and microscopy shows microblasts and reduced numbers of sideroblasts (page 229); there is an absence of stainable iron. The absorption of iron is stimulated by unknown mechanisms and may reach 40–90 per cent of the ingested iron. At the onset of iron lack, the marrow delivers normochromic and normocytic cells, but later the cells are hypochromic and microcytic. Symptoms usually appear when the haemoglobin concentration has fallen to approximately 10 g/100 ml. There has been an attempt to correlate the malaise and tiredness to a deficiency of the iron-containing respiratory enzymes, but this has not yet been substantiated.

Principles of Tests and Measurements

PERIPHERAL BLOOD MEASUREMENTS

The 2 most useful measurements are the estimation of *haemoglobin* concentration, after conversion to the stable cyanhaemoglobin compound (accuracy ± 5 per cent) and the *packed cell volume* (accuracy ± 2 per cent). The most useful index obtained from these 2 measurements is the *mean cell haemoglobin concentration* (MCHC) which is the ratio of haemoglobin concentration (g/100 ml) to packed cell volume (expressed as a fraction) and is characteristically reduced in iron deficiency. Estimates of red cell volume depend on estimates of red cell numbers, but the inaccuracy of the latter is high unless carried out by mechanical procedures. Size and shape of red cells can be more easily assessed by examination of a stained blood smear.

METHODS FOR ASSESSING RED CELL PRODUCTION AND DESTRUCTION

Moderate to marked degrees of haemolysis can be established by observing a persistently raised reticulocyte count and serum bilirubin concentration together with a reduced haemotocrit. When severe intravascular haemolysis is taking place free haemoglobin and met-haemalbumin appear in the plasma and haemoglobin is excreted in the urine. For a more complete assessment and for the provision of semi-quantitative or quantitative data, there are 6 tests that can be used for the evaluation of red cell production and destruction.

The erythroid-granulocytic ratio

Marrow hypo- or hyperfunction is directly reflected in the number of red cell precursors that it contains. Unfortunately the total numbers of red cell precursors cannot be estimated directly owing to the difficulty of measuring marrow volume but an indication of marrow activity is given by determining the ratio of erythroid to granulocytic cells, which is normally of the order of 1 : 3, depending on the particular technique used. This ratio is valid only if the number of granulocytic cells is normal and the only guide to this is a normal blood white cell count. This test can grade marrow activity into the following categories: hypoactive, normal, moderately (approx. 3 times normal) and extremely hyperactive, the latter being approximately 6 times normal activity.

Plasma iron turnover

There is a continuous turnover of iron bound to transferrin, and most of the iron turnover is the result of the metabolism of haemoglobin. Approximately 30 mg of iron is turned over each day (estimates vary from 0·35–0·55 mg/kg) and most of this (about 20 mg/day) is iron delivered to the marrow for haemoglobin production. Most of the remainder goes to the parenchymal cells of the liver. Thus about two-thirds of the iron turnover is dependent on the state of activity of the marrow, and this is high enough to allow the measurement to be used as an index of marrow function.

The rate of iron turnover can be estimated by injecting ^{59}FeCl intravenously and determining the rate of removal from the plasma. If the plasma iron concentration is measured at the same time, the results of these 2 estimates can be used to calculate the total iron turnover per day.

Owing to the large variation found in normals, hypoplasia of the marrow cannot be accurately assessed. On the other hand, increased erythropoietic activity can be assessed by this method and a 2-fold increase in plasma iron turnover (i.e. 60 mg iron through the plasma per day) is considered significant. This is the most accurate index of total marrow activity available at present.

Urobilinogen turnover

When red cells are broken down, either in the marrow (ineffective erythropoiesis) or at the end of their life span, haem is not reutilized but is converted to bilirubin in the reticuloendothelial system by the removal of iron and opening of the tetrapyrrolic ring by the splitting of a methene (=CH—) bridge with the production of carbon monoxide. Bilirubin is converted to urobilinogen by bacteria in the gut. Estimation of urobilinogen excretion is thus in the first place a measure of red cell destruction, but if the patient is in a state of equilibrium so that the red cell mass is constant, it is also a measure of the rate of production. The theoretical normal rate of excretion of urobilinogen in a 70 kg man is approximately 200 mg a day, but only about 75 per cent of this is found in the faeces on chemical analysis. Failure to obtain complete recovery suggests that there may be alternative pathways of metabolism but none is known at the present time. Alteration of the bacterial flora of the gut by antibiotics may also decrease the extent of the conversion to urobilinogen. Thus although urobilinogen excretion is usually found to be increased when the other indices also indicate increased production of haemoglobin, it is not a reliable or accurate measurement of red cell production. Increased urobilinogen concentration in the gut causes increased absorption and excretion in the urine, where it can be detected by using Ehrlich's reagent.

Liver disease and biliary obstruction also influence urobilinogen excretion (p. 452).

A rise in plasma unconjugated bilirubin (the 'indirect' fraction using Ehrlich's reagent) is a qualitative indication of increased pigment catabolism, but it cannot be used quantitatively because of the effect of liver function on bilirubin levels. It is not significantly raised until the red cell life span is reduced below 50 days.

Change in *total* erythropoietic activity of the marrow is thus reflected by the changes in the erythoid-granulocytic ratio, plasma iron turnover and pigment excretion. On the other hand *effective* erythropoietic activity, i.e. the number of viable cells which are delivered into the circulation, is reflected indirectly by the reticulocyte count and by iron utilization, and can also be calculated directly from an estimate of red cell volume and life span.

Reticulocyte count

The final maturation of the red cell takes place in the peripheral circulation and takes 1–2 days. Other things being equal, the number of reticulocytes in the blood should represent the rate of release of red cells from the marrow. The normal number of reticulocytes is 0·5–1·8 per cent of the total number of red cells, the value varying with the technique used and on the observer. In anaemic subjects the observed reticulocyte percentage must be corrected for the patient's haematocrit, otherwise the value will be too high. Alternatively, the reticulocyte count can be expressed as reticulocytes/cmm, the normal value being about 60,000. The reticulocyte count is the most practical way of determining the rate of red cell production but is not an accurate measure of viable red cell production under all conditions for two reasons: (1) red cells may remain in the marrow during the reticulocyte stage; this probably occurs in pernicious anaemia; (2) red cells may be released at a less mature stage, giving rise to an increase in the number of reticulocytes in the peripheral blood which does not represent an increase in production. These more immature cells have large aggregates of reticulum. The release of immature cells may be suspected if there are nucleated and large polychromatic red cells present; this situation occurs in certain types of haemolytic anaemia.

Red cell utilization of ^{59}Fe

When ^{59}Fe is injected intravenously into normals approximately 80 per cent or more normally appears as ^{59}Fe-haemoglobin in the red cell mass by 10–14 days. A decrease in the percentage of iron appearing in the peripheral circulation occurs under two circumstances. (1) Decreased erythropoiesis resulting from a diminution in stem cell activity; under these circumstances a greater proportion of the injected iron is diverted to iron stores and less iron is incorporated into red cells. (2) In the presence of ineffective erythropoiesis a proportion of the ^{59}Fe is incorporated into cells which are destroyed before they leave the marrow. The fate of the iron in these latter cells is not known,

9

but it appears that a fraction is diverted to iron stores; the final result is a decrease in the percentage of iron which is incorporated into viable red cells. Measurement of the rate of iron utilization cannot differentiate between these two possibilities.

Red cell life span and site of destruction

Severe haemolysis can be easily demonstrated by reticulocyte counts and by estimation of serum bilirubin. Minor degrees of haemolysis cannot be demonstrated with certainty with these tests and the greatest value of the determination of red cell life span is found when the rate of destruction of red cells is only 2–3 times normal. The life span can be determined using cells labelled with ^{51}Cr. A red cell volume determination can be carried out with the same injection of ^{51}Cr-labelled red cells. With a knowledge of the mean red cell life span and the red cell volume, the daily rate of red cell destruction can be calculated. If production and destruction are in equilibrium, this value also represents the rate of production. Furthermore, surface counting over the liver and spleen following injection of ^{51}Cr-labelled red cells indicates the main site of destruction.

^{51}Cr as $Na_2{}^{51}CrO_4$ is added to the red cells and the ^{51}Cr becomes attached to haemoglobin. The ^{51}Cr-haemoglobin bond is unfortunately not stable and after reinjection of the cells approximately 6 per cent of the ^{51}Cr elutes within the first day. Thereafter the elution rate is 1 per cent per day. A correction for this elution can be made and the corrected value for survival of radioactivity then represents the survival of the cells. The mean cell life can be obtained graphically by plotting the survival curve, drawing a tangent to the initial slope and extrapolating to the time axis. The point where it meets the time axis is the average life span.

When ^{51}Cr-labelled red cells are destroyed in the liver or spleen, the ^{51}Cr remains within the reticulo-endothelial cells of these organs and is only slowly lost at the rate of approximately 3 per cent per day. These ^{51}Cr deposits can be detected by surface counting over the heart, liver and spleen, but the results cannot be interpreted on an exact quantitative base because 50 per cent of the γ-rays produced by ^{51}Cr are absorbed by each 5 cm of path through which they travel in the tissues. Thus changes in the size of the liver and spleen and in the thickness of tissue overlying them alter the amount of radioactivity reaching the surface. Nevertheless, abnormal changes in the rate of accumulation of ^{51}Cr in the liver and spleen can be detected. Accumulation of ^{51}Cr exclusively in the spleen is a reasonably reliable indication that the patient will benefit from splenectomy. In normal individuals, radioactivity detected over the heart closely follows that of the blood; spleen and liver radioactivity is initially (within 30 min of injection) approximately 70 per cent of that over the heart and radioactivity from all areas falls progressively when measured daily. In patients who are destroying red cells in the spleen, radioactivity over the spleen is at first equal to or greater than that over the heart and rises progressively during the following 5–10 days to reach a value approximately 2–5 times as high as the heart radioactivity.

Surface counting can also be of value in detecting the presence of splenunculi after removal of the spleen. If ^{51}Cr-labelled red cells are either heated or coated with anti-D antibody they are removed from the circulation rapidly by splenic tissue, but only at a relatively slow rate by other tissues such as the liver or bone marrow. Thus if cells treated in either of these ways are injected into a patient with a splenunculus, they will accumulate in this organ over a period of 3–6 hours and their presence can be detected by surface counting.

^{51}Cr-labelling of red cells can also be useful in determining whether haemolysis is the result of an intrinsic or extrinsic defect of the red cell. Cells with an intrinsic defect normally also have a reduced survival in a normal recipient, whereas cells damaged by an extrinsic defect usually have a near normal survival in normal recipients.

Plasma haptoglobins

Haemoglobin released into the plasma combines with haptoglobins (MW, 100 000); the resultant complex is too large to be filtered through the glomeruli but is rapidly cleared by the reticuloendothelial system. Plasma haptoglobin concentration is measured indirectly by the ability to bind haemoglobin; normal plasma binds 100 mg haemoglobin per 100 ml plasma, i.e. all the haptoglobin in the plasma will combine with the haemoglobin released from approximately 10 ml of red cells. Haptoglobin levels are reduced even when red cell destruction is extravascular because some haemoglobin leaks into the plasma from engorged phagocytic cells. There is a correlation between plasma haptoglobin levels and mean cell life span. If the mean cell life is less than 30 days, the haptoglobin binding capacity is reduced to a barely detectable level.

When haptoglobin is used up, haemoglobin is broken down in the circulation and haem becomes attached to albumin to form methaemalbumin, which can be detected spectroscopically (*Schumm's test*). Free haemoglobin is filtered through the glomerulus and appear in the urine. Some is reabsorbed by the endothelium of the proximal tubules which later desquamate and the iron can be detected in the urine as *haemosiderin granules*.

TESTS USED IN DETECTION OF DEFICIENCY STATES

B_{12} deficiency

The most convenient and reliable single test for the detection of B_{12} deficiency is the determination of the serum B_{12} concentration. B_{12} levels are determined by microbiological or radio isotope techniques. Normal values usually range from 100–900 $\mu\mu$g/ml. Owing to the close interrelationship between B_{12} and folate in metabolic processes, B_{12} levels are low in folate deficiency. Thus levels at the lower limit of normal, 80–150 $\mu\mu$g/ml, are often due to folate deficiency alone; levels below 80 $\mu\mu$g/ml are the result of B_{12} deficiency or a combination of B_{12} and folate deficiency. There is some overlap however between the 'normal' and 'deficient' range and normal values do not exclude deficiency.

High levels of serum B_{12} are found in some patients with myelo-proliferative disorders due to high levels of a protein which binds B_{12}. In acute and chronic liver disease high levels are also found owing to release of B_{12} from the liver. If these conditions are present together with B_{12} deficiency, the serum level of B_{12} may be brought into the normal range.

B_{12} absorption. B_{12} deficiency is almost always the result of malabsorption. The most satisfactory test of the extent of absorption depends on measuring urinary excretion after giving ^{57}Co-labelled B_{12} (Schilling test). ^{57}Co-labelled B_{12} (1·0 μg) is given by mouth and at the same time a large dose (1 mg) of unlabelled B_{12} is given intramuscularly. This large dose of unlabelled B_{12} overburdens the storage mechanisms and brings about the urinary excretion in the 24 hours following administration of about $\frac{1}{3}$ of the ^{57}Co–B_{12} that is absorbed. In normals, 10 per cent or more of the administered dose is excreted. Values below 10 per cent may be taken as evidence of defective absorption; in pernicious anaemia it is usual to find values below 5 per cent. The test gives evidence of malabsorption both before and after B_{12} therapy. Its main disadvantage is that it requires an accurate 24-hour collection of urine.

Folate deficiency

Tests currently available for folic acid concentration and metabolism are not always reliable indicators of folate stores. Thus the diagnosis of folate deficiency as the cause of megaloblastic anaemia must rest principally on the exclusion of B_{12} deficiency. Megaloblastic anaemia in the presence of normal plasma B_{12} levels is almost always due to folate deficiency. However, serum B_{12} levels are sometimes low as a result of folate deficiency and exclusion of B_{12} deficiency then rests on finding a normal B_{12} absorption test. The following tests for folate deficiency should therefore only be used as confirmatory evidence.

Serum folate levels are measured microbiologically, using the growth rates of *lactobacillus casei* which measures the reduced co-enzyme forms as well as pteroylglutamic acid (p. 228). Normal values for serum folate are 5–16 ng/ml serum. In folate deficiency the majority of patients have values below 3 ng/ml although it is possible to have normal values. Serum folate levels may be reduced below normal values soon after the appearance of aetiological factors which lead to folate deficiency, such as diminished intake. Thus serum folate values may be low while stores are still adequate. Moreover serum folate levels are low in hospital patients with normoblastic haemopoiesis; 18–45 per cent of such patients may have low folate levels.

In pernicious anaemia, serum folate levels are usually normal; 15 per cent of patients have levels elevated above 16 ng/ml.

Red cell folate levels may also give an indication of folate stores. Normal values are 200–800 ng folate/ml red cells, i.e., 40–50 times the concentration in the plasma. Because of the slow turnover rate of red cells, folate levels may lag behind changes in total body folate. Red cell folate levels however will not distinguish between B_{12} and folate deficiency, as they are also low in B_{12} deficiency. In pernicious anaemia red cell folate levels return to normal soon after adequate therapy with B_{12}.

Small amounts of formiminoglutamic acid (FIGLU) are excretion in the urine in a proportion of folate-deficient subjects. FIGLU is a normal breakdown product of histidine but accumulates in the tissues in folate deficiency, because further breakdown is blocked as folate compounds are necessary for the removal of the formimino group. In order to demonstrate the abnormality in histidine breakdown with more certainty it is necessary to give a loading dose of 15 g of histidine and to collect urine over the following 8 hours. Normals excrete 1–17 mg FIGLU under this stress; folate deficient subjects excrete 20–1500 mg. FIGLU can be quantitatively estimated in the urine by a combined enzymatic and colorimetric method. Qualitative methods which merely state that FIGLU is present or absent in the urine do not give reliable results.

There are three situations where the results of the FIGLU excretion test must be interpreted with caution. (1) In pregnancy: half of all pregnant women with low folate stores have normal FIGLU excretion. This is the result of abnormal histidine metabolism in pregnancy when histidine is reutilized to a greater extent than normal for protein formation. (2) In megaloblastic anaemia resulting from anticonvulsant drugs, FIGLU excretion is usually in the normal range. (3) FIGLU excretion may be raised in vitamin B_{12} deficiency.

Folate absorption. Two tests are available for the assessment of folate absorption. (1) Estimation of folate excretion after giving folic acid first orally and then parenterally. Excretion after an oral dose should be at least 75 per cent of that after administration by the parenteral route. (2) After giving 40 μg folic acid orally, serum folate levels normally rise to 50 ngm in 2 hours. Folate levels in serum and urine are measured microbiologically in these two tests.

Plasma iron
There is a wide range of plasma iron concentration in normal subjects, from 60–200 μg/100 ml plasma with an average of about 125 μg/100 ml for men and 110 μg/100 ml for women. Plasma iron values show great lability; day-to-day variations are usually $\pm$ 30 per cent and there is a diurnal swing of about 50 per cent, values being highest during the early part of the day. Plasma iron values are normally below 100 μg/100 ml between 3 and 18 months of age and may be as low as 50 μg/100 ml. After this there is a steady rise until puberty is reached. As plasma iron is only present in trace amounts, care must be taken not to contaminate the blood with extraneous iron when obtaining the sample. Glass syringes and bottles may contain sufficient iron to contaminate the plasma appreciably unless these articles are acid-washed before use. Plastic syringes and containers are free from iron.

Increased plasma iron levels. Plasma iron levels represent a balance between the rates at which iron enters and leaves the circulation. Raised plasma iron levels may be considered under 4 categories. (1) Increased red cell destruction brings about the release of iron into the plasma but an increase in plasma iron level is usually only seen when there is also ineffective erythropoiesis as in pernicious anaemia and thalassaemia or when there is a block in the incorporation of iron into haem as in lead poisoning and pyridoxine deficiency. (2) When there is decreased production of red cells as in aplastic anaemia, less iron is removed from the circulation and elevated plasma levels are found. (3) When there is an increase mobilization from stores, as after an acute haemorrhage, more iron is mobilized than can be used by the marrow. Plasma levels are raised at the same time as the bilirubin in acute hepatitis. This is the result of the release of iron from damaged liver cells. (4) Plasma iron levels are raised when body iron stores are abnormally loaded, as in idiopathic haemochromatosis and in transfusion siderosis.

Decreased plasma iron levels. Plasma iron levels between 50 and 100 μg/100 ml are usually found in the presence of infection, neoplasm, chronic renal disease, rheumatoid arthritis and after tissue trauma. It is possible that plasma iron levels are controlled by the rate of release of iron from the reticuloendothelial system and this function appears to be impaired in these conditions, resulting in the release of less iron into the circulation.

Iron deficiency anaemia is usually associated with a reduction in plasma iron levels. Iron levels usually do not fall until there is total exhaustion of iron stores and may not fall even when there is a mild degree of anaemia present. When haemoglobin concentration falls below 9 g/100 ml low plasma iron levels are invariable; severe cases may have plasma iron levels below 20 μg/100 ml. On the other hand, in some individuals the plasma iron level may fall as soon as iron stores are depleted but before the haemoglobin concentration has fallen.

Total iron binding capacity (TIBC). Iron is transported in the plasma by transferrin and normally only about 30–40 per cent of the transferrin is saturated with iron. The total amount of transferrin present can be estimated in terms of the total iron binding capacity, which normally falls in the range 250–400 μg Fe/100 ml plasma, most estimates falling in the range 300–340 μg Fe/100 ml. An increase in TIBC is usually seen in iron deficiency anaemia although this is only a reliable diagnostic indicator when the haemoglobin concentration falls below 9 g/100 ml. This increase in TIBC in iron deficiency anaemia is to be contrasted with the fall seen in patients with infection, neoplasms and rheumatoid arthritis, and is thus a useful method of distinguishing the latter group from true iron deficiency.

Another cause of decreased transferrin level is hypoproteinaemia as seen in nephrosis, kwashiorkor and chronic liver disease.

TESTS USED FOR DETECTION OF INTRINSIC
RED CELL DEFECTS

Abnormal haemoglobins

The presence of abnormal haemoglobins can usually be demonstrated by electrophoresis on paper or starch gel. This results from the fact that the abnormal amino-acid in the molecule alters the total charge. In some cases, there is no alteration in charge but the presence of an abnormal haemoglobin can be demonstrated by heat precipitation ('heat-unstable haemoglobins'). It is necessary to use several buffer systems for electrophoresis as abnormal mobility sometimes only shows up in one particular system.

Heinz body formation. The haemoglobin and enzymes of the red cell contain atoms and groups, such as Fe^{++} and —SH, which can be oxidized, leading to a functional failure of the parent compounds. Oxidation is particularly likely to happen inside red cells because their internal Po_2 is higher than that of most other cells. The red cell contains a protective mechanism against this, namely the production of the compounds NADPH and GSH which reduce oxidized proteins. In the presence of certain abnormalities, maintenance of haemoglobin in the reduced form is not possible. Methaemoglobin is formed through oxidation of ferrous iron to the ferric form and then proceeds through oxidation of —SH groups to irreversible denaturation and precipitation. It is the agglomerations of precipitated denatured haemoglobin which stain with supravital dyes and which are termed Heinz bodies. Their appearance is seen with two types of abnormalities: (1) the presence of unstable types of haemoglobin (page 236), such as Haemoglobin H, Zurich, Koln and Seattle. These haemoglobins are more easily oxidized and denatured than Haemoglobin A. The so-called hereditary Heinz body anaemia is due to the presence of an abnormal but as yet unidentified haemoglobin. (2) Defects in the metabolic pathway for the production of NADPH and GSH, particularly defects in the oxidative pentose phosphate pathway, such as glucose-6-phosphate dehydrogenase deficiency.

Either of these abnormalities may be so severe that even under otherwise normal conditions *in vivo*, haemoglobin is denatured and Heinz bodies appear. This may be especially notable after splenectomy which allows red cells containing Heinz bodies to persist in the circulation for longer periods than in the presence of the spleen. On the other hand, it is more usual for Heinz bodies to appear after the exposure of red cells to drugs either *in vivo* or *in vitro*. These drugs (see page 234) are converted in the presence of oxygen into intermediaries which act as electron acceptors and can speed electron transfer (oxidation) away from Fe^{++} and —SH groups. In the initial period after the application of these drugs, NADPH and GSH act as electron donors for the drugs and thus protect the haemoglobin and enzymes from oxidation and destruction of the red cells. However, if either (a) NADPH and GSH replenishment is insufficient due to abnormalities in the oxidative metabolic pathway or (b) an unstable haemoglobin is present which is oxidized considerably more readily than Hb A, oxidation of the abnormal haemoglobin will proceed so far that denaturation and precipitation takes place.

Heinz bodies can be produced in normal cells by oxidizing reagents, but higher concentrations are required and fewer Heinz bodies appear than when there is an abnormality present. Formation of Heinz bodies *in vitro* by addition of acetylphenylhydrazine is used as a biological test for evidence of enzyme deficiency or haemoglobin abnormality.

TESTS USED IN BLOOD TRANSFUSION
Agglutination
Grouping within the ABO system and the detection of anti-A and anti-B is simple to carry out as these antibodies produce visible agglutinates when added to cells containing the appropriate antigen.

Anti-immunoglobulin reaction (Coombs' test).
Most blood group antibodies will not cause agglutination *per se*. Visible agglutination can be brought about by the addition of rabbit serum containing anti-human immunoglobulin to red cells coated with non-agglutinating antibodies, such as anti-D. This test can be used either to detect non-agglutinating antibodies already present on the surface of red cells, as in autoimmune haemolytic anaemia (p. 289, or it can be used to detect antibody in the plasma by first adsorbing it onto red cells containing the appropriate antigen.

Prior treatment of red cells with proteolytic enzymes such as papain or the addition of 20 per cent albumin allows 'non-agglutinating' antibodies to agglutinate. Both mechanisms probably act by reducing the effective negative charge on the red cell surface and thus diminishing the normal electrostatic repulsion between cells.

NEUTROPHILS

Normal function

Neutrophils develop from stem cells in the bone marrow. Myeloblasts, promyelocytes and myelocytes are dividing cells; thereafter maturation proceeds without division to polymorphonuclear leucocytes. The time taken for maturation from stem cell to adult neutrophil is approximately 12 days. Once in the circulation, neutrophils do not have a fixed life span as do red cells but they leave the circulation randomly irrespective of their age. Their average life in the circulation is approximately 10 hours. Neutrophils in the blood pool may be divided into two approximately equal populations: (1) a 'circulating' pool, and (2) a 'marginal' pool, in which neutrophils are attached to the vascular walls; there is a rapid exchange between these two pools. After administration of adrenaline or following exercise, the marginal pool is mobilized and neutrophils pass into the circulating pool. Bacterial products such as endotoxin also shift neutrophils from the marginal to the circulating pool and also have the effect of mobilizing marrow stores and bringing more neutrophils into the circulation. There are approximately twenty times as many neutrophils stored in the marrow as there are in the circulating blood. These stores of neutrophils can be rapidly mobilized as in the response to infection. The passage of neutrophils from the marrow through the blood to the tissues is unidirectional and there is no return of neutrophils to the circulation.

The number of granulocytes in the blood is usually maintained within close limits. The control mechanism is not known but there is evidence of a hormone which promotes leucocytosis and it is possible that this hormone may also regulate leucocyte production in a manner similar to the effect of erythropoietin on red cell production.

Leucocyte antigens and histocompatibility testing

As with red cells the chemical structure of the surface of leucocytes shows considerable variation amongst individuals and thus surface structures can act as antigens when transfused into recipients who lack the factors. Anti-leucocyte antibodies are produced following blood transfusion and it has also been found that 1 in 4 of all multiparous women contain anti-leucocyte antibodies, the result of the placental transfer of leucocytes from the foetus during pregnancy and labour.

It is now realized that some of the antigens present on leucocytes are common to many tissues and that they are probably identical to the transplantation antigens which lead to rejection of homografts. Identification of the presence of antigens and antibodies by histocompatibility testing requires exacting techniques and is still in its infancy, but should ultimately be valuable in the selection of donors for organ transplantation.

Abnormal function

ALTERED NEUTROPHIL COUNT

Neutrophilia

The total blood neutrophil content and turnover have been measured in chronic myeloid leukaemia in relapse. There is a 10 to 100-fold increase in the total neutrophil content and the life-span is of the order of 2–5 days compared with the normal of 10 hours. The reason for this prolongation of life-span is unknown, but the defect is certainly cellular. When normal cells are transfused into patients without leukaemia they survive for the normal period of 10 hours, whereas cells from patients with chronic myeloid leukaemia transfused into patients without leukaemia have a prolonged life-span. It has been suggested that the prolonged life-span in myeloid leukaemia is due to the delivery of immature cells into the circulation. In leukaemia there is no correlation between the increase in the total number of neutrophils and the prolongation in the mean cell survival in the circulation.

In contrast to this, neutrophilia in other conditions such as polycythaemia, myelofibrosis and bacterial infections is accompanied by only a slight increase of survival (up to 1 day) and there is a correlation between the extent of the neutrophilia and the prolongation of mean cell survival.

Neutropenia

In the small number of patients investigated it has been found that neutropenia is the result either of reduced production or increased rate of destruction or of both factors acting together. Reduced production of neutrophils is usually the result of drugs. The mechanism of increased destruction is not clear; the spleen undoubtedly plays a role in some patients. A case has been recorded with cirrhosis and splenomegaly in which the mean cell survival of neutrophils in the circulation was less than 1 hour and this returned to the normal value of 10 hours after splenectomy.

CHROMOSOME ABNORMALITIES IN BLOOD DISEASES

With the recent improvements in techniques for demonstrating chromosomes (p. 595) many reports have appeared on chromosome configuration in blood diseases. The most striking changes have been found in chronic granulocytic leukaemia. In nearly every case there is a loss of half of the long arm of the small chromosome No. 21; the abnormal chromosome is known as the Philadelphia chromosome. This abnormality is present only in red cell and granulocyte precursors and has not been found in skin cells or in lymphocytes, nor has it been observed in other diseases or in normal people. It has been seen in patients before the onset of the clinical disease and is present throughout the disease, even during remissions. Its limitation to leukaemic cells indicates that it is an acquired change, and its consistency and specificity suggests a causal relationship to the disease. This type of lesion can be produced by X-rays and viruses. The white cell alkaline-phosphatase level is also reduced in chronic granulocytic leukaemia and this suggests that chromosome 21 may be responsible for the level of this enzyme.

In contrast, chromosome abnormalities in acute granulocytic and lymphocytic leukaemia show no consistent pattern. In acute granulocytic leukaemia there is a reduced number of chromosomes and those that are missing are usually one of the following: Nos. 6–12, 21 and 22. On the other hand in acute lymphoblastic leukaemia there is an increase in the number of chromosomes up to 100, usually manifesting in chromosome Nos. 6–12, 21 and 22 but particularly in chromosome 9. These abnormal karyotypes disappear in remissions of these diseases. A small percentage of cases is seen in which there are no chromosome abnormalities. It is not known whether these chromosome abnormalities bear a causal relationship to the disease or not.

HAEMOSTASIS

Normal function

There are 3 mechanisms concerned with haemostasis: (1) contraction of the vessel walls which may itself be sufficient to obliterate the lumen; (2) plugging of the damaged vessel walls with platelets, and (3) the formation of a fibrin clot. The exact relationship of these mechanisms and their relative importance is obscure. When bleeding occurs from capillaries and venules, contraction of the arteriolar-capillary junction and the formation of a platelet thrombus are important in the initial stages; formation of a fibrin clot is then necessary to stabilize the platelet thrombus. In large vessels platelet thrombi alone are too friable to initiate haemostasis and firmer thrombi must be formed from a mixture of platelets and fibrin.

BLOOD COAGULATION

The details of blood coagulation are complex and difficult to elucidate experimentally, but there have been two recent developments which have considerably simplified our understanding of the processes involved. First, an International Committee has been formed to rationalize the nomenclature, which had become extremely diversified and confused; clotting factors are now designated by a Roman numeral. There are 12 established factors identified by I to XIII (excluding VI). Secondly, the apparent complexity of the process has been illuminated by the suggestion that the many stages in the clotting process are analogous to an electronic amplification system, each stage amplifying the preceding stage. Thus it has been suggested on good experimental evidence that each of the clotting factors is an enzyme normally present in the plasma in an inactive form. Clotting is initiated by the exposure of plasma to any foreign surface other than vascular endothelium.

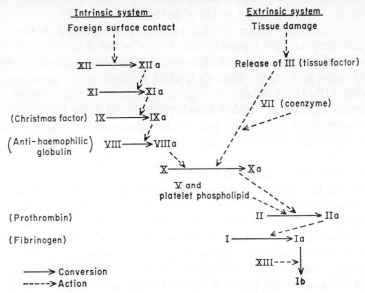

FIGURE 29. *Simplified version of clotting process (after McFarlane). Stage* $X \rightarrow X_a$ *onwards is common to both intrinsic and extrinsic pathways.*

By a process yet unknown, factor XII becomes converted to the active enzymatic form XIIa, which then acts on factor XI converting it to the active form XIa, and so on (Fig. 29). The amplification factor at each stage is not known, but if each enzyme activates 10 times the amount of the enzyme of the following stage, then as there are 6 stages following activation of factor XII there would be an amplification factor of 1×10^6 by the time the final stage was reached. Thus a trivial injury can bring about rapidly and efficiently the production of a fibrin clot involving many millions of molecules.

The complete sequence of reactions which occurs in clotting has not yet been elucidated, but the most probable sequence of events is shown in Fig. 29. There are 2 systems within the clotting process; the main system is termed the intrinsic system, as all clotting factors are contained in the plasma. The order in which the factors are activated is as follows: XII, XI, IX, VII, X, II and I. The other system is known as the extrinsic system because the initiating factor (factor III) is present in tissue and is released on injury and then feeds into the main intrinsic system by activating factor X using factor VII as a coenzyme. The intrinsic and extrinsic systems thus share a final common path from factor X onwards. Calcium (factor IV) is required for the activation process at several stages; the phospholipid components of platelets probably act as surface catalysts in the action of factor Xa on factor II.

The final stage in the clotting process is the splitting of factor I (fibrinogen) into 4 polypeptide units known as factor Ia (fibrin) by the proteolytic enzyme factor IIa (thrombin). The polypeptide units then polymerize to form the fibrin clot, which is stabilized by the action of factor XIII. Until the new Roman numeral nomenclature is generally accepted and widely used, it is still necessary to know the synonyms for some of the factors, but the clinician need only be concerned with the 4 which are given in Fig. 29.

FIBRINOLYTIC MECHANISMS

Although the existence of a mechanism in the plasma for the dissolution of fibrin clots (fibrinolysis) has been known for many years, it is only recently that it has been demonstrated that these fibrinolytic mechanisms are active in plasma under normal conditions. This finding has given rise to the concept that clotting may be proceeding slowly but continuously with deposition of fibrin on the vascular endothelium and that this is balanced by the fibrinolysis which removes the fibrin as it is formed. The fibrinolytic system is as yet ill-defined but the present working hypothesis is outlined in Fig. 30. It seems likely that the system may consist of a series of enzymes which are activated in a similar fashion to the clotting mechanisms. The plasminogen activator is the only substance so far identified which can act as the initiator in the reaction. There is considerable evidence that the activator is derived from vascular endothelium, particularly that of the capillaries and venules. Activator is being continuously released and its presence can be detected in the plasma. The plasmin that is being formed by the action of activator can break down fibrinogen as well as fibrin, and thus its continued presence in the plasma would soon lead to low levels of fibrinogen. Plasmin is therefore neutralized in the plasma by an inhibitor termed antiplasmin. A mechanism is thus necessary to overcome the effect of inhibitor when fibrinolysis is to take place. This mechanism is the absorption of activator and plasminogen onto the fibrin clot; the activator then converts the plasminogen to plasmin, which then acts directly on the fibrin. The plasmin produced on the fibrin is not accessible to inhibitor present in solution in the plasma.

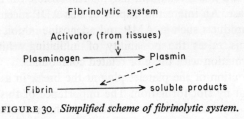

FIGURE 30. *Simplified scheme of fibrinolytic system.*

Thus fibrin concentrates the factors responsible for its disolution.

Plasminogen activator levels are physiologically increased by exercise and adrenaline and also by mental stress, which probably acts through the adrenaline mechanism. The fibrinolytic system is also activated by streptokinase from streptococcal filtrates, although the site of action of these agents is not yet known. Activator is also released from tissues following injury.

Plasminogen activator is present in all tissues, although its quantity varies considerably from site to site. It is present in the pleural and peritoneal cavities, where its function is to keep these areas free from adhesions.

PLATELETS

The 2 most important functions of platelets are the formation of platelet thrombi and the supply of a factor (phospholipid) involved in clotting. Platelets are essential in the initial stages of haemostasis.

Within seconds of a break in the vascular lining the platelets start to aggregate and form a thrombus to plug the hole. There are two related mechanisms which may be responsible for this sealing process: (1) platelets have the ability to adhere to exposed collagen fibres, and (2) adenosine diphosphate (ADP) causes platelets to become adhesive and to aggregate. ADP is a breakdown product of adenosine triphosphate (ATP), a compound present in all cells and platelets. As a result either of injury to tissue or of the contact between platelets with foreign surfaces or of proteolytic enzymes such as trypsin and thrombin, ADP is produced and released. This is known to be a rapid process. Clumping by this method is reversible and thus the extent of clumping is a result of the rate of production of ADP from ATP on the one hand and the rate of destruction to adenosine monophosphate and adenosine on the other hand. Following experimental injury to vessels, platelet aggregates increase in size to form white bodies which may break away from the surface to form emboli. The formation of these white bodies is probably due to ADP and this mechanism may be responsible for thrombosis in vascular disease. An interesting aspect of this ADP mechanism is that breakdown products such as AMP and adenosine inhibit the action of ADP and this raises the possibility of inhibiting white body and thrombus formation with these or related compounds.

The stabilization of the platelet plug at the break in a vessel wall is brought about by clot formation. The importance of this stabilization is illustrated by haemorrhage occurring in haemophilia where the initial formation of a platelet plug takes place satisfactorily but this is not stabilized by adequate clot formation. Phospholipids, of which the most important is phosphatidylethanolamine, have been extracted from platelets and these substances can take the place of platelets in the clotting mechanism. Platelets play an active role in bringing about clot retraction, and they also contain serotonin (5-hydroxytryptamine) which is released during the clotting process and aids haemostasis by causing contraction at the arteriolar-capillary junctions.

Details of the life span of platelets in the circulation are not yet completely elucidated. Platelets can be labelled with either ^{32}P (as di-isopropylfluorophosphate) or radioactive chromium; the survival curves obtained are variable in shape and usually are neither strictly linear nor exponential. The interpretation of the curves is difficult, but it is possible that platelets are endowed with a finite life-span (similar to red cells) upon which is superimposed a variable degree of random destruction. The life-span is of the order of 5–11 days, the value depending upon the method of analysis of the curves. It is not known at the present time why there should be this variation between different types of survival curves nor is the mechanism of destruction of platelets known. The life span of platelets is sometimes prolonged in diseases with hypocoagulability, that is, where there is a deficiency of haemophilia factor or Christmas factor. It might be expected that survival would be shortened in thrombocytopenia but although this is often found, other cases are seen with normal or even prolonged survival times.

The control of the number of platelets in the plasma is probably carried out through 2 mechanisms. First, there may be a hormone which acts on the marrow and stimulates platelet production. Secondly, the spleen may sequester and destroy platelets and the rate of destruction in that organ may be subject to control. It has been suggested that the hormone involved is erythropoietin, based on the fact that there is an increase in platelet numbers after haemorrhage or acute haemolysis when there is considerable erythropoietin release. Another pertinent observation is that patients who continue to be anaemic after splenectomy have exceptionally high platelet concentrations. It is suggested that in these patients the continuing anaemia stimulates erythropoietin production which leads to an increase in platelet production as well as red cells; the platelet numbers rise above normal levels owing to the absence of the splenic destructive mechanisms. There is a danger of thromboembolic phenomena after splenectomy under these conditions and this aspect is considered in deciding whether splenectomy should be carried out or not.

Abnormal function

BLOOD CLOTTING MECHANISM

Abnormalities in the blood clotting mechanisms may be conveniently considered in two categories, acquired and genetic.

The acquired changes result from vitamin K deficiency, from the action of the coumarin drugs, or in association with liver disease. These may all be considered together, because the first two produce an identical syndrome, and the changes seen in liver disease are very similar.

Vitamin K is a fat-soluble compound and hence it is not absorbed from the gastrointestinal tract in biliary obstruction or in steatorrhoea. Vitamin K is necessary for the production of 4 of the blood clotting factors, II, VII, IX and X. In vitamin K deficiency or following coumarin administration factor VII is the first to be affected and this is followed by a diminution in factor II (prothrombin) and in factors IX and X. It is probably the deficiency of factors VII, IX and X which contribute most to the clotting defect.

The genetic abnormalities are the hereditary and congenital deficiencies of the blood clotting factors. By far the most important are deficiencies of factors VIII and IX. Other deficiencies are rare and in some instances only a few cases are known; genetic deficiencies of factors V, VII, X, XI and XII have been found.

Deficiency of factor VIII (*anti-haemophilic globulin*)

Haemophilia is a sex-linked recessive disease in which a genetic defect on the X chromosome leads to deficiency of factor VIII. Quantitative estimates of factor VIII have shown different grades of deficiency. The severest haemophiliacs with frequent spontaneous bleeding do not have any detectable factor VIII; those with levels between 1–10 per cent are moderately severe and have some spontaneous bleeding; those with levels between 10–25 per cent only have serious bleeding following minor trauma, and those with levels between 25–50 per cent of normal only have serious bleeding following major trauma.

Platelets and vascular function are normal and hence the platelet count, tourniquet test and bleeding times are all normal. Most cases show a prolongation of the whole blood clotting time, but when the factor VIII level is 1–2 per cent or above, the whole blood clotting time is usually normal. The kaolin-cephalin and thromboplastin generation tests for the activity of the intrinsic clotting system are almost always abnormal.

Deficiency of factor IX (*Christmas factor*)

This deficiency cannot be separated clinically from factor VIII deficiency. It has only been recently recognized as a result of the development of the thromboplastin generation test (p. 264). This test was found to show normal factor VIII values in some cases which were diagnosed clinically as haemophilia. The abnormal factor came to be known as factor IX. In England the incidence is only about one-tenth that of haemophilia and it is inherited in the same manner. It can be differentiated from haemophilia by the thromboplastin generation test.

Acute defibrination syndrome

Fibrinogen deficiency may be the result of a congenital defect in fibrinogen production or may be an acquired condition resulting either from disease of liver tissue which impairs fibrinogen production, or from widespread clotting *in vivo*, which gives rise to the defibrination syndrome most frequently seen as an obstetric complication, but also seen after surgical operations, particularly those involving an extra-corporeal circulation. The initiating abnormality in the acute defibrina-tion syndrome appears to be the release of factor III from injured tissue. In obstetric cases, this may result from placental fragments released into the maternal circulation. This initiates the clotting process and results in the deposition of fibrin on vessel walls; the process may continue until most of the fibrinogen is gone. When this stage is reached, a generalized haemorrhagic state may ensue. Although in this syndrome fibrinogen is principally depleted, other plasma clotting factors such as II, V and VIII may also be deficient, and there is also thrombo-cytopenia. Despite low levels of the other clotting factors, the injection of fibrinogen alone appears to be adequate to halt the general haem-orrhagic state although it is also necessary to remove the source of factor III. Massive retroplacental haemorrhage and clot formation may also use up the fibrinogen and is a further cause of the low levels found in this syndrome.

Abnormal fibrinolysis
The fibrinolytic system and the clotting system have one feature in common, namely, that tissue injury leads to the release of initiating factors in both systems, plasminogen activator and factor III. Thus abnormal activation of the fibrinolytic mechanism is frequently present together with fibrinogen depletion resulting from excessive clotting, both processes often, but by no means always, resulting in abnormal haemorrhage. Activation of the two mechanisms do not necessarily occur equally and in any individual case of generalized haemorrhage either one or the other usually predominates.

Most cases of excessive fibrinolysis are due to the release of activator as a result of tissue trauma. Thus it is found in (1) obstetric complica-tions, usually associated with the acute defibrination syndrome, and (2) after extensive accidental or surgical trauma, particularly from thoracic operations, because lung contains large amounts of activator. Fibrinolysis also follows the use of the artificial heart-lung pump. Apart from tissue injury, plasminogen activator may also be released in abnormal amounts under the following circumstances: (1) In *carcinoma of the prostate*, especially with extensive metastases; excess activator probably arises from the neoplastic cells themselves. (2) After *transfusion with incompatible blood;* destruction of the red cells probably releases the plasminogen activator which they contain, as well as factor III, which initiates clotting with subsequent fibrinogen depletion. (3) In *cirrhosis of the liver*, in which excess fibrinolysis may agravate bleeding from oesophageal varices; this may be due to the failure of production of plasmin inhibitors in liver disease. (4) *Thrombocytopenia*, when excessive fibrinolysis may aggravate localized bleeding. Platelets contain antiplasmin which normally inhibits clot dissolution. When platelets are few, the reduced levels of antiplasmin in the clot may allow fibrinolysis to continue at an increased rate, resulting in local haemorrhage. (5) Bleeding from the urinary tract and prostate after operation may be due to the action of *urokinase*, a normal activator of fibrinolysis present in the urine. Urokinase normally keeps the urinary tract free from fibrin blockage.

PLATELET AND CAPILLARY ABNORMALITIES
Non-thrombocytopenic purpura
This is an ill-defined group of diseases in which purpura and haemorrhages are present in the absence of any change in platelet numbers. The evidence we have at the present time suggests that they can be classified into two categories: functional capillary defects and functional platelet defects.

Functional capillary defects (von Willebrand's disease).
This group is recognized at the present time by purpura and haemorrhages occurring in patients in whom the only consistent laboratory abnormality is a prolonged bleeding time. The nature of the primary defect is obscure; factor VIII is usually diminished, there is evidence of abnormal platelet adhesiveness, and also evidence of abnormal shape and contractility of the capillaries of the skin and mucous membranes but not of deep tissue.

Functional platelet deficiencies (thrombasthenia).
This category includes a group of diseases in which abnormal bleeding is associated with a prolonged bleeding time together with a functional defect in platelet activity. Several types of functional defect have been described: (1) failure to aggregate in the presence of ADP; (2) failure to release the phospholipids involved in clotting, giving rise to abnormal clotting tests; (3) failure to bring about clot retraction.

It must be emphasized that this classification into functional defects of capillaries and platelets is tentative.

Thrombocytopenic purpura
The exact relationship between thrombocytopenia and abnormal bleeding is obscure. The only well-established fact is that spontaneous

capillary haemorrhages occur when the platelet numbers are reduced. The concentration of platelets at which bleeding occurs varies considerably between patients, but is usually less than 50,000/cmm. Two functional abnormalities that may be involved are (1) reduction in the rate of production of fibrin, resulting from a decreased concentration of the phospholipid coenzyme; (2) a failure of clot retraction, dependent on an unknown platelet factor. There are undoubtedly other unknown factors involved in the relationship between platelets and the integrity of the vascular wall.

Principles of tests and measurements

TESTS USED IN CHARACTERIZING BLEEDING OR CLOTTING DEFECTS

Bleeding time
The cessation of bleeding from small vessels is dependent on vascular contraction and the formation of a platelet thrombus. Prolongation of the bleeding time is thus abnormal in the presence of thrombocytopenia and functional platelet and capillary defects, but it is usually normal in the presence of clotting abnormalities.

Capillary fragility (Hess's test)
This test consists of observing evidence of purpura after occlusion of the venous return from the forearm for 5 min. The test is usually positive in the presence of capillary and platelet but not clotting abnormalities; its diagnostic value is poor owing to considerable variation in the result obtained at different times.

BLOOD CLOTTING TESTS
There are 3 basic laboratory tests for the investigation of the integrity of the intrinsic clotting mechanism; (1) the whole blood clotting time, (2) the kaolin-cephalin clotting time and (3) the thromboplastin generation test. The test for the extrinsic system is the prothrombin time.

Whole blood clotting time
This method measures the clotting time of whole blood in glass test tubes; contact with the glass initiates clotting by activation of factor XII to XIIa. This test is relatively crude with a wide range of normal values and many instances of clotting deficiences give normal results.

The wide variation in normal clotting times is due both to variation in platelet activity and to variation in the initial contact reaction between glass and factor XII.

Kaolin-cephalin clotting time

The whole blood clotting time test has been considerably improved by the introduction of the kaolin-cephalin plasma clotting time. In this test, kaolin is preincubated with the plasma in order to activate factor XII. A crude cephalin extract which is a platelet substitute, is then added together with calcium. This method considerably improves the sensitivity although minor deficiencies of clotting factors still give results within the normal range.

Thromboplastin generation test

The term 'thromboplastin' in this test refers to the complex of factors Xa and V which activates factor II (see Fig. 29). The test was devised for detecting deficiency of factor VIII without relying on the use of plasma obtained from a patient with known haemophilia. Reference to Fig. 31 shows that the test consists of adding together a kaolin-adsorbed plasma preparation (containing factor VIII), serum (containing factors IX and X), platelets and calcium. The reaction starts with factor IXa present in the serum and proceeds up to factor Xa, but cannot proceed further as factor II is absent, having been adsorbed out of the plasma preparation by kaolin. The rate of production of factor Xa is then measured by adding aliquots of the mixture to citrated plasma and determining the clotting time. As factor VIII is in the adsorbed plasma and factor IX in the serum, the test can differentiate between haemophilia and Christmas disease by using either the patients plasma and a normal serum or vice versa. The mildest cases of haemophilia are not detected by this test and it is necessary to assay for factor VIII, which is carried out by a modification of the thromboplastin generation test in which the only variable is factor VIII.

Test for the extrinsic system (prothrombin time)

As is so frequently the case in this subject, the term prothrombin time is a misnomer as it is now known that the test is sensitive to abnormalities in factors I, II, (prothrombin), V, VII, X, and is relatively insensitive to changes in the prothrombin concentration alone. This test is simple to carry out and finds its greatest use in the detection of acquired deficiencies (p. 269). The test consists essentially of adding together plasma, calcium and an extract of tissue containing factor III, which initiates the clotting process, and estimating the time taken to clot (see Fig. 29). The addition of factor III means the first 4 stages of the intrinsic system are not involved.

The prothrombin time is the most suitable test for the control of anti-coagulant therapy with the coumarin drugs, but not for control of heparin therapy, for which the whole blood clotting time is the most suitable test. The prothrombin time is affected by calcium concentration, source and concentration of factor III (tissue extracts) and the extent of storage of citrated plasma samples. Normal values range from 12–24 sec. Because of this wide range of normal values estimates of a pathological plasma sample must be compared with a normal control. The simplest method of expressing results is to state the ratio between the prothrombin time of the pathological plasma and the normal. The aim of coumarin treatment is to maintain the maximum increase in prothrombin time without haemorrhage occurring. It is found in practice that an approximately 3-fold prolongation of prothrombin time is the maximum that can be tolerated. Thus a prolongation of 1·5–2·5 times normal is optimal. Because of the susceptibility of the prothrombin time estimation to minor changes in materials and techniques, it is necessary for each laboratory to determine for itself the maximum prolongation that is without danger to the patient. Moreover, patients differ in the safe maximum prolongation of pro-thrombin time and individuals also differ between one period of time and another. For instance, a patient may have a 3–5-fold prolongation of prothrombin time for 2 weeks with no untoward effect, and then start to bleed with no change in prothrombin time. This variation might be due to the fact that the coumarin drugs also decrease factor IX concentration, a deficiency which is not detected by the prothrombin time (see Fig. 29).

Tests for excessive fibrinolysis
There is no simple rapid test for estimating the rate of fibrinolysis. The difficulty in estimation results from the fact that both activator and plasmin are labile *in vitro* and from the presence of inhibitors in the plasma. Fortunately, a haemorrhagic syndrome usually develops only when there is a great increase in the rate of fibrinolysis, and very rapid rates of lysis are easy to detect. The simplest test is to clot whole blood and then to observe the clot for several hours, during which time partial or complete lysis will occur when fibrinolytic activity is excessive. Care must be taken not to confuse lysis with clot retraction. When fibrinolytic activity is very great, whole blood may not clot at

all due to lack of fibrinogen, destroyed by plasmin. Excessive fibrino-lytic activity is often indicated by observations made during blood clotting tests, such as the prothrombin time, when it will be seen that the clot partially or completely lyses soon after its formation.

If further investigation is required, 3 other tests may be helpful.

Dilute blood clot lysis time. If plasma is diluted the fibrinolytic inhibitors are inactivated to a greater extent than the fibrinolytic system itself. The presence of fibrinolysis can be demonstrated in normal plasma by this method, that is diluting the plasma and allowing it to clot and then observing the time taken for the clots to lyse which normally takes place in 2–10 hours. This time is reduced to less than 1 hour when fibrinolysis is excessive due to the presence of excess activator.

Plasminogen concentration. When plasmin has been formed at an excessive rate, plasminogen levels are always reduced and remain low up to 24 hours after cessation of excessive activator action. Plasminogen levels can be measured by converting plasminogen to plasmin with the activator streptokinase and then adding the substrate casein, which is broken down by plasmin. The amount of tyrosine released is used as a measure of the amount of plasmin formed from the plasminogen.

Plasma fibrinogen. Estimation of plasma fibrinogen concentration can be made by a simple biological test. Thrombin will convert fibrinogen to a visible fibrin clot when normal citrated plasma is diluted $\frac{1}{32}$ to $\frac{1}{128}$. When fibrinogen levels are reduced, the dilution at which a visible clot is formed is correspondingly reduced.

Practical Assessment

RED CELLS

Clinical observations
Haemoglobin concentration: colour of mucous membranes unreliable if Hb 9–17 g. Below 9 g./100 ml pallor reliable; above 17 g/100 ml plethora and peripheral cyanosis.

Identification of anaemia: Evidence of iron deficiency: brittle spoon-shaped nails (koilonychia); atrophy of tongue, especially at edges; cracks at corners of mouth; dysphagia (post-cricoid web). Evidence of B_{12} deficiency: atrophy of tongue; neurological damage (sub-acute combined degeneration of cord, peripheral neuropathy, psychosis).

Evidence of haemolysis. Severe: jaundice; haemoglobinuria. Moderate: excess urobilinogen in urine.

Routine methods
Haemoglobin: Normal values, 13·5 to 18·0 g/100 ml in men; 11·5 to 16·4 in women. Haematocrit + Hb allows calculation of mean cell haemoglobin concentration (MCHC). Normal: 32–36 g/100 ml; less than 32 indicates iron deficiency or defective Hb synthesis, especially thalassaemia (p. 237).

Stained smear: shape of red cells; reticulocytes. *Red cell count:* allows calculation of mean cell volume.

Marrow aspiration: cellularity; erythroid/myeloid ratio (p. 241); iron stores; megaloblasts with B_{12} or folate deficiency.

Haemolysis: Increased red cell destruction: plasma Hb and haptoglobin (p. 245); methaemalbumin (Schumm's test, p. 245); bilirubin (p. 451); total faecal pigment. If incompatible cells transfused, can be detected by Coombs' test (p. 251).

Increased red cell production: reticulocyte count; increased marrow erythroid/myeloid ratio; increased fragility of spherocytes; positive Coombs' test in autoimmune haemolysis.

Deficiency states: serum iron and iron binding capacity (p. 248); serum B_{12} and Schilling test for intrinsic factor; serum folate and FIGLU test (p. 247).

Special tests
Red cell destruction by ^{51}Cr-labelled cell survival; site of destruction can be identified by counting over involved organ.

Red cell formation by studies of ^{59}Fe turnover.

Abnormal haemoglobins by starch block electrophoresis; foetal Hb by denaturation resistance.

Red cell enzymes: identification of glucose-6-phosphate dehydrogenase deficiency or glutathione instability. Heinz bodies indicate defect in oxidative metabolic pathway or presence of an unstable haemoglobin.

WHITE CELLS

Routine methods
White cell counts and smear: Counts above 50,000/cmm rarely seen except in leukaemia; acute infections 15,000–40,000. Atypical cells in glandular fever; primitive cells in leukaemias.

Special stains: peroxidase staining for identifying cell type in acute leukaemia (lymphoblasts fail to take up stain); alkaline phosphatase deficiency may help in distinguishing myeloid leukaemic cells from normal.

Biopsy of marrow or lymph gland usually needed for firm diagnosis of leukaemia or lymphoma.

HAEMOSTASIS

Clinical observations
Capillary or platelet defects usually produce petechiae, later confluent purpura and bruises, and bleeding from mucous membranes. Clotting defects usually present with bleeding from cut surfaces, without purpura (unless after trauma), and haemorrhages into joints common (especially in haemophilia). Sometimes also haemorrhage from gut and renal tract. Family history may be important.

Routine methods (Fig. 31).

Prothrombin time (for extrinsic pathway)		Thrombin generation test (for intrinsic pathway)	
Plasma	Tissue extract	Adsorbed plasma	Serum
VII	III	VIII	IX
X			X
V and platelet phospholipid			
II			
I			

FIGURE 31. *Distribution of factors in the basic clotting tests.*

Platelet and vascular abnormalities: bleeding time prolonged, clotting time and prothrombin times normal. Thromboplastin generation test (p. 264) can reveal platelet abnormalities, even when stained film is normal.

Clotting disorders: bleeding time normal, but abnormal clotting ability can be shown in intrinsic and/or extrinsic system tests (thromboplastin generation test, and prothrombin time test, respectively). Certain drugs and liver disease may produce defects revealed in both tests.

Excessive fibrinolysis: by observation of clot lysis and plasmin concentrations; fibrinogenopenia can be shown by estimation of fibrinogen chemically or biologically.

References

HARRIS J.W. (1963) *The Red Cell.* Harvard University Press, Cambridge, Mass.

MOLLISON P.L. (1967) *Blood Transfusion in Clinical Medicine.* Oxford, Blackwell.

BORSOOK H. (1964) A Picture of Erythropoiesis at the Combined Morphologic and Molecular Levels. *Blood* 24, 202–7.

FINCH C.A. & NOYES W.D. (1961) Erythrokinetics in diagnosis of Anemia. *JAMA* 175, 1163–6.

BEUTLER E. (1965) Glucose-6-Phosphate Dehydrogenase Deficiency and Nonspherocytic Congenital Hemolytic Anemia. *Seminars in Hematology* 2, 91–138.

DACIE J.V. (1962) Haemolytic Mechanisms in Health and Disease. *Brit. Med. J.* ii, 429–36.

AMOROSI E. (1965) Hypersplenism. *Seminars in Hematology* 2, 249–85.

BAINTON D.F. & FINCH C.A. (1964) The Diagnosis of Iron Deficiency Anemia. *Amer. J. Med.* 37, 62–70.

HERBERT V. (1965) Drugs Effective in Megaloblastic Anaemias. Vitamin B_{12} and Folic Acid. In *The Pharmacological Basis of Therapeutics.* (1965) ed. GOODMAN L.S. & GILMAN A., New York, Macmillan, p. 40, 3rd edition.

BEUTLER, E., FAIRBANKS V. F. & FAHEY, J.L. (1963) *Clinical Disorders of Iron Metabolism.* New York, Grune and Stratton.

BIGGS, R. & McFARLANE R.G. (1962) *Human Blood Coagulation and its Disorders.* Oxford, Blackwell.

CARTWRIGHT G.E., ATHENS J.W. & WINTROBE M.M. (1964) The Kinetics of Granulopoiesis in Normal Man. *Blood* 24, 780–803.

LEHMANN H. & HUNTSMAN R.G. (1966) *Man's Haemoglobins.* Amsterdam, North Holland.

McFARLANE R.G. (1964) An Enzyme Cascade in the Blood Clotting Mechanism and its Function as a Biochemical Amplifier. *Nature* 202, 498–9.

WEATHERALL D.J. (1965) *The Thalassaemia Syndromes.* Oxford, Blackwell.

De Gruchy G.C. (1964) *Clinical Haematology in Medical Practice.* Oxford, Blackwell.

Wintrobe M.M. (1961) *Clinical Hematology* (5th ed.). London, Kimpton.

Dacie J.V. *The Haemolytic Anaemias,* Pr I (2nd ed.) *Congenital Anaemias* (1962): Pt II. *The Auto-immune haemolytic anaemias* (1962): Pt III. *Secondary or Symptomatic Haemolytic Anaemias* (1967). London, J. &. A. Churchill.

7

Immune Mechanisms

Normal function

The growth in knowledge concerning the physiology and pathology of immune mechanisms has brought confusion into the terminology. 'Immunology' was initially used to refer to the study of the process whereby an organism became 'immune' to a disease following exposure to bacteria or their products. In the early days of this study, it was thought that the process of immunization was always followed by a state of immunity. Later it became clear that exposure to a foreign substance sometimes gave rise to a state of 'hypersensitivity' rather than immunity. This led von Pirquet in 1906 to suggest that the term 'immunity' should be used only for those processes in which the introduction of a foreign substance caused no clinically evident reaction. He coined the word 'allergy' to refer to the 'changed state' that occurred after the initial exposure to a foreign substance; thus the 'allergic' state included both the state of 'immunity' and 'hypersensitivity'. In order to be consistent, the term 'immunology' should have become 'allergology', but this was not done, so that the meaning of the term 'allergy' became imprecise and its use restricted. It is now used synonymously with 'hypersensitivity'. In contrast the term 'immunology' has now expanded in meaning to cover the study of all aspects of the immune mechanisms activated by the entry of foreign substances into an organism; the term 'immunity' is used as a description of the protected state of the organism after the initial access of a foreign substance, and the terms 'hypersensitivity' or 'allergy' are clinical descriptions of the state where activation of immune mechanisms leads secondarily to disease.

All vertebrates from cyclostomes onwards have developed immunological methods of destroying foreign material. This function is associated with the presence of the thymus and cells of the lymphoid series. There are two different immune mechanisms within this system. (1) A mechanism whereby cells of the plasmacytic series produce free antibody which is distributed by the circulation and attacks the foreign substance at a distance. (2) A cell-mediated immunity which appears to rely on close contact between sensitized-lymphocytes and foreign material in order that destruction may take place. It has been suggested that the lymphocytes may react with foreign material by virtue of antibody bound to their surface. The evidence from phylogenesis and onto-genesis suggests that the sensitized-lymphocyte mechanism was the first to appear together with a limited ability to produce antibodies, which were those of high molecular weight. Later in evolution, the plasma cell series appeared and this was associated functionally with the ability to produce large amounts of free antibody.

FREE ANTIBODY SYSTEM
Sites and mechanism of production
This system is characterized by the production of immunoglobulins by cells of the plasmacytic series, found mainly in lymph nodes, spleen, liver, lung and bone marrow. Owing to the larger bulk of the bone marrow, it is probably the main organ of antibody synthesis against soluble antigens in the blood. The spleen plays an important part in the production of antibodies against particulate matter, and splenectomized subjects produce much less antibody after the injection of foreign red cells than do control subjects. The cytoplasm of plasma cells and their immature precursors contains a reticulum which can be demonstrated by electron microscopy and to which ribonucleic acid (RNA) granules are attached; it is at the surface of these granules that antibody is made, the exact structure being determined by messenger RNA. Antibody in high concentration can sometimes be demonstrated by conventional staining of plasma cells; the antibody appears as round hyaline eosino-philic structures, known as Russell bodies.

The following sequence of events occurs in the immune response. In the primary response, antigen reaches the lymph nodes via the lym-phatics, or reaches lymph tissue in the spleen, lung and bone marrow via the blood; it is then phagocytosed by the macrophages where it is processed in an unknown way. It is thought that substances (possibly small units of antigen) are then released and pass to the closely associated plasma cell precursors which are stimulated to mature into adult cells and to produce antibody against the antigen. Histological examination of a lymph node which is draining tissue containing antigen shows local areas of mitotic activity in the medullary cords associated with the production of cells of the plasmacytic series.

The time of appearance of antibody in the plasma in the primary response is variable but is usually of the order of 7 to 10 days after the initial exposure. The antibody is mainly IgM immunoglobulin (see below) in this initial phase. Following a second exposure of the organism to the antigen, there is a further rise in plasma antibody concentration beginning in 2–4 days after the stimulus. The antibody in this secondary response is usually IgG immunoglobulin. The earlier increase in plasma antibody compared to that seen in the primary response implies that there is an 'immunological memory'. The mechanism of this memory is unknown but it could be due to the persistence of antigen within reticulo-endothelial cells, or it may be due to the persistence of quiescent plasma cell precursors which are capable of responding immediately to a second exhibition of antigen. Plasma cells are found only in tissues or in lymph nodes and they release their antibody to attack the antigen at a distance. It is not known whether plasma cell precursors are small lymphocytes or whether plasma cells develop from a separate cell line.

Immunoglobulins
Following the development of the electrophoretic separation of plasma proteins into α-, β- and γ-classes, antibodies were located in the γ-globulin region. However, with the later development of immuno-electrophoresis, it was found that antibodies also travelled in the α- and β-globulin region and thus classification solely on the basis of electrophoretic properties was not possible. A new nomenclature was introduced and plasma proteins with antibody activity are now termed immunoglobulins and four classes are recognized, IgG (equivalent to γ-globulin on the old terminology) IgA, IgM and IgD in decreasing order of concentration. The 4 types of immunoglobulin differ in their electrophoretic mobility and in their antigenic specificity, that is, their ability to stimulate production of antibody specific for each class when injected into animals.

There is a basic structural design common to each class. The basic unit is a molecule (MW 140,000 to 180,000) composed of 4 polypeptide chains; 2 of these chains are 'heavy' chains (MW 50,000 to 70,000) and 2 are 'light' chains (MW approximately 20,000). There are 2 structurally different types of light chains, κ and λ, and both are found in all 4 classes; on the other hand the heavy chains are distinct for each class and these differences form the basis of the structural classification. The heavy chains are termed γ, α, μ and δ and belong to the IgG, IgA, IgM and IgD classes respectively.

Molecules of the IgG class always remain as single units of MW 140,000. They are Y-shaped and have a specific site at the end of each short branch to combine with antigen. Immunoglobulins of the IgM class always consist of 5 basic units held together by -S-S- bridges to give a molecular weight of approximately 900 000. It is because of their large size that this group is also descriptively termed macroglobulins.

TABLE 10. Immunoglobulins

Class	Molec. wt. (approximate)	Plasma conc. g/100 ml	Half life in plasma days	Placental transfer
IgG	140 000	1·2	21–28	Yes
IgA	140 000 or polymers	0·4	5	not known
IgM	900 000	0·12	5	No
IgD	140 000	0·003	not known	not known

Antibody molecules also have other specific functional areas on their surface apart from the sites which combine with antigen. There is a site for combining with complement (p. 275), and a site which is responsible for the active transfer of IgG across the placenta. The skin-sensitizing antibodies (p. 278) have a specific site for combination with mast cells.

The physiological significance of the different classes is not clear. Antibody of a single specificity may be found in all three classes. For instance, the blood group antibody anti-A of a group O person is mainly IgM, but some people also have small amounts of IgG anti-A. Following the injection of group A cells, IgG becomes the predominant type, but small amounts of IgA and IgM are also present.

There is considerable heterogeneity of structure within each immunoglobulin class; this is best exemplified by the IgG class on immunoelectrophoresis where the IgG runs from the α-globulin region to the end of the γ-globulin region. This variation in electrophoretic mobility indicates a wide range of electric charge, which is the result of the presence of molecules with different amino-acid sequences.

The capacity to form immunoglobulins is present from about the sixth month of intrauterine life. At birth IgM globulin is the main class that is actively produced; the IgG class of immunoglobulins is produced in significant amounts from about 2 months onwards.

Antigens

Foreign proteins and polysaccharides larger than a molecular weight of approximately 2000–5000 stimulate antibody production. These large molecules usually have many different discrete areas on their surface, each stimulating production of a different specific antibody; probably the size of each antigenic area is of the order of 1000–2000 Å^2. Chemical compounds smaller than MW 2000–5000 only stimulate antibody production when attached to large molecules and are known as haptens.

Antigen-antibody reactions
The association between antigen and antibody is a reversible chemical reaction. The forces involved are weak short range forces of several different types. These are (1) hydrogen bonds, where a H atom forms a weak link between 2 electronegative atoms (such as oxygen and nitrogen), (2) the electrostatic attraction between positive and negative charges, (3) van der Waal's forces (the non-specific attractive force every atom has for another atom when they approach close together), (4) the interaction of non-polar surfaces (the same phenomenon as that bringing about coalescence of oil drops in water). The specifity of the antibody is due to the fact that the contour enclosing the atoms at the binding site on the antibody closely approximates in a complementary manner the contour at the antigen binding site; thus the two sites come into such close apposition with each other that the intermolecular short range forces are powerful enough to hold antibody and antigen together.

The mode of destruction and disposal of antigen varies with different types of antigen. In the case of foreign inert particles or molecules, a lattice-work of antigen and antibody molecules is built up which eventually precipitates; this is followed by phagocytosis. Small soluble complexes (such as the combination of toxin and anti-toxin) are probably taken up by phagocytes by pinocytosis. Combination of antibody with bacteria and viruses may inhibit the action of important surface structures on these organisms. Alternatively, the complement system (see below) may be mobilized which, by unknown means, produces holes in the surface of the organism with subsequent release of the contents. This is the mechanisms of destruction of group A red cells by anti-A.

On the other hand, antibody may potentiate phagocytosis, as is shown in the case of Rh-positive red cells coated with anti-D which leads to their removal in the spleen without preceding lysis. Many bacterial exotoxins are enzymes and combination of antibody with these enzymes can inhibit the enzymic activity. In the case of viruses, attachment of antibody to the surface may prevent the penetration of the virus into the host cell.

The complement system
The complement system is a group of plasma proteins (9 have so far been identified) whose main purpose is to act in conjunction with antibodies and bring about lysis of bacteria or potentiate phagocytosis.

10

Antibodies (IgG and IgM) must first react with the bacterial cell wall and the first component of complement is then adsorbed on to a specific site on the antibody molecule. Following this, the other 8 components are activated successively by processes which are little understood at the present time. This activity takes place on the surface of the bacterial cell wall and when completed results either in the production of a hole in the cell wall with subsequent loss of intracellular components, or, by virtue of the presence of some of the components of complement on the cell surface, potentiates phagocytosis.

Lysis of red cells is also brought about in the same manner. For unknown reasons, complement is not always activated following antigen-antibody reactions. Thus, complement is bound following the reaction between anti-A and human red cells but not following the reaction with anti-D (anti-Rh).

Theories of antibody formation

Two theories are favoured at the present time, the selective and directive.

The *selective* theory states that the body contains a large number of groups of potential antibody-producing cells, each group genetically endowed to produce a certain specific antibody; following an antigenic stimulus those groups which produce antibody against that particular antigen will divide and develop into plasma cells and produce the specific antibody. Each group of precursor cells which can produce one type of specific antibody is known as a 'clone'. This theory implies that the body can only produce a finite number of different types of antibody the upper limit being set by the amount of genetic information that can be carried on the chromosomes.

The *directive* theory states that antigen enters a cell which is capable of producing immunoglobulin; the antigen then forms a template on which newly synthesized antibody can be correctly shaped so that its surface configuration is complimentary to the antigen molecule. Thus, antigen directs the formation of specific antibody and an infinite number of different types of antibody can be made.

There is so far insufficient evidence to decide firmly between these two theories, although the selection of genetically-endowed antibody producing cells is generally held to be the most likely mechanism.

CELL-MEDIATED IMMUNITY OR THE
SENSITIZED-LYMPHOCYTE SYSTEM

The preceding sections have dealt with the 'free antibody' system for the elimination of foreign substances. The other system, the sensitized-lymphocyte system, is imperfectly understood at the present time, although its importance may be greater than the free antibody system, especially in the aetiology of diseases associated with autoimmunity. Anatomically, the essential components of the system are the thymus and lymphocytes. The thymus plays an important role in the development of a competent immune system. The thymus is the first lymphoid tissue to develop, appearing after about 12 weeks of uterine life in man. Removal of the thymus in neonatal life in animals is followed by a profound depletion of small lymphocytes. The precise functional role of the thymus is not known but 2 roles are being considered at the present time. Firstly, the thymus may release a hormone which is responsible for the development of sensitized-lymphocytes. Secondly the thymus may be the main source of both short-lived and long-lived lymphocytes in the foetus and it may be the main source of long-lived lymphocytes in the adult.

Although it is certain that the thymus is essential for the full development and maintenance of the sensitized-lymphocyte system, it is not at all clear whether the thymus plays any part in the development of cells of the plasmacytic series.

It has been estimated that the total lymphoid tissue is equal in weight to the liver. There are approximately 40 times as many lymphocytes in the tissues as are found in circulation. Ninety per cent of the cells in the thoracic duct lymph are small lymphocytes which are undergoing continuous circulation from the lymph to the plasma and back to the lymph again. It appears that there are 2 populations of small lymphocytes, 1 population with a life span of approximately 5 days and the other with a far longer life span which has not yet been accurately estimated but may be 1 year or more. The relative functions of these 2 populations are not known; they cannot be distinguished by light microscopy.

Following the injection of antigen subcutaneously, 2 types of histological change can be seen in the draining lymph nodes. The first, the development of cells of the plasmacytic series in the lymph node medulla has already been discussed. The second type of activity occurs in the lymph node cortex, where areas of intense mitotic activity are associated with the production of lymphocytes and there is an increase in the number of lymphocytes leaving the node in the efferent lymphatics. Although no evidence has so far been produced, it seems probable that the cells leaving the node are sensitized-lymphocytes.

The mechanism of the sensitized-lymphocyte system can be exemplified by the homograft rejection reaction and by the response to the injection of tuberculin. The following plausible sequence of events has been suggested in graft rejection.

After a homograft has been applied, circulating small lymphocytes from the host make contact with antigen in the vascular walls of the graft; some of these lymphocytes are genetically endowed with recognition sites against the antigen and as a result of the contact migrate to the local lymph nodes where they multiply to produce a large number of sensitized-lymphocytes which leave the lymph node and migrate back to the graft where they become attached to the capillary walls and attack the endothelial cells. These are destroyed resulting in abolition of the blood supply to the graft. The mode of attack of antigen by sensitized lymphocytes is unknown. It appears to destroy the antigen by a direct attack through close contact. It has been suggested that its action may be mediated through cell-bound antibody or by soluble antibody which is released locally. This antibody may have high efficiency and be present in low concentrations and thus cannot be detected with existing methods.

Invasion by sensitized-lymphocytes is also seen in the reaction to the injection of tuberculin into subjects previously infected with the tubercle bacillus. The initial infection results in the production of sensitized-lymphocytes which are specifically active against components of this bacterium. When challenged with a subcutaneous injection of tuberculin, there is first an invasion by polymorphonuclear leucocytes but by 4 hours mononuclear cells predominate and by 24 hours there are closely packed perivascular masses of lymphocytes and macrophages. There is accompanying vasodilatation and thrombosis of capillaries. When the reaction is severe, necrosis results.

As the macroscopic appearance of the reaction to the injection of tuberculin does not appear for approximately 18 hours, and as the reaction, when severe, is deleterious in a manner analogous to anaphylaxis and serum sickness, it is termed the 'delayed hypersensitivity' reaction. A similar histological picture is seen in the lesions of tuberculosis and in such chronic infections as brucellosis, typhoid, syphilis and in various fungal infections; it is thought that it is the action of sensitized-lymphocytes against the bacilli starting secondary reactions which lead to the destruction of tissue in some unknown manner. The deleterious action on the body's own tissues is probably a different mechanism from that of graft rejection.

The activity of the sensitized-lymphocyte remains obscure because at the present time we have no insight into the central problem of how the lymphocyte reacts with the specific antigen against which it is sensitized. Following the reaction with antigen it is possible that a factor is released which damages the tissue and causes thrombosis in vessels, a mechanism analogous to the release of histamine following the reaction of tissue-adsorbed antibody and antigen (p. 283).

Does the reaction between sensitized-lymphocytes and antigen play a normal role in immunity without the appearance of deleterious manifestations of disease? This is a question which has never satisfactorily been answered. An experiment which suggests that it plays a normal role in immunity is as follows. It has been possible by varying both the amount and time relationships of the injection of both tubercle bacilli and tuberculin into animals to produce either delayed hypersensitivity or immunity to injections of tubercle bacilli. There is no convincing evidence that the free antibody system is responsible for immunity from tuberculosis and the sensitized-lymphocyte mechanism probably predominates. It is possible that the sensitized-lymphocyte normally destroys the bacillus and gives rise to 'silent' immunity but that under certain circumstances this mechanism breaks down and hypersensitivity with a consequent deleterious effect on the body is produced instead.

The sensitized-lymphocyte may also play a major role in counteracting virus and fungal infections, as individuals with thymic atrophy and lymphopenia are particularly susceptible to these diseases.

RELATIONSHIP BETWEEN THE TWO IMMUNE SYSTEMS
The following evidence suggests that the 'free antibody' and 'sensitized-lymphocyte' systems may be unrelated genetically. In birds lymphocytes and plasma cells are derived from separate sources; these sources are the thymus and the bursa of Fabricius, a cloacal lymphoid organ. Removal of the thymus in neonatal life in these animals leads to failure of small lymphocyte development and failure to reject skin grafts; removal of the bursa of Fabricius leads to failure to develop plasma cells and immunoglobulins in response to antigen injections. In man also there is evidence for a dual system; namely, that in the majority of sex-linked hypogamma-globulinaemias one immune mechanism is absent and the other is normal. In these patients there is an absence of plasma cells and a failure to develop immunoglobulin in response to antigen injection; on the other hand the thymus and small lymphocytes are present and a graft rejection by sensitized-lymphocytes is normal. It is possible that in man the precursor cells of both systems are derived from the thymus, but that they are under separate genetic control.

TOLERANCE
One of the remarkable facts about immune mechanisms is that antibodies are not made against the body's own tissues; that is, the antibody-forming mechanism can differentiate between 'self' and 'not-self'. The

understanding of the problem is the key to the understanding of auto-immune disease, but unfortunately the mechanism of tolerance, together with the mechanism whereby antibodies are formed are both unknown. The most important fact that has so far been established is that a state of tolerance towards a potential antigen is acquired during prenatal and early neonatal life. Thus during foetal development body compo-nents come into contact with cells concerned with immune mechanisms and these components are recognized as 'self'. After this critical period of 'immunological immaturity', any substance presented to the immune mechanisms is regarded as 'non-self'. This can be illustrated by 2 examples. Chimeras share a placental circulation and 'cross-trans-fusion' takes place *in utero*; thus a human chimera who is genetically group O and who has shared a placental circulation with a group A individual can tolerate group A red cells in the circulation and will not produce anti-A. Another example is the tolerance induced in animals by the injection of foreign antigen into the foetus *in utero* or into neo-nates within a few days of birth. Thus, bone marrow cells from one strain of mice injected at birth into mice of another strain will produce toler-ance in the recipient mice to skin grafts from the strain which donated the marrow cells.

At the present time, only the clonal selective theory of antibody formation can explain tolerance. It is suggested that during the period of immunological immaturity, 'self' components are presented to potential immunologically-competent clones of cells and that these clones are then suppressed and become 'forbidden' clones. There is evidence that the body component must continue to be presented to these clones throughout life in order for tolerance to be maintained.

Like other physiological functions, the induction and maintenance of tolerance can and does break down, allowing the immune mechanism to produce antibody or sensitized-lymphocytes active against 'self'.

Abnormal function

Abnormalities of immune mechanisms fall into 4 broad categories: (1) diseases in which there is a deficiency of either one or both types of immune mechanisms; (2) diseases in which there is an excessive pro-duction of immunoglobulins unrelated to antibody activity, as in myeloma; (3) allergic or hypersensitivity disease in which the reaction between antibody and antigen leads to harmful side effects; (4) auto-immune disease, where the immune mechanisms are directed against components of the bodies own tissues.

DEFICIENCY OF IMMUNOGLOBULINS

These syndromes have only recently been recognized and many details remain to be elucidated. On present evidence they can be divided into 3 categories. (1) A rare lymphoid aplasia involving thymic atrophy and absence of lymphocytes, plasma cells and immunoglobulins in the lymph nodes and blood (Swiss type of lymphopenia-agammaglobulinaemia). There is thus a deficiency of both the free antibody system and the sensitized-lymphocyte system, which results in susceptibility to infections. Affected children do not show the delayed hypersensitivity type of reaction and will not reject skin homografts. Such children do not live beyond the age of 2. (2) Hypoimmunoglobulinaemia, in which there is absence of plasma cells and low immunoglobulin level of all classes. (3) Dysimmunoglobulinaemia, in which there is selective failure of development of 1 class of immunoglobulins, i.e. low levels of IgG or IgA with a normal or increased amount of IgM, or a decrease in the level of IgA and IgM with a normal IgG concentration.

In categories 2 and 3, only the free-antibody system is affected and they are usually familial inborn errors of metabolism transmitted as sex-linked recessive traits. The disease is usually seen in boys, but a form occurring in girls has been described. These patients have an intact sensitized-lymphocyte system as they respond normally to the tuberculin test, develop contact sensitivity to chemicals, and will reject homografts. The main threat to these patients is frequent attacks of bacterial infection with pyogenic pathogens.

Deficiency of immunoglobulins may also appear as acquired diseases, either primary, or secondary to other diseases such as leukaemia.

Low immunoglobulin levels are also seen in protein-losing enteropathy (p. 407) when all classes of the serum immunoglobulins are reduced. In the nephrotic syndrome (p. 178) urinary loss of protein results in reduced levels of IgG and IgA; IgM levels are normal as this protein is too large to pass through the glomerulus.

EXCESS PRODUCTION OF IMMUNOGLOBULINS

Increased levels of immunoglobulins are found in 2 situations:

1. There is a general increase in all classes of immunoglobulins, either the result of hyperimmunization or in association with diseases such as systemic lupus erythematosus, sarcoidosis, hepatitis (various types), rheumatoid arthritis and certain neoplasms.

2. The other type of hyperimmunoglobulinaemia is associated with a neoplastic proliferation of plasma cells which are committed to the production of either IgG or IgA globulin, as seen in multiple myeloma,

or of IgM globulin, as seen in Waldenstrom's macroglobulinaemia. These abnormal proteins do not have demonstrable antibody properties, but this may be because they have not been tested against the right antigen. Abnormalities of protein production by neoplastic plasma cells fall into 3 categories: (a) Production of complete molecules of immunoglobulin, either of the IgA or IgG class. (b) Production of only the light chain polypeptide subunits, known as Bence-Jones proteins. As these chains are small, they pass through the glomeruli into the urine. (c) Production of both complete immunoglobulin molecules and the Bence-Jones protein.

Recently 'heavy chain disease' has been described in which the heavy polypeptide chains (MW 60,000) of the IgG class are produced. As the cells in these neoplastic diseases may be derived from a single abnormal cell, they produce protein which is structurally homogeneous and thus show a sharp peak on electrophoresis. This characteristic is useful in the identification of the abnormal plasma protein.

A homogeneous, myeloma type immunoglobulin is also occasionally found in individuals without any other evidence of disease; this has been termed 'asymptomatic monoclonal gammopathy'. However, clinical evidence of myeloma has later developed in a number of such patients.

ALLERGY

The term allergy is used now synonymously with hypersensitivity and refers to those situations where antibody-antigen reactions or the sensitized lymphocyte-antigen reactions are accompanied by secondary reactions which are inconvenient or harmful to the body. The term allergen refers to those antigens which bring about hypersensitivity reactions.

The growth in knowledge of the underlying mechanisms of the immune response have now advanced to the stage where a tentative classification of the different types of antigen-antibody reaction is possible on the basis of some aspects of their physiology. In *Type I reactions* the antibody is adsorbed on to tissue components and the antigen is free in solution before combining with antibody. In *Type II reactions*, the antigen is present on the surface of tissues and cells and the antibody is free in solution. In *Type III reactions* both antigen and antibody are initially free in solution and the antigen-antibody complex is formed in the plasma. In *Type IV reactions* the sensitized-lymphocyte mechanism is involved.

All of these 4 types of reaction can give rise to a state of hypersensitivity.

Type I, immediate or anaphylactic reactions

In this type of reaction, the initial introduction of antigen (allergen) stimulates the production of skin sensitizing antibodies, termed reagins, which are adsorbed to mast cells in the skin and mucous membranes. On a subsequent contact with the allergen, the formation of the antigen-antibody complexes sets a train of events in progress which leads to the release of histamine, serotonin and bradykinin from disrupted mast cells. These chemical substances cause contraction of smooth muscle and increased permeability of dilated capillaries, which account for the syndrome which is called anaphylaxis. This was so named in contra-distinction to prophylaxis because the immune response did not 'guard against' the injection of antigen but produced a secondary reaction which was harmful. The anaphylactic reaction is also termed the *immediate* reaction, because the signs develop within minutes of the reintroduction of allergen.

The basic defect in individuals showing anaphylactic reactions is not known but it has been suggested that they may inherit the capacity to produce reaginic antibodies. Opinions differ as to whether it is inherited through a single pair of genes or a number of pairs. Individuals in whom both parents have a history of allergy are likely to develop hypersensitivity before the age of 10, and those with only 1 parent affected develop symptoms at about puberty. Affected individuals without a family history usually develop symptoms in the third and fourth decades. Penetrance of the gene or genes is not complete and only a small proportion of children of affected parents develop the disease. It has been estimated that only 18 per cent of individuals with a heterozygous genetic make-up will be affected sometime in their lives. It is not known why individuals who are susceptible should develop reagins to certain allergens but not to others, or why the development of reagins should be delayed for so long in many cases.

Of the many different foreign substances to which an individual is exposed, only a few can bring about reagin formation. The common allergens are found in pollens, mould, spores, insect parts, animal dandruff, milk, eggs, fish, a few other foods and foreign serum proteins. Allergens that have been purified have been found to be small proteins of molecular weight, 3000–40,000, with which some carbohydrate is combined. There are only a few simple chemical allergens which provoke reagin formation and immediate anaphylactic reactions, the commonest in clinical practice being penicillin, organic iodides and local anaesthetics. These simple compounds, or their degradation products, react with tissue protein and form a haptenic group against which antibody

10*

is formed. Allergens act at extremely low concentrations, about 1 pg/ml being sufficient to release histamine from leucocytes.

Anaphylactic reactions in man may either be local or general. General reactions follow the injection of foreign serum, pollen extract, therapeutic and diagnostic agents, such as penicillin, organic iodides and local anaesthetics, or following insect stings. Laryngeal oedema and bronchiolar constriction predominate, but circulatory collapse may also occur. Local reactions are manifested as hay fever and asthma from inhalation of air-born substances; urticaria may be considered to be a local reaction resulting from ingestion of allergens in food, such as strawberries, nuts, milk, eggs or following the administration of penicillin and salicylates. Sudden cot death in babies is also a form of anaphylaxis resulting from inhalation of stomach contents containing cow milk. It has been shown that bottle-fed babies produce antibodies against cow's milk protein in the second week of life. This antibody is adsorbed in lung tissue and reacts with antigen following inhalation.

Desensitization can be brought about by the injection of allergens in gradually increasing amounts. This results in the production of IgG antibodies which react with the allergen and bring about its destruction, but do not cause skin sensitization. As the IgG antibody is present in much greater amounts than the reagin, it successfully competes for the allergen, thus diverting it away from the reagin adsorbed on to tissue sites. For this reason, the IgG antibody is known as 'blocking' antibody.

Type II or cytolytic reaction
In contradistinction to type I reactions, type II are characterized by the presence of antigen on cells. This group is dominated by the antibody responses to invasion by bacteria and viruses. The antibodies involved are of the IgG, IgA and IgM classes, and the combination with the antigens on the surface of the invading organisms leads to their immobilization and destruction by lysis or phagocytosis without harmful secondary effects from the antigen-antibody reaction. Transfusion reactions and haemolytic disease of the newborn are also due to type II reactions.

The most important group of type II reactions giving rise to allergic states are those following the ingestion of drugs. They may produce reactions which result in the shortening of the life span of red cells, white cells and platelets. When certain drugs are taken they may combine loosely with surface constituents of one of the formed elements of blood. The combination of the drug and surface constituent is now antigenic with the drug acting as a hapten. Antibodies are thus produced against the complex of hapten attached to the surface component in the normal way; when the antibody subsequently reacts at the cell surface, it brings about the destruction of the formed element by phagocytosis.

The classical example of this type of drug hypersensitivity is the thrombocytopenia resulting from the ingestion of Sedormid (allyl-isopropyl-acetyl-carbamide) and it is also seen following quinidine and sulphonamide administration. It can be demonstrated *in vitro* that the patient's serum will bring about agglutination of platelets in the presence but not in the absence of the drug. In a similar manner a variety of drugs (especially the phenothiazines) cause agranulocytosis and, less frequently, haemolytic anaemia.

Type III, antigen-antibody reaction in the plasma

The chief clinical representative of this type of reaction is serum sickness. This disease is the result of an antigen-antibody reaction but the mechanisms involved contrast notably with those concerned with anaphylaxis. In an anaphylactic reaction there is preformed antibody attached to skin cells and the antigen, by comparison, is present only in minute amounts. By contrast, in serum sickness there is no preformed antibody; the antigen (foreign serum protein) is first introduced into the plasma; antibody is formed in response to the antigenic stimulus and then reacts with the antigen still present in the plasma. It is the formation of antigen-antibody complex when the antigen concentration is greatly in excess of antibody that gives rise to the lesions of serum sickness. The signs and symptoms appear to be an unfortunate secondary manifestation of a system which is primarily designed to rid the body of foreign substances.

The disease appears approximately 7–14 days after serum therapy, usually the injection of horse serum containing tetanus antitoxin. The antigens are the α- and γ-globulins of the horse serum. It is a necessary condition that the antigens giving rise to this syndrome must remain in the plasma until the appearance of antibodies; only serum proteins will do this; other types of proteins are rapidly removed. The antibody (IgG) appears between 7 and 14 days after the injection of the antigen. At first only small antigen-antibody complexes are formed and antigen remains in the circulation but signs and symptoms appear at this stage; it is presumed that the circulating complexes are deposited in vessel walls and cause local inflammation. The lesion seen in this syndrome is a vasculitis with both an acute inflammatory exudate and a mononuclear infiltration around small arteries which leads to necrosis of arterial walls and myocardial fibres. The mechanism by which antigen-antibody complexes formed in antigen excess given rise to these lesions is entirely unknown.

The foreign serum proteins also stimulate the production of reagins which are absorbed to specific sites on the skin. The principal secondary manifestations of the reaction between allergen and the 2 types of antibody are fever, arthralgia, urticaria and a maculopapular eruption Nephritis, carditis, neuritis and peritarteritis nodosa are also occasionally seen.

During the first few days after the onset of the disease, the rate of antibody production rapidly increases and as plasma antibody levels rise so the complexes formed between antibody and antigen become larger and complement is bound to their surface; the complexes are then rapidly removed from the circulation and free antibody can then be detected in the plasma. The antibody concerned in this reaction can be detected by a haemagglutination reaction in which antigen is adsorbed on to red cells and addition of the antibody will then bring about agglutination (p. 300). It has been found that individuals who develop serum sickness usually have small amounts of this haemagglutinating antibody in the plasma prior to serum therapy and thus the likely occurrence of the disease can be predicted with some certainty. It is not known why these individuals should have these antibodies initially, but it could be due to the presence of a cross-reacting antibody formed in response to the ingestion of mammalian serum proteins, as it is known that serum proteins from different animals have some common antigenic sites. The value of detecting susceptible individuals lies in the possibility that corticosteroids could prevent the onset of the syndrome.

Drugs, especially penicillin, can also give rise to a serum-sickness type of syndrome. The initiating mechanism is the combination of penicillin or a penicillin derivative with serum proteins; penicillin thus acts as a hapten and a specific antibody is produced which will react with penicillin-protein present in the plasma to form the antigen-antibody complexes which give rise to the perivascular inflammatory exudate of serum sickness.

Glomerulonephritis. Much of our basic knowledge about serum sickness has come from experimental studies on animals. A finding of particular importance is the development of glomerulonephritis in which the lesion is a proliferation of the endothelium of the glomeruli similar to that found in glomerulonephritis in man. Further experimental work in rabbits has shown that a continuous injection of antigen (bovine serum albumin) just in excess of that needed to combine with all the antibody in the plasma leads to changes similar to those seen in human glomerulo-nephritis and systemic lupus. Electron microscopy has demonstrated irregular basement membrane thickening in these experimental animals; this thickening is thought to be due to deposits of antibody, antigen (bovine serum albumin) and complement, all of which have been demonstrated to be present in this area by fluorescent techniques.

There is little doubt that antigen-antibody complexes can cause lesions in animals which are almost identical to the lesions of human glomerulo-nephritis, but there is still no direct evidence that this is the cause of the disease in humans. The relationship between the disease and the preceding infection with β-haemolytic streptococci is still an enigma; there is no evidence of involvement of stretptococcal antigens in the formation of antigen-antibody complexes which might cause the renal damage. The only piece of indirect evidence which is relevant is the consistent finding of low serum complement levels which could result from a complement-fixing antigen-antibody reaction. The presence of complement in glomerular lesions has been demonstrated by immuno-fluorescence.

Type IV, delayed type hypersensitivity

Very little is known concerning the fourth type of reaction, which is that mediated by sensitized-lymphocytes. It is termed 'delayed hyper-sensitivity' as this describes one of the characteristics seen on skin testing, namely a delay of approximately 12–24 hours between the injection of antigen subcutaneously and the appearance of induration and erythema. Histologically, the induration is due to lymphocytes and macrophages and is classically exemplified by the response to the injection of tuberculin in people who have had a tuberculous infection. No free antibody has been consistently demonstrated and there appears to be a direct reaction between lymphocytes and antigen which leads through unknown mechanisms to the vascular damage and necrosis; the latter may be the result of the inadequate blood supply. In the case of the lesions of tuberculosis, there is considerable evidence that the pathogenesis results from hypersensitivity and not from endo- and exotoxins from the mycobacterium.

Delayed-type hypersensitivity develops as the result of contact with a wide variety of agents. Of the infectious diseases, it is particularly the chronic bacterial and fungal diseases in which it plays a part, such as typhoid, undulant fever, leprosy, coccidiodomycosis, blastomycosis and dermatomycosis, parasitic helminth infection, leishmaniasis and insect bites.

Contact dermatitis is also a manifestation of delayed hypersensitivity. The chemical concerned must be soluble and able to diffuse into tissue and also must be able to react with tissue protein. It is the complex between the chemical compound and tissue protein which is antigenic and provokes a delayed-hypersensitivity type of reaction. The same basic mechanism is also the cause of homograft rejection. Graft rejection has 2 factors in common with delayed hypersensitivity (1) infiltration with mononuclear cells, (2) failure of transference by serum from one animal to another. However, graft rejection can be transferred by a living cell suspension obtained from lymphoid tissue.

DRUG REACTIONS

It is to be noted that allergic drug reactions can appear as any of the 4 types of antigen-antibody reaction. The drugs which bring about reactions through immune mechanisms are all of low molecular weight and hence do not stimulate antibody production or activate the sensitized-lymphocyte system unless they are attached to a large molecule, almost invariably a protein. A wide variety of drugs is known to stimulate the immune mechanisms and many but not all are known to react with proteins. For instance, in a series of halogenated nitrobenzenes there is a relation between the ability to react with protein and the ease with which they provoke an immune response. The antibody produced by drugs not only reacts with the primary antigen but also with closely related compounds. Thus a patient with antibodies against streptomycin will also react against neomycin, and anti-benzocaine antibodies will also react against sulphonamides, as both benzocaine and sulphonamides have a common aminobenzene component.

The type of drug reaction depends partly on the reactivity of the drug and partly on the type of antibody produced in response to the hapten-protein complex. Thus drugs stimulating the production of reagins give rise to urticaria, bronchial asthma or severe anaphylactic shock. Drugs combining loosely with the formed elements of blood and giving rise to IgG antibodies bring about thrombocytopenia and haemolytic anaemia. Drugs combining with plasma proteins give rise to serum sickness though their reaction with IgG antibody. And finally, drugs can activate the sensitized-lymphocyte system, giving rise to contact dermatitis.

Drugs can give rise to many other signs and symptoms (exanthematic eruptions, erythema multiforme, liver, heart and kidney damage) but nothing is known of the underlying mechanisms as they cannot be classified at the present time.

AUTO-IMMUNE DISEASES

In the early years of immunological research, it was found that animals could not be immunized against their own body components and this phenomenon was expounded as the general law of 'horror autotoxicus' by Ehrlich. It is now known that, as with other rules, there are exceptions, and that an immune response is found against 'self' components in a number of diseases. The relationship between the presence of the immune response and both aetiology and pathogenesis of these diseases is however still uncertain. As far as aetiology is concerned, two fundamentally different mechanisms have been suggested. First, the primary defect may be a breakdown in tolerance mechanisms, so that certain body components may be recognized as 'not-self' and initiate an immune response, which leads to functional and structural changes. Secondly, the diseases may be due to agents which damage tissue and only lead secondarily to the appearance of the immune response. The activation of immune mechanisms in this case could be due to the release of slightly altered body components which are recognized as 'not-self'; the antibody and sensitized-lymphocyte which are produced may then react with unaltered body components as a result of their ability to cross-react with closely related antigenic structures.

There is some evidence for both hypotheses and it is possible that both mechanisms may exist, each giving rise to different diseases.

There is evidence that in auto-immune diseases both antibodies and sensitized-lymphocytes are produced. However it is generally agreed that, except in the case of the auto-immune blood diseases, antibodies are not the primary agents of the functional and structural abnormalities although they may play an aggravating secondary role. For instance, it is not possible to produce thyroiditis in animals by the prolonged injections of anti-thyroglobulin. Nevertheless, it is argued that the presence of antibodies against 'self' is evidence of an underlying disorder of the immune mechanisms and it is suggested that the sensitized-lymphocyte system is the primary agent responsible for the pathological changes. Until further light is thrown upon those problems, the definition of an auto-immune disease should be 'a disease in which there is evidence of the presence of an immunological response against apparently normal body components'.

Auto-immune haemolytic anaemia

Both IgG and IgM antibodies are found and the clinical syndrome is partly dependent on the distinct differences in the physico-chemical properties between the different types of antibodies.

IgG antibodies are found in acquired haemolytic anaemia; approximately one-third are specific against antigens of the Rhesus system, but the specificity of the remainder is unknown. These antibodies react at 37° and bring about the continual destruction of red cells in the reticulo-endothelial system.

The Donath-Landsteiner antibody, which gives rise to the syndrome of paroxysmal cold haemoglobinuria associated with syphilis, belongs to the IgG class and is specific against the blood group antigen P. The reaction between antibody and red cells only takes place to a significant extent below 20°, hence symptoms only appear after extensive lowering of the skin temperature. This antibody causes lysis of red cells, which gives rise to haemoglobinuria.

A third type of antibody which is well characterized is the macro-globulin (IgM) causing the cold agglutinin syndrome. This antibody is specific against the blood group antigen I or i, and reacts with the red cells below 30–32° and hence causes symptoms on mild cooling of the skin. This antibody brings about agglutination which blocks small vessels and gives rise to Raynaud's phenomenon.

Auto-immune thrombocytopenia and leucopenia
The existence of platelet auto-antibodies is uncertain, partly because the demonstration of platelet agglutination due to antibodies is a difficult technical procedure. Moreover, there is evidence that the concentration of antibody which will cause thrombocytopenia *in vivo* is far below the concentration that can be detected by *in vitro* tests. A further complication is the difficulty of obtaining adequate numbers of platelets for investigation from patients with thrombocytopenia. Nevertheless, it is almost certain that auto-immune antibodies may develop in association with thrombocytopenia in a small number of cases.

These remarks on the difficulty of demonstrating auto-antibodies against platelets apply similarly to the demonstration of auto-antibodies directed against leucocytes. Nevertheless, it is now well established that auto-immune antibodies are found in many patients with leucopenia.

Thyroid disorders
Activation of immune mechanisms appears to be responsible for certain thyroid disorders, especially Hashimoto's thyroiditis and primary myxoedema (p. 554). The presence of anti-thyroglobulin and anti-thyroid microsomes can be demonstrated in the plasma. These antibodies may play a part in the pathogenesis of this disease since babies born to mothers may show transitory signs and symptoms during the

time of persistence of IgG antibodies derived from the mother. Invasion of thyroid tissue by lymphocytes and plasma cells suggests that there is also activation of the sensitized-lymphocyte system.

In a small proportion of patients, anti-thyroid antibodies are associated with antibodies against one or more of the following: nuclei, intrinsic factor, gastric parietal cell, liver cell and red cells. This suggests that these thyroid disorders may be part of a general breakdown of tolerance to certain tissue components.

Rheumatoid arthritis

Both the antibody producing and the sensitized-lymphocyte mechanisms are probably activated in rheumatoid arthritis. The antibodies are the so-called rheumatoid factors. These are antibodies which specifically react with antigen sites on the patient's own IgG immunoglobulins. The antigen sites are hidden when IgG is free in the plasma, but they become exposed when IgG is adsorbed to inert particles, such as bentonite, or when IgG antibody has reacted with antigen to form an antigen-antibody complex. It is generally accepted however that rheumatoid factors do not bring about the lesions in the synovial membranes; this is suggested by the fact that rheumatoid factor is not found in all patients, and also because patients with low concentrations of immunoglobulins have rheumatoid arthritis indistinguishable from that of other people. Despite this, it is generally held that the presence of auto-immune antibody in so many patients with rheumatoid arthritis suggests that the disease is due to some other derangement of immune mechanisms. The mechanism that is postulated to be active is the sensitized-lymphocyte system, partly on the basis that the infiltration with lymphocytes in the synovial membrane is closely akin to that seen in the delayed hypersensitivity type of reaction. Although this view may prove to be correct, the evidence for it which we have at the present time is tenuous.

Sjögren's syndrome

There is evidence of widespread involvement of immune mechanisms in this disease. No antibodies have been demonstrated which are active against salivary glands, but the glands show considerable lymphocytic infiltration suggesting activation of the sensitized-lymphocyte system. The presence of the following antibodies has been demonstrated: anti-nuclear, anti-liver extract, anti-thyroid, anti-gastric antibodies and rheumatoid factors. This disease thus bears a resemblance to systemic lupus erythematosus and to rheumatoid arthritis.

Pernicious anaemia
Both anti-intrinsic factor and anti-gastric parietal cell antibody are
found in patients with pernicious anaemia. It is unlikely that these
plasma antibodies bring about the gastric atrophy or are the primary
cause of intrinsic factor deficiency as large amounts of anti-intrinsic
factor are found in some patients with thyroiditis who have normal
B_{12} absorption. Moreover antibodies are not found in all cases of pernicious anaemia as would be expected if they bore a causal relationship
to the intrinsic factor defect. Activation of the sensitized-lymphocyte
system has again been suggested as the factor bringing about the pathological changes.

Systemic lupus erythematosus
This disease is characterized by the presence of a variety of auto-antibodies active against nuclear components, cytoplasmic constituents
such as mitochondria and microsomes, and against cell membranes.
   As with other auto-immune disease, the precise role played by antibodies in the aetiology and pathogenesis is obscure. Pregnant women
with systemic lupus transmit the antibodies to the foetus who is nevertheless unharmed by their presence. On the other hand, the multiplicity
of the antibodies and the fact that they act against antigens common to
many tissues argues in favour of a fundamental fault in tolerance mechanisms. Several reports have now appeared of the appearance of the
delayed hypersensitivity reaction following injection of the patients own
white cells, indicating activation of the sensitized-lymphocyte system.

Adrenocortical failure
There is now evidence that some patients with Addison's disease (p. 528)
have auto-immune antibodies active against cells of the adrenal cortex.
Antibodies have also been found against the thyroid antigens in some
of these patients, suggesting that there may be a general breakdown of
tolerance.

Rheumatic heart disease
Two facts of an immunological nature have now been established in
relation to rheumatic heart disease. First, an attack of rheumatic fever is
almost invariably preceded by an infection with β-haemolytic streptococci, and is accompanied by a rise in titre of antibodies against one or
more of the streptococcal antigens, such as streptolysin O. Secondly,
auto-immune antibodies against heart tissue have been demonstrated
to be present in certain cases. The question is whether these auto-immune

antibodies are the cause or the effect of the cardiac lesion. Auto-immune antibodies against cardiac tissue can be demonstrated following cardiac surgery and myocardial infarction. Thus, antibodies in rheumatic fever could be the result of the release of cardiac antigens following damage to the heart by some other agent. On the other hand, it has recently been found that there is a common antigenic determinent in streptococci and in cardiac tissue and it is suggested that streptococcal antigens give rise to specific antibodies which then cross-react with cardiac antigens.

Principles of tests

From a clinical point of view, investigations on immune mechanisms fall into 3 categories: (1) the determination of the plasma concentration of each of the 3 classes of immunoglobulin; (2) the detection of the presence of a specific antibody in the plasma; and (3) the detection of the antigen-antibody reactions seen in hypersensitivity syndromes.

PLASMA IMMUNOGLOBULIN CONCENTRATION
Total serum proteins
As the immunoglobulins form only a part of the total serum proteins, measurement of the total protein content or total globulin content is clearly a crude method for determining either deficiency or excess and will only detect grossly abnormal deviations. The normal range of concentration depends on the method used for the estimation. The biuret method which is commonly used, gives a total protein content between 6·2 g and 7·7 g/100 ml. The globulin content (α-, β- and γ-globulins) is found by precipitating the globulins with sodium sulphate, measuring the concentration of albumin remaining in solution and calculating the difference between total protein and albumin content; normal values for globulins range from 1·4–2·9 g/100 ml.

Paper electrophoresis
Different types of plasma globulin molecules are characterized by having differing overall surface charge and hence move at different rates in the presence of a voltage gradient; this is the basis for the classification into α-, β-, and γ-globulin classes. The γ-globulin region contains only the IgG immunoglobulin, but the α- and β-globulin regions both contain a number of different proteins; IgA and IgM immunoglobulins are found in the β-globulin region. Thus, the separation of proteins by electrophoresis on filter paper followed by staining gives useful information.

A deficiency of IgG globulin can easily be demonstrated, but IgA and IgM globulins do not show as separate peaks and deficiency of these proteins cannot be recognized by this method. However, the presence of abnormally high concentrations of IgG and IgA proteins as in myeloma, can be recognized by paper electrophoresis. As these abnormal proteins are homogenous, abnormal IgA usually shows a sharp peak in the region between the normal β- and γ-globulin, varying slightly in position for each patient. Abnormal IgG travels more slowly and is usually found as a sharp peak at the end of the normal γ-globulin region. Differentiation into IgG or IgA types cannot however be made with certainty by this method. Normal IgG globulin is usually reduced in amount in the presence of either type of myeloma protein.

Abnormal IgM macroglobulin cannot be well assessed by this method as it often precipitates on the filter paper and remains at the site of origin. When a satisfactory electrophoretic pattern is obtained, it cannot be distinguished from the IgG and IgA myeloma proteins.

Starch gel electrophoresis
When electrophoresis of serum is carried out on starch gel, the pores are too small to allow the large IgM globulin molecule to enter and abnormal IgM macroglobulin therefore remains at the origin. However, if the reducing agent, 2-mercaptoethanol, is incorporated in the gel, the IgM molecule is broken down into 5 subunits about the size of an IgG molecule, which can penetrate the gel and staining demonstrates the presence of the abnormal protein.

Sia water test
IgM immunoglobulins usually have the property of precipitating out of solution when the ionic strength is reduced. Thus, if serum containing abnormal IgM is diluted with distilled water a precipitate rapidly forms. A precipitate is also obtained if large amounts of IgM antibody are present as in malaria or Leishmaniasis, but this precipitate only appears very slowly. The presence of most but not all abnormal IgM macroglobulins can be demonstrated this way.

Immunological methods
The qualitative differentiation of immunoglobulins into IgG, IgA and IgM is based on the fact that each type possesses its own distinctive antigenic groupings. Thus, after injection of purified IgG, IgA or IgM into a rabbit, the animal produces specific antibodies against these immunoglobulins. The reaction between these antibodies and antigen

to form a complex results in the precipitation of the complex out of solution.

The precipitation reaction can be elegantly demonstrated by the method of immunodiffusion in which the specific antibody is incorporated into a thin layer of agar gel on a glass plate. If serum containing the antigen is placed in a hole in the agar, the antigen diffuses into the agar, reacts with the antibody and forms a ring of precipitate around the hole. Precipitates only form when the ratio of antibody to antigen is correct (usually of the order of 2 : 1 to 10 : 1); in excess of either one or other component, the antigen-antibody complex remains soluble. Thus, the diameter of the ring of precipitate is proportional to the concentration of antigen in the solution placed in the hole; as the concentration of antigen increases so the correct conditions for precipitation will be found further from the hole. By using agar places containing either anti-IgG, anti-IgA or anti-IgM, the concentration of the corresponding immunoglobulins can be estimated in human serum, using purified preparation of these proteins as standards. This method can be applied to any protein present in serum, once a specific antiserum has been produced in animals. The accuracy of the method is reasonable, the coefficient of variation of repeated determination on the same sample probably being about 10–20 per cent. For this reason, precise normal limits for the three classes of immunoglobulins cannot be given, but should be established in each laboratory for each particular batch of antisera that is used. Average values for the immunoglobulins in adults that may be expected are as follows: IgG, 1·2 g/100 ml, IgA, 0·4 g/100 ml, IgM, 0·12 g/100 ml.

In assessing IgG concentration account must be taken of the age of the patient. Very little IgG is produced by the newborn, but is provided by the mother so that, at birth, levels are approximately the same as maternal concentrations. The level falls to reach a value of 0·3–0·8 g/100 ml by 6–12 weeks, when IgG globulin production becomes significant and the level then rises to adult values by 5–7 years.

There is no sharp dividing line between normal and abnormally low levels of IgG, but the majority of patients with clinical symptoms resulting from deficiency have levels below 0·2 g/100 ml.

DETECTION OF SPECIFIC ANTIBODIES

The only way of recognizing the presence of a specific antibody is by detection of its reaction with the antigen. The reaction between antigen and antibody may be divided into two phases. The first is the primary chemical reaction between antigen and antibody, a phase which cannot be detected by any simple method. In the second phase, the formation of the antigen-antibody complex results in such reactions as precipitation, agglutination, complement-fixation, and phagocytosis. It is these secondary manifestations which are utilized in detecting the presence of antibody. The relative concentration of antibody is usually expressed in terms of titre, which is the reciprocal of the highest dilution of antiserum that gives rise to a just-detectable reaction.

The LE cell factor

This factor is one of several antibodies specific against the DNA-histone complex. Serum containing the factor is added either to a white cell preparation containing damaged cells or to whole nuclei and the antibody becomes attached to the nuclei. The nuclei swell and become sensitized to phagocytosis by neutrophils; it is the appearance of altered nuclear remnants in the leucocytes that characterize the LE cell. The test is positive in approximately 90 per cent of cases of systemic lupus but it is also positive in some cases of rheumatoid arthritis, sclerodema, dermatomyositis, polyarteritis, Sjögren's syndrome, and chronic active hepatitis.

The antinuclear factor

This factor is a collection of antibodies specific against nuclei and which includes the LE cell antibodies. This collection of antibodies is demonstrated by the method of immunofluorescence. The technique is as follows: (1) A section or smear of tissue is exposed to the antiserum; antinuclear antibody (IgG) becomes attached to the nuclei. (2) An antiserum containing fluorescin-labelled anti-IgG is added; this anti-IgG becomes attached to the anti-nuclear antibody and its presence on the nuclei can be established by microscopic observation of the fluorescence. Sera from different patients bring about different patterns of fluorescence, suggesting different types of antibody in different cases. This test is positive in the majority but not all cases of systemic lupus but it is also positive in some cases of 'juvenile' cirrhosis, chronic active hepatic and primary biliary cirrhosis.

The autoimmune complement fixation test (AICF)

Many IgG and IgM antibodies have specific sites on their surfaces to which complement is bound once antigen-antibody complexes have been formed. The utilization of complement can be used as an indication of the presence of an antigen-antibody reaction, particularly when no visible secondary reaction occurs, such as precipitation.

The AICF is a test for the presence of antibodies against cytoplasmic constituents. The antigen is a saline extract of human liver which is added to serum suspected of containing antibodies. If there is formation of an antigen-antibody complex, complement is subsequently bound and the diminution in serum complement concentration can be detected by the sensitized sheep red cell method (p. 301). This test is positive in most cases of systemic lupus and is also positive in certain cases of 'lupoid' hepatitis, post-viral hepatitis, alcoholic cirrhosis, primary biliary cirrhosis, and in approximately 10 per cent of patients with rheumatoid arthritis.

Rheumatoid factor

There are two basic methods for determining the presence of this factor, depending on the antigen used; one method uses human IgG as antigen and the other uses rabbit IgG. When human IgG is used, this is first adsorbed on to bentonite, latex particles or tanned red cells (normal red cells do not adsorb protein but they will do so after treatment with tannic acid). The adsorption procedure exposes the antigenic sites on the IgG against which rheumatoid factor acts and the addition of sera containing anti-IgG (rheumatoid factor) then brings about agglutination of the coated particles or red cells. This method can give rise to a false-positive reaction, as human IgG has other antigenic sites on its surface, which will react with 'non-rheumatoid factor' antibody such as is found in syphilis, sarcoidosis and viral hepatitis. The other method of detecting rheumatoid factor is more specific and relies on the cross-reactivity of the rheumatoid antibody with rabbit IgG. This is the *Rose-Waaler* test and consists of adding the patient's serum to sheep red cells sensitized with sub-agglutinating amounts of an anti-sheep red cell antibody obtained from a rabbit. The anti-sheep cell antibody, when reacted with sheep cells, has sites exposed on its surface against which the rheumatoid antibody will react and bring about agglutination.

Anti-thyroid antibodies

The presence of anti-thyroglobulin may be demonstrated by two methods. (1) A precipitate will form on addition of human thyroglobulin to the patient's serum; this is not a sensitive test and low levels of anti-body cannot be detected but it is usually positive in cases of Hashimoto's thyroiditis. (2) A test of high sensitivity is the agglutination of tanned red cells coated with thyroglobulin. Very high titres (greater than 25,000) are obtained in the majority of cases of Hashimoto's thyroiditis and primary myxoedema. The test is positive in about half the cases of thyrotoxicosis, but with low titres, usually between 5 and 25 000. Low titres are occasionally seen in non-toxic colloid goitre and in carcinoma.

TESTS USED IN ALLERGIC REACTIONS

Detection of the 4 different types of immune reaction requires basically different tests in each case. Diagnosis of the reactions of type I and IV can only be detected by *in vivo* skin tests in man at the present time; antibodies associated with type II and III reactions can be detected *in vitro*.

Type I, immediate or anaphylactic reaction

There is no laboratory test available at the present time for detecting reagins (skin-sensitizing antibodies) and resort must be made to *in vivo* tests. Skin tests are available for determining whether reagins are present in patients with asthma, rhinitis, urticaria, and gastro-intestinal abnormalities. These skin tests are the local manifestation of the anaphylactic reaction. Suspected antigen (extracts of pollen, house dust etc.) is introduced into the skin and if reagin is present adsorbed to skin tissue, the antigen reacts with it and this leads to the release of histamine from mast cells. The release of histamine gives rise in a few minutes to an urticarial weal and erythematous flare.

Negative reactions do not exclude hypersensitivity; failure to obtain a response may be the result of the arbitrary nature of the antigen, which may differ considerably in potency from different sources and with different batches. Moreover patients with negative reactions may be found to respond when tested a few years later.

Skin testing with drugs suspected of causing allergic reactions are only occasionally positive. The reason for this is that the antibody is formed against the drug or drug derivative complexed with protein and the combining site on the antibody reacts not only with the drug but also with a small area on the protein surface immediately surrounding the site of attachment of the drug. The drug alone does not combine adequately with the antibody, and when the drug is injected into the skin, there may not be any of the correct protein present for complex formation.

Skin testing for penicillin hypersensitivity can be successfully carried out using the synthetic polypeptide, penicilloyl-polylysine. Approximately half the patients with a history of penicillin allergy give a positive skin test. A small number of individuals with no history also give a positive test, and these individuals have a chance of developing penicillin allergy. The skin test with penicilloyl-polylysine becomes negative for a time following a therapeutic dose of penicillin, which is presumably due to competition by the penicillin for the antibody.

Passive transfer test (Prausnitz–Küstner test). Patients with type I reaction have reagins in the plasma which can be demonstrated by subcutaneous injection of the plasma into a normal individual. Reagin is adsorbed on to specific tissue constituents, and histamine is released with subsequent weal formation and erythema when challenged with the antigen 24 hours later. The use of this test is limited by the danger of the transfer of serum hepatitis.

Blocking antibody. The presence of IgG antibody which competes with the reagins for the allergen can be demonstrated by an agglutination reaction using tanned red cells to which the allergen has been adsorbed. Unfortunately, there is no relationship between the titre of the IgG antibody demonstrated in this way and the concentration of reagins, so that the presence of IgG antibody in the serum is only evidence of an immune response to the allergen but not that reaginic antibodies are present and are responsible for the symptoms. Antibodies against the following antigens have been demonstrated by this technique—grass pollens, protein hormones, penicillin, coffee bean, horse serum, milk and egg-white proteins.

Tests for type II hypersensitivity drug reactions
Antibodies specific against the complex of drug and protein on the surface of platelets and red cells can often be detected *in vitro*. Anti-leucocyte antibodies cannot be detected with certainty.

Antibodies causing thrombocytopenia. The simplest test is the addition of the patient's serum to normal plasma to which a saline solution of the suspected drug has been added; clot formation is then allowed to take place. The combination of antibody, drug and platelets brings about inactivation of the function of the platelets in promoting clot retraction. Thus, if clot retraction is poor in the presence of the drug compared to a control to which only saline is added, then this is an indication of a relation between the bleeding manifestations and administration of the drug.

The presence of antibodies can also be demonstrated by observing either agglutination of platelets or complement fixation when the patients serum, drug and platelets are added together.

These tests are not positive in every case and thus as many as possible should be carried out; the complement-fixation test is the most reliable.

Antibodies causing haemolytic anaemia. If the drug is added to normal red cells, it will combine with sites at the red cell surface. The addition of the patient's serum containing the suspected antibody may bring about agglutination as the result of the reaction between antibody and the drug–red cell complex. If agglutination does not occur, this may be because the concentration of antibody is insufficient, and the sensitivity of the test can be enhanced by the addition of an anti-immunoglobulin serum.

Type III, antigen-antibody haemagglutination reactions
Antibodies of the IgG type specific against penicillin derivatives and against the foreign serum proteins which cause serum sickness can be demonstrated by haemagglutination techniques, in which the penicillin or foreign serum proteins are adsorbed on to tanned red cells and the addition of the patient's serum produces agglutination.

Type IV, delayed or tuberculin-type reaction
This type of reaction involves the action of sensitized-lymphocytes which invade the tissues and attack the antigen by direct contact. This results in the secondary manifestations of erythema, thrombosis and necrosis. This reaction is particularly suitable for demonstrating hypersensitivity to bacteria (in tuberculosis, leprosy, brucellosis), fungi (in dermatomycosis, coccidiomycosis, histoplasmosis), viruses (in psittacosis, lymphogranuloma inguinale), hydatid disease and leishmaniasis. The reaction is brought about by the subcutaneous injection of extracts containing a protein derivative from these infecting agents. The protein remains at the site of injection sufficiently long to allow the invasion of sensitized-lymphocytes in those subjects who are already sensitized. The typical reaction is a raised red indurated area which becomes visible after 18–24 hours, reaches a maximum in 48 hours and takes a week to subside. If a large dose of antigen is given, the area may become necrotic. On histological examination the area is found to be infiltrated with lymphocytes and macrophages. A positive reaction indicates past or present infection but cannot differentiate between the two. Hypersensitivity may persist for months or years after destruction of the infecting agent. A negative reaction indicates absence of the infecting agent, with the exception that hypersensitivity does not arise until several weeks after the initial invasion, and may also be negative in the acute phase of the disease.

Allergic contact dermatitis. Delayed type IV sensitivity-reactions are also seen in contact dermatitis where the hapten is some well-defined chemical substance. The patch test in which the suspected allergen is placed on a small area of skin is the simplest to use and positive reactions are shown by redness, swelling, papules, vesicles and if severe, by a confluent blister. Although this reaction is macroscopically different from the tuberculin-type reaction, histologically it is basically the same, both showing monocyte infiltration. The reaction appears in 24–48 hours but may occasionally be delayed for 96 hours. False positive reactions are given by chemicals which are irritants; the character of the reaction may be different (irritants usually cause pustules, necrosis and bullae) but the hypersensitivity lesion may be simulated. Hypersensitivity lesions can be repeatedly and consistently produced, whereas irritant lesions are variable in response. False positives may also be seen if the skin is in a highly reactive state after an acute attack of eczema. Plaster sensitivity may also cause confusion. False negatives are seen when inadequate concentrations of the chemicals are applied to the patch or when there is inadequate contact with solid materials.

Estimation of complement activity
A biological test is available for the determination of complement activity which depends on the fact that a rabbit anti-sheep red cell antibody requires complement to bring about the lysis of sheep red cells. For any given concentration of antibody, the rate of lysis and liberation of haemoglobin is dependent on the concentration of complement. The rate of lysis brought about by the unknown source of complement is thus compared to that brought about by a serum containing normal complement levels.

Activation of the complement system only occurs following an initial antigen-antibody reaction. Thus low complement levels are an indication that an antigen-antibody reaction has taken place. However, not all antigen-antibody reactions result in complement-fixation so that the presence of normal levels of complement does not exclude an antigen-antibody reaction.

Practical assessment

Clinical observations
Deficiency of immunoglobulins may be suspected in underweight children suffering from multiple and recurrent infective diseases.

Excessive production of immunoglobulins by plasma cells are associated with multiple small bone tumours and pathological fractures.

Allergic reactions. Type I or immediate reactions (cell-bound antibody): local manifestations of erythema and weal formation in the skin; conjunctivitis and rhinitis, as in hay fever; generalized anaphylactic reaction, as asthma and circulatory collapse.

Type II reactions (cell-bound antigen) (commonest type): rarely produces functional disorder; when antigen is on the surface of one of the formed elements of blood, the reaction with antibody results in diminution in numbers of the formed element; can cause spontaneous allergic haemorrhage and anaemia.

Type III reactions (antigen-antibody reaction in plasma): fever, lymphadenopathy, and joint swelling 7–14 days after the parenteral administration of a foreign protein or drug.

Type IV reactions (sensitized-lymphocyte system): contact dermatitis due to allergic mechanisms suspected when lesions develop only after prolonged contact with the causative agents.

Autoimmune reactions. No characteristic signs and symptoms with the immune response itself. The clinical abnormalities are those associated with the functional and pathological changes in the tissue or organ involved in the disease.

Routine investigations
Deficiency or excess of immunoglobulins in the plasma: evaluated crudely by the biochemical estimation of total serum globulins or more accurately by electrophoretic analysis on paper. Excess immunoglobulin production may be associated with the presence of light chains (Bence–Jones protein) in the urine.

Allergic reactions. Type I reactions: agent responsible for both local and general reactions may be identified by skin testing, and observation of the local immediate anaphylactic response.

Contact dermatitis due to a type IV reaction: diagnosed by elicitation of a delayed response on intradermal injection of the suspected agent. There are also many diseases due primarily to an infecting agent (bacteria, fungi, tape worms etc.) in which the pathological changes may be due at least in part to type IV reactions. Infection with these agents, either past or present, may be diagnosed by elicitation of delayed hypersensitivity reactions following subcutaneous injection of extracts of the infecting agents.

Autoimmune diseases. Diagnosis depends on the demonstration of antibodies in the patient's plasma. Anti-immunoglobulin test (Coombs' test) demonstrates antibodies on red cells in haemolytic anaemia. Other tests include those for macroglobulin in cold agglutinin syndrome, Donath-Landsteiner antibody (haemolytic test), rheumatoid factor (Rose-Waaler test), and LE cell test (p. 296).

Special investigations
Plasma concentration of immunoglobulins in deficiency diseases or in cases of excessive production determined by immunodiffusion on agar plates.

Allergic reactions. Type I. The presence of reagins can be demonstrated by the passive transfer of serum from the patient into a normal recipient (Prausnitz–Küstner test).

Type II reactions. Antibodies acting against drugs (sedormid, quinidine, penicillin) adsorbed to platelets or red cells and causing thrombocytopenia and haemolytic anaemia can be detected by agglutination reactions, using the suspected drug adsorbed to tanned red cells. Anti-white cell and anti-platelet antibodies can also be detected by agglutination techniques.

Type III reactions. Antibodies causing serum sickness detected by a haemagglutination technique in which penicillin or foreign serum proteins are adsorbed to red cells.

Autoimmune diseases. The presence of antibodies on certain cells of the thyroid, adrenal cortex, stomach (gastric parietal cells) and white cell nuclei can be demonstrated on biopsy material by the technique of immunofluorescence.

References

BOYD W.C. (1956) *Fundamentals of Immunology.* New York and London, Interscience.

BURNET F.M. & FENNER F. (1949) *The Production of Antibodies.* London, Macmillan.

BURNET F.M. (1959) *The Clonal Selection Theory of Acquired Immunity.* London, Cambridge University Press.

GELL P.G.H. & COOMBS R.R.A. (ed.). (1963) *Clinical Aspects of Immunology.* Oxford, Blackwell.

HOLBOROW E.J. (1967) An ABC of Modern Immunology. *Lancet,* **i,** 833, 890, 942, 995, 1049, 1098, 1148, 1208.

HUMPHREY J.H. & WHITE E.G. (1964) *Immunology for Students of Medicine.* Oxford, Blackwell.

RAFFEL S. (1953) *Immunity, Hypersensitivity, Serology.* New York. Appleton-Century-Crofts.

TOMASI T.B. (1965) Human Gamma Globulin. *Blood,* **25,** 382–403.

Topley and Wilson's Principles of Bacteriology and Immunity revised by WILSON G.S. & MILES A.A. (1964) London, Arnold, 5th edition.

SAMTER M. & ALEXANDER A.L. (ed.) (1965) *Immunological Diseases.* London, Churchill.

ZWEIFACH B.W., GRANT L. & McCLUSKEY R.T. (ed.) (1965) *The Inflammatory Process.* London, Academic Press.

HOLBOROW E.J. (Scientific editor) (1963) Antibodies. *British Medical Bulletin,* **19,** No. 3.

BRENT L. (Scientific editor) (1965) Transplantation of Tissues and Organs, *British Medical Bulletin,* **21,** No. 2.

TURK J.L. (Scientific editor) (1967) Delayed Hypersensitivity: Specific Cell-Mediated Immunity, *British Medical Bulletin,* **23,** No. 1.

8

Bone

Normal function

The solid matter of bone is made up of an orderly array of minute mineral crystals lying on a dense web of collagen fibres bound together by a mucopolysaccharide cementing substance (the organic matrix or osteoid). The remarkable strength and resilience of bone is probably due to this complex arrangement. Mineral salts—chiefly calcium and phosphorus—make up nearly 37 per cent of bone by weight, but over 19 per cent is organic matter and the rest is water (44 per cent).

Ninety-five per cent of the organic matrix of bone (osteoid) is collagen. It provides the scaffolding or trabeculae upon which the mineral crystals are deposited, but it also provides a local chemical and structural environment which favours the orderly precipitation of calcium salts to form bone. Only native collagen, which has a specific helical structure and is synthesized by osteoblasts, can initiate nucleation from metastable solutions of calcium phosphate. By using a calcium-chelating agent such as ethylenediamine tetra-acetic acid (EDTA), decalcified bone sections can be made which show a lattice of collagen fibre bundles on electron microscopy. These bundles are prominent along lines of stress and in the cortex of the long bones. The ground substance between the fibres is a complex polymerized mucopolysaccharide containing chondroitin, chondroitin sulphate and hyaluronic acid. Small amounts of muco-protein are also present.

The cells found in bone consist of (1) the osteocytes which maintain the life and structure of bone, (2) the osteoblasts which appear at the sites of new bone formation and are intimately concerned with the production of new matrix and its calcification, and (3) the osteoclasts which are multinucleated giant cells seen at sites of bone resorption. Osteoblasts, therefore, are numerous in conditions such as rickets or healing fractures associated with the rapid new formation of matrix; whereas osteoclasts are seen particularly in conditions associated with excess resorption of bone such as hyperparathyroidism.

The mineral crystals of bone are extremely small but can be seen under the electron microscope as flat tablets about 200 Å long and 25–50 Å thick. The crystals appear to be formed along the collagen fibres in a regular way, and the spatial configuration of collagen molecules determines the sites on which crystals can form. Bone crystals are composed of a compound of calcium, phosphate, hydroxyl ions and water. In many ways, they closely resemble the larger crystals of synthetic basic calcium phosphate or hydroxyapatite ($3Ca_3(PO_4)_2 . Ca(OH)_2$), the only known form of calcium phosphate which is stable at physiological ECF hydrogen ion concentrations (40 mμ-equiv/l. or pH 7·4). However, crystals of bone also contain carbonate, citrate and small quantities of other ions (particularly sodium, magnesium, strontium, chloride and fluoride). They are surrounded by a hydration shell which increases their effective size and allows the free exchange of ions. The ions at the surface of the crystals equilibrate rapidly with the surrounding medium (and, therefore, with the extracellular fluid) and slowly with the ions in the centre of the crystal. Thus the crystal structure of bone resembles an ion-exchange column, and surface exchanges have been demonstrated with many different ions. For example, the Ca^{++} near the surface is readily exchanged for Na^+ or for H_3O^+ (hydronium ion). In general, cations displace Ca^{++}, multivalent anions displace phosphate, and F^- displaces OH^-. The presence of the organic matrix greatly slows the rate of ion exchange presumably because the crystals are intimately mixed with matrix and all exchanging ions must permeate through it. But there must still be a very large area in equilibrium with the comparatively small volume of extracellular fluid, even if a relatively small proportion of the total crystal surface (estimated at over 100 acres for a normal man) is available for ion exchange. Bone is thus important in contributing to and reflecting the composition of the extracellular fluid. Foreign elements such as lead or strontium gain ready access to bone. These substances, which are deposited in bone by exchange with Ca^{++}, can usually be removed from the body if chelating agents such as EDTA are administered soon after ingestion. After a few weeks, however, it is impossible to remove every trace of the foreign element because by this time it has penetrated deep into the crystal structure.

THE PROCESS OF CALCIFICATION

The formation of hydroxyapatite crystals cannot take place until the solubility product of Ca and P ions exceeds a certain value. Under normal physiological conditions, the concentration of total calcium in the body fluids is considerably greater than the concentration of calcium ions available for chemical reactions. About half the total plasma calcium is loosely bound to protein (mainly albumin) and some of the remainder is chelated to citrate and other anions. But in addition only 30 per cent of the ions themselves are *specifically active* at the temperature, concentration and [H⁺] of body fluids. The reason for this is that the movement, and hence the 'activity', of large multivalent ions is restricted in solution by mutual attraction and repulsion, according to ionic charge. Only when infinitely dilute do ions exert their full, calculated effects on osmotic pressure, freezing-point depression, and electrical conductivity. However, although many factors tend to reduce the solubility product of calcium and phosphate ions in the body fluids, the blood plasma (and hence interstitial fluid) still appears to be supersaturated with respect to bone mineral even if we allow for the additional fact that carbonate, magnesium, citrate and other ions increase the effective solubility of bone mineral. A more conventional view of the calcification process considers that $CaHPO_4 . 2H_2O$ (secondary calcium phosphate) is laid down initially and is then hydrolyzed to hydroxyapatite. The evidence for this is indirect and is based on the fact that under many different experimental and clinical conditions, a simple product of $[Ca] \times [P]$, which corresponds closely to the solubility product of Ca^{++} and HPO_4^{--} ions, gives the best expression of the effect on bone calcification of varying phosphorus and calcium concentrations. In this case, the plasma would appear to be undersaturated with respect to bone mineral. The difficulty with this view is that $CaHPO_4 . 2H_2O$ can probably never exist in the body because it spontaneously hydrolyzes to hydroxyapatite at physiological hydrogen ion concentrations. Therefore, the only way in which secondary calcium phosphate can be implicated is to assume that the hydrogen ion concentration at the bone surface is considerably greater (about 150 mμ-equiv/l., or pH 6·8) than the rest of the extracellular fluid.

Thus there is a basic problem which will remain unsolved until somebody manages to measure the [H⁺] at the mineral surface. If the body fluid is supersaturated, then clearly there must be mechanisms which prevent unrestricted mineral deposition in bone and also other tissues. Alternatively, if the body fluids are undersaturated there must be local mechanisms which increase the solubility product of calcium and phosphate ions. This second approach has dominated most past research. Whatever the answer, the initiation of calcification almost certainly involves both alkaline phosphatase and some sort of 'seeding' process (epitaxy) related to the specific molecular structure of bone

11

collagen. Views on the role of alkaline phosphatase in the calcification process will clearly depend on whether the extracellular fluid is super-saturated or undersaturated with respect to bone mineral. If the latter, more conventional, view is held, then the high concentration of alkaline phosphatase in bone provides a ready mechanism for a booster system by which the local concentration of phosphate can be raised so that the critical ion product of calcium and phosphate needed for precipitation is exceeded. Alternatively, it has been suggested that alkaline phosphatase promotes calcification by hydrolyzing a hypothetical coating of phosphate esters which normally protects bone mineral from being exposed to the full concentrations of calcium and phosphate in the extracellular fluid. This would fit well with the idea that the extracellular fluid is normally supersaturated. However, the necessity for alkaline phosphatase in the process of calcification has been questioned because, *in vitro*, rachitic cartilage will still calcify in normal serum even if the enzymes have been destroyed by heating. The fact that the disorder, hypophosphatasia, produces a calcification defect similar to rickets does, however, suggest that alkaline phosphatase is important.

BONE GROWTH AND REPLACEMENT

New bone is formed continuously—and the old destroyed—at a rate which changes with age and varies greatly in different parts of the same skeleton. The effect of ageing on the relative rates of bone formation and resorption is not clearly understood, but at both extremes of life bone is normally less compact than in middle life. This steady replacement involves the formation of new matrix as well as new mineral crystals so that physiological and pathological factors which influence the availability of protein are probably as important as calcium and phosphorus in the manufacture of bone. The net result of new bone formation (accretion) and its simultaneous destruction (resorption) can be measured by means of tracer elements, either radio-active ones such as ^{47}Ca (which has a half-life of about 5 days), or inert ones like strontium which bone does not appear to distinguish from calcium. By this means the normal adult rate of calcium turnover in bone has been estimated at 10 mg/kg body weight/day: it is raised in hyper-parathyroidism and diminished in hypoparathyroidism. About 0·05 per cent the whole skeleton is renewed each day in adults, 0·3 per cent in adolescents and 1 per cent in infants.

The formation of new bone is associated with the appearance of osteoblasts by which the process is probably controlled. The dissolution of bone is accompanied by the appearance of osteoclasts, but it is not clear whether they actually destroy the bone or whether they simply remove the products of matrix destruction. Youth, injury, mechanical stress and the sex hormones stimulate new bone formation: old age, disuse and protein deficiency allow the matrix to degenerate.

Bone growth, in contrast to bone replacement, ceases after puberty. Long bones grow from the ossification of cartilage (endochondral bone formation); the flatter bones grow from connective tissue (membranous bone formation). The growth of the skeleton depends upon an adequate rate of secretion of growth hormone and of the thyroid hormones (see page 549). Although pre-pubertal growth depends on the presence of growth hormone, the spurt of growth at puberty is not associated with an increase of the plasma growth hormone concentration. It is, of course, associated with an increased secretion of androgens and oestrogens but these hormones also promote fusion of the epiphyses of long bones and children whose puberty is precocious are usually stunted. Other factors, such as nutrition, also affect growth. Skeletal dwarfism often accompanies severe chronic illnesses in infancy or childhood, especially those associated with intestinal malabsorption.

The maximum rate of growth of an individual occurs during infancy, and on the average a child acquires half of his or her adult stature at the age of 2 years. The rate of growth falls later, and between the ages of 5 and 12 years growth proceeds at a constant rate of about 5 cm (2 in.) each year. Boys normally develop a rapid spurt of growth coinciding with puberty, between the ages of 12 and 15 years, amounting to 7·5 cm (3 in.) or more each year. They also become increasingly muscular at this time. The rate of growth usually reaches its maximum between 14 and 15 years of age. Thereafter it rapidly falls again, and after the age of 18 years it almost ceases because the epiphyses close. Girls show a similar but less pronounced spurt of growth which starts a little earlier, owing to the earlier onset of puberty. Growth also ceases earlier than in boys, usually at about 17 years of age. The differences are commonly accounted for by the differences between androgens and oestrogens in their relative growth-promoting and epiphyseal-closing actions, but genetic differences may also be important.

BONE AND THE EXTRACELLULAR FLUID

In addition to containing nearly all the body's calcium and about 88 per cent of its phosphorus, bone contains about 58 per cent of its magnesium, 35 to 40 per cent of its sodium and 6 per cent of its potassium.

By themselves, however, these figures do not mean much physiologically. We really need to know the proportion of each mineral which is freely and rapidly available to contribute to the homeostasis of the electrolyte composition of the extracellular fluid. A reasonable estimate of this can be obtained by isotope dilution and is often considerably less than the value obtained by carcass analysis. The total 'exchangeable' quantity is obtained by estimating, at equilibrium, the radio-activity per unit mass (specific activity) in a representative sample of body fluid after the administration of a suitable radio-isotope (see also p. 35). With this type of method, about 30 per cent of the sodium and 20 per cent of the magnesium in bone mineral has been shown to be in rapid equilibrium with the extracellular fluid. In contrast, the proportion of the total skeletal calcium which is readily exchangeable is surprisingly small (less than 0·5 per cent in adults). Nevertheless, it probably represents a considerable fraction of the total exchangeable calcium in the whole body, and changes in the rate of turnover of this compartment form the basis of many recent studies concerning the relative rates of bone formation and destruction in disease.

Since about one-third of the sodium in bone mineral is freely exchangeable, bone may act as a buffer to protect the electrolyte composition of the extracellular fluid against sudden change. About 300 m-equiv. is potentially available to act in a homeostatic capacity but salt depletion does not appear to cause mobilization of much bone sodium. It seems more likely that newly-formed bone merely reflects the composition of the extracellular fluid bathing it. A change in the composition of the extracellular fluid (e.g. hyponatraemia) will soon result in the formation of new bone crystals whose hydration shell has a different composition from normal.

CALCIUM AND PHOSPHORUS METABOLISM

Body content
A 70 kg man contains about 1100 g of calcium; 1000 g (99 per cent) is present as bone, 10 g is intracellular and 1 g is extracellular. Whether intracellular calcium can be mobilized in hypocalcaemia is unknown. There is roughly one-half as much phosphorus in the body as calcium; 90 per cent of it is in bone.

Absorption
Although diets vary greatly, about 800 mg or more of calcium and 1100 mg of phosphorus are usually consumed each day, chiefly in the form of milk and milk products. In addition about 200 mg of calcium

is secreted in the digestive juices each day and this mixes with the dietary calcium in the small intestine. Of this mixture 200–300 mg of calcium are absorbed and the rest excreted in the faeces.

Calcium absorption from the intestine depends on the presence of vitamin D, but local factors, such as the dietary Ca/P ratio, the amounts of phytic acid in the meal (calcium phytate is almost insoluble), the acidity of the upper gut (where the bulk of Ca is absorbed) and the amount of magnesium present, probably determine day-to-day variations of Ca absorption. Whether changes of vitamin D activity are ever involved facultatively is unknown but in the absence of circulating vitamin D the quantity of calcium excreted in the faeces equals or exceeds the intake, however high the intake of calcium. Conversely, if an adequate amount of vitamin D is available, then calcium absorption will usually be sufficient even if the diet contains very little calcium. It is probably only during periods of rapid growth, pregnancy or lactation that clinical evidence of calcium deficiency can occur without coincident deficiency of vitamin D.

Most of the *phosphorus* in the diet is well absorbed unless there is an excess of some poorly absorbed metal such as aluminium, or a gross excess of calcium. $Al(OH)_2$ is given as a means of reducing the absorption of phosphorus for diagnostic purposes. The faecal excretion of phosphorus is comparatively small whatever the intake: it ranges from 20–40 per cent of the amount in the diet.

Calcium and phosphorus in the blood

In the plasma the total *calcium* concentration varies within the narrow limits of 9·0–10·5 mg/100 ml in normal people. Even a slight fall affects neuromuscular transmission and any prolonged rise jeopardizes the kidneys. About 40 per cent of the total plasma calcium is loosely bound to protein (mainly albumin), but despite its importance little is known about the factors which influence the calcium binding properties of the plasma proteins. The calcium not bound to protein (i.e. the ultrafiltrable calcium) is almost all ionized and it is this fraction that is physiologically important. A small proportion—usually about 0·5 mg/100 ml—is ultrafiltrable, but unionized: it is complexed with citrate and other organic substances. The level of ionized calcium in the plasma is largely independent of the overall calcium balance of the body. It is regulated by the circulating concentrations of parathyroid hormone and vitamin D, and also, possibly, by those of thyrocalcitonin (p. 316). Without the parathyroid glands or vitamin D, the plasma calcium concentration varies with dietary calcium intake to a far greater extent than normal.

At the hydrogen ion concentration in blood, 85 per cent of the plasma *inorganic phosphate* is in the form of HPO_4^{--}. The plasma concentration varies proportionally more than that of calcium (3·2–4·2 mg/100 ml), because there are so many factors which affect it. Parathyroid hormone and vitamin D are important influences and normally they act in opposite directions (see p. 317). In addition the plasma concentration is influenced by the amount of phosphorus in the diet, by the adequacy of renal function and by the metabolic activity of muscle. After a meal glucose enters the cells together with phosphate and the plasma phosphate concentration falls. In chronic renal failure with azotaemia there is phosphate retention and a rise in plasma concentration, whereas in renal tubule disease there is often an excessive loss of phosphate in the urine with resulting low plasma concentrations. Adrenocortical steroid hormones, particularly cortisol, and many other substances increase renal phosphate clearance and so reduce the circulating phosphate level.

Urinary excretion of calcium and phosphate

The urinary excretion of *calcium* reflects the plasma concentration and, like it, is largely determined by endogenous factors (see p. 328). This contrasts with the urinary excretion of other common electrolytes such as sodium or potassium which depends rather precisely on their intake. However, this may be an oversimplification because when calcium intake is reduced rapidly and considerably (from say 1000 to 100 mg/day), the urine calcium excretion falls within days. On the other hand with smaller changes of Ca intake it may take weeks or months to achieve equilibration.

The factors which influence renal handling of calcium are poorly understood because it is so difficult to estimate the filtered load, but calcium almost disappears from the urine when the plasma concentration falls below 7–8 mg/100 ml. About 90 per cent of the calcium filtered at the glomeruli is ionic and the rest is unionized calcium complexed with citrate and other organic substances. In the urine, however, a much higher proportion of the total calcium is in the complexed form. Despite a filtered load of about 6 mg/min or 10 g/day, only 1–2 per cent of this appears in the urine (100–200 mg/day).

In contrast to calcium the urinary *phosphate* excretion is normally determined largely by the rate of intestinal phosphate absorption. The urine phosphate output is, therefore, a relatively high proportion of the intake (60–80 per cent). Nearly all the plasma phosphate is ultrafiltrable under physiological conditions so the amount of phosphate filtered at the glomeruli can be determined with an accuracy comparable to that of glomerular filtration rate measurements. About 5–10 per cent of the filtered load appears in the urine, the exact proportion depending largely on the plasma phosphate concentration. There is a 'threshold' of plasma phosphate concentration (about 2 mg/100 ml) below which very little phosphate appears in the urine. Despite a widespread assumption that, like sodium, the urine phosphate is filtered phosphate which has not been reabsorbed, the exact renal mechanism by which phosphate is excreted is not known. It has been claimed that active tubular phosphate secretion can be demonstrated in dogs loaded with acid-phosphate, but whether, as in the case of potassium (p. 158), tubular secretion is the normal physiological means by which phosphate is excreted remains obscure. The relationship between the plasma phosphate concentration (whether spontaneous or raised by infusions of phosphate) and the simultaneous rate of urine phosphate excretion varies in many conditions. Based on this, many diagnostic tests have been devised in an attempt to differentiate between hyperparathyroidism and other causes of hypercalcaemia and hypercalciuria (p. 328).

VITAMIN D

This vitamin was the first to be identified and the syndrome of vitamin D deficiency was well described over 50 years ago, but the mechanism of its biological action and its interrelationship with parathyroid activity are still far from clear.

The most obvious and sensitive action of vitamin D is to promote calcium absorption from the upper gastrointestinal tract. As mentioned already, very little calcium is absorbed in the absence of vitamin D, however high the calcium intake. The vitamin also has an important direct action on bone. It increases the resorption of bone mineral, so raising the plasma calcium concentration. With the right experimental conditions it is possible to produce a rise of plasma calcium without an increase in calcium absorption from the bowel. Studies with radio-isotopic calcium show that vitamin D facilitates both resorption and deposition of bone mineral. Mineral deposition usually appears to predominate over resorption during the correction of vitamin D deficiency and the Ca^{++} concentration in the plasma may fall and even provoke tetany. In vitamin D poisoning resorption of bone predominates, causing hypercalcaemia, hypercalciuria and metastatic soft tissue calcification, even in the absence of calcium in the diet.

Vitamin D was thought to have a direct effect on renal tubular phosphate handling, acting in the opposite direction to parathyroid hormone. In the rachitic infant, vitamin D does cause phosphate retention but this is probably mediated through changes of parathyroid activity. An increase of plasma Ca^{++} concentration as a result of giving vitamin D reduces the production of parathyroid hormone which, in turn, causes phosphate retention and a fall of urine phosphate excretion. In patients with hypoparathyroidism vitamin D reduces the plasma phosphate concentration, and so acts like parathyroid hormone.

As well as increasing the plasma concentration of calcium and phosphate, Vitamin D also increases the plasma concentration of citrate. This does not happen if the plasma concentrations of Ca^{++} and P are increased by direct infusion. Therefore vitamin D may act by increasing the concentration of citrate in bone; a high local citrate concentration at the crystal surface may dissolve the bone mineral by chelation and lowering pH.

THE PARATHYROID GLANDS

Although two distinct types of cells can be seen histologically in human parathyroid glands (the chief and the oxyphil cells), the only function of these minute organs known at present is to secrete adequate amounts of parathyroid hormone. This regulates the concentration of ionized calcium in the extracellular fluid by directly influencing (1) the amount of ionized calcium reabsorbed from bone, (2) the amount of phosphate excreted by the kidney. The existence of two types of cells, two main biological actions of parathyroid extracts and two clinical syndromes of hyperparathyroidism, the one associated with bone dissolution and the other with renal stones, has led, in the past, to the idea that there may be two separate parathyroid hormones. Evidence for this is, so far, lacking. Animal experiments based on the relative calcium-mobilizing and phosphaturic properties of crude parathyroid extracts are inconclusive and we now know that parathormone, isolated in pure form from extracts of the parathyroid glands, still has both calcium-mobilizing and phosphaturic properties. It is a straight or slightly folded polypeptide with a molecular weight of about 9000. *In vitro*, it may influence the rate of exchange of Ca and P in mitochondria. Other polypeptides have also been purified from parathyroid extracts which stimulate glycolysis or which promote the uptake of P but they have no effect on Ca^{++} or P *in vivo*. The discovery of calcitonin and thyrocalcitonin (see below) helps to explain the confusing physiological effects of crude parathyroid extracts.

Mobilization of calcium from bone

Removal of the parathyroids causes a fall of plasma Ca^{++} concentration to 5–7 mg/100 ml, a level which is subsequently maintained by skeletal mineral without parathyroid intervention. The parathyroids, therefore, cause bone mineral to support higher levels of calcium in the extracellular fluid than would be expected from simple solubility considerations. Excess parathyroid activity causes a dissolution of bone by a primary direct action; for example, parathyroid tissue will slowly dissolve the surrounding bone if grafted on to it. How this happens is unknown, but osteoclasts accumulate and these cells may be directly stimulated by parathyroid hormone. On the other hand, they may appear secondarily to serve some sort of scavenger function. The precise biochemical change in bone induced by the parathyroid hormone is unknown but recent theories include an action on bone citrate similar to the effect of vitamin D (see above), a depolymerizing effect on the ground substance and an action on subcellular fractions, particularly mitochondria. The difficulties of *in vitro* techniques and the use of impure parathyroid hormone makes interpretation difficult but the evidence is now against an action on organic acid production.

Renal actions of parathyroid hormone

Parathyroid extracts have a considerable, swift and direct effect on the kidney to increase phosphate excretion in the urine. This is distinct from its effect on bone because it appears immediately after injection of hormone, before there is an increase of plasma calcium concentration. Although impure preparations of parathormone increase the rate of glomerular filtration, the pure hormone does not. Therefore it must act directly to increase tubular phosphate secretion or, as more conventionally considered, to inhibit tubular phosphate reabsorption (see p. 157). Parathormone may also influence directly the rate of tubular calcium reabsorption.

The rapidity by which parathyroid extracts increase urinary phosphate excretion was used by Albright to develop a unifying concept of parathyroid action. The hormone was presumed to act by inducing phosphaturia, calcium being affected only indirectly. The fall of plasma phosphate as a result of urine phosphate loss would then stimulate bone dissolution and so produce hypercalcaemia. However, it is now clear that parathyroid extracts will raise the plasma calcium in nephrectomized animals; and, in otherwise intact dogs, hypocalcaemia precedes hyperphosphataemia after removal of the parathyroid glands. Nevertheless, the renal action of parathyroid hormone may be important in the

11*

normally functioning organism even though an important direct effect on bone is demonstrable in experimental animals.

Parathyroid hormone also has other renal effects. It reduces sensitivity to vasopressin (ADH) and renal hydrogen ion secretion is diminished (p. 164). The urine becomes alkaline and there is a tendency to acidosis. These effects may be a simple consequence of hypercalcaemia or phosphaturia rather than a specific effect of the hormone itself.

The control of parathyroid hormone production

The production of parathyroid hormone appears to be directly controlled by the concentration of ionized calcium in the extracellular fluid. Low values for [Ca^{++}] in the blood reaching the parathyroid glands increase the rate of secretion of parathormone and high values depress it. This is reminiscent of the way in which insulin production by the pancreas is controlled by the concentration of glucose in the arterial blood (p. 473). We do not know by what reference standard this control is set, but all cells throughout the body are very sensitive to slight variations of the [Ca^{++}] of the fluid bathing them. Suggestions that changes of plasma phosphate concentration also influence parathyroid activity, but in the opposite direction to that of Ca^{++}, are based on indirect evidence which can equally well be interpreted on the basis of coincident changes of plasma Ca^{++} concentration. Recent studies show that when P is infused into cattle, the plasma concentration of immuno-reactive parathyroid hormone is unchanged unless plasma Ca^{++} also changes.

There is no conclusive evidence for the existence of a parathyroid stimulating hormone from the pituitary or elsewhere, and patients with hypopituitarism do not suffer from hypocalcaemia. But there may well be other factors apart from reduced plasma Ca^{++} concentration which can stimulate parathyroid hormone or at least influence the 'setting' of the direct control of hormone production by [Ca^{++}]. For example, it appears that the considerable increase of urine calcium excretion seen following injections of growth hormone depends upon the presence of intact parathyroid glands.

Thyrocalcitonin and the regulation of plasma calcium

When parathormone is injected intravenously or when the parathyroid glands are removed, the concentration of Ca^{++} in the plasma changes slowly. When the plasma Ca^{++} is raised by infusions of calcium salts or lowered with EDTA, it changes rapidly. Therefore a negative feedback system involving only Ca^{++} and parathormone does not explain the very small fluctuations of plasma Ca^{++} seen normally (p. 326); and, another system, with a more rapid rate of equilibration, must be involved. It may be that parathormone acts more swiftly on the kidney than on bone but the recent discovery of a hormone from the thyroid-parathyroid complex which lowers plasma Ca^{++} swiftly by reducing the rate of Ca^{++} resorption from bone, is probably a more likely mechanism. It now seems reasonably certain that this rapidly-acting hormone, called thyrocalcitonin, is secreted by the thyroid gland in response to hypercalcaemia. Like parathormone it is a polypeptide but it is probably only about half as big. Because it cannot yet be measured in plasma, its intimate physiological role is still speculative but the plasma Ca^{++} may be more difficult to control after total thyroparathyroidectomy than after parathyroidectomy alone.

INTER-RELATION BETWEEN PARATHYROID ACTIVITY AND VITAMIN D

We have seen that parathyroid hormone and vitamin D share one important biological effect—they both mobilize calcium and phosphate from bone. But there the similarity ends. The extra-skeletal effects of the two principles are very different. Vitamin D promotes calcium absorption from the bowel whereas parathyroid hormone has little, if any, effect. Renal phosphate excretion is profoundly affected by the parathyroid hormone, whereas vitamin D probably has no direct action on the kidney. Even the bone effects are dissimilar in other ways. In the early stages of vitamin D poisoning (i.e. before the development of secondary hyperparathyroidism as a result of renal failure) bone becomes rather more dense, whereas as soon as 12 hr after the injection of parathyroid extract into animals, increased bone resorption can be demonstrated histologically. Clearly, therefore, the vitamin and the hormone have different, if not almost opposite, effects and act at different sites, even though both tend to raise the solubility product of calcium and phosphate in the plasma.

Nevertheless, in the whole organism there is obviously a close physiological association between the two substances. This is well illustrated by considering the confusing and variable effects of vitamin D deficiency on the plasma levels of calcium and phosphate. A fall of plasma calcium level is usually checked by increased activity of the parathyroids. This will tend to prevent the rise of phosphate concentration which would otherwise occur as a result of the fall of plasma calcium concentration. But this is variable and in some individuals very little change of parathyroid activity occurs; ionized calcium levels in the plasma fall considerably and the 'classical' picture of tetany and rickets is seen. Thus, vitamin D deficiency will always cause some fall of plasma calcium concentration, but the extent of the fall, and whether the plasma phosphate (and hence phosphate excretion in the urine) falls, rises or remains unchanged will depend largely on the associated changes of parathyroid function. However, changes of responsiveness to parathormone may be equally relevant because there is some evidence that vitamin D deficiency reduces the response to parathormone.

Disordered function

The common patterns of metabolic bone disease can be conveniently discussed under four headings: parathyroid diseases, defective mineralization (osteomalacia or rickets), deficiency of new bone formation (osteoporosis), and the skeletal effects of other diseases such as renal failure.

HYPERPARATHYROIDISM

Hyperparathyroidism means, essentially, a disorder which is caused by oversecretion of parathyroid hormone. Overactivity of the parathyroid may be the primary lesion, in which case the cause is usually a tumour. Hormone production is inappropriate for the body's needs and cannot be changed by alterations of calcium or phosphate in the extracellular fluid, i.e. there is a breakdown of the normal feedback mechanism. Alternatively hyperparathyroidism may be secondary to any other condition which causes disordered calcium and phosphate metabolism, e.g. renal failure or osteomalacia. Occasionally persistent stimulation of the parathyroid glands causes adenomatous transformation of grossly hyperplastic glands and this may then resemble primary hyperparathyroidism functionally, in the sense that hormone production is largely autonomous ('tertiary' hyperparathyroidism).

Clinical features of hyperparathyroidism

The clinical features of primary hyperparathyroidism are varied, ranging from severe bony manifestations to recurrent renal stone formation without bony changes, but most of the features can be explained in terms of the underlying biochemical defect. As we have seen this is characterized by a high ionic calcium and low phosphate concentration in the extracellular fluid. Hypercalcaemia leads to hypercalciuria which, in turn, often causes recurrent renal stone formation and deposition of mineral in renal tissue (nephrocalcinosis) with subsequent impairment of renal function. The increased circulating calcium comes from both the diet and from dissolution of bone. If the latter predominates, there are bone pains, deformities and pathological fractures (sometimes at the site of an 'osteoclastoma') but often bone is barely affected, so that renal stones are the only feature.

The bone changes are fairly typical radiologically and consist of patchy rarefaction, often with bone cysts. The teeth may loosen because the lamina dura tends to break up. Subperiosteal erosions, particulary in the finger bones, are early signs which may exist without other evidence of bone involvement. Histologically the bone mass is diminished and there is excessive fibrosis; cysts may form (*osteitis fibrosa cystica*) and osteoclasts accumulate. Because the bones are softer than normal (and therefore more vulnerable to mechanical stresses), osteoblasts also accumulate. As a result the plasma alkaline phosphatase concentration is usually raised.

Hypercalciuria due to hypercalcaemia is associated with thirst and polyuria. This is partly caused by resistance to antidiuretic hormone and partly by the fact that calcium reduces tubular absorption of many other electrolytes by some unknown mechanism. Potassium and sodium are readily lost and magnesium deficiency is probably more common than recognized, because magnesium excretion tends to parallel that of calcium. Anorexia and vomiting as a result of the hypercalcaemia contribute to these electrolyte deficiencies and will, in severe cases, add a 'pre-renal' element to already poorly functioning kidneys. Severe muscle weakness with hypotonia (constipation is a common complaint) is probably the result of hypercalcaemia and also hypokalaemia (when present). The common association with duodenal ulcer and the rare association with pancreatitis are unexplained.

The main diagnostic difficulties arise in patients with renal failure or idiopathic hypercalciuria. In renal failure phosphate retention will tend to depress plasma calcium, and hypercalciuria is usually absent, so masking the characteristic biochemical defect. Many cases of primary hyperparathyroidism (a correctable form of renal failure) are misdiagnosed as having a primary (and therefore uncorrectable) chronic renal lesion and secondary hyperparathyroidism. Adenomatous transformation of hyperplastic parathyroid glands may then produce an autonomous hyperparathyroidism akin to the primary form.

In patients with renal stone formation due to idiopathic hypercalciuria it is very difficult to exclude hyperparathyroidism because hypercalcaemia may be slight and intermittent even in patients with an obvious parathyroid tumour. More complicated metabolic studies, such as calcium infusion and phosphate deprivation tests, may be required to test the sensitivity of the parathyroid glands to alterations of plasma calcium and phosphate concentration, but often surgical exploration of the neck (and if no tumour is found, the mediastinum) is the only way to be sure that no tumour is present although angiography may be useful.

HYPOPARATHYROIDISM

Accidental removal of the parathyroid glands during total or partial thyroidectomy is the most common cause of hypoparathyroidism, although cases of unknown aetiology do occur rarely (idiopathic hypoparathyroidism). The clinical manifestations are the direct consequence of hypocalcaemia and hyperphosphataemia. Chronic tetany with total plasma calcium levels of 5–7 mg/100 ml is associated with the virtual absence of calcium from the urine. The plasma phosphate concentration is elevated; the solubility product of calcium and phosphate ions tends to be elevated, and osteoclastic activity is reduced so that there may be some increased calcification of bone, although this is rarely evident radiologically. For the same reason, soft tissues tend to show metastatic calcification. When present, this seems to be confined to the basal ganglia.

Finally, a variety of ectodermal defects develop if the condition remains untreated for long enough. Cataracts are common, the skin is dry and scaly, the nails are brittle and prone to monilia infection, the hair is sparse, and the teeth underdeveloped.

There is another, genetic, disorder of calcification which is probably related to the parathyroid hormone in some way. It is characterized by achondroplasia (manifested particularly in the form of short metacarpal bones), a short, stocky stature with 'mooning' of the face, mental retardation, and extensive deposition of calcium in soft tissues which may proceed to actual ossification. Epilepsy is a common clinical presentation, and may be due partly to brain damage (the basal ganglia are nearly always calcified) and partly to the hypocalcaemia itself. Biochemically most of the cases show hypocalcaemia and hyperphosphataemia indistinguishable from hypoparathyroidism. Because parathyroid extract often fails to induce phosphaturia (the Ellsworth-Howard test) and because hyperplasia of the parathyroid glands has been observed, the biochemical manifestations may be the result of a failure of the renal tubules to respond to parathyroid hormone. However, the renal tubules do respond to vitamin D. Arguing that hyperplasia meant hypersecretion of parathyroid hormone, Albright called the disorder 'pseudo-hypoparathyroidism', meaning that the parathyroids were normal (or possibly overactive) but that the response to parathyroid hormone was not. There are no striking changes of bone texture so that, since parathormone also affects bone directly, a similar lack of response must be present in bone. Possibly the parathyroid in pseudo-hypoparathyroidism produces a chemical variant which inhibits the biological action of normal parathormone. Other patients with this widespread genetic skeletal abnormality are not hypocalcaemic. This condition has been flippantly termed 'pseudo-pseudo-hypoparathyroidism', but until we know more of the aetiology of this peculiar disorder it would be better to use a term which implies no specific aetiology.

OSTEOMALACIA AND RICKETS

Osteomalacia may be defined as a failure of mineralization of new bone, i.e. already formed bone is unaffected but any new matrix is not calcified. In growing children osteomalacia is called rickets, which only differs from adult osteomalacia in showing a typical pathology and X-ray appearance at the growing ends of long bones. Histologically the bone trabeculae are thickened by increased growth of uncalcified matrix or osteoid. Special techniques for cutting sections without decalcification are needed to show this clearly. In rickets the normal orderly sequence of calcification of the epiphysial cartilage is disrupted and the epiphysial line greatly widened.

Clinical features of osteomalacia
As with osteoporosis, low back pain is a frequent presenting symptom. Muscle weakness is, however, a common feature and this gives rise to a characteristic waddling gait. In contrast to osteoporosis, bones are often tender and their texture is soft rather than brittle. Consequently gross fractures are unusual, but instead partial cracks tend to appear at stress points. These are the so-called 'pseudo-fractures' (Looser's zones) which are often bilateral. In growing children the bony deformities characteristic of rickets develop. The bone ends swell, particularly the radius and costochondral junctions (producing the 'rickety rosary'); the legs bend, producing either knock-knee or bow-legs; the pelvis is compressed into a 'triradiate' deformity; and the frontal and parietal bones of the skull become bossed. Tetany due to hypocalcaemia may occur especially when vitamin D deficiency is due to intestinal malabsorption.

Aetiology of osteomalacia

Patients with osteomalacia as defined above fall roughly into two groups—those with a very low urine calcium output and those with a normal or high urine calcium output.

The first type of osteomalacia is due to a primary defect of calcium absorption from the bowel, and it has been variously termed simple osteomalacia, deficiency osteomalacia or vitamin D-sensitive osteomalacia. Simple dietary deficiency of vitamin D, calcium or phosphate is a very rare cause in the western hemisphere and virtually all the cases are due to absorption defects associated with steatorrhoea or coeliac disease. Although patients with a simple dietary deficiency of vitamin D respond adequately to relatively small amounts of the vitamin when given by mouth those with absorption defects may be highly resistant to oral vitamin D. It is only when vitamin D is given parenterally with enough oral calcium (say 15–30 g. calcium lactate per day) to counteract the tendency to form insoluble calcium soaps in the gut that relatively small amounts of vitamin D are likely to be adequate.

The second type of osteomalacia is more complex. Patients with this disorder do not have any clear cause for vitamin D deficiency, and relatively large doses of vitamin D (over 4 mg or 160,000 international units daily) are needed to heal the bones. The plasma phosphate concentration tends to be particularly low and the urine phosphate excretion excessively high. In other words, there is a high renal phosphate clearance. Clearly then, patients with this type of osteomalacia do not suffer from vitamin D deficiency but rather from a defect in their renal phosphate handling. This condition is often termed 'vitamin D-resistant rickets'. Although the bones may heal, the defect of phosphate metabolism does not. The defect may be a primary renal tubular lesion involving excessive phosphate loss or to some other factor which promotes increased phosphate excretion. One well-recognized cause of this 'phosphate diabetes' is renal tubular acidosis. In this condition the plasma bicarbonate and potassium concentrations are low, and renal excretion of hydrogen ions is defective (p. 176). Because of the failure to excrete hydrogen ions adequately, calcium is probably excreted in excess to cover the excretion of urinary anions. Another renal cause is cystinosis (p. 174). This is a congenital disorder, characterized by aminoaciduria, glycosuria, hypokalaemia and metabolic acidosis. It usually becomes clinically manifest in infancy or early childhood, but very rarely adult cases do occur.

OSTEOPOROSIS

In osteoporosis there is a reduction of bone mass per unit volume without any change in the nature and mineralization of the bone tissue present. In other words the bone is quantitatively deficient but qualitatively normal. This is essentially a histological definition and does not preclude the existence of more subtle functional abnormalities. In the past there has been considerable confusion about nomenclature. This arose principally because of the habit of calling all bones 'osteoporotic' which were rarefied or abnormally translucent radiologically. It is very difficult, however, to make a pathological diagnosis radiologically unless there are other characteristic features apart from a mere loss of bone density on X-ray.

In osteoporosis the bones are brittle, break easily, and are readily compressed so that patients with osteoporosis usually present with a chronic low backache or with a bone fractured following minimal trauma. Trabecular bone is principally affected, particularly in the vertebral column. Kyphosis with consequent loss of height is common. In contrast to osteomalacia the bones are not tender unless they are broken. Radiologically there is loss of bone trabeculation and fine structure particularly in the femoral neck and vertebral bodies. The plasma concentrations of calcium, phosphate and alkaline phosphatase are normal. In the early stages of rapidly progressive osteoporosis there will be a demonstrably elevated urinary calcium excretion, but usually this is normal at the time most patients are seen.

Generalized osteoporosis can be conveniently classified as either primary or secondary. The primary or idiopathic cases, which are the most common, occur chiefly amongst the elderly, particularly postmenopausal women. Osteoporosis may, on the other hand, be secondary to impaired supply of protein to the bone. This may be the result of an inadequate diet, intestinal malabsorption, excessive protein loss, impaired protein synthesis (as in chronic liver disease) or excessively rapid protein breakdown (as in diabetes mellitus, Cushing's syndrome and hyperthyroidism). In these examples there are many other factors apart from protein deficiency which also contribute to the development of osteoporosis but little is known about them. Osteoporosis may, in addition, be secondary to lack of stimulation by mechanical stress as in any cause of prolonged bed rest (particularly extensive muscle paralysis) or to lack of stimulation by the sex hormones. Castration in either sex may be accompanied by osteoporosis. In these cases of secondary osteoporosis it is fairly easy to understand how deficient bone matrix formation, whether the result of poor protein supply to the bone, sex hormone deficiency, or of lack of mechanical stimulation, may lead to thin bones with normal mineralization. But in the case of primary or idiopathic osteoporosis the position is more difficult. Bone atrophy (or osteoporosis) must be the result either of an abnormally slow rate of new bone formation or of an abnormally rapid rate of bone resorption. The Albright school argue, by analogy with known causes of osteoporosis, that the rate of new bone formation is reduced because of defective bone matrix formation. Certainly no primary abnormality of calcium or phosphorus metabolism has been demonstrated and treatment with the appropriate sex hormone may apparently ease bone pain and reduce the tendency to bone fractures. Bone density, however, remains unchanged.

More recently the suggestion has been made that a mild, prolonged calcium deficiency—possibly operating through a combination of mildly reduced calcium and vitamin D intake, and a tendency to intestinal malabsorption—may lead to osteoporosis. The stimulus to this idea comes from experimental work which shows that rats fed a calcium deficient diet, which is nevertheless adequate in vitamin D, develop a histological picture similar to that seen in human osteoporosis. However, in contrast to the human disease, this type of osteoporosis is rapidly corrected by feeding calcium. Only further investigation will solve this important problem, but it is already fairly clear from isotopic studies that the rate of bone formation in human osteoporosis falls within the normal range, but because the bone mass is reduced this is difficult to interpret. Quantitative histological studies on the femur suggests that there is a considerable increase of the rate of bone resorption in the elderly.

OTHER GENERALIZED BONE DISORDERS

RENAL OSTEODYSTROPHY

Renal disease is associated with metabolic bone disease in three main situations: (1) azotemic renal osteodystrophy, (2) primary hyperparathyroidism with renal failure due to nephrocalcinosis (p. 318), and (3) osteomalacia due to a renal phosphate leak (p. 322).

Azotemic renal disease, if of long enough duration, will nearly always lead to renal osteodystrophy. The condition is most commonly seen in children whose more rapid bone growth is more liable to show it, but all adults will develop bone lesions in some form if they live long enough. These patients presumably always have some degree of secondary hyperparathyroidism because of a tendency to hypocalcemia, but this does not wholly explain the bone lesions themselves. In different patients, one or other of the following manifestations are seen: (*a*) osteomalacia (usually mild), (*b*) subperiosteal erosions (suggesting hyperparathyroidism), and (*c*) excessive bone destruction with increased fibrosis and accumulation of osteoclasts. This latter is called osteitis fibrosa and resembles the bone lesions of hyperparathyroidism, but cysts are virtually never seen. Finally there may be (*d*) patchy areas of increased bone density (osteosclerosis) affecting particularly the vertebral and the subperiosteal region of the shafts of the hand bones. Metastatic soft tissue calcification is common although in contrast to the nephrocalcinosis of primary hyperparathyroidism the kidneys themselves are rarely involved. A rising plasma alkaline phosphatase concentration is a useful early sign and may appear before there is any clear change in plasma concentrations of calcium or phosphorus. Azotaemic renal osteodystrophy can be readily distinguished from osteomalacia due to renal tubular lesions by the fact that the plasma phosphate concentration is raised rather than lowered. As mentioned on p. 319 differentiation from the renal failure of primary hyperparathyroidism may give trouble. Nephrocalcinosis, a high normal or elevated plasma calcium concentration, and hypercalciuria should always lead to strong suspicion of parathyroid tumour.

MALIGNANT INVASIVE BONE DISEASE
Carcinomatosis (commonly from breast or bronchus), multiple myeloma, lymphomas and acute leukaemias may produce dissolution of bone, and symptoms difficult to distinguish from hyperparathyroidism, osteomalacia or osteoporosis. The bone matrix is replaced by malignant tissue, which can no longer support a mineral structure. Hypercalcaemia sometimes occurs in such conditions and is particularly seen during treatment of metastatic carcinoma of the breast with sex hormones. New bone formation by malignant invasion is rare, except in carcinoma of the prostate.

MALIGNANCY NOT ASSOCIATED WITH BONE DISEASE
Rarely certain malignant tumours, notably those of the bronchus or kidney, cause hypercalcaemia and hypophosphataemia indistinguishable from hyperparathyroidism without bone lesions. Removal of the offending tumour cures the condition. The tumour produces a substance which is immunologically identical with parathormone itself.

PAGET'S DISEASE (OSTEITIS DEFORMANS)

The cause of Paget's disease is unknown. Pathologically there is very greatly increased vascularity of the affected bones, proliferation of osteoblasts and irregular deposition of coarse new bone. In very extensive disease a hyperdynamic circulatory state may occur, since the areas of diseased bone represent a substantial arterio-venous shunt. In most cases only a few bones are affected, and there are few symptoms. Bone pain may occur, however, and is sometimes very intense. Pathoorgical fractures sometimes appear, and there is often enlargement of the head, and bowing of long bones. The disease never affects the entire skeleton—it usually selects the pelvis, skull, spine, femur or tibia. Radiologically the appearances are characteristic; and biochemically there is nearly always an increase in alkaline phosphatase concentration in plasma and often an increased urinary output of calcium. Plasma calcium and phosphate concentrations are normal.

SARCOIDOSIS

Sarcoidosis occasionally causes hypercalcaemia and hypercalciuria, sometimes with renal stones, nephrocalcinosis and patchy skeletal rarefaction. These complications of the disease closely resemble vitamin D intoxication and patients with sarcoidosis seem to be abnormally sensitive to vitamin D.

Principles of tests and measurements

PLASMA CALCIUM CONCENTRATION

Calcium is present in three forms in the plasma: ionized, complexed and protein-bound. The physiologically important component is the ionized fraction, but the estimation of this is tedious and liable to considerable error. The total plasma calcium concentration is therefore commonly used to provide an index of the ionized fraction. Fortunately high levels of total calcium nearly always signify high levels of ionized calcium, and low levels of total calcium signify low ionized calcium levels provided that the plasma protein concentration is normal. But where there is doubt about whether the total calcium concentration is an adequate index of the ionized level then a direct measurement of the ionized calcium may help.

As mentioned on p. 311 the plasma calcium concentration is normally maintained within narrow limits. This means that considerable clinical significance can and should be placed on relatively small deviations from the normal range provided that the technical difficulties of measuring the calcium concentration to within about 0·2 mg/100 ml can be overcome. The range of normal is narrow (9·0–10·5 mg/100 ml) providing that the plasma protein concentration is taken into account (see below).

The protein-bound fraction (40 per cent of the total) varies according to the plasma protein concentration (mainly the albumin concentration). The total calcium concentration varies correspondingly, and nomograms are available to help deduce the normal total calcium concentration for a given plasma protein concentration. For example, in the nephrotic syndrome it tends to be low because the plasma albumin concentration is reduced. Conversely an increase of the plasma albumin concentration increases the calcium concentration. This is illustrated by the usual recommendation that venous blood taken for the estimation of the plasma calcium should be collected without the use of a tourniquet because venous stasis increases the plasma protein concentration. The significance of minor deviations of total plasma calcium concentration from normal is increased if the specific gravity of the plasma is known. For every point above or below 1027, 0·25 mg/100 ml should be subtracted or added, respectively.

With these provisoes, hypercalcaemia suggests hyperparathyroidism, bone dissolution (as with multiple myeloma or carcinomatosis) or vitamin D intoxication (as with sarcoidosis or an excessive vitamin D intake). Hypocalcaemia suggests hypoparathyroidism, osteomalacia, or azotaemia.

PLASMA PHOSPHATE CONCENTRATION

The phosphate present in the plasma is almost all in the free ultra-filtrable form; but, rarely, when the plasma calcium concentration is very high (over about 16–17 mg/100 ml), a colloidal calcium-phosphate complex may form. As mentioned on p. 312 the range of normal plasma phosphate concentration is considerable, being influenced not only by the continual release and deposition of bone phosphate, but also by the amount in the diet, by the metabolic activity of muscle, by changes of renal function and by the rate of deposition of glucose to form glycogen. Plasma phosphate measurements, therefore, should always be made in the fasting state as a routine. Renal disease may affect the plasma phosphate concentration either way; chronic renal failure with azotaemia is associated with a high plasma level, whilst renal tubular disease is often associated with low plasma phosphate concentrations. Increased parathyroid activity reduces the plasma phosphate concentration and diminution of parathyroid activity raises it. Many agents, such as cortisol, tend to lower the plasma phosphate level by increasing renal phosphate clearance; and in general a low plasma phosphate concentration alone must not be taken to imply a metabolic bone disorder unless other factors can be excluded.

URINARY CALCIUM EXCRETION

The rate of calcium excretion in the urine is relatively independent of the amount in the diet and depends mainly on the circulating levels of vitamin D and parathyroid hormone. Nevertheless, over a matter of weeks or months the urine calcium excretion will reflect the intake and after 1–2 weeks on a low calcium diet (100–150 mg daily) the urinary calcium excretion provides a clinical guide of the individual's capacity to conserve calcium. A daily urinary calcium excretion rate of over 200 mg on this diet is probably always abnormal. Deficiency of vitamin D and reduced parathyroid activity reduces urine calcium excretion, and vitamin D poisoning and increased parathyroid secretion raises it. Any condition associated with increased bone destruction such as invasion of the bone by malignant cells, osteoporosis in its active phases, and sudden skeletal immobilization also increases urinary calcium output.

URINE PHOSPHATE EXCRETION

The rate of urine phosphate excretion is normally determined mainly by the rate of intestinal phosphate absorption and by the many factors which affect renal phosphate clearance. The latter, in turn, is normally directly related to the plasma phosphate concentration. Urine phosphate excretion is influenced by many different factors in addition to parathyroid activity, but nevertheless many diagnostic tests based on renal phosphate handling have been described in an attempt to differentiate between hyperparathyroidism and other causes of hypercalcaemia and hypercalciuria. Those most commonly used either give a direct measure of the spontaneous renal tubular phosphate reabsorption or relate this to the plasma phosphate concentration (the 'phosphate excretion index'). These tests do not depend on thoroughly accurate bladder emptying, as do simple measurements for the renal phosphate clearance alone or of the phosphate Tm (p. 185). But they do depend upon the accurate chemical estimation of both phosphate and some substance which is filtered at the glomeruli and not handled by the tubules. Ideally inulin should be used for the latter purpose, but in practice reliance is nearly always placed on a measurement of endogenous creatinine, which is a somewhat uncertain chemical determination liable to be distorted by non-specific chromogens. Nevertheless, these tests can be very useful despite their imperfections. In the absence of a primary renal lesion producing a tubular phosphate leak, a low rate of tubular phosphate reabsorption and a high urinary excretion rate for the observed plasma level usually signify hyperactivity of the parathyroid glands or vitamin D intoxication. Although many other conditions can affect this relationship, most of them are easily recognized by other means. The value of tests of tubular phosphate handling can be improved by trying to suppress parathyroid activity. The administration of aluminium hydroxide by mouth to reduce intestinal phosphate absorption, or the infusion of calcium gluconate to raise the plasma calcium concentration normally leads to an increase of tubular phosphate reabsorption, whereas in the presence of an autonomously functioning parathyroid tumour little change occurs.

PLASMA ALKALINE PHOSPHATASE CONCENTRATION

The plasma alkaline phosphatase concentration reflects both osteoblastic activity and the excretory capacity of the liver because the enzyme is normally excreted in the bile. Providing that liver disease can be excluded, the plasma alkaline phosphatase concentration is a most useful index of the rate of bone turnover. It is raised whenever osteoblastic activity is increased. Except in growing children and during the healing of bone fractures a value above the adult range of 3–13 King-Armstrong units/100 ml suggests metabolic bone disease, e.g. osteomalacia or hyperparathyroidism. Paget's disease, of unknown aetiology, is specially characterized by high plasma concentrations of alkaline phosphatase.

Practical assessment

CLINICAL OBSERVATIONS

Symptoms accompanying bone rarefaction

Bone pain, usually symmetrical, relieved by rest and aggravated by weight-bearing. Loss of height signifies vertebral collapse; sudden collapse of vertebrae is not common, but may mimic an acute chest or intra-abdominal catastrophe.

Reduced spinal mobility usually accompanies skeletal rarefaction, and a freely mobile spine virtually excludes any serious generalized bone disease.

Certain specific clinical features may help in assessing the type of rarefaction present. Defects in mineralization of bone are usually accompanied by general effects on the body. Muscular weakness may give rise to a waddling gait, and if severe may prevent patients rising out of a chair without assistance. Latent tetany demonstrable by Trousseau's or Chvostek's signs (p. 358) sometimes occurs in osteomalacia, and signifies a reduced plasma ionized calcium concentration. Bony tenderness is common in osteomalacia, but also occurs in malignant bone disease.

Symptoms of hypercalcaemia
Anorexia, vomiting, constipation, vague abdominal pain, polyuria and thirst may occur with bone disease, and suggest hypercalcaemia. Such symptoms may be the only clinical evidence of hyperparathyroidism. In longstanding and severe cases signs may appear in the eyes. A diffuse haziness may extend inwards from the limbus on to the cornea, as a band. This resembles the common arcus senilis, but may be distinguished from it because calcium is deposited mainly at the sides while the arcus senilis is better defined at the top and bottom of the cornea. The arcus senilis is separated from the limbus by a definite gap, whereas hypercalcaemic 'band keratitis' extends inwards from the limbus with no interruption. A slit-lamp is required for proper assessment. Small triangular white deposits may also be seen on the exposed sclerae at either side.

Urine testing
The Sulkowitch test can be used to give an approximate estimate of urinary calcium excretion. A concentrated early morning specimen of urine is used. If this shows no turbidity there is good evidence for a mineralization defect. Glycosuria is associated with renal tubule defects; albuminuria with glomerular lesions; and Bence-Jones protein with multiple myeloma.

Growth
In either sex growth is estimated by serial measurement and comparison with those obtained from surveys of children and adolescents of similar age in the general population. Total stature is a reflection of the genetic, nutritional and endocrine influences on growth which have been discussed on p. 309. In normal adults the span of the outstretched arms approximately equals the total height and the measurement of the lower limbs from the heels to the pubic symphysis equals that from the pubic symphysis to the vertex of the skull. Disproportionate lengthening of the limbs as compared with the trunk, head and neck is a feature of

hypogonadism (pp. 615–617), whereas relatively short limbs are a feature of normal childhood, pituitary infantilism or achondroplasia.

The development of the epiphyses is a measure of the secretion of growth hormone and thyroid hormone in childhood. Maturation and closure of the epiphyses reflects the action of sex hormones (pp. 309) but is also influenced by genetic factors.

ROUTINE METHODS

X-rays	Chiefly valuable in assessment of:
Lateral skull:	Multiple myeloma, Paget's disease, post-menopausal osteoporosis (skull unaffected).
Chest PA:	Metastatic deposits, sarcoidosis, Looser's zones in ribs.
Both hands and wrists:	Hyperparathyroidism, sarcoidosis, rickets.
Straight abdomen:	Nephrocalcinosis, radio-opaque renal stones, kidney size.
Lateral lumbar spine:	Severity of bone rarefaction, vertebral collapse, metastatic deposits, renal osteodystrophy, osteoporosis, osteomalacia.
Pelvis and hips:	Chronic osteomalacia (tri-radiate deformities), acute osteomalacia (Looser's zones), Paget's disease.
Both knees AP:	Rickets and osteomalacia.

There is often a difference between bone texture in osteoporosis and osteomalacia best seen in the lateral lumbar spine. Irregular vertebral collapse and loss of fine structure with coarse vertical reticular markings suggests osteoporosis, whereas severe chronic osteomalacia may produce even loss of density, a 'ground-glass' appearance and evenly deformed biconcave vertebrae. Renal osteodystrophy sometimes produces bands of sclerosis alternating with translucent bands.

Bone age is estimated by radiographs of various epiphyses, according to the age of the subject, and comparison with those of average individuals.

Chemical estimations

Assessment requires estimations of plasma or serum calcium, phosphate, alkaline phosphatase, carbon dioxide content or bicarbonate (p. 215) and blood urea. Plasma protein estimation is helpful in assessing the amount of protein-bound calcium (p. 327). Reduced 24-hr urinary calcium excretion (on a normal diet) is the most sensitive index of vitamin D deficiency: and characteristic changes occur in other disorders. These can conveniently be summarized in tabular form (see Table 11).

Cortisone test in hypercalcaemia

If cortisone (50 mg 8-hourly) is given for 10 days to a patient with hypercalcaemia, the plasma calcium concentration will usually fall in cases of sarcoidosis and multiple myeloma, and will frequently fall in disseminated bone carcinoma. By contrast little change occurs in hyperparathyroidism.

Prednisone is probably equally effective (although results have not yet been standardized), but there is some evidence that the more potent synthetic glucocorticoids may not necessarily have the same effect.

SPECIAL TECHNIQUES

Plasma ionized calcium concentration. Apart from its value in research studies, estimation of ionized calcium concentration may be of value in the diagnosis of hyperparathyroidism, particularly when the plasma calcium concentration is not clearly elevated.

Bone biopsy. There is no surgical difficulty in bone biopsy; but special facilities are necessary for cutting undecalcified sections unless the bone is extremely soft. Biopsy can be very useful, particularly in the diagnosis of malignant disease.

Calcium balance. Calcium balance requires special laboratory facilities' and is mainly a research investigation since most cases of generalized bone disease can be diagnosed, assessed and treated adequately without this aid, provided that urinary calcium excretion can be measured.

Other tests. The effect of phosphate deprivation and calcium infusion can be useful in the diagnosis of hyperparathyroidism, but they require special metabolic facilities. Calcium turnover can be studied with radio-active ^{45}Ca or ^{47}Ca or with stable strontium, but these are research procedures. The assay of plasma parathyroid hormone concentration by immunochemical techniques is now possible in cattle and will doubtless soon become available in humans.

TABLE 11. Usual biochemical changes in some generalized bone diseases

(*modified by Dent, after Dent and Hodson, Brit. J. Radiol.*, **NS 27**, 605, 1954)

	Plasma Ca (mg/100 ml)	Plasma inorganic P (mg/100 ml)	Plasma HCO_3^- (m-equiv./l.) (venous blood)	Alkaline phosphatase (K-A units)**	Urine Ca (mg/24 hr normal diet)	Blood urea (mg/100 ml)
Normal adult ..	9–10·5§	3·2–4·2	23–29	3–12*	120–250	15–35
Normal child (over 1 year)		4·0–6†		12–25†	10–100	
Osteoporosis ..	Normal	Normal‡	Normal	Normal	Normal¶	Normal
Primary hyperparathyroidism (uncomplicated)	10·5–16	1–3	Normal	15–100‖	150–600	Normal
Primary hyperparathyroidism with renal failure; renal failure with secondary hyperparathyroidism	May be normal	May be normal or even increased	May be low	15–100	50–200	50–400
Osteomalacia and rickets (any origin, non-acidotic)	5–9	1–3	19–29	15–100	10–100	Normal
Osteomalacia and rickets (any origin, acidotic)	7–10	1–4	10–22	15–100	150–350	30–80
Hypophosphatasia	9–15	4–8	19–29	1–2 in adults; 3–8 in infants	Normal	
Hypoparathyroidism	4–8	6–12 >7 in children	Normal	Normal	Normal or low	Normal

* 3–10 in women: 5–12 in men
† during active growth
‡ may be low in Cushing's syndrome
§ 4·5–5·2 m-equiv./l.

¶ raised in active phase
‖ only increased if bone lesions are present—otherwise normal
** for Bodansky equivalents divide by 3

References

ALBRIGHT F. & REIFENSTEIN E.C., Jr. (1948) *The parathyroid glands and metabolic bone disease.* Baltimore: Williams & Wilkins.

FOURMAN P. (1960) *Calcium metabolism and the bone.* Oxford: Blackwell.

STANBURY S.W. & LUMB G.A. (1966). Parathyroid function in chronic renal failure. *Quart. J. Med. New Series* xxxv, **137**, 1–23.

FRASER R.T. & KING E.J. (1964) Diseases of bone and the parathyroid gland. *In Biochemical disorders in human disease* (Ed. THOMPSON R.H.S. & KING E.J.) London: J. & A. Churchill, pp. 492–547.

COPP D.H. (1964) Parathyroids, calcitonin and the control of plasma calcium. *Rec. Prog. Horm. Res.* **20**, 59–88.

MUNSON P.L. (1966) Thyrocalcitonin. *Ann. Intern. Med.* **64**, 1353–7.

COMAR C.L. & BRONNER F. (ed.) (1964). *Mineral Metabolism: an advanced treatise in.* Vol. II Part A. Academic Press, pp. 341–482.

HAWKER C.D., GLASS J.D. & RASMUSSEN H. *Biochemistry* (1966). Further Studies on the isolation and characterization of parathyroid polypeptides. **5**, 344.

POTTS J.T., AURBACH G.D. & SHERWOOD L.M. (1966). Parathyroid hormone: chemical properties and structural requirements for biological and immunological activity. *Rec. Prog. Horm. Res.*

NEUMAN W.F. & NEUMAN M.W. (1958) *Chemical dynamics of bone mineral.* Chicago: Univ. of Chicago Press.

FANCONI A. & ROSE G.A. (1958) The ionized, complexed, and protein-bound fractions of calcium in plasma. *Quart. J. Med.* **27**, 463–494.

DENT C.E. (1952) Rickets and osteolmalacia from renal tubule defects. *J. Bone Jt. Surg. (British)*, **34**, 266–274.

BARTTER F.C. (1957) Osteoporosis. *Amer. J. Med.*, **22**, 797–806.

HARRISON H.E. (1959) Physiology of Vitamin D. *Helv. paediat. Acta*, **14**, 434–446.

Skeletal Muscle

Normal function

STRUCTURAL ORGANIZATION OF STRIATED MUSCLE FIBRES

A muscle fibre is an aggregate of longitudinally orientated myofibrils surrounded by a surface membrane, the sarcolemma, outside which is a connective tissue layer, the endomysium. Each fibre contains numerous nuclei which lie immediately underneath the sarcolemma. Viewed with a conventional light microscope, the myofibrils show cross-striations lying at corresponding levels on each fibril: optically dense bands (anisotropic or A bands) alternate with optically less dense bands (isotropic or I bands). The central regions of the A bands are slightly lighter than the rest of the band (H zones) and are divided by a dark M line. The I bands are bisected by dark Z lines. Electron microscopy has contributed much towards explaining the significance of these structural features, and the basic organization of the striated muscle fibre revealed by this means is illustrated in Fig. 32. The dense A bands are produced by filaments composed of myosin; these interdigitate with finer filaments composed of actin situated in the I bands. The actin filaments extend into the A bands, the regions of overlap representing the darker outer portions of these bands. The sarcoplasm between the myofibrils contains mitochondria and a system of tubular structures, the sarcoplasmic reticulum.

Although in some species there is a clear-cut difference between 'red' and 'white' muscles, this difference is not so apparent in man, most muscles containing both types of fibre. Red muscle fibres contain a relatively greater amount of myoglobin. Myoglobin, like haemoglobin, is a ferrous-porphyrin-protein complex which combines reversibly with oxygen. Its dissociation curve differs from that of haemoglobin in that little oxygen is yielded until relatively low partial pressures of oxygen are reached. It is thus capable of acting as a reservoir supplying oxygen under conditions of temporary oxygen lack. Functional differences between red and white muscle fibres are not entirely clear but, in general, red muscles occur at sites where long-maintained contraction is required, as in postural muscles or in the flight muscles of birds. It has been suggested that muscles that frequently accumulate a large 'oxygen debt' tend to be red.

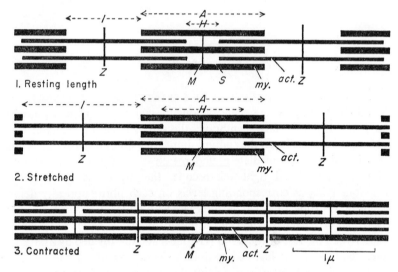

FIGURE 32. *Diagram of the organization of striated muscle in longitudinal section as revealed by electron microscopy, showing the changes occurring during stretch and contraction.*

1 shows the elements at resting length in the body, 2 after passive stretch, and 3 after isotonic contraction to about 40% of maximum.

A. anisotropic (dark) band; *act.* actin filament; *H.* H zone; *I.* isotropic (light) band; *M.* M line; *my.* myosin filament; *Z.* Z line.

During passive stretch the actin filaments are partly withdrawn from the A band. In contraction the actin filaments are drawn into the *A* band. With further shortening the filaments crumple.

(Modified from J. Z. Young, *The Life of Mammals.*)

In some species there is also a well-marked difference between 'fast' and 'slow' muscles, this distinction depending upon the rapidity of contraction. Histological differences exist between the two types of muscle fibre. Fast muscles tend to be used predominantly for phasic movements and slow muscles in the maintenance of posture. In man, this difference is again not so apparent (p. 364).

INNERVATION

The motor nerve fibres to a muscle branch repeatedly a short distance from the muscle, each nerve fibre innervating a number of muscle fibres. A motor unit consists of the muscle fibres controlled by one anterior horn cell. In some muscles, such as those of the limbs, each motor unit contains numerous muscle fibres, at times as many as several hundred; in others, such as the extrinsic eye muscles, where fine adjustments of movement are required, each unit contains only a few fibres.

Functional contact between the nerve and muscle fibres is achieved through the motor end-plates where there is intimate contact between the respective surface membranes, although they remain separated by a narrow synaptic cleft (Fig. 33). Immediately before reaching the motor end-plate, the nerve fibre loses its myelin sheath and the enveloping connective tissue sheath of the nerve fibre becomes continuous with the endomysium. The muscle substance in the region of the end-plate forms a specialized grooved structure, in which the terminal portions of the axon are embedded (see Fig. 34). Electron microscopy has revealed that in the region of the groove the muscle membrane is profusely and finely folded: histochemical staining shows that cholinesterase activity is localized to these folds.

NEUROMUSCULAR TRANSMISSION

It is now accepted that transmission at the neuromuscular junction is mediated by acetylcholine, which may be stored in small vesicles in

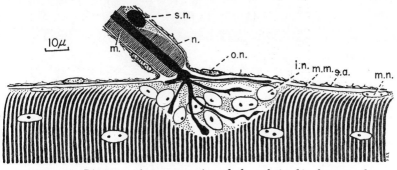

FIGURE 33. *Diagrammatic representation of the relationship between the nerve and muscle fibres at the motor end-plate.*

i.n. inner nuclei of end-plate; *m.* myelin; *n.* neurilemma; *m.m.* surface membrane of muscle fibre; *m.n.* nuclei of muscle fibre; *o.n.* outer nuclei of end-plate (? fibrocytes); *sa.* sarcolemma; *s.n.* Schwann cell nucleus.

(From E. Gutmann and J. Z. Young, *J. Anat.*, **78**, 15, 1944.)

the presynaptic nerve terminals from which it is released at the surface membrane. Acetylcholine causes the electrical depolarization of the motor end-plate. At this time the end-plate has a greatly increased ionic permeability. The acetylcholine, once released, is rapidly destroyed by cholinesterase. Activity at the end-plate, as measured by the electrical end-plate potential, must reach a threshold value before excitation is propagated over the muscle membrane.

MUSCULAR CONTRACTION
Activation

The muscle membrane acts as an apparent diffusion barrier, there being a high intracellular concentration of potassium with a low concentration of sodium, the reverse obtaining in the extracellular fluid. The membrane is electrically polarized with a resting potential of approximately 90 millivolts (mV), the interior being negative with respect to the exterior. This potential difference depends upon the ionic distribution across the membrane. The function of the membrane is to distribute the muscle action potential, initially arising at the motor end-plate region, over the

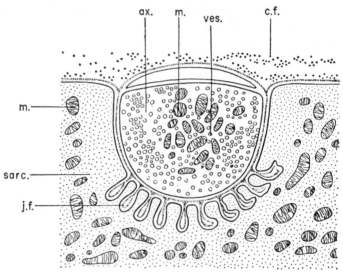

FIGURE 34. *Schematic drawing of a synaptic groove seen in cross-section.*
The axon contains numerous synaptic vesicles and is embedded in a trough in the end-plate, the floor of which is profusely folded.

ax. axoplasm; m. mitochondria; ves. vesicles; sarc. sarcoplasm; j.f. junctional fold; c.f. collagen fibres.

(From Couteaux, R., in *Structure and Function of Muscle* (Ed. G. H. Bourne), 1960, London: Academic Press, Inc.)

whole of the fibre. The excitatory process developed at the end-plate spreads in both directions at a rate of 3–4 m/sec. The action potential begins as a brief reversal of the potential across the membrane, the interior becoming approximately 40 mV positive to the exterior, this probably being associated with a sudden increase in permeability to sodium ions. The rising phase of the action potential is thus of the order of 130 mV. During the falling phase there is probably an outward passage of potassium ions. Propagation of the impulse occurs in a way analogous to that in non-myelinated nerve fibres. The accumulation of sodium ions within the muscle fibre is thought to be prevented by the action of a metabolically-driven 'sodium pump'.

Other ions, particularly the divalent calcium and magnesium ions, are concerned in stabilizing the electrical potential across the muscle membrane. However, the membrane of the peripheral nerve fibre is more sensitive to alterations in these ions than is that of the muscle fibre; consequently, the changes in neuromuscular excitability which occur in conditions of altered ionic concentration of calcium and magnesium in the extracellular fluid (see p. 349) are mainly due to the effects of these ions on the peripheral nerves. Reduction of the extracellular concentration of calcium ions renders the membrane more excitable by causing the exchange of other ions across the membrane in both directions to become more rapid. Conversely, a high extracellular concentration of calcium ions inhibits ionic exchange, increasing the stability of the membrane and decreasing its excitability. Magnesium ions have a similar but smaller effect.

Little is known about the way in which the activation process is transferred from the muscle membrane to the contractile mechanism, but the membrane potential may be conducted to the interior of the fibre by the tubules of the sarcoplasmic reticulum. Initiation of contraction is probably mediated by calcium ions.

Shortening

During muscular contraction the I bands shorten whereas the A bands remain unaltered in length (Fig. 32). The supposition is that during this process the actin threads are pulled into the A bands, sliding alongside the myosin threads; this is thought to occur by the action of 'cross-bridges', although the nature of these is uncertain. *In vitro* experiments have shown that adenosine triphosphate (ATP) will cause the shortening of actomyosin (actin+myosin) filaments. This action sufficiently resembles the behaviour of intact muscle to make it a plausible basis for muscle contraction.

During passive stretching the changes are the reverse of those occurring during contraction, elongation of the I bands taking place (Fig. 32).

Under certain circumstances it is possible for contraction to occur without this being accompanied by a propagated muscle action potential. This is referred to as contracture (to be distinguished from the use of the term in its clinical sense, when it implies a fibrotic shortening of muscle).

Energy release

The dephosphorylation of ATP to adenosine diphosphate (ADP) results in a considerable release of energy and this is probably the immediate energy source for muscular contraction. Myosin may act as an enzyme in this process. Resynthesis of ATP is thought to occur initially by the reaction of ADP with creatine phosphate and later by energy derived from carbohydrate breakdown. The carbohydrate store in muscle is glycogen, which yields energy by anaerobic breakdown to lactic acid and pyruvate, via hexose and triose phosphates; pyruvate can then enter the tricarboxylic acid cycle for oxidative breakdown (p. 472).

This scheme accords with observations that have been made on the heat production during muscular contraction, the larger part of which is released after the contraction is over. Heat is released during contraction (initial heat) but a larger quantity (heat of recovery) is produced after contraction has ceased and only under aerobic conditions.

Muscle is also able to use sources of energy other than carbohydrate, for contraction is still possible when glycolysis is prevented by poisoning with iodoacetate.

Force of contraction

When a motor unit is activated it normally contracts with a standard (maximum) force. Alteration in the force of muscular contraction is produced by variation in the number of units in action and by variation in the frequency with which each unit contracts. This frequency varies between 5 and 50 times per second. The force of the contraction developed by each fibre is related to the quantity of calcium entering per contraction.

Fatigue

Although it was long thought that muscular fatigue was a neural phenomenon, it is now clear that it is due to changes in the muscle fibres. Electrical stimulation of the nerve to a muscle completely fatigued by exercise, although giving rise to a muscle action potential, does not produce a contraction. It is probable that the failure lies in the contractile mechanism itself, although there may be a failure of the 'coupling' process between the muscle action potential and the contractile mechanism.

MUSCLE TONE

There is no motor unit activity in resting muscle. Muscle tone is assessed clinically as the degree of resistance felt by the examiner during passive extension of a muscle. This depends partly upon the elasticity of the muscle, but mainly upon the contraction of muscle fibres excited reflexly through stretch receptors in the muscle spindles. The most important factor influencing this tone is the activity of the fusimotor (gamma efferent) system which innervates the muscle spindles (see Chapter 10).

Disordered function

This account will be restricted to a consideration of muscular weakness and of hyperexcitability due to dysfunction of the motor unit. Disorders of muscle tone and the control of movement are discussed in Chapter 10.

Weakness
This may arise from a number of different functional defects. In the first place the disorder may involve the process of *excitation*:
- (*a*) disease of the anterior horn cells or failure of conduction in the motor nerve fibres;
- (*b*) failure of acetylcholine production or release from the nerve terminals;
- (*c*) excessively rapid destruction of acetylcholine by excess cholinesterase;
- (*d*) failure of the end-plate to respond because of competitive (curariform) block;
- (*e*) failure of the end-plate to respond because of persistent depolarization (depolarization block);
- (*f*) failure of excitation of the muscle membrane;
- (*g*) failure of the 'coupling' process between the membrane action potential and the contractile mechanism.

Secondly, the fault may lie in the *contractile mechanism* itself:
- (*a*) failure of the contractile elements;
- (*b*) failure of the energy processes.

Muscular hyperexcitability

This may involve discharges arising in the muscle fibre, as in

(*a*) myotonia;

(*b*) fibrillation.

Or in neural structures, as in

(*a*) fasciculation;

(*b*) muscle cramps;

(*c*) tetany.

WEAKNESS

DENERVATION

After acute denervation in man, the distal portion of the nerve remains electrically excitable for 3–4 days until Wallerian degeneration proceeds to the stage where conduction fails. Progressive atrophy of the muscle fibres then ensues but they remain directly excitable, although increasingly strong stimulation is required, until atrophy has proceeded to complete loss of striation. This usually occurs after about 3 years.

The functional recovery possible after a peripheral nerve lesion is considerably influenced by the length of the period of denervation: the longer re-innervation is delayed, the less likely is it that a good functional result will be achieved. Reasonable recovery is possible for periods of up to a year, but from then on a satisfactory result becomes increasingly less likely, the outlook being very poor after 3 years. Although it has been shown that electrical stimulation during the period of denervation can retard the degree of muscular atrophy, it has not yet been demonstrated with certainty that the ultimate functional recovery is improved.

It has been questioned whether the occurrence of fibrillation in denervated muscle increases the rate of wasting. If fibrillation is suppressed by the administration of quinine, no reduction in the rate of wasting is observed.

DISORDERS OF NEUROMUSCULAR TRANSMISSION

Acetylcholine lack

Deficient production or release of acetylcholine from the motor nerve terminals is a possible cause for failure of neuromuscular transmission. The substance hemicholinium prevents the synthesis of acetylcholine, and it has been shown that the weakness produced by the toxin of *Clostridium botulinum* arises from a fault in the release of acetylcholine.

Once released, the acetylcholine might be destroyed too rapidly by excessive amounts of cholinesterase, although no clinical instance of this is known.

Competitive block

Neuromuscular transmission may be blocked by substances that compete with acetylcholine for the receptors on the end-plate and thus prevent its depolarization. This is termed competitive inhibition and curare and gallamine tri-ethiodide (Flaxedil) are examples of agents that act in this way. Increasing the concentration of acetyl choline in the neighbourhood of the end-plates by anticholinesterases (which prevents the normal destruction of acetylcholine) tends to overcome competitive inhibition.

Depolarization block

Prolonged depolarization of the end-plate will also block neuro-muscular transmission. This may result from excess acetylcholine caused, for example, by the administration of anticholinesterases, and is seen in poisoning with certain insecticides. A depolarization block is also produced by decamethonium iodide and succinylcholine (Scoline). Anticholinesterases, in contradistinction to their effect in competitive block, potentiate a depolarization block.

Myasthenia gravis

The recognition that myasthenia gravis is a disorder of neuromuscular transmission began with the observation that it resembled the paralysis produced by curare, in that the anticholinesterase physostigmine produced a temporary beneficial effect. However, it has since been demonstrated that the neuromuscular block in myasthenia gravis shows certain differences from that produced by curare, but is more similar to that produced by hemicholinium. This suggested that the fault in myasthenia gravis may be a failure in the synthesis or release of acetylcholine from the nerve terminals. Recent intracellular recordings made on muscle biopsies from patients with myasthenia gravis have also suggested that the failure is proximal to the myoneural junction.

Recently observations have been made which indicate that there is also abnormality in the response of the end-plate to acetylcholine or its degradation products. This was first suggested on the basis of the effect of decamethonium in myasthenia and later shown for acetyl choline itself. Instead of simply producing depolarization, in myasthenia gravis acetylcholine produces a dual effect, depolarization being followed by competitive inhibition. Furthermore, it is now known that the end-plates are histologically abnormal in myasthenia gravis. Possibly a long-continued deficiency of acetylcholine may lead to secondary changes in the end-plates.

In normal subjects, decamethonium gives rise to a depolarization block after an initial brief stimulation. In clinically weak muscles in myasthenia, decamethonium produces an initial brief improvement. This is immediately followed by a block showing all the features of competitive inhibition. This dual type of response (i.e. depolarization followed by competitive inhibition) has been shown to occur normally in certain species of animal.

In normal subjects and in patients with myasthenia, the response to an intra-arterial injection of acetylcholine is a brief period of stimulation which is immediately followed by a transient depolarization block. This is then succeeded by a late prolonged block, probably produced by choline resulting from hydrolysis of acetylcholine. In normal subjects, this late prolonged block has the features of a depolarization block, but in myasthenia gravis it is of competitive type.

The response of clinically unaffected muscles to decamethonium in patients with localized myasthenia gravis is also of interest. In myasthenic patients there is usually an increased tolerance to decamethonium. This probably represents a stage in the transition between the normal response of depolarization and that of competitive inhibition found in myasthenia.

The relationship between the thymus, neuromuscular transmission and myasthenia gravis remains obscure, but may involve auto-immune mechanisms. Claims reporting the existence of a neuromuscular blocking agent in thymic tissue remain unsubstantiated. Myasthenia is well known to occur in the presence of thymic tumours and some patients are reported to improve after thymectomy, although, apparently paradoxically, these are usually patients in whom a thymoma is not present. A myasthenic syndrome, differing in certain respects from myasthenia gravis, is also encountered at times in patients with broncho-genic carcinoma.

DISORDERS OF THE MUSCLE MEMBRANE
Muscular weakness resulting from a disturbance in the activity of the muscle membrane, including that of the end-plate, occurs in disorders of potassium metabolism. The importance of the role of potassium in the production of the muscle action potential has already been stressed.

Hyperkalaemic and hypokalaemic weakness

Generalized muscular paralysis is occasionally met with in hyperkalaemic and hypokalaemic states (see p. 18). The muscles are electrically inexcitable either directly or through the motor nerve, the inference being that the muscle membrane is inexcitable. It is unlikely that this depends simply upon an elevation or depression of the concentration of potassium ions in the extracellular fluid since, under clinical conditions, these changes probably only develop when alterations in the intracellular concentration of the ion have also occurred. It is known that the muscle membrane potential depends upon both the external and internal concentrations of potassium.

Hyperkalaemic familial periodic paralysis. This rare disorder is characterized by attacks of muscular weakness that tend to occur during periods of rest after exercise. Myotonic phenomena may also be observed. The plasma potassium concentration is usually raised during attacks and the urinary excretion of potassium is increased. Potassium probably leaks out of the muscle cells, although the reason for this is not known. The muscle membrane potential is reduced, especially at the time of an attack. The weakness may be related to the depolarization of the muscle membrane although it does not seem possible to explain the change in membrane potential directly in terms of the alteration in the extracellular concentration of potassium.

In *hypokalaemic familial periodic paralysis*, attacks of muscular weakness occur during rest after exercise or following a carbohydrate meal. The muscles are inexcitable to direct electrical stimulation. The plasma potassium concentration characteristically falls in the attacks and the urinary excretion of potassium is reduced, potassium migrating into the muscle cells. Yet the paralysis does not depend directly upon a reduction in the extracellular concentration of potassium because weakness may occur at times in the absence of hypokalaemia. Moreover, it does not depend upon hyperpolarization of the muscle membrane. Its precise mechanism has still to be explained.

FAILURE OF THE COUPLING PROCESS BETWEEN THE MEMBRANE ACTION POTENTIAL AND THE CONTRACTILE MECHANISM; DISORDERS OF THE CONTRACTILE MECHANISM ITSELF

Patients with *osteomalacia* may develop muscular weakness in which the pelvic girdle muscles are predominantly affected. Since the weakness is not closely related to the plasma calcium concentration and is relieved by vitamin D administration, it has been suggested that the disorder is the result of vitamin D deficiency. As this vitamin possibly influences the transfer of calcium across the muscle membrane, the process of activation of muscular contraction may be defective.

In *muscular dystrophy*, abnormalities of the myofilaments have been demonstrated by electron microscopy so that a disturbance of the contractile elements probably contributes to the weakness.

DISORDERS OF ENERGY PROCESSES

Glycogen storage disease occasionally involves skeletal muscle, giving rise to hypotonic weakness. It represents one cause of the syndrome of 'amyotonia congenita'. The muscle fibres are infiltrated with glycogen. The condition depends upon a fault in the enzymatic breakdown of glycogen.

Hereditary myophosphorylase deficiency (*McArdle's syndrome*) represents a defect confined to muscle glycogen breakdown; no accompanying defect in liver glycogenolysis has been detected. In this disorder, muscular weakness, pain and stiffness occur following exercise. The muscles exhibit sustained painful localized contractions that electromyographically show no electrical activity and which therefore presumably represent contractures in the true physiological sense. On ischaemic exercise, the normal rise in blood pyruvate and lactate levels does not occur. Muscle phosphorylase, necessary for the initial stage of muscle glycogen breakdown, is absent. Attacks may be associated with myoglobinuria, and the patients may exhibit a slowly progressive muscular wasting.

In *idiopathic paroxysmal myoglobinuria*, exercise is followed by muscular weakness and stiffness and the excretion of myoglobin in the urine. This is the result of destruction of muscle fibres with consequent release of myoglobin. In some instances it has been found that this is the result of a glycolytic defect leading to the intracellular accumulation of excessive quantities of acid metabolites.

CONDITIONS CAUSING WEAKNESS IN WHICH
THE PHYSIOLOGICAL DISTURBANCE IS EITHER
UNKNOWN OR IS DUE TO A GENERAL DESTRUCTION
OF THE FIBRES

The *muscular dystrophies*, *polymyositis* and *dermatomyositis*, and *thyrotoxic myopathy* all involve diffuse degeneration of muscle fibres. A myopathy occurs in rabbits after administration of large doses of *cortisone* and is associated with a general destruction of muscle fibres.

This is probably equivalent to the myopathy that may occur in man, predominantly affecting the pelvic girdle muscles, after the administration of certain cortisol derivatives (e.g. triamcinolone). *Vitamin E deficiency* has been shown to cause muscle disease in a wide variety of experimental animals, producing a diffuse necrosis of muscle fibres. There is no evidence that deficiency of this vitamin is ever responsible for muscle disease in man.

INCREASED EXCITABILITY

MYOTONIA

The phenomenon of myotonia is mainly encountered in myotonia congenita (Thomsen's disease) and dystrophia myotonica. The most prominent disturbance is a delay in muscular relaxation after sustained forceful contraction. The muscles are abnormally sensitive to mechanical stimulation and percussion of an affected muscle gives rise to a persistent localized contraction lasting several seconds.

The phenomenon is greater in the cold and may only appear under such circumstances (paramyotonia). It is usually reduced by repeated activity, but may be increased (myotonia paradoxa).

Electromyographic examination of myotonic muscle reveals that the primary discharge arises both from individual muscle fibres and from groups of fibres. The abnormal sensitivity to mechanical stimuli is manifested by the fact that movement of the exploring needle or percussion of the muscle results in a myotonic discharge.

The occurrence of congenital myotonia in goats has helped in the understanding of the functional disorder present. Here it has been possible to show unequivocally that the myotonia occurs because of an abnormality of the muscle fibres, since it persists after nerve section and complete curarization. It has also been demonstrated that myotonia in human muscle continues after nerve block and local curarization. The reason for the tendency to repetitive activity of muscle fibres in myotonia is not known. That no essential nervous system component is involved is shown by the persistence of the myotonia after nerve section or block, although it has been suggested that reflex discharges induced by activation of stretch receptors by the abnormal myotonic contraction may also play a part. Myotonia may be observed in hyperkalaemic familial periodic paralysis when it is probably related to partial depolarization of the muscle membrane (see p. 345).

Quinine and procaine amide, which reduce myotonia, presumably act by increasing the stability of the muscle membrane.

12*

Sluggish relaxation after muscular contraction is at times seen in hypothyroidism, and myotonia may be elicited by percussion. This 'myxoedematous myotonia' is not associated with an electrical discharge in the muscle. It is thought to be due to an alteration in the contractile mechanism which interferes with lengthening after muscular contraction. A similar phenomenon may be seen in amyloidosis involving skeletal muscle.

FIBRILLATION AND FASCICULATION

Denervated muscle fibres often show 'spontaneous' contractions, known as fibrillation, the origin of which is at present uncertain. This phenomenon does not appear until 2–3 weeks after severance of the nerve supply. Since the contraction is of individual muscle fibres or of very small groups of fibres it is not visible through the skin, except perhaps in the tongue, and electromyographic methods have to be used for its detection. Denervated muscle fibres are abnormally sensitive to acetylcholine.

Spontaneous motor unit activity may also be encountered in partially denervated muscles. This is termed fasciculation and, in contra-distinction to fibrillation, may be visible externally and therefore constitutes a valuable physical sign. It is usually observed as a fine rippling movement of the skin overlying the muscle, although at times the movement may be coarser. It has been shown that fasciculation may arise either centrally —i.e. from the anterior horn cell—or peripherally: section of the nerve to a fasciculating muscle may not immediately abolish it completely. When arising peripherally, it seems likely that the discharge arises at some point in the terminal arborization of the motor nerve fibre and then spreads throughout the motor unit by a 'motor axon reflex'.

Spontaneous motor unit activity may occur in normal subjects, particularly under conditions of emotional stress or fatigue, and has been referred to as myokymia. The contractions are often coarser than in the fasciculation associated with denervation, and electromyographically there is, of course, no concomitant evidence of denervation.

MUSCLE CRAMPS

These may be defined as involuntary, localized, painful contractions of muscle which may be protracted in duration but are often capable of being relieved by stretching the affected muscle, probably by activation of the Golgi tendon receptors, the afferent pathway from which has an inhibitory action on the large (α) motoneurons (see p. 364). They occur in normal subjects, most frequently after vigorous exercise or nocturnally, and during pregnancy. They are also encountered in various disease states such as affections of the anterior horn cells (acute anterior poliomyelitis, motor neurone disease) and sodium deficiency.

Electromyographic examination of cramps has demonstrated that the discharge is of motor units, indicating a neural origin. The level of origin is as yet uncertain.

TETANY

Clinical tetany is not a muscle disorder: it has been shown to arise through overexcitability of the peripheral nerves. It appears that tetany in man is in nearly all cases associated with a reduction in the ionized calcium concentration in the extracellular fluid. This applies to the tetany of respiratory and metabolic alkalosis as well as to that associated with frank hypocalcaemia. A few patients with tetany have recently been recognized in whom the ionized calcium concentration is normal; the explanation of these cases of 'idiopathic tetany' is uncertain. Tetany also occurs occasionally with, and particularly during correction of, potassium deficiency, but the mechanism for this is also obscure. It remains disputed whether magnesium deficiency causes true tetany in man (p. 21).

Principles of tests and measurements

CREATINE AND CREATININE EXCRETION

Creatine is derived both from the diet and by synthesis within the body. Although the precise manner of its synthesis is not certain, it is likely that it is derived initially from glycine which is converted, possibly in the kidney, to guanidoacetic acid by receiving an amidine group from arginine. Guanidoacetic acid is then transmethylated in the liver to creatine, methionine being a possible source for the methyl group. Creatine is delivered from the liver into the bloodstream and taken up by the muscles. Most of the creatine in the body, about 98 per cent, is present in muscle, mainly as creatine phosphate. The role of creatine phosphate in muscle metabolism has already been mentioned (p. 340).

Negligible quantities of creatine are excreted in the urine in the male, but in women and children small quantities (up to 50 mg/day) are eliminated. Creatinuria may be produced in diseases of muscle by two separate mechanisms. In the first place, the rapid destruction of muscle tissue leads to its release and loss in the urine. Secondly, if the total bulk of muscle is sufficiently reduced, the normal quantities of creatine produced by the liver and delivered into the bloodstream are not fully taken up by the muscles and the blood level of creatine rises. If the renal threshold for creatine is exceeded, creatinuria results. This also provides the basis of the creatine tolerance test. If a normal individual is given a creatine load of about 1 g, this is taken up by the muscles and does not appear in the urine. If the total muscle bulk is sufficiently reduced, the creatine is not removed from the blood and any quantity above the renal threshold is lost in the urine. The creatine tolerance test, although illustrating the physiology of creatine metabolism, is not of very great clinical importance.

Creatinine is the anhydride of creatine and is probably an end product of muscle metabolism. The daily excretion of creatinine is 1–2 g/day and is approximately constant for any one individual, the actual amount being proportional to muscle mass. The excretion of creatinine therefore falls in muscle-wasting diseases.

SERUM ENZYMES

The concentration in the serum of a number of muscle enzymes such as creatine kinase and aldolase may be increased in muscular dystrophy. This is considered to be due to a generalized leakage of enzymes from the muscle cells rather than any specific metabolic defect. Disorders in which destruction of muscle fibres occurs, such as polymyositis, may also give rise to elevated serum enzyme levels.

MEASUREMENT OF THE ELECTRICAL EXCITABILITY OF MUSCLES

The relationship between the strength and the duration of the electrical stimulus required to activate nerve or muscle fibres is a convenient measure of their excitability. If a muscle is stimulated over its motor point (the site at which the nerve enters the muscle and at which contraction is most readily evoked) with electrical pulses of varying duration, and the strength of the stimulus necessary to cause a just visible contraction determined, the resulting relationship represents the strength-duration (or intensity-time) curve of the muscle. The strength of the stimulus may be varied by altering either the current or the voltage. When a normally innervated muscle is activated in this way, it is in reality being stimulated through its nerve supply, since nerve fibres are excited far more readily than muscle fibres. The stimulus durations normally employed range between 300 and 0·01 milliseconds (msec) and a normal curve is shown in Fig. 35. There is little change in the stimulus strength required for stimulus durations of 300 to 1 msec, but the curve rises fairly steeply between 1 and 0·01 msec. Two other measures of excitability that have been employed are the rheobase and the chronaxie. The rheobase is the minimum stimulus strength required to activate the muscle with a stimulus of infinite duration (in practice, over 100 msec); the chronaxie is defined as the minimum stimulus duration required to activate the muscle with a stimulus strength of twice the rheobase.

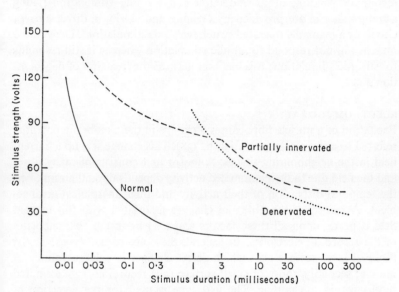

FIGURE 35. *Typical appearance of strength-duration curves for normal, denervated and partially innervated human muscles.*

The lines on the graph indicate the least stimulus strength and duration required to produce muscular contraction.

(From Ritchie, 1954; reproduced by kind permission of the author and the Controller of H.M. Stationery Office.)

In a completely denervated muscle, the muscle fibres must be activated directly and the muscle is considerably less easily stimulated. The strength-duration curve (see Fig. 35) shows a progressive increase in the strength of stimulus required for stimulus durations between 300 and 1 msec with no response to the shorter shocks. This difference between the electrical excitability of normally innervated and denervated muscles forms the basis of the diagnostic use of strength-duration curves for clinical purposes. In partially denervated muscle, the curves may show 'kinks' (see Fig. 35) and it has been demonstrated by electromyographic recording that these result from the combination of two curves, one derived from the innervated and the other from the denervated muscle fibres.

In the so-called faradic-galvanic testing, the response of the muscle to stimuli of widely differing duration is assessed and, in effect, the two ends of a strength-duration curve are obtained. Short duration shocks are provided by an interrupted current delivered from the secondary winding of an induction coil (faradic stimulation); long duration shocks are provided by opening and closing a direct current circuit by a manually operated switch (galvanic stimulation). Denervated muscle will not respond to faradic stimulation whereas it still responds to galvanic stimulation; this has been termed the 'reaction of degeneration'.

ELECTROMYOGRAPHY

Excitation of a muscle fibre causes a change in the membrane potential referred to as an action potential (p. 338). This change sets up a current field in the neighbouring tissues. A motor unit consists of many fibres and the field due to their summated activity depends upon their number, the temporal dispersion of their activity and their anatomical arrangement. A record of the potential changes associated with this current field depends upon all these factors and also upon the characteristics of the recording electrodes. In general, these are of two types: firstly, those of large surface area which detect changes in a large volume of muscle; secondly, those of small surface area recording from a limited radius within the muscle. The first type is used for the detection of muscular activity or for the study of the summated excitation of many units in a bulk of muscle. The second type (such as the concentric needle electrode) is used for studying the detailed electrical characteristics of individual motor unit potentials and is of more value in clinical physiology.

The concentric or coaxial needle electrode is a bipolar electrode, one pole being formed by the shaft of a hypodermic needle, the other by a wire threaded through the shaft; an insulating layer is provided between the two. The electrode just records at its tip, thus sampling a restricted area within the muscle. The needle tip is bevelled and this bestows on it considerable directional properties. The potential differences recorded between the two poles of the electrode are amplified and displayed on a cathode ray oscilloscope. Since the frequencies happen to be within the audio-frequency range, they are also fed into a loudspeaker, a procedure which appreciably assists in the interpretation of the electromyogram.

The normal electromyogram as recorded with
a concentric needle electrode

In a normal subject, the muscle is electrically silent when it is at rest. Movement of the needle may provoke momentary discharges termed insertion activity.

On muscular contraction, the propagated action potentials of the muscle fibres are recorded. The size of the potential obtained depends considerably upon the position of the recording needle in relation to the active muscle fibre or fibres, the size of the potential falling exponentially with the distance between the source of the potential and the electrode. With the size of needle electrode ordinarily used, the potentials recorded approximate to those produced by individual motor units and are termed 'motor unit action potentials'.

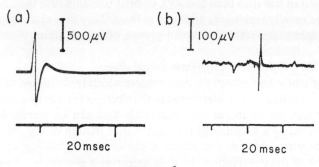

FIGURE 36.

A. Normal motor unit potential from human muscle. B. Fibrillation potential from denervated muscle. Records obtained from a concentric needle electrode. Note the smaller size and shorter duration of the fibrillation potential.

Normal motor unit potentials in the limb muscles are usually bi- or triphasic, about 0·5–2 mV in amplitude and 5–10 msec in duration (Fig. 36A). A small proportion are polyphasic in form. In the facial muscles they are smaller in size and briefer in duration. It has been shown that the rate of spread of the propagated action potential over the constituent fibres of the unit is too rapid to account for the observed duration of the motor unit potential. Its duration probably depends largely upon the scatter of the end-plates within the innervation zone, so that activation of the fibres occurs at varying distances from the point at which the potential is recorded. This will also largely determine the way in which the potentials of the individual fibres summate and hence the form of the total potential, although differences in the rate of conduction along individual muscle fibres presumably contribute to this.

On slight voluntary contraction, small numbers of motor unit potentials are recorded, but with increasingly vigorous contraction, more and more units are recruited and their discharge rate is augmented. The potentials run into one another and the resulting confused oscillographic picture is termed the 'interference pattern' of the muscle. The motor units first to appear on slight voluntary contraction are of smaller size than those appearing later when the contraction is more vigorous. The latter survive longer on fatigue.

The activity of single muscle fibres is not seen in normal muscles by this recording technique, but it is observable in the fibrillation potentials that may appear in denervated muscles. Such potentials (Fig. 36b) are small in size (less than 200 μV), of brief duration (less than 2 msec) and are usually biphasic or triphasic in form. They may also result from the synchronous activity of small groups of muscle fibres.

Alterations in the electromyogram during disease
Loss of motor unit potentials. Any process which leads to loss of motor nerve fibres to a muscle is reflected in the electromyogram as a reduction in the number of motor unit potentials that can be recruited. This is observed as a thinning of the interference pattern of the muscle on voluntary contraction, the extent of the change depending upon the severity of the denervation. Loss of motor unit potentials also occurs in the advanced stages of primary muscle disorders such as muscular dystrophy, although such a process, which diffusely affects muscle fibres, initially causes changes in the appearance of individual units without substantial change in their numbers.

Alterations in the amplitude of motor unit potentials. If the number of muscle fibres in a motor unit is reduced, there is a reduction in the amplitude of its electrical potential. This occurs in diffuse primary affections of muscle such as muscular dystrophy or polymyositis. Alternatively, if the number of fibres in the unit increases, the amplitude of the potential is augmented. In chronic partial denervation, motor unit potentials of considerably larger size than normal may be encountered. 'Giant' units of 15–20 mV are at times recorded. In partially denervated muscles, sprouting of the remaining nerve fibres and the re-innervation by these branches of muscle fibres that have lost their nerve supply has been observed histologically. It is thus likely that these large units result from the surviving nerve fibres extending their territory in this way, although other mechanisms may also be involved.

Alterations in the duration of motor unit potentials. The importance of the spatial dispersion of the end-plates in the innervation zone in determining the duration of the motor unit potential has been stressed. Normally, activation occurs more or less simultaneously at the different end-plates. If, however, temporal dispersion in the spread of the excitation process throughout the terminal arborization of the nerve fibre were to occur, the result would be a lengthening of the potential. It is likely that such a process accounts for the long duration units seen during re-innervation and in polyneuritis where abnormally slow nerve conduction exists.

A reduction in the duration of motor unit potentials occurs if the number of fibres in the unit is reduced to a sufficient extent, and this is seen in primary muscle disorders.

Changes in the form of motor unit potentials. A polyphasic motor unit potential results if the action potentials in the constituent fibres of the unit arrive at the recording electrode sufficiently asynchronously. At present, the precise way in which this occurs is not certain. Polyphasic units are met with in primary muscle disease (Fig. 37), in chronic partial denervation and during re-innervation. Temporal dispersion of activation is again a possible explanation for the polyphasic potentials in polyneuritis and during re-innervation.

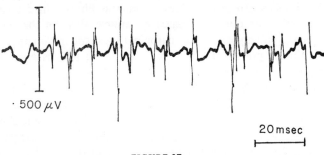

500 μV

20 msec

FIGURE 37.

Electromyographic recording obtained by a concentric needle electrode from a patient with polymyositis, showing low voltage, short duration polyphasic motor unit potentials.

Changes in muscular excitability. Denervated muscle fibres are abnormally sensitive to many forms of stimulation. 'Spontaneous' discharges (fibrillation) may be observed. These potentials occur independently of volition and often with a very constant frequency between 2 and 10 per second. Fibrillation can at times be brought out by the administration of an anticholinesterase such as edrophonium (Tensilon).

Denervated muscle fibres are abnormally sensitive to mechanical stimuli. Movement of the needle electrode may provoke prolonged fibrillary discharges which slowly die away. The so-called 'positive sharp' waves may also occur in which an initial rapid positive potential is followed by a prolonged decline; these potentials are not propagated and are thought to arise from damaged regions of muscle fibres.

The potentials recorded in myotonia are of single fibres (fibrillary) or of groups of fibres, the latter often having bizarre shapes. Myotonic discharges induced by needle movement or percussion of the muscle take the form of high frequency repetitive potentials which at first may be at the rate of 100–150/sec, falling rapidly to a tenth of this rate

The spontaneous motor unit discharges of fasciculation occur at an irregular rate. They are not infrequently polyphasic, suggesting an abnormal spread of excitation throughout the motor unit.

Practical assessment

ASSESSMENT OF TYPE OF DISORDER

DISORDERS PRODUCING WEAKNESS
Clinical observations
Wasting implies atrophy or loss of muscle fibres either secondary to denervation or due to diseases of muscle such as the muscular dystrophies, polymyositis and chronic thyrotoxic myopathy. When fasciculation is present it indicates denervation; it does not occur in primary muscular disorders.

Aggravation of the weakness by *fatigue* suggests myasthenia; exercise precipitates attacks in paroxysmal myoglobinuria; rest following exercise, or meals, may do so in hypokalaemic familial periodic paralysis; and rest following exercise in hyperkalaemic familial periodic paralysis.

The *distribution of the weakness* may be characteristic, as in the muscular dystrophies (e.g. facio-scapulo-humeral and limb-girdle forms), in myasthenia gravis where the external ocular and bulbar muscles are often selectively involved, or in polymyositis and chronic thyrotoxic myopathy where there is a tendency for the limb girdle and proximal limb muscles to be affected. The age of onset, the rate of progress and the presence or absence of fluctuation in severity are frequently helpful.

Associated clinical features may suggest the nature of the weakness as in disturbances of potassium metabolism, thyrotoxic myopathy and the various causes of denervation.

A family history of similar disorder may be obtained in the muscular dystrophies, in familial periodic paralysis, and in other metabolic myopathies.

Routine methods
Electrical reactions (strength-duration curves). Abnormal in denervation.

Electromyography. In denervation, the important changes are increased mechanical irritability and spontaneous fibrillation, and reduction in the number of motor units under voluntary control. In chronic partial denervation the motor unit potentials may be large. Primary muscle disease (e.g. the muscular dystrophies) is manifested by the presence of low amplitude, short duration, polyphasic motor unit potentials; in polymyositis there may in addition be increased excitability of muscle fibres of the type occurring in denervation.

Anticholinesterase test for myasthenia. The use of prostigmine has largely been superseded by edrophonium (Tensilon) in view of the rapidity of the response and the relative absence of side effects. 10 mg of edrophonium is injected intravenously; if positive, an improvement in the muscular weakness is observed within a minute. (An unequivocal result is not always obtained.)

Urinary creatine excretion. Increased in the presence of wasting whether this is due to muscle disease or denervation.

Serum enzymes. The level of serum creatine kinase and other enzymes may be elevated in muscular dystrophy and disorders such as polymyositis that produce destruction of muscle fibres.

Muscle biopsy. May be required at times in the diagnosis of conditions where there is structural damage.

Plasma potassium concentration and *ECG* in potassium disturbances, including familial periodic paralysis of hyper- and hypo-kalaemic types.

Special techniques
Electromyography in myasthenia gravis. The size of the compound action potential of an affected muscle may be diminished on rapid repetitive stimulation of the motor nerve and the administration of an anti-cholinesterase may lessen or reverse this effect. A pronounced post-tetanic potentiation in the size of the muscle action potential evoked by nerve stimulation is a feature of the myasthenic syndrome associated with bronchogenic carcinoma.

Provocation of attacks in hypokalaemic familial periodic paralysis by a carbohydrate load, with or without insulin, causing a shift of potassium into the cells; and in hyperkalaemic familial periodic paralysis provocation of attacks by the administration of potassium.

DISORDERS PRODUCING INCREASED MUSCULAR EXCITABILITY
Clinical observations
Slowness in relaxation after forcible muscular contraction and on percussion of the muscle belly indicate myotonia. Associated *dystrophic changes* are present in dystrophia myotonica and a family history is often obtained both in this condition and in myotonia congenita.

Attacks of *muscular spasm* in the extremities with associated paraesthesiae suggest tetany. Hyperventilation may be the cause or there may be clinical evidence of a disorder that produces hypocalcaemia (p. 327) or hypokalaemia.

Latent tetany may be demonstrated by the following simple tests which depend upon heightened excitability of the peripheral nerves:

Chvostek's sign: percussion of the facial nerve in front of the tragus gives rise to a twitch of all the facial muscles on that side.

Trousseau's sign: ischaemia of the forearm and hand produced by a sphygmomanometer cuff inflated above systolic pressure for 5 min results in stiffening of the muscles (particularly the thenar muscles) and the hand may take up the *position d'accoucheur*.

Routine methods
Electromyography—diagnostic in myotonia (p. 356).

Plasma calcium, potassium, and bicarbonate concentration—may be altered in tetany (p. 326).

Special techniques
Plasma ionized calcium concentration in tetany (p. 326).

ASSESSMENT OF FORCE OF CONTRACTION

Clinical observations
A good assessment of the force of muscular contraction can be obtained by the routine clinical methods. This is particularly true of the limb muscles where comparison between sides may be helpful.

The following semiquantitative scheme (MRC Scale) is useful for recording muscle power:

Grade 0 complete paralysis
       1 flicker of contraction
       2 contraction with gravity eliminated
       3 contraction against gravity
       4 contraction against gravity and some resistance (subdivision of this grade is possible)
       5 full power.

Routine methods
A variety of devices, such as dynamometers for measurement of the strength of the hand grip, is available; none is very useful for clinical purposes. The vital capacity is a convenient measure for the respiratory muscles, but they must be considerably weakened before the vital capacity is reduced.

Special techniques
For research investigations in which it is wished to compare the number of motor units in action in the same muscle in different conditions, the integrated electromyogram is of value. It does not permit comparison between muscles or between individuals.

References

ADAMS R.D., DENNY-BROWN D. & PEARSON C.M. (1962) *Diseases of muscle: a study in pathology* (2nd Ed.). New York: Hoeber.

ADAMS R.D., EATON L.M. & SHY G.M. (ed.) (1960). *Neuromuscular disorders. Res. Publ. Ass. nerv. ment. Dis.*, **38.** Baltimore: Williams & Wilkins.

BOURNE G.H. (ed.) (1960). *Structure and function of muscle* (vols. i, ii and iii). New York: Academic Press.

WALTON J.N. (ed.) (1964). *Disorders of voluntary muscle.* London: J. & A. Churchill.

The Nervous System in the Control of Movement

Normal function

Willed movement of skeletal muscle is superimposed on a background of muscle tone, and is accompanied by alterations in both the amount and extent of such tone. Indeed, so intimately are changes of tone associated with willed movements that abnormalities of tone are sometimes revealed because of their interference with the execution of willed movement. The word tone has been used with somewhat different connotation by different groups of workers. To the physiologist the word tone is almost synonymous with the static reaction of the stretch reflex, while to the clinician tone means the resistance offered by the muscles to passive movement. Such different meanings for the word tone may lead to difficulty, and a return to this point will be made in a later section.

THE SPINAL ORGANIZATION OF THE STRETCH REFLEX

The monosynaptic reflex arc. As its name implies the stretch reflex is the reflex contraction of skeletal muscle which follows stretch. The physiologist divides the total reflex response into two parts, the phasic stretch reflex for which the afferent discharge is initiated during the period of actual stretching, and the static stretch reflex which is the reflex contraction resulting from a constant maintained stretch. The phasic stretch reflex may be studied in isolation by using short lasting stretches, as is done clinically in eliciting the tendon reflexes. The motor response to such short-lasting stimuli is, in the normal individual, well localized, and produces almost exclusively contraction of only those muscles—or even parts of muscle—that have been stretched. The sensory end organs chiefly concerned are the primary endings of the muscle spindles (Fig. 38). These nerve fibres originate from the equator (nuclear bag region) of the muscle spindles, which are themselves embedded in the skeletal muscles effectively in parallel with the striated or extrafusal muscle fibres. The primary afferent (group IA) fibres from the muscle spindles are large diameter myelinated fibres and therefore rapidly conducting (70 m/sec). These afferent fibres enter the spinal cord via the dorsal root, and make monosynaptic connections with the motoneurone pool of the parent muscle. Many of the incoming IA afferents also make inhibitory connections with antagonist muscle motoneurone pools via interneurones. There are no monosynaptic inhibitory connections. The efferent motor fibres arise from the large (α) anterior horn cells and pass to innervate the extrafusal muscle fibres as described in Chapter 9. This reflex arc is obviously capable of rapidly responding to stretch of the primary ending, since both the afferent and efferent nerve fibres are amongst the most rapidly conducting in the body, and the central delay is reduced to a minimum by the presence of only one synapse (synaptic delay 0·5–1 msec).

Role of the gamma motor system

The sensitivity to stretch of the primary sensory ending is not fixed. The muscle spindles contain specialized muscle fibres, the intrafusal fibres, which by their shortening are able to stretch the primary ending. Since it is immaterial to the primary ending whether the applied stretch is due to stretch of the muscle as a whole, or to shortening of the intrafusal fibres, the afferent discharge is similar in the two cases, and the central results identical. The intrafusal muscle fibres receive a special motor innervation from the small (γ) anterior horn cells, and this system (consisting of the small anterior horn cells, their small diameter— and therefore slowly conducting—motor fibres, and the specialized intrafusal muscle fibres which they innervate) constitutes a method of varying the sensitivity of the primary sensory ending to applied stretch. Thus the size of the reflex muscle contraction following a transient stretch depends primarily upon the setting, or bias, of the primary sensory ending. If the tonic gamma motoneurone discharge which is present in the wakeful state is blocked, the tendon jerk will be abolished, whereas if the gamma motoneurone discharge is increased—as is thought to occur during clinical reinforcement of the tendon jerks—the reflex response will be increased. It should be noted that these changes are chiefly due to alterations in the sensitivity of the sensory end organ and not to changes in excitability of the large (α) anterior horn cells. During sleep the discharge from the gamma motoneurones to the intrafusal fibres ceases, and the tendon jerks are lost.

Other neuronal pathways concerned in the stretch reflexes

The majority of mammalian muscle spindles contain in addition to a primary sensory ending, one or more secondary sensory endings. These secondary endings are also in close contact with the intrafusal muscle fibres and are sensitive to stretch but differ from the primary endings in giving rise to smaller diameter and therefore more slowly conducting afferent nerve fibres. The central connections of these group II afferent fibres are not yet known in detail but all appear to influence large anterior horn cells only through interneurones (see Fig. 38).

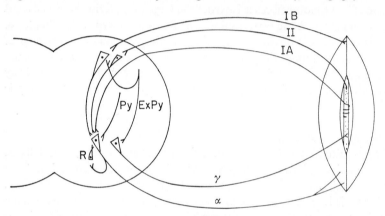

FIGURE 38. *Diagram of the spinal reflex arcs concerned in posture.*

The spinal cord is shown in transverse section on the left: a skeletal muscle is shown at the right. α represents a nerve fibre passing from a large anterior horn cell to the extrafusal muscle fibres, γ one passing from a small anterior horn cell to supply the intrafusal muscle fibre. IA represents an afferent fibre from the primary spindle ending, IB a fibre from the golgi tendon organ, and II a fibre from the secondary spindle ending. Py=descending pyramidal tract; ExPy=descending extrapyramidal tracts; R=recurrent Renshaw loop and Renshaw cell.

While both the primary and the secondary endings within the muscle spindle are sensitive to stretch there appear to be differences in their relative sensitivities to the speed of stretching and to maintained stretch. In general the primary endings give the major information on the rate of change of length and the secondary endings the major information on the absolute length at any instant.

It is also now known that the intrafusal muscle fibres may be divided into two types, the larger nuclear bag fibres which are characterized by a central bag of nuclei, and the smaller nuclear chain fibres which have their nuclei arranged linearly along the length of the fibre. The primary sensory ending is wound round the equatorial region of a nuclear bag fibre, while the secondary endings are in contact with the nuclear chain fibres. There is also some, less direct, evidence that the two types of intrafusal muscle fibre have separate motor innervations. The implication of this is that the spindle may have its sensitivity to degree of stretch and rate of change of stretch set independently. If this is so it goes a long way to explaining the remarkable stability of the stretch reflexes in the face of changing loads.

As has been stated above the afferent nerve fibres from the secondary sensory endings terminate centrally on interneurones. The extrapyramidal descending tracts are known to exert their dominant influence on small (γ) anterior horn cells and interneurones. It is therefore apparent that the discharge from the secondary sensory endings may be modified centrally by extrapyramidal activity before it influences the large (α) motoneurones.

The role of the Renshaw cell

The large (α) motoneurones give off collateral branches from the intramedullary parts of their axons. These collaterals form synapses with the Renshaw cells (Fig. 38) which are also found in the anterior horn. The Renshaw cell axons then pass to form inhibitory synapses on the surface of the anterior horn cells of the same motoneurone pool. Thus a nerve impulse generated by an α motoneurone passes via the motor nerve fibre to the muscle, but also passes via the recurrent Renshaw loop back to the same motoneurone pool, where it produces an inhibitory or damping effect. By this means all but the initial impulses arriving at a motoneurone pool during a maintained discharge from the spindle endings will find the anterior horn cells partially inhibited, and will therefore produce a smaller reflex motor discharge than the initial excitatory volley.

It seems probable that the tendon reflex (or phasic reaction of the stretch reflex) is due to the conduction of a volley of impulses over the most rapid (monosynaptic) pathway, the motor volley leaving the spinal cord before the inhibitory Renshaw loop has had time to come into action, while the reflex response to slower and more prolonged stretch (the static reaction of the stretch reflex) is the resultant response of the motoneurone pool to impulses reaching it from muscle stretch receptors over both monosynaptic and polysynaptic spinal pathways and also via the Renshaw loop.

Summarizing the neuronal organization of the stretch reflex at the spinal level, it may be said that at least three types of afferent nerve fibres are involved. First there is the primary spindle afferent (Group IA). Second is the secondary spindle afferent (Group II, Fig. 38), transmitting its impulses to the cord along smaller diameter and therefore more slowly conducting fibres. Thirdly there is the Golgi afferent (Group IB), producing autogenetic inhibition at high tension. The central connections between the incoming afferents and the parent motoneurone pool may be direct (monosynaptic excitatory) or via interneurones. Descending impulses may modify the excitability of these interneurones. The motor output is in two parts: the gamma outflow(s) to the intrafusal muscle fibres by means of which the sensitivity of the spindle afferents to stretch may be modified; and the alpha motoneurone output—the final common path—by which contraction of the extrafusal muscle fibres is ultimately achieved. In addition to the afferents from muscle, other reflex pathways converge on the α-motoneurones and may modify the stretch reflex. Cutaneous sensations and particularly pain are important examples.

'Fast' and 'slow' muscles

In some animals there are two distinct populations of striated muscles: the rapidly contracting (fast) muscles and the slowly contracting (slow) muscles. In such species there is some evidence that the slow muscles play a major part in the maintenance of the static stretch reaction and that their motoneurones, which are functionally distinct from those of fast muscle, receive a disproportionately large monosynaptic inflow. The present evidence suggests that there are not two distinct muscle populations in man (though some muscles may consist of an intimate mixture of two functionally different types of fibre) and there is little evidence of specialization of the stretch reflex in any particular muscle.

The relation between muscle length and force of contraction

The tension developed by a muscle during an isometric contraction depends upon the initial length of the muscle fibres. Thus, within certain limits, as the muscle is stretched the tension developed in response to a given nerve activity is increased. Therefore, the tension developed by a muscle contracting reflexly in response to a certain (fixed) afferent inflow will depend upon the initial length of the extrafusal muscle fibres.

SUPRASPINAL CONTROL OF THE STRETCH REFLEX

The discharge of the small anterior horn cells (determining the bias of the spindle sensory end organs) and the excitability of spinal interneurones are under supraspinal control. This controlling mechanism may be termed the extrapyramidal system. Like muscle tone, the term extrapyramidal system has been variously defined in the past. It is here used to include the basal ganglia, their associated nuclei and the brain stem reticular formation, together with their descending spinal pathways. Intimately connected functionally with this system are the vestibular nuclei and part of the cerebellum. This total group of structures represents a functional unit, and at present it is unrewarding to attempt to delineate an exact and unique function for each of the component parts. A pertinent analogy may be drawn with a complex electronic circuit in which it may be difficult to state a precise and unique function for a particular component. The function of the component may vary according to the state of another part of the circuit, or, indeed, a particular component may not be functionally in circuit at all until certain conditions prevail elsewhere in the apparatus. It is then obviously only possible to define the function (as opposed to the form and connections) of the component in terms of the working of the whole. Similarly, it may be noted that the failure of a component in such complex apparatus may produce a defect in the operation of the whole which may be far removed from the normal function of the single component.

The extrapyramidal system exercises its influence on spinal neurones by virtue of the descending extrapyramidal pathways. The exact anatomy of these tracts is not well known in man, nor it is possible to assign a particular function to any of them. Rather may they be considered as a mixture of excitatory and inhibitory fibres, impulses in the former leading to an increased excitability of the postsynaptic cells on which the fibres terminate and impulses in the latter leading to a decreased excitability.

By these descending pathways the extrapyramidal system exercises its control over the stretch reflexes throughout the spinal cord, and normally sets the excitability in each segment at a level which is most appropriate to the functioning of the body as a whole. In order to compute the most appropriate setting, the extrapyramidal system requires an adequate inflow of information. Such a concentration of information appears to occur in the reticular formation of the brain stem, and it is dominantly from this region that the descending extrapyramidal tracts take origin. Largely from work on animals two functional areas of the brain stem named respectively the inhibitory reticular formation and the facilitatory reticular formation have been demonstrated. Stimulation of the former against a background of spinal stretch reflex activity reduces the reflex response. Stimulation of the latter (facilitatory) region enhances the reflex response. Into these two regions passes information which allows computation of the pattern of descending excitatory and inhibitory impulses which will set optimal spinal reflex excitability (Fig. 39).

The inflow into the smaller inhibitory reticular formation is from cortical inhibitory areas, the corpus striatum (particularly the caudate nucleus) and the anterior lobe of the cerebellum. The inflow into the facilitatory reticular formation is from the middle lobe of the cerebellum

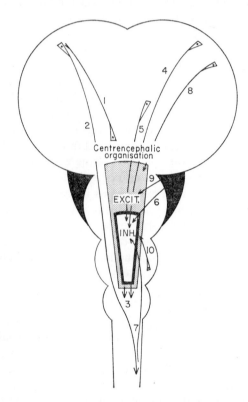

FIGURE 39. *Diagram of central organizing areas and tracts.*

Longitudinal section of brain. EXCIT=excitor reticular formation. INH=inhibitor reticular formation. Black shading=cerebellum. Tracts: 1=ascending pathways from centrencephalic centre to cortex; 2=pyramidal tract; 3=descending extrapyramidal tracts from excitor and inhibitor reticular areas; 4, 5, 6 and 7=pathways to the inhibitor reticular formation from the inhibitory cortex, caudate nucleus cerebellum and ascending sensory pathways respectively; 8, 9 and 10=pathways to the excitor reticular formation from the motor cortex, cerebellum and vestibular nuclei respectively.

and from the vestibular nuclei. The brain stem reticular formation also receives collateral branches from ascending sensory pathways, impulses in which are used by the ascending reticular activating system. This sensory information from the periphery may also be used by the reticular formation in determining the best pattern of descending extrapyramidal impulses. Thus the reticular formation acts as a coordinating centre or headquarters of the extrapyramidal system, collecting information from a variety of sources and on the basis of this information directing the distribution and extent of the stretch reflexes throughout the cord.

Viewed in this manner the postural reflexes such as the tonic neck reflexes, the tonic labyrinthine reflexes and the righting reflexes become special examples of the total activity of the extrapyramidal system, with the difference that these reflex activities may extend further than simply altering the sensitivities of spinal reflex arcs and may lead to the contraction of extrafusal muscle fibres. However, this represents no true discontinuity in the functioning of the system, for there is ample evidence that the contraction of the extrafusal fibres is produced as a reflex following on imposed alterations in the length of the intrafusal muscle fibres. This simply means that the descending extrapyramidal excitatory impulses have increased the small anterior horn cell discharge (and hence intrafusal muscle fibre shortening) to such a level that the discharges from the spindle sensory endings are sufficient to activate the large anterior horn cells and hence cause shortening of the extrafusal muscle fibres. Such activity of the extrafusal muscle fibres will continue until the stretch on the sensory endings (imposed by the intrafusal muscle fibres) is removed, with the resultant cessation of the afferent discharge.

While this appears to be the most common method of producing postural reflex activity in the normal animal, postural adjustments can also be obtained by direct descending extrapyramidal activation of the large anterior horn cells. In the experimental animal the anterior lobe of the cerebellum appears to play a part in determining by which route (gamma or direct alpha) the extrafusal muscle fibres shall be activated. One determining factor in deciding which route to use might be the speed with which the desired postural adjustment is required, since transmission over the gamma fibres and reflex arc imposes a delay on the initiation of the skeletal muscle movement. In this context it may be noted that at least some of the descending extrapyramidal tracts are composed of large diameter, and therefore rapidly conducting nerve fibres.

In summary, the extrapyramidal system may be considered the controlling mechanism determining the setting of the stretch reflexes. The set includes the sensitivity of the primary spindle ending to stretch and the excitability of the appropriate interneurones. Note that this is a sensitivity of the reflex arc *to stretch*. If a limb is completely at rest, with all sources of muscle stretch removed, the muscle will be electrically silent with no motor unit activity. However, any stretch will result in a reflex contraction, the extent of which will be determined by the setting imposed on the sensory end organs by the extrapyramidal system. It seems that the static response of the stretch reflex can be voluntarily inhibited presumably by inhibiting interneurones. The extrapyramidal system can also potentiate the response to superadded stretch, and also increase the afferent discharge from the sensory endings to an extent such that actual reflex contraction of the extrafusal fibres is brought about (postural reflexes). The inflow of information to the reticular formation which allows it continuously to adjust tone throughout the body during the waking hours comes from a wide variety of sites, and correct action by the reticular structures depends upon a full and accurate inflow from these sources.

THE CONTROL OF WILLED MOVEMENT

Willed movements are superimposed upon a background of tone and postural reflexes. A willed movement will itself inevitably bring about alterations in tone in order that the movement may be optimally performed. In other words, a normal willed movement involves simultaneous correct functioning of both the pyramidal and extrapyramidal systems. This fact leads to discussion of the 'co-ordination' of willed movements in many textbooks, but from what has been said concerning the normal function of the extrapyramidal system it should be apparent that imposed willed movements are only one of the variables with which the brain stem reticular formation has to deal, and that the postural changes accompanying a volitional act are in no essential way different from those described above. In other words, prior knowledge of intended willed movements constitutes an additional inflow of information to the reticular formation which must be taken into account as much as any other when the optimal postural adjustments are computed. The anatomical pathway for this inflow is not known, but Penfield has postulated a 'centrencephalic integration system' at the level of the higher brain stem, in which situation it might overlap with the facilitatory reticular formation. This postulated centrencephalic system is envisaged as a functional area, anatomically ill defined, which as well as acting as a sensory integrating area, serves as the site for the initiation of willed movements. The will to initiate a movement is thought to originate in this area, and nerve impulses pass from the centrencephalic region to the motor cortex. From the motor cortex impulses pass down in the pyramidal tract to the anterior horn cells. Although the concept of the centrencephalic system has no strict anatomical reality, some such centrally placed structure must be implicated in the organization of simultaneous bilateral willed movements. Furthermore, observations made while stimulating the exposed motor cortex of conscious man suggest that there is some inflow to the motor cortex from lower centres. Liminal stimulation of a point on the motor cortex may lead to a fragmentary contraction of a muscle or muscle groups (excitatory points) or simply to the inhibition of willed movements in a particular part of the musculature (inhibitory points). Finally, stimulation of certain sites of the motor cortex appears to fire off inborn bilateral (probably brain stem) mechanisms responsible for such acts as sucking and swallowing.

The two primary motor cortices possibly furnish a method of obtaining a larger store and variety of willed movements than could otherwise be acquired, and this bilateral repertoire of movements may be called upon at will by the centrencephalic system. It should be noted that the Rolandic motor cortex is not the only area of the cortex capable of giving rise to activity in skeletal muscle when stimulated. Movements may also be produced from the supplementary motor area and possibly from the second sensory and mesial temporal areas. The organization of the Rolandic motor cortex is well known and the relative distribution of cortical area to different regions of the body musculature is well illustrated by many cortical maps. The large Betz cells which characterize area 4 give rise to only some 4 per cent of fibres of the pyramidal tract, and the vast majority of the descending fibres are of small diameter and therefore slowly conducting. The pyramidal fibres terminate either directly on the surface of anterior horn cells, or indirectly via interneurones.

From what has been stated previously, it may be seen that the pyramidal tract terminations might be with either large (α) motoneurones or small (γ) motoneurones. In the former case willed contraction of skeletal muscle would be brought about by directly activating the α motoneurones and the final common path, while in the latter case the contraction would be brought about by a reflex following such as was described for postural movements. Under these conditions the descending pyramidal impulses would increase the discharge of the small (γ) anterior horn cells. This would lead to intrafusal fibre shortening and a resultant increase in afferent discharge from the muscle spindles. The increased afferent discharge, reaching the large (α) motoneurones over the fast monosynaptic pathway, would produce a reflex ('following') contraction of the extrafusal fibres. The contraction of the extrafusal fibres would then be maintained as long as the increased discharge from the γ-motoneurones continued. It has become fashionable to stress the similarity of such behaviour to that of certain servo mechanisms and to describe such a contraction of the extrafusal fibres as a 'follow-up length servo', i.e. a system controlled by negative feedback. At the present time there is no evidence on which to decide which of these two possible mechanisms, the direct or indirect, is used under specified circumstances. That willed movements can occur in de-afferented limbs in which the indirect method could not be operative is well authenticated, though the execution of such movements is not precise. The apparent advantage of the follow-up method would seem to be that it offers a more accurate control of the movement, since information is inevitably being fed back from the muscle spindles about the progress being made as the movement is executed. It must be emphasized, however, that there is no definite evidence whether the follow-up is commonly—or ever—used in willed movements.

Summarizing the genesis of a willed movement we may say that the will to initiate a movement originates in a functional area named the centrencephalic region. From here impulses pass out to the motor cortex and to the brain stem reticular formation. The latter structure—on the basis of its sensory inflow—gives rise to a pattern of descending excitatory and inhibitory extrapyramidal impulses which set the excitability of the various stretch reflexes. Meanwhile, the motor cortex discharges down the slowly conducting pyramidal tract a pattern of impulses, which, acting initially either on large or small anterior horn cells, leads to the ultimate activation of the 'prime mover' muscles.

Disordered function

DISTURBANCES OF TONE

Hypertonia

Hypertonia, or increased tone, may exist in one of two forms, as spasticity or as rigidity. Both are due to excessive reflex motor discharges to maintained stretch, but the pattern of the motor discharge differs. In spasticity the excitability of the static stretch reflex arc is certainly increased at the muscle spindles and probably also at the spinal inter-neurones. This means that the reflex contraction to stretch is excessive, and as the degree of stretch is increased, more and more motor units are recruited. If the stretch to the muscle is continued sufficiently, the reflex tension developed by the muscle is sufficient to fire off the Golgi tendon organs. Impulses from these sensory endings inhibit the anterior horn cells and lead to a sudden inhibition of the static stretch reflex with the result that the muscle suddenly relaxes and 'gives'—the 'clasp knife' phenomenon. In rigidity the sensitivity of the static stretch reflex to stretch is also excessive, but the number of motor units contracting at any time remains the same whatever the degree of stretch. The reason is that as additional motor units are recruited others cease contracting. The resistance to stretch felt by the examiner is therefore constant throughout a movement—lead pipe rigidity. Why the number of active motor units remains constant during stretch instead of increasing as in spasticity is not known. If tremor coexists with rigidity, it may be felt during the examination of tone, and is appreciated as a 'cog-wheel' rigidity, the synchronized motor unit activity of the tremor being super-imposed on the lead pipe rigidity.

Hypotonia

Hypotonia, or decreased tone, may occur with an anatomically intact static stretch reflex arc if the excitability of the spinal interneurones is lowered. This may occur in cerebellar disease and chorea. More com-monly, however, hypotonia is produced by an interruption of the stretch reflex arc. If the lesion is on the motor side then flaccidity is accom-panied by wasting of the muscles whose motor supply has been cut. If the lesion is on the sensory side, as in tabes dorsalis, then the hypo-tonia occurs with no, or very much less, wasting.

Tremor

Tremor is due to the synchronized rhythmical involuntary contraction of a sufficient number of motor units to move the part. It must be differentiated from fasciculation (p. 348) and myokymia. In the normal individual, a slight tremor with a frequency of 9–10 c/s is often present which may be due to purely chance beating of several motor units, or to instability in the stretch reflex arc. Tremor of a comparable frequency is seen in hyperthyroidism and psychoneurotic states. The tremor of extrapyramidal disease is slower and coarser. Its presence may sometimes be more easily felt—as 'cog-wheel' rigidity—than seen. Its causation is not known. Intention tremor is a disorder of willed movement (p. 368).

13

ALTERATIONS OF TENDON JERKS
Hyperreflexia
Increased tendon jerks may be due to excessive bias of the muscle spindles. Such is the case in the hyperreflexia of hemiplegia, in which the excitability of the α-motoneurones remains normal. Hyperreflexia might also be due to hyperexcitability of the α-motoneurones with normal spindle bias, and this may be the mechanism of the increased tendon reflexes below the level of the lesion following spinal transection.

Hyporeflexia
Decreased tendon jerks are most commonly due to an interruption of the monosynaptic stretch reflex arc. A selective loss of the large IA afferent fibres appears to be present in Adie's syndrome in which there is loss of tendon jerks with retention of normal tone. This again emphasizes the functional separation of the phasic and static stretch reflexes. It has recently been shown that the loss of tendon reflexes in Friedreich's ataxia is due to a loss of spindle bias as well as to degeneration of posterior roots at their entry zone. Whether the loss of spindle bias is due to diminished gamma drive or to primary dysfunction of the intrafusal muscle fibres is not known.

The loss of tendon jerks which occurs in tabes is due to destruction of the large afferent fibres. The similar, but temporary, loss of ankle jerk which may occur in sciatica is probably due to a block in conduction caused by pressure on the nerve fibres.

SPINAL LESIONS
Local lesions
Lesions of the spinal cord may present very different clinical states depending upon the nature, the site and the rate of development of the lesion. Disease processes may involve specific groups of cells as in the destruction of α-motoneurones in poliomyelitis or motor neurone disease which causes a clearly recognizable loss of the final common path. Or the disease process may interfere with a particular spinal function as in the case of tetanus toxin and inhibitory synaptic processes. The spasms of tetanus are due to a 'paralysis' of inhibition, probably at the anterior horn cells of the spinal cord. In this respect, tetanus toxin resembles strychnine. The discharge of Renshaw cells and the monosynaptic stretch reflex are unaffected in the early stages of the disorder.

Most spinal lesions are non-specific as regards the cells or functions with which they interfere, and while such lesions may be accurately identified as to site, the function defects produced will be simply a result of their particular anatomical location.

Spinal transection

Immediately following sudden complete spinal transection in man there is a period of motor paralysis below the level of the lesion. This period, which may last for two or three weeks, is known as the stage of spinal shock. The complete section of all descending pathways effectively silences the motoneurones so that no activity, reflex or volitional, is produced in the final common path. Gradually the spinal segments below the section assume a degree of automatic functioning which progresses to a state of augmented reflex excitability. The stretch reflexes, both phasic and static, pass from a state of total absence during spinal shock to hyperactivity in the chronic spinal state. However, the stretch reflexes are not the only reflex arcs to show heightened excitability, and in many cases practically any cutaneous or other stimulus below the level of the lesion will lead to a massive withdrawal reflex, the repeated performance of which may lead to the state of paraplegia in flexion. The increased reflex excitability is due to the inherent activity of spinal centres, though this activity may be enhanced by discharges from adhesions and distortions of the distal cord at the site of the transection.

Incomplete transection of the cord may occur suddenly or slowly. In the latter case the limbs below the lesion become spastic and initially are often extended. This condition is known as paraplegia in extension, and its mechanism is not understood. It usually proceeds to paraplegia in flexion, the terminal stage mentioned above.

PYRAMIDAL LESIONS

Pure lesions of the pyramidal pathway are rare. In some animals excision of the motor area (area 4) alone is reported to give a flaccid paralysis of the affected limbs. The one unequivocal sign of a pyramidal tract lesion is an extensor plantar response (p. 379).

Clinical hemiplegia

The commonest form of 'pyramidal damage' is that due to a vascular accident in the internal capsule. Such a lesion affects not only the descending corticospinal fibres, but also fibres passing down to the reticular formation (extrapyramidal fibres) from higher centres. Many of the resultant signs often attributed to upper motor neurone damage are in fact due to concurrent damage to the descending extrapyramidal fibres which leads to a resultant imbalance of excitatory and inhibitory descending extrapyramidal impulses from the reticular formation.

Immediately following a capsular haemorrhage consciousness is usually lost. During this state the affected limbs may be hypotonic and the tendon reflexes lost. If consciousness is recovered, a period of up to several weeks may ensue during which time the hemiplegic side exhibits hyperreflexia with hypotonus. During this time the spindles are excessively biased, but the interneurones of the static stretch reflexes must be inhibited. Spasticity is slowly added to the hyperreflexia, and the picture of chronic hemiplegia emerges. The plantar response on the hemiplegic side is extensor throughout. Willed movements of the limbs of the affected side are impaired to a greater extent distally than proximally, and what remnants of willed movements remain may be further impaired at the later stages by the presence of spasticity. From what has been stated earlier it will be appreciated that the alterations of tendon jerks and tone are due to dysfunction of the extrapyramidal system, while the defect of willed movement and the extensor plantar response are due to disruption of the 'pyramidal tract'.

EXTRAPYRAMIDAL LESIONS
Experimental lesions of the extrapyramidal system (as defined on p. 365), while producing a wide variety of abnormalities, have not yet been shown to mimic clinical syndromes. As has been indicated, isolated lesions within a complex control system like the extrapyramidal system are not likely to yield complete explanations of the system's normal functioning, and similarly it is not surprising that they throw little light on the mechanisms of clinical disorders. They will not be further discussed.

Parkinsonism
This syndrome, which may be the end result of a variety of pathological causes, is characterized by rigidity, with or without tremor, and a poverty of willed movements.

The tendon jerks remain normal, and the plantar responses are flexor. There may be a variety of anatomical lesions, but almost always the basal ganglia are involved. It appears that these damaged structures give rise to an abnormal afferent inflow into the reticular formation which leads to an imbalance in the descending extrapyramidal spinal pathways. This in turn leads to an increase in the sensitivity of the static stretch reflexes, and also sometimes to tremor. The rigidity is itself the cause of the poverty of willed movements which may be very marked. Surgical destruction of the pallidofugal fibres may result in a great reduction of the rigidity and in the return of a surprising degree of willed control, a return which emphasizes the integrity of the pyramidal pathways in Parkinsonism.

Involuntary movements

Various types of involuntary movement may be produced by disease of the basal ganglia. Athetosis and hemiballismus are two examples. The latter, like Parkinsonism, may be greatly improved by destruction of the pallidofugal fibres, but the mechanism of the involuntary movements is not known. For example, are some or all of these involuntary movements produced via a route similar to the majority of normal postural reflexes, namely the gamma motor system, or by direct descending activation of the large anterior horn cells? What part does the cortex play in maintaining such movements? Great care must be exercised in interpreting the results of various surgical remedies. For example, the cessation of an involuntary movement following the extirpation of some cortical tissue does not necessarily mean that the abnormal activity passed that way, still less that it originated there. It may simply indicate that the region of tissue excised formerly provided an excitatory inflow into the reticular formation, the removal of which inflow lowered the excitability to a level at which the discharge ceased. Furthermore, the excitatory inflow itself may be the result of damage elsewhere.

Notwithstanding the difficulties of interpretation, certain generalizations may be made. Pathological disorders of the basal ganglia lead dominantly to changes in muscle tone and to the production of involuntary movements. The former is characteristic in form and distribution and the total sum of the various striatal and pallidal syndromes suggests that the basal ganglia are normally concerned with the distribution of tone, and with postural adjustments not directly connected with willed movement. This appears so since volitional activity is unimpaired except in so far as it is impeded by rigidity or involuntary movements. It further appears that the functional outflow to the reticular formation from the basal ganglia is concentrated into the fasciculus lenticularis and ansa lenticularis. By destroying these pathways in the vicinity of the lateral nucleus of the thalamus any abnormal activity of the basal ganglia (including the subthalamic nucleus and substantia nigra) may apparently be prevented from reaching the final integrating area of the extrapyramidal system. Whether the abnormal activity represents a release of uncompensated discharge or the equivalent of an injury discharge remains undecided. In either case, such a destructive lesion reduces many functional disturbances due to disease of the basal ganglia, and in the most successful cases returns the patient to normality. Since in such circumstances the main efferent pathway from the basal nuclei is severed it remains problematical what information and instructions are carried by this tract in the normal individual.

DISORDERS OF THE CEREBELLUM

It has been stated above that diseases of the basal ganglia leave willed movements unimpaired except in so far as they may be burdened by hypertonus or involuntary movement. Acute cerebellar dysfunction on the other hand is most apparent during willed movement. Such movement becomes ill-controlled or ataxic. Thus the inability to produce smooth rapid alternating movements of pronation and supination, the intention tremor, scanning speech and nystagmus are all examples of cerebellar ataxia. It is tempting to imagine that the connections between the cerebral cortex, the midbrain and the cerebellum indicate that the primary normal function of this organ is to harmonize the simultaneous activity of the motor cortex and reticular formation during the execution of a willed movement. One is, however, faced with the problem of how well an individual may manage after the surgical removal of a cerebellar hemisphere. Residual disability may be very small, and the reason for this—when compared with the full-blown picture of an acute cerebellar lesion—is obscure.

Disorders of equilibrium may possibly be due to local disease of the middle lobe of the cerebellum but are more commonly due to abnormal functioning of the vestibular nucleus and the pathways connecting it to this part of the cerebellum.

DISORDERED CONTROL OF WILLED MOVEMENT

Since at the present time the centrencephalic system is only conceptual, no lesions of it can be studied. However, some akinetic states may be due to an inability to initiate willed movements rather than to an inability to execute them after they have been initiated. Here again the evidence necessary for a decision is not available. Akinetic states are often associated with slow delta waves in the EEG such as occur in sleep, suggesting that the ascending reticular activating system is inoperative, causing a functional disconnection of the initiating region and the motor cortex. Certainly the centrencephalic system, if it exists, must anatomically overlap the brain stem activating system.

Rarely, altered activity of willed movement may occur in lesions of the frontal lobe. This defect is known as tonic innervation or perseveration, and is seen in a slow relaxation following a willed contraction. This is to be distinguished from myotonia, which is discussed in Chapter 9.

JACKSONIAN EPILEPSY

Excessive discharge, initially from a circumscribed region of the motor cortex, may give rise to a focal or Jacksonian fit. Willed control of the part is lost during the convulsive movements, as it is also lost during electrical stimulation of the cortex. Following the attack there may be some temporary weakness of the affected muscles. Whether the movements are produced by direct activation of the α motoneurones is not known.

Principles of observations and tests

MUSCLE TONE AND REFLEXES

Although the phasic and static reactions of the stretch reflex share the final common path, they are largely under separate supraspinal control. Translating to the approximate clinical equivalents, namely tendon jerk and muscle tone, this implies that the findings of these two examinations should be treated as independent variables. For example, while it is usual to find hyperreflexia associated with hypertonus, this is by no means invariably the case, and hyperreflexia may coexist with hypotonus.

The tendon jerk

In examining the tendon jerk one is both sensing the bias of the muscle spindles which has been imposed by the gamma motor system and also testing the integrity of the segmental monosynaptic reflex arc.

The gamma motor system is normally controlled by descending extrapyramidal pathways, but in the same way that the final common path determines the ultimate activity in the extrafusal muscle fibre, it is the gamma motoneurone which finally determines the shortening of the intrafusal muscle fibre. During deep sleep the tonic discharge of the gamma motoneurones ceases and tendon jerks are lost. A similar loss of tendon jerks may be produced in the waking state by a selective block of the gamma motor fibres with procaine.

The bias of the muscle spindle may be increased by enhanced activity of the small anterior horn cells. This occurs normally during the procedure of reinforcing the tendon jerks, the increased reflex response being due to a larger afferent discharge. A similarly increased biasing of the spindles appears to occur in hemiplegia and has been demonstrated following cerebrovascular accidents at a time when the limbs are hypotonic. The hyperreflexia under such conditions is due to the increased sensitivity of the primary spindle ending to transient stretch, which in turn is due to increased discharge from the small motoneurones. This increased discharge is presumably due to an altered pattern of descending extrapyramidal impulses. The excitability of the large α-motoneurones remains the same as on the normal side. Under such conditions the patient is 'permanently reinforced' on the affected side and can further increase tendon jerks either very little or not at all by forceful willed movement of the normal side.

Although it may be that enhanced or diminished tendon reflexes can be due to altered excitability of the large anterior horn cells, such changes in excitability have not so far been shown. It seems rather that the final common path maintains fixed excitability while the ability to modify responsiveness is bestowed on interneurones. Since the tendon jerk is monosynaptic such modifications at the interneurones play no part in determining this reflex response.

The changes discussed above concern the size of the reflex contraction, which should be considered apart from the speed of the contractile process. For example, in long-standing hypothyroidism the muscle response shows a characteristic slow relaxation (p. 348), while in hyperthyroidism the mechanical response may be very rapid. Similarly, the presence of irradiation, i.e. contraction of muscles not actually stretched, should be ignored while examining the tendon jerk.

Changes in the tendon jerks which are due to lesions of the final common path and striated muscle will not be further discussed, as they have already been considered in Chapter 9.

Muscle tone

The static stretch reflex is the most important cause of resistance to passive movement offered by the muscles during the clinical estimation of tone, but at least two other factors must be borne in mind. First there are the physical characteristics of the muscle fibres themselves. Muscle fibres have inherent elasticity and offer a certain degree of resistance to stretch. There is now overwhelming evidence that human muscle completely at rest is electrically silent: there is no evidence of an asynchronous motor unit activity. There is also reason to believe that a co-operative subject can inhibit the static response of the stretch reflex at least over part of a muscle's passive range. This being so it may be that the physical characteristics of the muscle play an appreciable part in the resistance offered to passive movement in the normal subject, and also that the alteration so noticeable in a flaccid limb is largely due to alterations in these purely passive (non-reflex) characteristics. Secondly, it must be remembered that some or all of the motor unit activity which may be present during the examination of tone in a hypertonic limb may be due to direct descending activation of the α-motoneurones from higher centres, and not at all due to sensory discharge from the muscle spindles.

Changes in the static reaction may result from either altered excitability at interneurones, such that more or less impulses are passed on to the α-motoneurones for a given afferent inflow, or from an altered discharge of impulses from the muscle spindle in response to transient and maintained stretch. At the present time there is no evidence on which to decide the relative importance of these two mechanisms in various clinical situations. However, in both cases the deviations from normal must represent an alteration in the descending pattern of extrapyramidal impulses to either (or both) the small anterior horn cells or the interneurones. That the abnormal pattern of descending impulses is capable of a variety of forms is well appreciated clinically. Thus as has been pointed out above, the hypertonus of spasticity in its florid state is easily distinguished from rigidity, but one is forced to admit that at the spinal level the exact mechanisms of hypertonus and hypotonus in various clinical conditions is not known.

Clonus

Sustained clonus is frequently associated with the hypertonus of spasticity. It is probably due to increased excitability of the static stretch reflex. A poorly sustained clonus may be observed in individuals having very rapid relaxation of the mechanical response, e.g. hyperthyroidism.

The plantar response

Normally a light stroke applied to the skin of the outer border of the sole of the foot produces plantar flexion of the toes accompanied by dorsiflexion of the ankle. This is known as the flexor plantar response. The extensor plantar response consists of a dorsiflexion of the large toe accompanied by a fanning or spreading of the outer toes.

The presence of an extensor plantar response (Babinski's sign) is an unequivocal sign of damage to the pyramidal tract, except in the first year of life, during deep sleep or coma or immediately following an

13*

epileptic fit. The reason for this abnormal response, which appears to be part of a general flexion reflex, is not known. It has been suggested that some spinocortical fibres run with the pyramidal tracts and that it is damage to these afferents which leads to the appearance of the abnormal response.

The loss of the abdominal reflexes which often accompanies an extensor plantar response has not been satisfactorily explained.

Co-ordination

Tests of co-ordination of the motor system aim at demonstrating any failure to harmonize the activities of the pyramidal and extrapyramidal systems during a willed movement. Such a test is the finger-to-nose test, in which the patient is requested to touch alternately his nose and the examiner's finger. The execution of the movement is judged against the usual performance of a normal individual. A failure on the part of a patient to achieve a satisfactory result—in the presence of a normal sensory system and adequate muscle power—suggests a lack of co-ordination, possibly due to a cerebellar defect. It must be stressed that tests of co-ordination in this sense assume normal proprioception. If the patient is unable to appreciate the position of his limbs in space, then movements may become ataxic due to this sensory loss. The patient may compensate for such a sensory loss by watching his performance, but a request to close the eyes will usually reveal a proprioceptive deficiency.

Power

Motor power as tested clinically depends upon the number of motor units active in the muscle being examined and the frequency at which the units are working (see Chapter 9).

Practical assessment

Clinical observations

Extrapyramidal system: extent and distribution of stretch reflexes; abnormal posture; involuntary movements; tremor; muscle tone; spasticity and clonus.

Pyramidal system: strength of volitional contraction in various muscle groups (provided that lower motor neurone is intact); range of movements; distribution of weakness (e.g. pyramidal lesion between internal capsule and C5 produces hemiplegia, but cortical pyramidal lesion may produce monoplegia because cortical representations of arm and leg widely spaced); Jacksonian fits; reduction of willed movement in Parkinsonism. True pyramidal damage is always associated with abnormal plantar response and loss of abdominal reflexes.

Cerebellar function: inco-ordination of willed movement in absence of sensory loss; nystagmus; intention tremor uninfluenced by visual information; hypotonia.

Routine methods
Anatomical site of lesions: Lumbar puncture and Queckenstedt's test; myelography; angiography; ventriculography; EEG; ultrasound; brain scan.

Pathological process: CSF microscopy and chemistry.

Identification of functional disorders: EEG applied to diagnosis of epilepsy; electromyography.

References

HOLMES G. (1952) *Introduction to clinical neurology.* (2nd ed.) London: Livingstone.
FIELD J. (ed.) (1959, 1960). Neurophysiology, *Handbook of Physiology*, Section 1. Washington: Amer., Physiol. Soc. (particularly Vol. 2).
Physiology of voluntary muscle. *Brit. Med. Bull.* (1956), **12**, No. 3.
DENNY-BROWN D. *The basal ganglia and their relation to disorders of movement* ii *Lancet* (1960) 1099–1105; 1155–1162.
PENFIELD W. (1958) *The excitable cortex in conscious man.* Liverpool: Univ. Press.
MATTHEWS P.B.C. (1964), Muscles Spindles and Their Motor Control. *Physiol. Rev.* **44**, 219–288.
RAGNAR GRANIT (ed.) (1966). Muscular afferents and motor control; proceedings, *1st Nobel Sömposium*, 1965. John Wiley and Sons, London.

The Gut

MOTILITY

Normal function

PROPERTIES OF INTESTINAL SMOOTH MUSCLE

Between the mid-oesophagus and the external anal sphincter the musculature of the alimentary canal is composed of smooth muscle. This
differs from striated muscle in both its electrical and mechanical
properties. For example, it has innate tone whereas skeletal muscle can
relax completely (p. 341). This 'tonus' permits sustained and sometimes
powerful contraction over long periods of time with a very small
expenditure of energy. It also accounts for the fact that the ante-mortem
length of the alimentary tract (250 cm) is considerably less than its
length post-mortem (650 cm). Furthermore, smooth muscle is capable
of complex variations in tone even after denervation. For example,
quick stretching may evoke depolarization of the surface membrane
potential and result in muscular contraction. On the other hand the
muscle may respond to more gradual stretching by a decrease in tension
and an increase in length. This response explains the facility with which
the stomach and colon can vary their volume within wide limits, and
thereby accommodate large amounts of material with no increase in
intraluminal pressure.

The response of smooth muscle to neuro-humoral transmitters and
to pharmacological agents varies considerably between species and in
different parts of the alimentary tract. In man, the dominant response to
adrenergic drugs is relaxation. Oesophageal muscle, however, may
respond by either contraction or relaxation, and only in the circular
muscle at the lower end is relaxation the predominant response. Muscle
from the internal anal sphincter is also atypical in that it contracts in
response to noradrenaline. Differences in smooth muscle depending
upon its anatomical source are also demonstrated by the response to

5-hydroxytryptamine (5HT, serotonin), of which large amounts are found in the gut. Both *in vivo* and *in vitro* small intestinal and internal anal sphincter smooth muscle is stimulated but large intestinal smooth muscle is inhibited.

Peristalsis is produced by intestinal distension, and consists of contraction of circular muscle behind a mass of intestinal contents, preceded by a zone of muscular relaxation. Although it is not abolished by extrinsic denervation it can be prevented by local anaesthesia, asphyxia, or removal of the mucous membrane. Both sensory and motor components of an intrinsic reflex are therefore in existence within the bowel wall, and although peristalsis can be modified by the extrinsic autonomic nerves, only the intrinsic nervous plexus is essential for the local co-ordination of smooth muscle activity. In fact total extrinsic sympathetic denervation has no demonstrable effect on bowel motility. The apparent unimportance of the sympathetic system is also indicated by the fact that the inhibition of tone which follows sympathetic stimulation in animals is delayed, and probably due to the adrenergic mediators liberated either from adjacent nerve endings on blood vessels or the adrenal medulla, rather than to a direct action of the sympathetic system on muscle. The parasympathetic system, on the other hand, appears to be of considerable importance. Although, in man, vagotomy has no demonstrable effect on small intestinal motility, it results in marked delay in gastric emptying. Bilateral high vagal section in animals is followed by almost total oesophageal paralysis, but the low vagal section performed at the diaphragm in man does not permanently affect oesophageal peristalsis.

SWALLOWING

The initiation of swallowing is voluntary, the muscles concerned being the striated muscles of both the jaw and pharynx whose motor nuclei are in the medulla and upper cervical cord. Their activity is co-ordinated in the medulla. Swallowing is initiated by the tongue, which compresses the bolus against the hard palate. The jaw closes, and the mouth is separated from the nasal cavity by elevation of the soft palate and contraction of the palato-pharyngeal muscles. As the base of the tongue propels the bolus backwards into the pharynx the larynx is elevated and displaced forwards under the posterior part of the tongue.

The entrance to the oesophagus is normally tightly closed by tonic contraction of the crico-pharyngeus muscle, but as the co-ordinated wave in the pharynx reaches this sphincter, it relaxes. A 'primary' wave of peristalsis then smoothly conveys material to the lower end of the oesophagus, any reflux into the pharynx being prevented by the crico-pharyngeal sphincter, which for a few seconds is closed very tightly. Material introduced directly into the oesophagus by a tube initiates a similar 'secondary' peristaltic wave, which under physiological conditions is concerned in the complete clearing of food from the oesophagus. The pharyngeal phase of swallowing is very rapid, being completed within one second, whereas the oesophageal phase occupies about ten seconds.

THE COMPETENCE OF THE CARDIA
At rest, supine, the intra-abdominal (and intra-gastric) pressure is 15 cm higher than the intra-thoracic (and oesophageal) pressure, and this pressure difference can be considerably accentuated by straining and by positional changes. In spite of this, reflux of stomach contents into the oesophagus does not occur when the stomach lies in its normal position below the diaphragm. The cardia therefore functions like a valve, and two factors probably work together to maintain its 'competence'.

1. *The cardiac sphincter.* Under resting conditions the lower 2–5 cm of the oesophagus, part of which is above and part below the diaphragm, is the site of a high pressure zone, and constitutes the physiological gastro-oesophageal sphincter. It relaxes at an early stage of oesophageal peristalsis to allow food to pass, but otherwise remains contracted. The pressure it exerts is only about 10 cm of water, so that unaided this sphincter is not an effective barrier to reflux.

2. *The intra-abdominal oesophagus.* The lower 2 cm of the oesophagus lies below the diaphragm. Any rise in intra-abdominal pressure will compress this segment as much as it raises intragastric pressure so that there is no net pressure tending to cause regurgitation.

Other factors which have been invoked as aids to the cardiac sphincter include a pinching action of the diaphragm, and the normal acute angle of entry of the oesophagus into the stomach. Any 'pinchcock' action of the diaphragm is almost certainly unimportant; the delay in flow of barium into the stomach which occurs on inspiration is probably due to the increase in intra-abdominal pressure. Clinical and experimental evidence on the importance of the oesophago-gastric angle is conflicting.

GASTRIC MOTILITY AND REGULATION OF GASTRIC EMPTYING

The stomach is never completely at rest, for even in the fasting state weak waves of peristalsis begin at a pacemaker near the cardia and sweep towards the pylorus. At variable intervals much stronger contractions occur, but contrary to earlier opinions there is little evidence that these bear any relationship to the sensation of hunger.

Swallowing is accompanied by a relaxation of the stomach muscles, and for some time after a meal gastric motility is inhibited: waves of peristalsis then reappear at their usual frequency of 3-4 per minute, and thereafter steadily increase in amplitude. They do not completely occlude the lumen, but each one sweeps a small amount of antral contents into the duodenum. The pylorus, in contrast to the upper and lower oesophageal sphincters, is not normally in a state of contraction. It does however remain contracted for a short period at the end of each peristaltic wave, and as duodenal contractions are not synchronized with those of the stomach this reduces reflux back into the stomach.

Gastric emptying is normally regulated in such a way that the secretory and absorptive capacity of the small gut is not overloaded, and the intrinsic capacity of the duodenum to regulate the tonicity and pH of its contents not overwhelmed. This regulation is mediated to a considerable extent by receptors in the duodenal wall. On stimulation these inhibit gastric motility either by initiating nervous reflexes, or by releasing the hormone enterogastrone.

Accurate information on the rate at which a normal meal leaves the stomach is difficult to obtain, but there is no doubt from X-ray studies that liquids leave the stomach more quickly than solids. Liquid entering a stomach already containing food can be seen to pass around the solid material and enter the duodenum. The emptying of liquid meals has been thoroughly studied, and follows a regular pattern, the volume remaining in the stomach falling in a smooth almost exponential curve when plotted against time. The receptors in the duodenal wall are sensitive to the osmotic pressure of fluid leaving the stomach, but they are not equally sensitive to all ions. Thus, as the concentration of potassium chloride or glucose in an instilled test meal is raised from zero, the rate at which it leaves the stomach becomes progressively slower. On the other hand, as the concentration of sodium bicarbonate, sodium chloride, or urea in a test meal is raised, the rate of emptying of the meal increases at first, but above about 200 m-osmole/l. becomes progressively slower. Any grossly hypertonic fluid therefore delays gastric emptying considerably, and the fluids which leave the stomach most rapidly are slightly hypotonic solutions of sodium chloride, sodium bicarbonate, or urea. The most potent inhibitor of gastric emptying, however, is the presence of fat in the duodenum.

INTESTINAL MOTILITY AND DEFAECATION

Small intestine. The most common movements are non-propulsive, segmenting contractions, whose main function is the mixing of intestinal contents. Peristaltic waves propel food along the lumen, but little is known about the factors which control their strength and frequency. A pacemaker near the bile duct analogous to that of cardiac muscle has been suggested, but it seems likely that local pacemakers exist throughout the length of the gut which influence the segment of bowel distal to them. The rate of passage through the duodenum is usually rapid, and if hypertonic fluids are introduced directly into the duodenum vigorous peristalsis rapidly spreads the solution over a long length of intestine and facilitates its dilution. On the other hand, rate of transit in the ileum may be very slow, and food remnants reaching this region may be static for some time.

Small intestinal activity increases after eating, and ileal activity may be increased by both the psychic stimulation of food preparation, or by introducing food directly into the duodenum. It may be accompanied by relaxation of the ileocaecal valve and discharge of ileal contents into the caecum. This reflex is abolished by atropine, but occurs normally after vagotomy. Its anatomical basis is not known.

Large intestine. As in the small intestine, most contractions are non-propulsive, and these segmenting contractions are responsible for some of the haustrations of the colon (others are mucosal folds). A general increase in tonus tends to follow food, but the pathway of this 'gastro-colic reflex' is not known. It may occur merely at the sight of food, and occurs normally in patients with transection of the spinal cord. True peristalsis occurs infrequently. When these 'mass movements' of colonic contents do occur, they involve the transverse and left colon. Haustrations disappear, and there is rapid synchronous contraction of a considerable length of bowel.

Defaecation

Continence is maintained by two sphincters. The internal sphincter reflects the activity of the circular muscle of the intestine, of which it is a part. Normally it is in tonic contraction, and accounts for most of the pressure which can be recorded from the anal canal. The external sphincter also shows continuous resting activity, in contrast to striated muscle elsewhere in the body (p. 341). Both the external sphincter and the pubo-rectalis muscles electromyographically show heightened activity with effort, coughing, and voluntary sphincteric contraction, and are inhibited on defaecation and micturition.

Distension of the rectum produces the conscious call to stool, and a moment later inhibition of the external sphincter and pubo-rectalis muscles occurs. The glottis is closed, and a rise in intra-abdominal pressure produced by contraction of the diaphragm and muscles of the abdominal wall helps the colon to expel its contents. The extent of bowel cleared at defaecation varies widely. It may be the rectum alone, or the whole of the left colon up to the splenic flexure.

Disordered function

DYSPHAGIA (difficulty in swallowing)
This symptom may result from organic obstruction or may be psychogenic, but in an appreciable proportion of patients it is due to neurological or muscular dysfunction.

Obstructive dysphagia is usually caused by neoplasms of the pharynx or oesophagus, or by stricture formation after inflammatory lesions. Iron deficiency causes atrophic and inflammatory changes in the mucosa lining the upper part of the oesophagus (Plummer–Vinson syndrome), and this may be followed by fibrosis and obstructive dysphagia. The precise sequence of events is not known.

Disordered function of striated muscle
Dysphagia due to lesions of the medulla oblongata. The twelfth cranial nerve nucleus supplying the tongue, the nucleus ambiguus supplying the pharyngeal muscles, and the dorsal vagal nucleus supplying the cricopharyngeal sphincter and oesophagus lie in the medulla, and lesions in this region frequently cause dysphagia. For example, poliomyelitis, motor neurone disease, and posterior inferior cerebellar artery thrombosis are common causes of this type of dysphagia. In each this follows a similar pattern.

Paralysis of the palatal muscles prevents the closing off of the nasopharynx during swallowing and allows regurgitation through the nose. These patients learn to swallow only in the erect position when gravity aids the passage of the bolus, which they cautiously allow to flow off the back of the tongue instead of forcing it rapidly into the pharyngeal cavity, and so causing regurgitation through the nose. Paralysis of the pharyngeal constrictors converts the pharynx into a flaccid-walled cavity through which the bolus flows slowly under the influence of gravity alone. After swallowing, residua are left in the valleculae and pyriform sinuses.

A remarkable feature of the distribution of paralysis in medullary lesions is the sparing of the crico-pharyngeal sphincter which continues to function normally. This may be explained by its innervation from the dorsal nucleus of the vagus which is less commonly affected by poliomyelitis and motor neurone disease than is the nucleus ambiguus.

Dysphagia due to cranial nerve damage. Damage to cranial nerves may produce difficulty in swallowing by interference with the afferent side of the reflex (IXth nerve) or by paralysis of the tongue (XIIth nerve) or palatal and pharyngeal muscles (Xth and XIth nerves).

Myopathic dysphagia. Weakness of all the muscles of deglutition may occur in myasthenia gravis, and the resulting dysphagia differs from that seen in bulbar disorders in that the tongue and crico-pharyngeus are always involved in myasthenia. Paralysis of the tongue may lead to difficulty in initiating swallowing, the patient tilting his head backwards to allow the bolus to run off the back of the tongue.

A similar type of dysphagia occasionally occurs in other muscle disorders notably dystrophia myotonica.

Disordered function of smooth muscle
Achalasia. In this condition peristalsis occurs normally in the upper oesophagus, but when it reaches the smooth muscle of the lower oesophagus it stops and is replaced by irregular, unco-ordinated, non-propulsive contractions. These are called 'tertiary' contractions, to distinguish them from the normal primary and secondary peristaltic waves. The intrinsic sphincter at the lower end of the oesophagus is not unduly contracted, as is implied by the synonym 'cardiospasm', but it does fail to relax normally on swallowing. Food accumulates in the oesophagus, and only enters the stomach when the gravitational pressure of the column exceeds the tone of the sphincter. Symptoms include dysphagia, substernal pain, and regurgitation of food into the mouth and trachea.

The physiological disturbance in achalasia is complex. The failure of peristalsis is probably due to the loss of ganglion cells in Auerbach's plexus, and destruction of this plexus in South American trypanosomiasis (Chagas' disease) produces a similar condition. In addition, cholinesterase is diminished in the body of the oesophagus, and the injection of a cholinergic drug such as methacholine (Mecholyl) results therefore in violent and painful contraction. Failure of the sphincter to relax appears to be due to loss of the adrenergic pathway which normally mediates its relaxation (p. 382). Octyl nitrite relaxes the spincter by its general action on smooth muscle, and although its effects are transient it may be useful if taken before meals.

Diffuse spasm. In this condition normal peristalsis is defective only in the lower oesophagus, and the intrinsic sphincter relaxes normally. 'Tertiary', non-propulsive contractions are recognizable radiologically by the narrow crenated barium outline, and in some cases as a tortuous and elongated 'corkscrew' oesophagus. It may be associated with oesophageal pain which in its localization and character can resemble angina pectoris. Assessment is complicated by the fact that this disturbance of motility is often seen in elderly patients who are symptom free, and may also occur in reflux oesophagitis.

Systemic sclerosis. This condition can affect smooth muscle anywhere in the gut, and results in weakened peristalsis. Oesophageal involvement is particularly common. The lower oesophageal sphincter becomes defective, and reflux oesophagitis and stricture may follow.

INCOMPETENCE OF THE CARDIA
This is one of the commonest disorders in the gastro-intestinal tract. It is usually associated with a hiatus hernia, in which condition reflux occurs as a result of the absence of the intra-abdominal oesophagus. Any rise in intra-abdominal pressure results in acid reflux as the unaided intrinsic sphincter is incompetent (p. 384). Stooping, bending and the recumbent posture aggravate the symptoms. Obesity commonly precipitates a hernia, and the heartburn of pregnancy may be at least partly due to a temporary hiatus hernia and consequent oesophagitis. Division of the oesophageal sphincter as in Heller's operation for achalasia is not usually followed by reflux if the anatomical arrangement is not otherwise disturbed, i.e. if a segment of oesophagus remains in the abdomen, and the oesophago-gastric angle is preserved.

DISTURBANCES OF GASTRIC MOTILITY
Delay in gastric emptying
Obstruction to outflow by pyloric carcinoma or duodenal scarring is much the commonest cause of delay in gastric emptying. Gastric atony almost always follows the operation of vagotomy, and this procedure

has therefore to be combined with a procedure such as pyloroplasty or gastro-jejunostomy to facilitate emptying. Hypertonic glucose solutions may leave the stomach slowly (p. 385) and variable gastric emptying is one factor responsible for the poor reproducibility of glucose tolerance tests.

Rapid gastric emptying

This can occur after any of the operations performed for peptic ulcer although partial gastrectomy with gastro-jejunal anastomosis ('Polya' gastrectomy) is the worst offender. The term 'early dumping' is applied to symptoms of flushing, sweating, and weakness which immediately follow a meal. Sudden distension of the small bowel is responsible for some of these symptoms. A reduction in plasma volume caused by loss of fluid into the lumen of the gut to reduce the tonicity of the contents is another factor. The vasomotor symptoms may be due to the release of a bradykinin-like polypeptide into the circulation. 'Late dumping' is due to hypoglycaemia 1–3 hr after a meal, and results from a failure of the liver to resume glucose production sufficiently quickly after the inhibition of hepatic glucose output which follows oral glucose. Normally gastric emptying is regulated in such a way that entry of glucose into the portal circulation decreases gradually at the end of a meal and the liver is able to maintain normoglycaemia by resuming glycogenolysis and gluconeogenesis.

Vomiting

This can be induced by a wide variety of stimuli, including metabolic disturbances, middle ear disorders, and raised intra-cranial pressure, in addition to disease of the gastro-intestinal tract. Nausea is associated with profound relaxation of the stomach musculature, including the gastro-oesophageal sphincter, and by increased and reversed peristalsis in the duodenum. Ejection of gastric contents is then achieved by strong contractions of the abdominal wall and diaphragm, with a closed glottis. Incompetence of the cardia is probably achieved by induction of a temporary hiatus hernia. The pressure gradient across the cardiac end of the stomach during vomiting is considerable and may cause longtitudinal muscle tears at the lower end of the oesophagus, which can result in profuse bleeding ('Mallory-Weiss' syndrome), and, rarely, in spontaneous rupture of the oesophagus.

DISTURBANCES OF INTESTINAL MOTILITY

Symptoms of disordered intestinal movement, particularly of the colon, are very common, but are poorly understood.

Constipation

The normal call to stool occurs when the rectum is distended to a certain critical volume, which is normally 100–150 ml. This call can be resisted by voluntary contraction of the external sphincter, and further distension may then be necessary before evacuation can begin. Ultimately the full rectum may no longer lead to sphincteric relaxation, and resort is had to purgatives to induce evacuation. Eventually these also fail to act, and the result is dyschezia, or rectal constipation. Colic constipation occurs if food passes slowly through the colon, without evidence of retention in the rectum, and is a normal reaction to illnesses associated with fever, vomiting and dehydration. In addition, neuromuscular dysfunction causing constipation occurs in the following conditions.

Irritable colon syndrome. This condition occurs as a result of abnormal responses of colonic muscle to food, stress and drugs. Patients with this disorder can be separated into two main groups. Those with spastic colon have pain, often after meals, as their main symptom, and a tendency to constipation. Those with functional diarrhoea have this as their main complaint, pain being infrequent. Intraluminal pressure records show that compared with normal subjects patients with spastic colon have high levels of activity in the distal colon, whereas patients with functional diarrhoea have low levels of activity. Emotion, food, and prostigmine enhance colonic motility to an abnormal degree in both groups of patients.

Diverticulosis. There is increasing evidence that this condition is partly a muscular disturbance. Pronounced muscular thickening is usual, and although intraluminal pressure patterns are normal under resting conditions abnormally high pressures are recorded in the sigmoid colon after meals, or after injection of morphine or prostigmine.

Neurological lesions. Destruction of the lumbo-sacral cord results in constipation. Decreased cholinergic activity is presumably responsible, but the physiological disturbance is complex.

Hirschsprung's disease

In this congenital abnormality the intramural nerve plexus is absent in the last few inches of the rectum, and occasionally also in the lower sigmoid colon. Bowel proximal to the contracted aganglionic segment is dilated and hypertrophied. This condition must be distinguished from idiopathic and also from acquired megacolon, in which the dilated segments extend right down to the anal sphincter. True Hirschsprung's disease is relieved by resection of the aganglionic segment.

Drugs

Ganglion blocking drugs, and also anticholinergic agents such as atropine, decrease motility of the stomach, small intestine, and large bowel, and can cause constipation. Morphine and codeine increase the tone of smooth muscle, and therefore cause constipation by an entirely different mechanism. Pethidine does not have this effect.

Diarrhoea

This means the passage of excessive amounts of soft or fluid stools. Apart from a group of disorders characterized by steatorrhoea (p. 422) this symptom must be due to a failure of the ileum and colon to absorb a normal quantity of water, and impies either rapid intestinal transit or impaired water and electrolyte absorption. This may be due to the following causes.

An osmotic purge. Any non-absorbable solute retains water in the bowel lumen. The resultant increased bulk of intestinal contents promotes peristalsis and induces diarrhoea. Examples are magnesium sulphate when used as a purgative, and lactose in the condition of intestinal lactase deficiency (p. 425).

Failure of electrolyte absorption. In cholera, the profuse watery diarrhoea is due to failure of normal sodium and water absorption. This also is a feature of other inflammatory diseases of the bowel, including gastro-enteritis, Crohn's disease, and ulcerative colitis, although increased bowel irritability also contributes to the diarrhoea of these patients.

Intestinal resection. Rapid gastric emptying after partial gastrectomy, and any intestinal resection, by-pass, or fistula may cause diarrhoea. Vagotomy, with any of the gastric drainage operations with which it is always combined, usually increases stool frequency. The cause is unknown.

Increase in intestinal peristalsis

This occurs in the irritable colon syndrome (p. 391), as a result of anxiety, and in thyrotoxicosis. In metastasizing argentaffinoma peristalsis is stimulated by 5-hydroxytryptamine secreted by secondary deposits of tumour in the liver. Non-β-cell pancreatic islet tumours can produce diarrhoea, usually as a result of gross gastric hypersecretion (p. 405), but also, rarely, by another mechanism, perhaps the secretion of an as yet unidentified hormone.

Principles of tests and measurements

OVERALL GUT TRANSIT

The time taken for an orally administered non-absorbable marker such as carmine to appear in the stools is a crude test. A better method is to follow the appearance in the stool of a non-absorbable radioactive marker, e.g. chromium compounds. High residue diets cause more rapid transit than low residue diets, and all studies agree that there is repeated mixing of colonic contents so that when a stool is passed it represents a blend of the residues of what has been eaten over several days.

GASTRIC EMPTYING

The serial test meal has been used extensively to investigate the factors controlling the emptying by the stomach of a liquid meal. The same meal, containing phenol red, is administered on successive days to the same individual, and the volume remaining in the stomach is determined by aspirating after a different time interval each day. The amount of dye recovered is an indication of the amount of the administered meal remaining in the stomach, and dilution of the dye an indication of gastric secretion.

Emptying of a non-liquid meal has been studied by a variety of radio-logical techniques, all of which involve mixing a contrast medium with the food. The barium sulphate suspension usually used is not ideal, because of its high specific gravity. A more physiological method is to scan the abdomen with counting equipment at varying intervals after the ingestion of a meal containing a γ-emitting radio-isotope.

MOTILITY MEASUREMENTS

Intraluminal pressure measurements

Our present knowledge of oesophageal peristalsis and the lower oeso-phageal sphincter has been largely obtained by the use of narrow open-ended polyethylene tubes connected to manometers. Gradual with-drawal of a tube from stomach to oesophagus enables the position of the diaphragm (reversal of respiratory pressure swings) and the intrinsic sphincter (a zone of increased pressure) to be detected. Simultaneous use of several tubes with their tips at different levels makes possible the detection of orderly peristaltic waves, and of abnormal 'tertiary' contractions (Fig. 40).

Intraluminal pressure can also be recorded from small balloons attached to manometers, or by pressure-sensitive radio-telemetering capsules. It is important to realize that many of the pressure waves thus recorded, particularly those from telemetering capsules, are not the intermittent transmitted waves which result in movement of intestinal

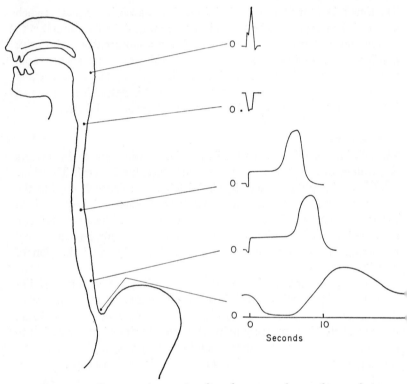

FIGURE 40. *Pressure changes in the pharynx and oesophagus during swallowing.*

Note the elevated resting pressure in the sphincteric zones at the cricoid level (second record) and the oesophagogastric junction (lowermost record). Relaxation of these sphincters during swallowing results in a fall in pressure. The passage of the bolus gives rise to the initial peak in intrapharyngeal pressure and the positive plateau in the intra-oesophageal records. The final steep wave of pressure in these records is caused by the contraction of the pharyngeal constrictor muscles and the muscular wall of the oesophagus respectively.

(Reproduced by kind permission of Dr M. Atkinson).

contents, but are solely due to the non-transmitted local contractions which serve to promote mixing. This accounts for the paradox that these pressure waves recorded in either the small or large intestine are diminished in diarrhoea and increased in constipation.

Interpretation of intraluminal pressure records can be aided by simultaneous cine-radiography.

In vitro techniques
The contractile response to pharmacological agents of strips of intestinal smooth muscle removed at operation is proving a valuable tool in clinical investigation. Smooth muscle from different parts of the gut has been shown to have different properties (p. 382).

Practical assessment

SWALLOWING AND GASTRO-OESOPHAGEAL REFLUX
Clinical observations
Pharyngeal dysphagia indicates search for weakness or anaesthesia of tongue, palate (nasal regurgitation), larynx; difficulty in swallowing liquids when supine. Overall test for swallowing: ability to drink a glass of water in 20 seconds.

Incompetence of cardia: postural retrosternal burning pain, acid regurgitation.

Routine methods
Barium swallow: obstruction, inco-ordination, loss of peristalsis, reflux. Edrophonium test for myasthenia gravis (p. 357). Infusion of N/10 HCl into oesophagus to differentiate oesophageal pain from other pains.

Special techniques
Intraluminal pressure records (p. 393).

GASTRIC EMPTYING
Clinical observations
Unhelpful except in gross pyloric obstruction; copious vomiting of food swallowed many hours before; distended stomach with visible peristalsis.

Routine methods
Gastric aspiration: more than 50 ml after overnight fast suggests pyloric obstruction. Barium meal: stomach should empty in 6 hr.

Special techniques
Serial test meal (p. 393).

INTESTINAL MOTILITY
Clinical observations
Constipation may indicate decreased (drugs) or increased (spastic colon, some other drug) contraction of colonic muscle, in addition to obstruction. Colicky central abdominal pain (peri-umbilical if small intestine, hypogastric if large intestine) indicates powerful contractions.

Stools: hard and difficult to pass in true constipation; 'rabbitty' in spastic colon; watery in hypermotility; bulky, greasy and difficult to flush in steatorrhoea (p. 422); mucus and blood in inflammatory lesions. Daily weight should not exceed 150 g.

Auscultation: silence in paralytic ileus; hypermotility difficult to judge.

Routine methods
Plain X-ray supine and erect reveals dilated gas filled loops in obstruction; mucosal pattern and position differentiates large bowel from small. Barium meal: information on motility and obstruction.

Special techniques
Intraluminal pressures (p. 393).

GASTRO-INTESTINAL SECRETION

Normal function

SALIVARY GLANDS

Structure. Most of the saliva is secreted by the three main pairs of glands. The acinar cells of the parotid are of a pure 'serous' type, whereas those of the submandibular and submaxillary are of mixed 'mucous' and 'serous' types. Fluid from the acini is conducted to the mouth first along short 'intercalary' ducts lined by small cuboidal cells, and then along intralobular ducts with lining cells which histologically appear to have a secretory role, and finally along collecting ducts.

Secretion. The primary secretion elaborated by the acini resembles a plasma ultrafiltrate in its sodium and potassium composition. During its passage down the duct sodium is removed, potassium is added, and the saliva becomes hypotonic. This sodium/potassium exchange across the ducts is partially influenced by aldosterone. As the secretion rate rises, e.g. in the human parotid from o to 4 ml/min, the sodium and bicarbonate concentration and the pH gradually increase, and the potassium concentration falls. Iodide can be secreted by the ducts to a concentration of ten or more times the plasma level, and bicarbonate to twice the plasma level.

The main enzyme of saliva is the α-amylase 'ptyalin' (p. 416). Mucoproteins are also secreted, particularly by the sublingual and submaxillary glands.

Control. This is unique among the gastro-intestinal glands in that it is exclusively nervous. Both parasympathetic and sympathetic stimulation can cause a flow of saliva. Conditioned reflexes are particularly important, but mechanical contact with the buccal mucosa and taste also excite secretion.

THE STOMACH

Structure

The differing physiological roles of the body and antrum are reflected histologically. *The mucosa of the body* contains glands which are long, tortuous and often branched. They contain oxyntic (parietal) cells and zymogenic (chief) cells, and only a few mucous cells. The parietal cells are found predominantly near the neck of the gland. There is strong presumptive evidence that they are responsible for the secretion of hydrochloric acid, and in man, of intrinsic factor. The chief cells, containing pepsinogen, are the most numerous. *The antral mucosa* is less thick, and the glands contain neither parietal nor chief cells. Its precise extent is variable and does not necessarily correspond to the antrum as defined anatomically—very often it extends into the body of the stomach, especially along the lesser curvature. The hormone 'gastrin' is produced by the antral mucosa, but the cells responsible have not been indentified.

Secretion

The body of the stomach secretes a juice whose main constituents are hydrochloric acid, pepsin, and intrinsic factor. Small amounts of other proteolytic and lipolytic enzymes and a urease are also present. Pepsin, the major proteolytic enzyme of the stomach, is probably a mixture of several similar enzymes. The active form is produced in the lumen from its inactive precursor, pepsinogen, either by contact with acid, or autocatalytically. The parietal cell has the remarkable ability of raising the concentration of hydrogen ions from 10^{-7} M in plasma to 0.16 M in gastric juice, and this involves considerable energy expenditure. One bicarbonate ion is released into the blood for each hydrogen ion secreted in gastric juice. These bicarbonate ions are formed within the cell from CO_2 and water under the influence of the enzyme carbonic anhydrase. Their release into the blood after a meal may be reflected by an 'alkaline tide' in the blood and urine.

The pyloric mucosa produces a scanty non-acid viscid solution. This, with the mucus produced elsewhere in the stomach, contributes to the neutral or slightly alkaline layer of mucus which covers the entire gastric surface. The mucoproteins secreted by the stomach and other parts of the gastrointestinal tract include, in some individuals, the blood group antigens A, B, and H.

Control

Gastric juice is secreted in three phases, which are normally integrated so that secretion is smooth and continuous, and, equally important, is stopped after a suitable time. The first, or cephalic phase is nervous, and is similar to that involved in salivary secretion. It produces a juice rich in both enzymes and acid, and is abolished completely by vagotomy. The second or gastric phase, is hormonal. Distension of the antrum, or contact of the antrum with food, results in production of the polypeptide hormone gastrin (p. 409) which stimulates the body to secrete a juice rich in acid. Gastrin release is strongly inhibited when the antral contents are acid. The third, or intestinal phase of secretion is probably hormonal, but its relative importance is difficult to assess for technical reasons.

The duodenum, like the antrum, also has an inhibitory mechanism, which is evoked by the presence of acid, fat or carbohydrate in the duodenum. This is usually attributed either to 'enterogastrone', a hormone which has not been purified but is present in duodenal extracts, or to a vagal mechanism.

The extreme complexity of the interrelationships between the vagal and hormonal control of gastric secretion has only recently been appreciated. It is now known, for instance, that vagal innervation of the antrum allows the marked potentiation of gastrin release in response to mechanical stimulation. Furthermore an intact vagal supply to the body allows the potentiation of the acid secretory response to injected gastrin. The operation of vagotomy, therefore, in addition to eliminating the psychic phase, also interferes with both the release of gastrin and its action on the oxyntic cell.

THE PANCREAS

Structure

The secretory acini are uniformly composed of pyramidal zymogen-containing cells. From the acini secretion passes into long 'intercalary' ducts and then into excretory ducts lined with cuboidal epithelium. Small mucous glands open into the largest ducts, the walls of which contain smooth-muscle cells and can contract. Preganglionic parasympathetic fibres of the vagus nerve synapse with ganglion cells within the pancreas. Unmyelinated postganglionic fibres innervate the acinar cells and smooth muscle of the dusts. Some post-ganglionic cholinergic secretory fibres are also present in the splanchnic nerves. The pancreas also contains islets of α- and β-cells, which secrete glucagon and insulin *internally*. These islets, and the acini which form the *external* secretion, are served by separate arterioles.

EXOCRINE SECRETION

The secretion of enzyme juice and aqueous juice is more clearly separable than in the case of the stomach, and the two secretions, although always mixed to some extent, can be considered separately.

The aqueous juice is distinguished by a high concentration of bicarbonate. As the secretion rate increases, the concentration of bicarbonate rises steadily from a minimum of 70 mM to as high as 140 mM, and the concentration of chloride, the other main anion, correspondingly falls. The concentrations of sodium and potassium remain approximately those of plasma. The cellular source of the bicarbonate is not clear, and the relative contribution made by acini and ducts to the water and electrolyte content of pancreatic secretion is quite unknown.

The enzyme juice is entirely a product of the acini and contains major enzymes for the digestion of each of the three major classes of foodstuffs. The proteolytic enzymes (trypsin, chymotrypsin and carboxypeptidase) are secreted as inactive zymogens and become enzymatically active only after intraluminal contact with enterokinase, an enzyme secreted by the duodenal mucosa, or with trypsin itself. This device for the prevention of pancreatic auto-digestion is aided by a specific trypsin inhibitor in pancreatic juice. Pancreatic amylase is an α-amylase similar to that of saliva. Pancreatic lipase is indispensable for the normal digestion of fats. Many other enzymes are also present, including an elastase, a ribonuclease, and a desoxyribonuclease.

Control

The secretion of the pancras, like that of the stomach, is controlled by both neural and hormonal mechanisms. The first, or psychic phase, resembles the corresponding phase in the stomach, in that it is rapid in onset, vagally mediated and produces a juice rich in enzymes. The second or humoral phase is due to two distinct hormones. *Secretin*, although the first hormone to be discovered, has still not been isolated in pure form. It is released from duodenal mucosa in response to the presence of acid and to a lesser extent, of soaps and the products of protein digestion. It causes a profuse flow of pancreatic juice with a high bicarbonate but low enzyme content. It also stimulates bile flow (p. 410). *Pancreozymin* is released from duodenal mucosa in response to the presence of a wide variety of food products. It causes an increase in secretion of enzymes, but not in the volume of secretion or its bicarbonate concentration. Like secretin, it has not been isolated, and the purest extracts available also stimulate gallbladder contraction (p. 410). The complexity of the situation in the intact animal is illustrated by the fact that chemically pure gastrin also potentiates the volume and enzyme output of the pancreas in response to secretin.

ENDOCRINE SECRETION

Insulin is secreted in response to a rise in blood glucose concentration. For an equivalent rise in blood glucose concentration, the rise of plasma insulin is much greater when glucose is given orally or intrajejunally than when given intravenously. This is due to the release by glucose of a humoral substance from the intestinal mucosa. Secretin, pancreozymin, and glucagon are all present in the intestinal mucosa, but although each of these can stimulate insulin secretion under certain conditions the intestinal hormone normally involved in insulin release remains to be identified.

THE SMALL AND LARGE INTESTINE

The only true *exocrine* glands of the small intestine are Brunner's glands in the duodenum. These produce a small quantity of highly viscid, alkaline fluid which is probably purely protective in function. The 'secretion' of succus entericus by the remainder of the intestine is confined to the desquamation of surface epithelial cells and their contained enzymes. The anatomical site of the *endocrine* cells which produce hormones such as secretin and pancreozymin has not been located.

The ionic composition of intestinal contents

Although no glandular secretion occurs in the gut there is a rapid exchange of water and electrolytes across all parts of the mucosa. Water moves in response to osmotic gradients, a hypertonic solution being rapidly diluted by movement of water from blood to lumen, and a hypotonic solution rapidly concentrated by absorption of water. Intestinal contents are thereby maintained isotonic with blood. The pH in the ileum (about 7·6) is more alkaline than that in the jejunum (about 6·8) partly because the bicarbonate concentration in the ileum is relatively high (30 m-equiv/l. in the ileum compared to 5 m-equiv/l. in the jejunum). The bicarbonate concentration in the colon is also quite high (30 m-equiv/l.), but here the major anions are organic acids formed by bacterial action.

Sodium is actively absorbed in both small and large intestine, and water absorption in both organs follows the osmotic gradient set up by this sodium transport. Net water absorption is considerable, as it includes 7 l. per day contributed by the digestive glands in addition to $1\frac{1}{2}$ l. per day taken by mouth. Most of this is absorbed by the small intestine, but about 400 ml each day is absorbed by the colon. Potassium is absorbed by the small intestine but is secreted by the large intestine. The net result is that the volume of normal stool water is approximately 100 ml/24 hr, with a Na^+ and K^+ concentration of 25–49 and 80–132 m-equiv/l. respectively. For comparison, the volume of a normal ileostomy discharge is approximately 500 ml/24 hr, with concentrations of Na^+ and K^+ of 100–126 and 8–13 m-equiv/l. respectively.

Protein loss in the gastro-intestinal secretions

Under normal conditions an unknown but significant quantity of albumin leaks into the gut lumen, in various secretions such as saliva, gastric juice, succus entericus, and bile. The exuded albumin is digested and re-absorbed, and it is estimated that up to one half of the normal daily catabolism of albumin may be accounted for in this way.

Disordered function

SALIVARY SECRETION

Dry mouth (*xerostomia*) may be caused by either mouth breathing (which evaporates the saliva) or by deficient salivary secretion. This may be caused by destruction of the glandular cells, as after irradiation or in Sjögren's syndrome. More commonly it is a temporary phenomenon, as for example, in fluid depletion. It may follow fear, anxiety, and the administration of a wide variety of drugs, including ganglion blocking, anti-cholinergic, and sympatholytic agents.

Excessive salivation (ptyalism) is usually reflexly produced by irritation of the mouth or oesophagus by local disease. It may follow iodide administration and poisoning by mercury.

GASTRIC SECRETION
Achlorhydria
Complete failure of gastric acid secretion (p. 397) indicates severe gastric mucosal degeneration. It is invariable in pernicious anaemia, but is also found in a few patients with hypochromic anaemia or gastric carcinoma, and in apparently healthy relatives of pernicious anaemia patients. Deficient hydrochloric acid secretion causes no disability, but the associated intrinsic factor deficiency can result in failure of vitamin B_{12} absorption.

Auto-immune factors have been implicated in the gastric atrophy of pernicious anaemia. More than 60 per cent of pernicious anaemia sera contain intrinsic factor antibodies, and nearly 90 per cent contain parietal cell antibodies. Parietal cell antibodies are also found in the sera of a third of all patients with Hashimoto's disease, primary myxoedema, and thyrotoxicosis and although they can occur in 'control' subjects they always indicate the presence of chronic gastritis histologically. Intrinsic factor antibody is much more closely associated with the more complete gastric atrophy of pernicious anaemia, and although it is also present in the sera of some patients with thyrotoxicosis and adrenal insufficiency these are found on investigation to have severe gastric atrophy. As in other 'auto-immune diseases' (p. 289) the aetiological significance of autoantibodies has not been established.

Peptic ulcer
Although the pattern of acid secretion in patients with duodenal ulcers tends to be different from that in patients with gastric ulcer, there are certain common features. Benign peptic ulceration occurs when mucosal resistance to attack by acid and pepsin breaks down. It never occurs in the absence of gastric acid secretion, as in pernicious anaemia. All surgical procedures for the relief of peptic ulcer are directed to the reduction of acid secretion, either by removal of the antrum, the source of gastrin, or by vagotomy, and there is abundant evidence that their success in the healing of ulcers and prevention of recurrence is related to the degree in which this aim is achieved. On the other hand, gastric

acid secretion is often normal in patients with peptic ulcer, indicating the importance of other factors.

The tendency to high secretion found in duodenal ulcer patients is associated with a large area of acid-bearing fundic mucosa and the output of acid in response to maximal dose of histamine correlates well with the number of parietal cells. The fundamental physiological disturbance remains obscure. In the past the observation that vagotomy reduced the basal and nocturnal secretion has been adduced as evidence that this is nervous in origin. Current knowledge of the complexity of the role of the vagus (p. 398) makes this explanation too naive, as vagotomy also interferes with the hormonal phase of gastric secretion.

Gastric ulcers can be divided into three types: two of these, prepyloric ulcers, and the gastric ulcer occurring with duodenal ulcers are associated with normal or greater than normal gastric acid secretion. The third type of gastric ulcer is most commonly situated in antral type mucosa near the incisura, and the rate of gastric acid secretion is low. This is associated with a reduced parietal cell mass and atrophic gastritis in the acid-bearing mucosa.

Patients with duodenal ulcer, and to a lesser extent those with gastric ulcer, belong more commonly to Group O than to any of the other blood groups, and, independently of this tend to be non-secretors of ABH blood-group substances in their alimentary mucous secretions. The mechanism of the association between blood group, secretor status, and peptic ulceration, is unknown.

The physiological basis of peptic ulcer therapy

This is unsatisfactory, as it has not proved possible to demonstrate conclusively that any regime of diet and drugs directed to reduction of gastric acid concentration has any influence on the healing of gastric and duodenal ulcers. On the other hand there is no doubt that reduction in gastric acid concentration, even for brief periods, is the most effective means of pain relief, and it is clear that pain occurs at a time when intragastric and intraduodenal acidity are greatest, i.e. 1–3 hr after meals (Fig. 41). Two-hourly feeding has been shown to reduce the maximum acidity below that found with four-hourly feeding, but sloppy foods such as milk are ineffective in maintaining reduction of gastric acid concentration because of the speed with which they leave the stomach. Anticholinergic drugs, although they depress gastric secretion under experimental conditions, have little effect on gastric acidity under conditions of clinical use. Antacids reduce gastric acidity for only a very short time, and although this may be adequate for pain relief they must

14

be administered continuously to maintain the reduction in acid concentration. 'Rational' therapy in ulcer treatment is therefore at the present time based on a combination of measures which have been shown empirically to speed healing but to have no effect on gastric

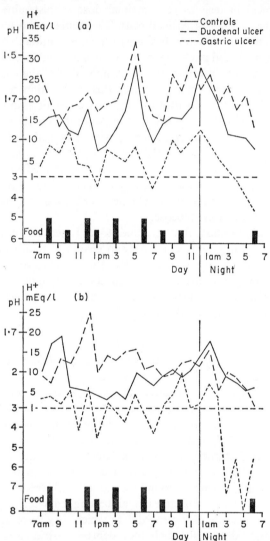

FIGURE 41. *Changes in the acidity of the contents of the stomach and the first part of the duodenum during the 24 hours.*

(From Atkinson, M., and Henley, K. S., *Clin. Sci.*, **14,** 1 1955.)

secretion (bed rest, cessation of smoking), and measures which relieve pain and reduce acidity but have not been shown to influence healing (frequent feeds and antacids).

Effect of surgery on gastric secretion
The effectiveness of any operation for peptic ulceration, particularly of the duodenum, depends largely upon the efficiency with which it reduces gastric acid secretion. All operations for duodenal ulcer rely on either removal of the antrum, the source of gastrin, or section of the vagus nerves, or both. In man, vagotomy alone abolishes the psychic phase of gastric secretion, and in addition it considerably reduces the hormonal phase, while leaving the duodenal inhibitory phase intact.

Endocrine disorders associated with changes in the rate
of gastric secretion and the incidence of peptic ulcer
The only condition in which there is direct and unequivocal evidence of an association between hormonally induced gastric hyper-secretion and peptic ulceration is the Zollinger–Ellison syndrome, due to non-insulin secreting islet cell tumours of the pancreas. The continuous release of a hormone apparently identical to gastrin results in a basal acid output of more than 200 ml, or 20 m-equiv/hr. This is associated with intractable duodenal and jejunal ulceration, and often with steatorrhoea due to inactivation of lipase by the low pH of intestinal contents.

Adrenal corticosteroids influence gastric secretion, but endogenous hypersecretion of cortisol in Cushing's syndrome, although often associated with hypersecretion of acid, is not associated with an increased incidence of duodenal ulcer. High doses of exogenous steroids also increase gastric secretion after they have been given for 3 days or more, but again good evidence that this results in duodenal ulcer is lacking, although the incidence of haematemesis and of gastric ulcer is increased.

Hyperparathyroidism is associated with an increase in basal acid output, perhaps due to hypercalcaemia, and the incidence of duodenal ulcer is also probably increased.

Spontaneous hypoglycaemia due to insulin-secreting β-cell tumours of the pancreatic islets results in hypersecretion, and is occasionally associated with duodenal ulceration. Conversely diabetes mellitus is often associated with a diminished secretion of acid, and the incidence of duodenal ulcer is low.

Secretion of acid is lower in women of reproductive age than in older women or in men, and peptic ulcer is correspondingly less common. Stilboestrol therapy speeds the healing of duodenal ulcers in men although it does not measurably affect acid secretion.

PANCREATIC SECRETION

Impairment of secretion

A severe reduction in the output of pancreatic enzymes results in steatorrhoea. It may be due to chronic pancreatitis, resection of the pancreas, or, in childhood, to fibrocystic disease of the pancreas. Although pancreatic juice normally neutralizes the gastric effluent in the duodenum, peptic ulcer is uncommon in patients with chronic pancreatitis. In contrast, chronic biliary obstruction does seem to predispose to duodenal ulcer.

Autodigestion of the pancreas

Acute pancreatitis occurs when the pancreatic enzymes, normally activated within the duodenal lumen (p. 399) become activated within the gland itself. Experimentally a similar condition can be induced by pancreatic duct obstruction especially if bile is also introduced into the ducts. Pancreatic enzymes escape into the tissues and peritoneal cavity, causing necrosis in both the gland itself and in adjacent organs. Patchy fat necrosis is induced by escaped lipase, and hypocalcaemia occasionally follows the formation of calcium salts of the resultant fatty acids. Transient hyperglycaemia and glycosuria may also be present, but more valuable in diagnosis is the raised serum amylase concentration. The impairment of pancreatic exocrine and endocrine function is only temporary.

Chronic relapsing pancreatitis is usually associated either with alcoholism or gall stones. The presenting features in any particular case may be either pain, steatorrhoea, or diabetes mellitus.

INTESTINAL SECRETION

The ionic composition of the fluid inside any particular part of the bowel is normally maintained constant by large bidirectional fluxes of ions and water across the mucosa (p. 401), but there is evidence that the precise ionic composition achieved is influenced by aldosterone and perhaps other hormones. In a sodium depleted patient, for example, ileal contents drained from an ileostomy have a low Na^+/K^+ ratio, and the faecal Na^+/K^+ ratio is low in patients with an aldosterone secreting tumour. The most common condition to change the stool water Na^+/K^+

ratio, however, is diarrhoea. The normal stool Na^+/K^+ ratio of 0·3 gradually rises with increasing stool volume. The explanation of this may simply be that with the decreased time of contact between intestinal contents and colonic mucosa, there is less opportunity for normal Na^+ and K^+ exchange, so that the Na^+/K^+ ratio of ileal contents, which is greater than 10, is approached. Even so, the Na^+/K^+ ratio of plasma is never attained, so that diarrhoea inevitably leads to potassium depletion (p. 18). Hypokalaemia due to faecal potassium loss is a particular feature of some villous adenomas of the colon which actually secrete potassium. Cholera is a special case, in that the stool water has approximately the same electrolyte content as plasma. Stool water content in this condition may be anything from 2–20 l. in 24 hr, and it is possible that intestinal sodium and hence water transport is specifically depressed by the cholera vibrio.

Protein loss through the gastro-intestinal tract
The normal loss of serum albumin into the gastro-intestinal tract may be increased in a variety of conditions such as ulcerative colitis, idiopathic steatorrhoea, neoplasms, and giant rugal hypertrophy of the stomach.

The reserve capacity of the liver for albumin synthesis is limited (p. 436) so that although the albumin is digested and absorbed the serum albumin may fall and result in oedema. Many cases of what was formerly called idiopathic hypercatabolic hypoproteinaemia have been shown to be due to increased gut albumin loss, sometimes due to an anatomical abnormality of the lymphatics in the small intestine (intestinal lymphangiectasia).

Principles of tests and measurements

GASTRIC SECRETION
Tests of acid secretion are in practice confined to measuring either the total amount of secretion evoked by standard parenteral stimuli, or the concentration of acid in small volumes of aspirated juice. Measurements of other components of gastric secretion, such as chloride, pepsin, and intrinsic factor, are not in routine use.

Acid secretion is assessed in terms of (i) volume (in millilitres) of gastric juice (ii) the concentration of hydrogen ions (as pH), and (iii) the titratable acidity (m-equiv of hydrogen ion per litre). This is determined by titration with N/10 NaOH to neutrality either electrometrically, or colorimetrically using phenol red as an indicator. The concept of 'free' and 'combined' acid arose because the titration curves of gastric contents following a test meal were found to follow that of pure hydrochloric acid only from pH 1–3. The titration curve of uncontaminated gastric juice does not in fact differ significantly from that of hydrochloric acid, so that nothing is gained by the traditional separate titration of 'free acid' to pH 3·5 (Töpfers reagent) and 'total acid' to pH 8 (phenolphthalein).

For all tests it is essential that the sampling tube is radiopaque, of adequate bore, and is adjusted under radiological control so that the tip lies in the most dependent portion of the stomach. If mechanical suction is used the patency of the tube must be repeatedly checked by the use of a syringe.

The serial test meal (p. 393)

This is not suitable for routine use, but does enable the amount of acid, chloride, and pepsin secreted in response to an artificial meal to be calculated.

Basal gastric secretion

The interdigestive, basal, or nocturnal secretion can be collected by continuous overnight gastric suction. Similar information can be obtained by collecting a one hour basal secretion in the morning after an overnight fast, as is done before an augmented histamine test. The normal basal output of acid is less than 5 m-equiv/hr.

The augmented histamine test

Histamine is widely distributed in the tissues of the body, including gastric mucosa. It is a very potent secretory stimulus to the stomach, producing a juice rich in acid and poor in pepsin, although no physiological role has been established. Antihistamine drugs antagonize all the actions of histamine other than its effect on the parietal cells, and their use enables such a large dose of histamine to be given that a maximal and reproducible acid response is obtained. Gastric juice is collected for a basal one hour, in the middle of which 50 mg of mepyramine ('Anthisan') is given. Histamine (0·04 mg/kg body weight) is injected subcutaneously, and secretion is collected for a further four 15 min periods. The maximum acid output is usually attained in the second and third 15 min periods. The volume, pH and titratable acidity (m-equiv/hr) are measured.

The one hour maximal output

This is an estimate of the number of parietal cells in the gastric mucosa, although due to the sensitizing action of cholinergic innervation on the parietal cell (p. 398) it is reduced by vagotomy or anti-cholinergic drugs. Normal values are up to approximately 25 m-equiv/hr in a man, and rather less in a woman. Failure to secrete acid, i.e. achlorhydria, is present if the pH fails to fall below 6·0 in any specimen.

The normal range of both basal output and maximal acid output is wide, and the significance of an observed result in terms of the probability of duodenal ulcer or gastric ulcer and carcinoma is limited. Gastric secretion studies are of unequivocal value only in the detection of complete anacidity or gross hypersecretion. Elevation of basal acid output to at least 50 per cent and often nearer 100 per cent of the maximal acid output is characteristic of the presence of a tumour secreting a gastrin-like substance (Zollinger–Ellison syndrome).

The clinical use of histamine in tests of gastric acid secretion is now being superseded by the use of Pentagastrin. Gastrin itself is a 17-amino acid polypeptide, but the tetrapeptide chain Try. Met. Asp. Phe. NH_2 which occupies positions 14–17 has all the physiological properties of the entire gastrin molecule. Pentagastrin, a synthetic polypeptide, contains the same C-terminal tetrapeptide. A dose of $6\mu g/kg$ subcutaneously stimulates maximal acid output, and side effects are less frequent and less severe than those following histamine. After vagotomy the maximal acid output in response to subcutaneous Pentagastrin is reduced by 60%, a result very similar to that seen when histamine is used as the stimulus to acid secretion.

The insulin hypoglycaemia test

Hypoglycaemia induced by insulin stimulates gastric secretion of acid and pepsin by a central mechanism mediated through the vagus nerves. After vagotomy this secretory response is lost, and so this test is used as a measure of the completeness of vagal section. A suitable dose of insulin is 15 units intravenously, and for the test to be valid the blood sugar should fall to 50 mg/100 ml or below during the 2 hr collection of gastric juice.

Twenty-four hour gastric analysis

This is the only technique which gives some indication of gastric secretion under relatively physiological conditions. The patient swallows a tube which is left in the stomach for 24 hr. Meals are taken normally, but about 5 ml of gastric contents are aspirated hourly for determination of pH (Fig. 41).

Tubeless gastric analysis

These methods depend on the displacement by hydrogen ions of quininium or a dye from a cation exchange resin given by mouth. The excretion of quininium or dye in the urine indicates the presence of acid in the stomach. False negative results may arise from defective absorption or excretion of the cation, and compounds containing barium, calcium, magnesium, aluminium and iron may give rise to false positive results.

Blood and urine pepsinogen

A small fraction of the pepsinogen produced by the chief cells is secreted into the blood, and there is some association between blood and urinary pepsinogen levels and the capacity to secrete acid. After total gastrectomy and in pernicious anaemia blood and urinary pepsinogen values are very low, but otherwise their diagnostic value is limited.

Intrinsic factor secretion

This can be measured by immunological assay. In general its secretion closely parallels that of acid, although, as is the case for pepsin, continuous histamine infusion intravenously results only in a temporary increase in output, whereas acid output is maintained indefinitely.

PANCREATIC SECRETION

Duodenal aspiration

The response to intravenous secretin and pancreozymin. These two hormones are available in preparations suitable for clinical use. All preparations of pancreozymin also contain cholecystokinin, and so stimulate the gall bladder to contract, in addition to stimulating pancreatic enzyme output. Duodenal contents are aspirated continuously during the test, contamination with gastric juice being prevented by continuous gastric aspiration through another tube. The volume, bicarbonate, enzyme, and bilirubin concentration are measured basally, for 60 min after 1 u/kg body weight of secretin and for a further 20 min after 1·5 u/kg body weight of pancreozymin. This test requires considerable care in its execution. The normal range is wide, and its reproducibility has not been studied.

The response to a standard meal. This simpler test involves the determination of the concentration of pancreatic enzymes in duodenal juice during the two hours after a standard meal. Abnormal results are found if pancreatic insufficiency is causing steatorrhoea.

Serum enzyme provocative tests

These depend upon a combination of secretory stimulation by secretin and closure of the sphincter of Oddi by morphine derivatives. A rise in amylase and lipase levels occurs in the majority of normal subjects, but is absent in advanced pancreatic disease. If secretin and pancreozymin are injected without morphine little or no rise in enzyme levels takes place in normal subjects, but a significant elevation occurs in obstruction of the pancreatic duct.

Fibrocystic disease of the pancreas

There is an increased concentration of sodium and chloride in the sweat of individuals with this condition. Sweat can be collected in a weighed swab placed in contact with the skin and the sodium concentration measured after it has been eluted from the gauze. A screening test can be performed by pressing the finger tips upon an agar place impregnated with silver nitrate, and observing the precipitate of silver chloride. Sweat electrolyte concentrations are unreliable in detection of fibrocystic disease over the age of 30, as false positives are very frequent.

Scanning after radio-isotopes

The pancreas has a high rate of protein turnover, and therefore accumulates large amounts of the amino acid methionine, which can be labelled with selenium 75, a potent γ-ray emitter. Its anatomical extent and any gross filling defect can then be assessed by a sensitive external scanning device over the abdomen. The liver also accumulates significant radioactivity and a preliminary scan of this organ may be necessary using another isotope.

TESTS FOR GASTRO-INTESTINAL PROTEIN LOSS

Albumin can be labelled with ^{131}I and its metabolism followed after intravenous injection. If albumin synthesis is diminished as in starvation or liver disease, catabolism is decreased, and the $T\frac{1}{2}$ (time for catabolism of half the body albumin pool) is increased. If the $T\frac{1}{2}$ is short, on the other hand, this suggests increased catabolism, possibly by leakage into the gut. Unfortunately ^{131}I albumin loss into the gut cannot be quantitated by counting faecal radioactivity after intravenous injection, as the ^{131}I is digested off the albumin, absorbed, and excreted in the urine. Direct demonstration of increased leakage of macromolecules into the gut can be achieved by counting stool radioactivity after the intravenous injection of the inert polymer polyvinyl pyrrolidine (PVP) (MW 40 000 approximately) labelled with [131]I. Normally less than 1 per cent of the

14*

injected dose is found in the 4 days following injection. Alternatively 100 to 200 μC of ^{51}Cr labelled chromic chloride can be given intravenously. The plasma proteins are labelled *in vivo* and normally less than 1 per cent of the radioactivity is excreted in a 5 day stool collection. This test is only valid because chromium, unlike iodine, is not reabsorbed from the bowel after leaking into the lumen. Unfortunately chromium labelled albumin is denatured and cannot be used to measure albumin turnover rates.

Practical Assessment

SALIVA
Clinical examination is adequate to assess xerostomia or ptyalism. Collection of pure parotid secretion can be made by a capsule which fits over the opening of the parotid duct. Determination of the sodium/potassium ratio may be useful in suspected hyperaldosteronism.

GASTRIC SECRETION
Clinical observations
Not possible.

Routine methods
Basal 1 hr acid output (BAO) and 1 h maximal acid output after histamine (MAO) is adequate; insulin test only for assessing vagotomy. Most useful for extremes of secretion: true achlorhydria (p. 402) in pernicious anaemia, high basal output (more than 60 per cent of MAO) in Zollinger–Ellison syndrome. MAO more than 40 m-equiv/hr very suggestive of duodenal ulcer, MAO greater than 25 m-equiv/hr very suggestive of anastomotic ulcer. BAO and MAO both normal in most gastric ulcers, low in most carcinomas.

Appearance of barium meal quite useful rough indication: bald mucosa in pernicious anaemia.

Special techniques
Twenty-four-hour test meal (p. 409); shows lower nocturnal pH in duodenal ulcer (Fig. 41). Most useful for assessing dietary regimes and drugs on gastric acid concentration. Intrinsic factor can be measured during histamine test; absent in pernicious anaemia, low in atrophic gastritis; in general I.F. secretion parallels that of acid.

PANCREATIC SECRETION
Clinical observations
If very low: steatorrhoea, perhaps diabetes, and abdominal pain.

Routine methods
Normal mucosal function (xylose, B_{12}, folic acid, and iron absorption; normal biopsy) incriminates pancreas as cause of steatorrhoea; also impaired glucose tolerance, pancreatic calcification.

Special techniques
Duodenal aspiration (p. 410).

INTESTINAL SECRETION
Clinical observations
Volume, elecrolyte concentration of all losses (vomit, aspiration, ileostomy discharge, faeces). Gastro-intestinal protein loss: oedema, gastro-intestinal symptoms, sometimes lymphoedema in legs, arms.

Special techniques
Five day stool excretion of radioactivity after intravenous PVP ^{131}I, or $^{51}CrCl_3$.

DIGESTION AND ABSORPTION

Normal function

Digestion consists of the intraluminal breakdown of complex foodstuffs into simpler molecules or complexes which can be absorbed.

Absorption is the transfer of this material across the intestinal epithelium into the blood or lymph. Although this epithelium is complex, the problems of absorption can best be discussed using the nomenclature developed for describing the transport processes observed in simpler biological membranes, e.g. that of the erythrocyte. The phenomena observed can be most readily explained if all such membranes are considered as composed mainly of lipid, but penetrated by small water-filled pores. The broadest subdivision of these phenomena is into passive diffusion, and special mechanisms (including active transport and pinocytosis).

Passive diffusion is the passage of a substance across the cell membrane down an electro-chemical gradient. In the case of non-electrolytes this simplifies into passage down the concentration gradient.

Active transport is the passage of a substance across the cell membrane against an apparent electro-chemical gradient. It differs from diffusion in being energy dependent.

Pinocytosis is the term applied to the uptake of intact macromolecules by a process of vesicle formation, analogous to phagocytosis. Electron microscopic evidence suggests that it may be responsible for the capacity of the newborn of many species to absorb antibody from ingested colostrum, but pinocytosis probably does not occur in man. It has however been claimed that it is partly responsible for absorption of fat.

The ease with which any substance penetrates a biological membrane depends largely on three factors, (i) lipid solubility, (ii) molecular size and (iii) whether or not it is ionized.

Highly lipid-soluble (non polar) compounds readily enter all cells, including those of the intestinal tract, by virtue of their ability to dissolve in the cell membrane and diffuse through it. In the case of ionized compounds, only the unionized molecule is absorbed, being lipid soluble, as the intestinal mucosa is relatively impermeable to charged particles. The absorption of weak acids and weak bases is therefore a function of their pK and of the intraluminal pH. This explains the relatively rapid absorption from the stomach of weak acids such as acetyl-salicylic acid.

Water-soluble (polar) compounds do not readily traverse cell membranes, but if sufficiently small (MW < approx. 100) will diffuse through the aqueous pores. Larger water-soluble compounds are thought to be absorbed by attaching themselves to mobile 'carriers', which have been postulated to act as ferry-boats across the lipid membrane. Carrier-mediated, or 'facilitated' transport is characterized by a high degree of substrate specificity and by a limited capacity. It is probably responsible for absorption of monosaccharides and of amino acids.

THE SITE OF ABSORPTION

In general, absorption is limited to the specialized epithelium of the small intestine. Within the small intestine the site of absorption depends both on the capacity of particular segments of gut for absorption, and on the length of time for which a substance is present in a digested, assimilable form in the different segments of intestine. The site of maximum absorptive capacity for most substances is the jejunum, but appreciable amounts may remain for absorption in the ileum. The absorption of bile salts and vitamin B_{12} occurs almost exclusively in the ileum.

Highly lipid soluble compounds, particularly drugs such as alcohol and trinitroglycerine, can be absorbed from any part of the gastro-intestinal tract. Very limited amounts of water soluble compounds such as glucose can be absorbed by diffusion from concentrated solutions placed within the stomach or rectum.

STRUCTURE OF THE SMALL INTESTINE

The villi of the small intestine are slender, finger-like processes 0·2–1 mm in length, which project into the lumen (Fig. 42). They are covered by an epithelium consisting of two cell types: the columnar absorbing cells and mucus secreting goblet cells. The crypts of Lieberkühn, which are gland-like structures between the villi, contain argentaffin cells and the eosinophilic cells of Paneth, whose function is unknown, and also a large number of actively dividing cells. Cells produced in the crypts migrate up the walls of the villi and are finally extruded at the tip, and by this means the entire small intestinal epithelium is continuously renewed. These cells probably have a higher rate of turnover than any other cells in the body, their life span being only two days.

The ultrastructure of the columnar absorbing cell is shown in Fig. 43. The luminal border of each cell is covered with approximately 600 minute microvilli which greatly increase the absorptive area and constitute the 'brush border' when seen by the light microscope. Hydrolytic enzymes including peptidases and dissaccharidases are located in the microvilli, and it is in this region of the cell that active transport of monosaccharides and amino acids occurs. The reactions which yield the large amounts of energy required for the numerous transport and metabolic processes involved in absorption take place in the mitochondria. The function of the endoplasmic reticulum is less well understood. It constitutes an extensive intracellular vacuolar system involved in lipid synthesis and transport and is the major site of cell protein synthesis.

Absorbed materials pass through the basement membrane of the epithelial cells and enter the extracellular fluid. Their passage into either lymphatic or blood vessel capillaries is then governed by the particle size.

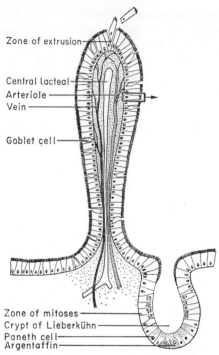

Zone of extrusion

Central lacteal
Arteriole
Vein

Goblet cell

Zone of mitoses
Crypt of Lieberkühn
Paneth cell
Argentaffin

FIGURE 42. *Diagrammatic representation of a small intestinal villus.*

Sugars and amino acids can enter both capillary systems, but are chiefly absorbed into the blood capillaries where the flow rate is considerably greater. Chylomicra are too large to enter the small pores of the blood capillaries and are therefore absorbed exclusively into the lymphatics.

CARBOHYDRATE DIGESTION AND ABSORPTION

Most dietary carbohydrate is in the form of starch, which is composed of straight and branched chains of glucose molecules. The branch points are composed of $1,6'$-α glucoside linkages, the straight chains being held together by 1-$4'$-α glucoside linkages. The α-amylases of saliva and the pancreatic juice split the 1-$4'$-α glucoside bonds, the result being a mixture of the disaccharides maltose ($1,4'$-α link) and isomaltose (1-$6'$-α link) with only some 15 per cent as free glucose. These disaccharides, together with dietary sucrose (glucose plus fructose) and lactose (glucose plus galactose) are split by disaccharidases (maltase, iso-maltase, invertase, and lactase) in the outer region of the brush border.

Monosaccharides are absorbed in identical fashion whether ingested as such, or produced within the brush border from disaccharides. Glucose and galactose are rapidly absorbed by the same active carrier mediated transport system. This carrier system is specific for sugars with certain common structural features, the essentials of which are a *d*-pyranose ring structure with a hydroxyl group of the glucose configuration at carbon 2. No chemical reaction such as phosphorylation occurs during their absorption and certain non-metabolizable synthetic sugars which share this general formula are also actively absorbed by this transport system, e.g. 3–*o*–methyl glucose.

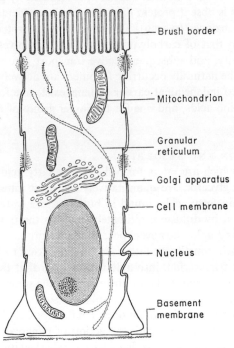

FIGURE 43. *Diagrammatic representation of a columnar absorbing cell of the small intestine.*

Fructose is absorbed less efficiently than glucose and galactose, and *in vitro* active transport cannot be demonstrated. Xylose, a pentose sugar, is absorbed in the jejunum like the hexoses, but to a lesser extent than fructose, so that the large amounts used in tests of absorption may result in diarrhoea due to the osmotic effect of unabsorbed sugar. Most other monosaccharides, e.g. sorbose and mannose, are absorbed very poorly, and their oral administration even in small doses provokes diarrhoea.

Disaccharides and their constituent monosaccharides can be absorbed throughout the small intestine but both the disaccharide splitting enzymes and the monosaccharide transport systems are most active in the jejunum.

PROTEIN DIGESTION AND ABSORPTION

Protein derived from desquamated cells and gastro-intestinal secretions (about 50 g daily) in addition to dietary protein, is normally completely absorbed in the small intestine. Digestion is initiated by gastric pepsin, but even if this is absent protein digestion can be efficiently carried out by pancreatic enzymes (p. 399). The final stage in protein absorption is analogous to that of carbohydrates, in that it involves intracellular peptidase activity, and subsequent active transport of the amino acids formed. Only the naturally occurring *l*-isomers are actively transported, and at least two independent carrier systems exist, one for cystine and the dibasic amino acids, and one for the larger group of neutral amino acids.

FAT DIGESTION AND ABSORPTION

Triglycerides, which are esters formed between fatty acids and the trihydric alcohol glycerol, are quantitatively the most important dietary fats. Short chain fatty acids, found in butterfat, are water soluble and can be absorbed by diffusion, ultimately entering the portal vein (Fig. 44). Most dietary lipids however, pose a special problem to the intestine because their constituent fatty acids, e.g. stearic or oleic acid, are, like the parent triglyceride, insoluble in water, so that they cannot be dispersed into molecular units for absorption in the same way as sugars or amino acids.

Some initial emulsification of fat occurs in the stomach, but the critical phase of fat digestion starts with the action of pancreatic lipase. This splits off the outer (α) ester bonds of triglyceride, leaving a mixture of fatty acids and β-monoglycerides. This mixture is insoluble in water, but in the presence of an adequate concentration of bile salts forms an optically clear solution. This is due to the detergent-like activity of the bile salts, which form polymolecular aggregates called 'micelles'. These micelles are able to incorporate fatty acids and monoglycerides, and the products of fat digestion are all therefore incorporated in a clear micellar solution, a process known as 'micellar solubilization'. Under physiological conditions the bile salt micelle is the final common path of dietary fat, and indeed of all other water insoluble molecules. However, other mechanisms of absorption must exist, since fat is absorbed to some extent in the absence of bile.

The constituents of the micelle penetrate the microvilli of the intestinal epithelial cell by a mechanism which is poorly understood, and within the cell are resynthesized into triglyceride (Fig. 44). This triglyceride, together with some phospholipid and cholesterol ester, is then aggregated into particles approximately 1 μ in diameter. After these have been coated with a fine layer of lipoprotein, they are discharged as chylomicrons into the lacteals (lymphatics).

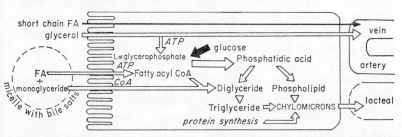

FIGURE 44. *The pathways and major biochemical reactions involved in fat absorption.*

Most dietary fat is absorbed in the duodenum and jejunum. Bile salts, on the other hand, pass on down the intestine to be absorbed by a specific active transport system in the ileum.

THE ABSORPTION OF VITAMINS

The fat soluble vitamins A, D and K are usually associated with lipids in the diet, and, in the lumen of the small intestine, are incorporated with fat in the bile salt micelle. Indeed, the absorption of vitamin D, in contrast to triglyceride, is completely dependent upon bile salts. The intestinal mucosa is the main site of conversion of carotene to vitamin A.

Most of the water soluble vitamins, e.g. nicotinamide, ascorbic acid and biotin are probably absorbed by passive diffusion. The form in which they are present in the diet may however profoundly influence their absorption, e.g. pyridoxine, when in the form of its free alcohol, diffuses readily, but in the diet it is probably present as a bound form of aldehyde or amine. Thiamine dissociates into large charged ions in solution, and hence would not be expected to diffuse easily. It has its own active transport system. A special mechanism for the absorption of folic acid (another large ionized molecule) is also probably present in the upper jejunum. Vitamin B_{12} is unique as it is not absorbed in the absence of intrinsic factor, a secretion of gastric parietal cells. Intrinsic factor is probably a mucoprotein, with a molecular weight of approximately 50 000, and it binds vitamin B_{12} very strongly. The vitamin B_{12}–intrinsic factor complex passes down the small intestine and is absorbed intact by a specific active transport system in the ileum.

THE ABSORPTION OF MINERALS

Calcium is absorbed mainly in the duodenum and jejunum, where there is an active transport system which needs vitamin D and probably parathormone for full activity. The transport system is more active if the subject has had a low dietary intake of calcium. The higher pH in the ileum favours the precipitation of insoluble calcium salts, and so is less favourable to calcium absorption. If there is malabsorption of fat unabsorbed fatty acids may also hinder calcium absorption due to the formation of insoluble calcium soaps. Faecal calcium is a mixture of unabsorbed dietary calcium, and of 'endogenous' calcium arising from gastro intestinal secretions.

Iron has an active transport system for ferrous (Fe^{++}) ion in the upper small intestine. It is unique in that absorption from the diet varies inversely with body stores of iron, and directly with the degree of erythropoiesis. Absorption is therefore increased considerably in iron deficiency anaemia, to a lesser extent in haemolytic anaemia, and not at all in aplastic anaemia. Furthermore, absorption is decreased for some time after a dose of oral iron. This so-called 'mucosal block' which can also be demonstrated in the iron-overloaded animal, is now known not to be due to saturation of the protein 'apoferritin' in the mucosa. The mechanism may be that transfer of absorbed iron from mucosal cells to the blood stream is very slow and if body iron stores are high is even further delayed. Iron freshly absorbed into the mucosal cells may therefore be shed with these cells into the gut lumen (p. 415) before it can be transferred to the blood stream. The availability of iron in different foods varies from 5 to over 50 per cent of that of inorganic iron salts. Liver, muscle, and haemoglobin iron are as well absorbed as iron salts added to food, but the iron of vegetables and eggs is poorly absorbed.

Disordered function

Malabsorption can be caused by a wide variety of disorders. In some of these, symptoms due to malabsorption will predominate (e.g. coeliac disease). In others, malabsorption may only constitute one facet of a

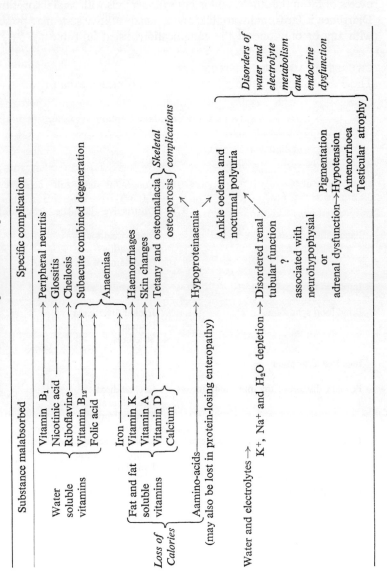

TABLE 12. Malabsorption and its sequelae

Substance malabsorbed	Specific complication
Water soluble vitamins { Vitamin B$_1$ → Peripheral neuritis	
Nicotinic acid → Glossitis	
Riboflavine → Cheilosis	
Vitamin B$_{12}$ → Subacute combined degeneration	
Folic acid →	
Iron → Anaemias	
Loss of Calories Fat and fat soluble vitamins { Vitamin K → Haemorrhages	
Vitamin A → Skin changes	
Vitamin D → Tetany and osteomalacia } *Skeletal complications*	
Calcium → osteoporosis ↗	
Aamino-acids → Hypoproteinaemia → Ankle oedema and nocturnal polyuria	
(may also be lost in protein-losing enteropathy)	
Water and electrolytes → K$^+$, Na$^+$ and H$_2$O depletion → Disordered renal tubular function ? associated with neurohypophysial or adrenal dysfunction → Hypotension	*Disorders of water and electrolyte metabolism and endocrine dysfunction*
Pigmentation	
Amenorrhoea	
Testicular atrophy	

disorder e.g. carcinoma of pancreas. 'Steatorrhoea' means only an excess of fat in the stools, and is not synonymous with 'malabsorption'. Diarrhoea is far from invariable, and a malabsorptive state may present with any or only one of the complications listed in Table 12.

CAUSES OF MALABSORPTION
These are listed in Table 13, which is by no means exhaustive.

TABLE 13. Causes of Malabsorption.

Disturbances of digestion	
Deficiency of bile	Congenital bile salt deficiency (rare)
	Obstructive jaundice (common)
Pancreatic disease	Mucoviscidosis
	Pancreatitis
	Carcinoma of the pancreas
Impaired mixing.	After gastric surgery
Blind loop syndrome.	Jejunal diverticula
	Fistulae
	Strictures
Impaired absorption	
Primary disease of the intestinal mucosa	Coeliac disease
	Idiopathic steatorrhoea
	Tropical sprue
Involvement of mucosa or mesenteric lymphatics in systemic diseases.	Crohn's disease
	Whipple's disease
	Lymphoma
Intestinal resection	
Miscellaneous	Neomycin
	Irradiation
Specific transport or metabolic defects	Pernicious anaemia
	Cystinuria and Hartnup disease
	Acanthocytosis
	Disaccharidase deficiency
	Glucose/galactose malabsorption

Disturbances of digestion

Malabsorption of fat or of the fat soluble vitamins D and K is the dominant defect, so that these disorders present with steatorrhoea, osteomalacia, or a bleeding tendency. Anaemia due to deficiency of iron, vitamin B_{12}, or folic acid is rare except after gastric surgery. Indeed, iron absorption tends to be excessive in the presence of pancreatic insufficiency.

Gastric surgery is now the commonest single cause of malabsorption from disturbances of digestion. The most severe disturbances result from a Polya type of operation, but no form of operative procedure for peptic ulcer is immune from this complication. By-passing the duodenum results in poor mixing of food with pancreatic juice and bile,and inadequate stimulation of secretin and pancreozymin release (p. 399). An associated vagotomy may also disturb pancreatic function. Steatorrhoea is mild unless there is associated pancreatic disease or a blind-loop syndrome, and any weight loss is largely due to reduced food intake. Absorption of inorganic iron is normal, but food iron is poorly absorbed, resulting in hypochromic anaemia. In addition, megaloblastic anaemia may occur because with the passage of time the mucosa of the gastric remnant tends to atrophy, causing intrinsic factor deficiency. Bone disease is the other major complication, and may take the form of either osteomalacia or osteoporosis (p. 321).

Disturbances of absorption
Blind-loop syndrome

A wide variety of pathological processes may result in this condition, e.g. strictures, jejunal diverticula, fistulae between different parts of the small intestine, gastro-colic fistula and, to a variable extent, partial gastrectomy. Common to all of these is stasis and consequent bacterial invasion of the normally sterile small bowel lumen. The resultant malabsorption affects particularly vitamin B_{12} and fat. Defective fat absorption is probably due to bacterial hydrolysis of conjugated bile salts to free bile acids and consequently to deficient micelle formation (p. 418). Vitamin B_{12} deficiency is probably due to direct competition between the host and the intestinal bacteria for the available vitamin. Both steatorrhoea and vitamin B_{12} absorption are improved by treatment with a broad spectrum antibiotic.

Primary disease of the intestinal mucosa.

In coeliac disease of children, and idiopathic steatorrhoea in adults the small bowel mucosa is abnormal in the duodenum and jejunum, and the ileum is normal or less severely affected. Any combination of the possible deficiencies indicated in Table 12 may be present, but folic acid deficiency is particularly common. A variable degree of functional and anatomical recovery follows the withdrawal of wheat gluten from the diet. Tropical sprue shows many similarities to idiopathic steatorrhoea, but the histological lesion, though usually less severe, extends throughout the whole length of the small bowel, and folic acid deficiency is invariable. A poor dietary intake of folic acid predisposes to the development of tropical sprue, and in its early stages the disease can be cured by additional folic acid. It does not respond to a gluten-free diet.

Involvement of mucosa or mesenteric lymphatics in systemic diseases. Here the primary disease often dominates the clinical picture. The precise absorptive defects vary according to the anatomical site and extent of the disease. In *Whipple's disease* the lamina propria and mesenteric lymph nodes are infiltrated by macrophages containing PAS positive material. This condition responds to a prolonged course of antibiotics and is probably due to a specific bacterial infection. *Intestinal lymphangiectasia* may be associated with abnormalities of lymphatics elsewhere in the body, such as lymphoedema of a limb: sclerotic lesions of the abdominal lymphatics cause dilatation of lacteals in the villi. Rupture of these into the bowel lumen can cause a protein-losing state (p. 407) and their rupture into the abdominal cavity may cause chylous ascites. There may also be malabsorption of fat, vitamin D, and calcium.

Intestinal resection

Limited resections of small bowel can be tolerated well, because the small bowel has a large reserve capacity, and because, with time, the remaining bowel increases its absorptive capacity. Resection of a sufficient amount of terminal ileum, however, results in complete inability to absorb vitamin B_{12}. Occasionally ileal resection also results in steatorrhoea, perhaps by interrupting the entero-hepatic circulation of bile salts (p. 434). Massive resection of small bowel results in considerable steatorrhoea, voluminous stools, and serious malnutrition. Although life can be maintained with 30–60 cm of small bowel, permanent restriction of dietary fat and supplementary vitamins will be needed. Crohn's disease may produce a similar result by its direct involvement of the mucosa in addition to affecting the mesenteric lymphatics and causing blind loops.

Miscellaneous

Antimitotic drugs and irradiation may seriously damage the small intestinal mucosa. Malabsorption is usually transient, but occasionally a chronic malabsorption syndrome results. Neomycin commonly induces steatorrhoea and other drugs, e.g. phenindione, do so rarely.

SPECIFIC TRANSPORT AND ENZYMATIC DEFECTS

These are rare with the exception of pernicious anaemia and perhaps disaccharidase deficiency, and their importance is chiefly because of the light they throw on normal mechanisms of absorption.

Transport defects

Several diseases are now known to be caused by the absence of specific active transport systems. Absence of the transport system for glucose and galactose results in profuse osmotic diarrhoea from birth, and is rapidly fatal unless fructose is substituted as the sole dietary carbohydrate. In cystinuria the small bowel shares with the renal tubule the inability to absorb dibasic amino acids. In Hartnup disease, both the kidneys and the small intestine fail to absorb neutral amino-acids. Even more rarely the small intestine may be unable to absorb tryptophan ('blue diaper syndrome'), or methionine ('oast-house syndrome').

Enzyme defects

Lactase deficiency is the commonest of these, and its frequency shows considerable racial variation. Sucrose and isomaltose intolerance always occur together for some reason, although these two disaccharides are split by separate enzymes. In adults lactase deficiency may be an acquired condition but its precise frequency and significance is disputed. Other enzymatic deficiencies can be shown in the small intestine, for example of aldolase in hereditary fructose intolerance, and of glucose-6-phosphatase in Type i glycogen storage disease. Enzyme determination in biopsy specimens may be useful diagnostically, but the clinical picture results from absence of the enzyme in the liver. Acanthocytosis is an excessively rare cause of fat malabsorption. The steatorrhoea probably occurs because there is a defect in lipoprotein synthesis so that the intestinal cell cannot make normal chylomicrons (p. 419). As a result absorbed triglyceride cannot escape from the mucosal cells and these are laden with fat. This condition is also characterized by crenated red cells (acanthocytes) and central nervous system abnormalities.

Principles of tests and measurements

TESTS OF ABSORPTION

METHODS INVOLVING STOOL COLLECTION

All methods based on stool measurements suffer from the difficulty of obtaining complete collections. Substances which are metabolized by bacteria in the colon, e.g. sugars, cannot be studied in this way.

Balance studies

The daily intake and daily excretion are measured, and the difference between the two taken as a measure of absorption.

Calcium absorption measured thus is a net figure as this element is secreted into the bowel as well as absorbed.

Fat absorption can be assessed adequately without accurate measurement of the intake, because due to the considerable absorptive reserve most normal individuals will excrete less than 5 g daily (of which about half is due to desquamated cells, bacteria, etc.) on fat intakes varying widely between 50–250 g. A borderline result can be clarified by repeating the test on a high (150 g) fat diet, but normally a 3–5 day stool collection on the usual ward diet (50–100 g fat) is adequate.

Radio-isotope studies

A radioactively labelled compound is given by mouth, and the amount excreted in the stools is subtracted from the oral dose. This technique has been successfully used to study calcium and iron absorption, but the result can vary widely according to the salt used, and whether it is given fasting or with a meal. For technical reasons, particularly the purity of the labelled compound used, the absorption of triolein labelled with radioactive iodine has proved unsatisfactory as an indication of fat malabsorption.

OTHER METHODS

Measurement of blood concentrations after an oral load

The glucose tolerance test is the most familiar example of this method, and also illustrates its drawbacks. As a test of absorption it is very dependent on variables such as gastric emptying and tissue uptake.

Nevertheless similar tests have been used to study the absorption of vitamin A, iron and radioactively labelled vitamin B_{12}. Normal increases in blood sugar after 50 g of the appropriate disaccharide orally rules out deficiency of the corresponding disaccharidase. If a flat curve is obtained the test must be repeated using the constituent monosaccharides to ensure that the mucosa is capable of absorbing these.

An ingenious and accurate modification for the study of iron absorption which overcomes variations which might be due to variable iron utilization can be performed by giving known doses of two different isotopes (Fe^{55} and Fe^{59}) simultaneously, one orally and one intravenously. The assumption that absorbed iron and intravenously administered iron are utilized identically enables absorption to be accurately calculated by determining the relative quantities of the two isotopes incorporated in red cell haemoglobin after an interval of 10 days.

Measurement of excretion in the urine after an oral dose
The ideal substance for this test should be neither metabolized nor stored in the body, and should be rapidly excreted in the urine. The amount excreted in the urine would then equal the amount absorbed from the gut. The pentose sugar xylose (p. 417) is not ideal, as it is to some extent metabolized and is partially reabsorbed in the renal tubule but the excretion of less than 4·5 g in the 5 hr after an oral dose of 25 g is in practice a valuable indication of malabsorption. In an unmodified form this type of test cannot be applied to vitamin B_{12} absorption, as the vitamin is largely taken up by the liver. In the Schilling test, liver deposition is minimized by giving a very large (1 mg) intramuscular 'flushing' dose of non-radioactive vitamin B_{12} at the same time as the small (0·5 μg) oral dose of radioactive vitamin. Under these circumstances more than 15 per cent of the oral dose is excreted in the urine in 24 hr in normal people. In pernicious anaemia the low or absent absorption can be corrected by giving intrinsic factor orally. In the blind-loop syndrome (p. 423) the low absorption may be partially corrected by a course of antibiotics. As B_{12} excretion depends on the glomerular filtration rate, a low result must always be checked by measuring the creatinine clearance, even if the blood urea is normal. Another modification of this type of test is used to study folic acid absorption. The urine excretion of an oral dose is compared with that of a parenteral dose given on another day.

All tests of this type are invalidated by poor renal function, and for this reason are often unreliable in elderly subjects.

External and whole body counting after oral administration of an isotope
An alternative method of assessing absorption of Co^{59}–vitamin B_{12} is
to count the radioactivity over the liver after oral administration. A
quantitative measurement of absorption can only be made by measuring
the retained radioactivity in the whole body, and this has also been used
to study absorption of calcium and iron. This method has the advantage
of being independent of the hazards of incomplete stool collection
and abnormal renal function, but needs costly apparatus.

Direct sampling of intestinal contents
Intubation of the small intestine enables the disappearance of nutrients
from the lumen after a standard meal to be studied directly. If a double

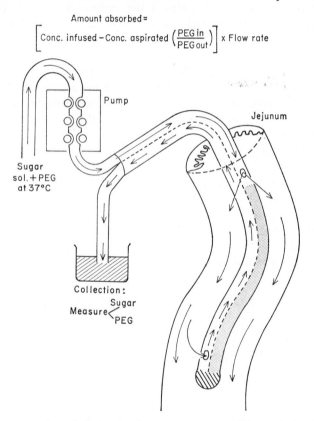

FIGURE 45. *A method for the direct measurement of intestinal absorption
in man.*

(From Holdsworth C.D. and Dawson A.M. *Clin. Sci.* 27, 371, 1964.)

lumen tube is used, a short length of intestine can be perfused, and absorption measured directly (Fig. 45). A non-absorbable solute such as polyethylene-glycol(PEG)(MW 4000) must be included to correct for net water absorption in any investigation of this type. As no non-absorbable marker has yet been developed which is miscible with fat, the application of these techniques is limited to water-soluble nutrients such as sugars and amino acids.

Practical assessment

Clinical observations

Diarrhoea, nutritional disturbance (Table 12). History: onset at weaning, remission at puberty (idiopathic steatorrhoea), abdominal pain, diabetes (pancreatitis), operations (gastric surgery, blind loops).

Routine methods

Assess deficiencies: blood film, serum B_{12}, folic acid, calcium, phosphorus, alkaline phosphatase, proteins, iron, and bone X-rays. Test absorption: faecal fat, xylose excretion. Exclude anatomical abnormality: Biopsy, barium follow through.

Special techniques

Absorption of folic acid, vitamin B_{12}, iron, calcium. Pancreatic and liver function tests. Biochemical assay of biopsy specimens. Urinary indicant for small gut bacterial activity.

References

General:
DAVENPORT H.W. (1965) *Physiology of the Digestive Tract.* (2nd. ed.). Chicago: Year Book Med. Publs. Inc.

JONES F., AVERY & GUMMER J.W.P. (1960) *Clinical Gastro-Enterology.* Oxford: Blackwell.

TRUELOVE S.C. & REYNELL, P.C. (1963) *Diseases of the Digestive System.* Oxford: Blackwell.

INGELFINGER F.J. (1958) Esophageal Motility. *Physiol. Rev.* **38,** 533–584.

CODE C.F. (1958) *An Atlas of Esophageal Motility in Health and Disease.* Springfield, Ill: Thomas.

HUNT J.N. (1959) Gastric Emptying and Secretion in Man. *Physiol. Rev.* **39,** 491–533.

TRUELOVE S.C. (1966) Movements of the Large Intestine. *Physiol. Rev.* **46,** 457–512.

Secretion:
BABKIN B.P. (1950) *Secretory Mechanisms of the Digestive Glands.* (2nd. ed.). New York: Hoeber.

430 *Clinical Physiology*

JAMES A.H. (1957) *The Physiology of Gastric Digestion*. London: Arnold.

GREGORY R.A. (1962) *Secretory Mechanisms of the Gastro-Intestinal Tract*. London: Arnold.

BARON J.H. (1964) Measurement and Nomenclature of Gastric Acid. *Gastroenterology*, **45**, 118–121.

KAY A.W. (1953) Effect of Large Doses of Histamine on Gastric Secretion of HCl. *Br. Med. J:* ii, 77–80.

DE RUIECK A.V.S. & CAMERON M.P. (1962). *The Exocrine Pancreas*. London: Churchill.

Absorption:

WILSON T.H. (1962) *Intestinal Absorption*. Philadelphia: Saunders.

WISEMAN G. (1964) *Absorption from the Intestine*. London: Academic Press.

BADENOCH J. (1960) Steatorrhoea in the Adult. *Br. Med. J*. ii, 879–887; 963–974.

LASTER L. & INGELFINGER F.J. (1961) Intestinal Absorption: Aspects of Structure, Function and Disease of the Small-Intestine Mucosa. *New Engl. J. Med.* **264**, 1138–1148; 1192–1200; 1246–1253.

DAWSON A.M. (1965) Malabsorption. *Abst. World Med.* **38**, 361–381.

The Liver

Normal function

ANATOMY

The liver is a mass of cells traversed by a labyrinth of tunnel systems. Eighty-five per cent of cells are parenchymal in type. The life of rat liver cells is between 200 and 450 days. Rapid cell-replication occurs after partial removal of the liver in man and animals. This may be controlled by a circulating hormonal regulator.

There are two main tunnel systems in the liver. Portal and hepatic central canals run at right angles and do not communicate. Portal canals contain bile ductules, hepatic arterioles, and radicles of portal veins which connect through thin-walled sinusoids to central veins. These veins and surrounding connective tissue form the central canals. Hepatic arterioles form plexuses around bile ductules and supply portal tracts, thereafter entering sinusoids at different levels. In man, the portal triad of hepatic arteriole, portal venule and bile ductule together with surrounding liver cells make up a functional unit. If the liver is injured by hypoxia or poisons such as carbon tetrachloride damage is first seen at the periphery of such units. Lobules consisting of a central vein surrounded by liver cells and portal areas are seen in certain animals such as the pig but do not occur in man.

The walls of hepatic sinusoids are formed by endothelial cells and phagocytic cells of the reticulo-endothelial system called Küpffer cells (see Chapter 7).

The excretory system of the liver starts with bile canaliculi. These are intercellular spaces bounded by two or more liver cells from whose cytoplasm they are separated only by a single membrane. Protrusion of this membrane into the canaliculus results in the formation of a microvillus which augments the area available for interchange. Canaliculi form networks around individual liver cells and drain into thin-walled cholangioles which enter bile ductules in portal canals.

The portal areas are surrounded by connective tissue which joins up with the liver capsule.

HEPATIC AND PORTAL CIRCULATION

The total liver bloodflow in hepatic artery and portal vein is about 1·5 l./min. Between a third and a fifth of this blood is carried by the hepatic artery and is 100 per cent saturated with oxygen. The remaining fraction is carried by the portal vein and is 80–90 per cent saturated. The total oxygen consumption of the liver is 55 ml/min of which 70 per cent is provided by the portal system. During digestion, portal venous oxygenation decreases due to increased intestinal utilization of oxygen and flow increases by one third.

Approximately 60 per cent of portal venous blood is derived from the superior mesenteric vein which drains the small and part of the large intestine and the head of the pancreas. The remainder comes from the splenic vein which drains the stomach, pancreas and spleen and part of the large bowel. These two main streams are well mixed in man so that all parts of the liver receive the same blood. In animals only partial mixing occurs; blood from the superior mesenteric vein passes mainly to the right lobe of the liver and that from the splenic to the left. Para-umbilical veins in man run from the anterior abdominal wall to the left main branch of the portal vein. They are the counterpart of the foetal umbilical vein. The pressure in the portal system is normally between 5 and 13 mm Hg. It depends upon the relative resistances at either end of the venous bed and the flow through it. Portal venous blood mixes freely with high pressure arterial blood in hepatic sinusoids.

The hepatic veins are formed from central veins. These join sublobular veins which then merge into the hepatic veins proper. Hepatic venous pressure is about 6 mmHg and the blood is normally two-thirds saturated with oxygen.

Sphincters exist in all vascular components in the liver. They regulate the local contributions of hepatic artery and portal vein as well as total liver bloodflow and the capacity of the portal venous bed. This can accommodate up to one-third of the total blood volume. The splanchnic vessels may therefore play a major part in regulation of the general circulation. Despite these vascular regulating mechanisms, total liver bloodflow is not as well protected from changes in the systemic circulation as renal bloodflow because renal autoregulation is more effective (p. 151).

The liver produces 0·75 ml of lymph/min. Its protein content is 90 per cent of that of plasma. Forty per cent of the total plasma protein pool is returned to the blood each 24 hr. through hepatic lymphatics. These vessels communicate freely with the sinusoids.

METABOLISM AND EXCRETION OF BILE

Bile is an isotonic, viscous, golden-yellow fluid. Some 500–1000 ml are secreted by the liver every 24 hr. It is essential for the digestion and absorption of lipids (see Chapter 11) and is the route of excretion for some substances which are poorly excreted by the kidney.

The main constituents of bile can be grouped according to the degree to which they are concentrated. Bile pigments and salts and excretory products of steroid and other hormones (see Chapter 15) are present in concentrations up to a thousand times greater than in blood. They are secreted by an active transport mechanism whose energy requirements are derived from the metabolism of glucose. A large number of different substances, notably organic anions, are probably also actively secreted into the bile. These include various phenolphthalein derivatives (including bromsulphthalein: p. 457), salicylate, a number of antibiotic drugs, and indocyanine green (p. 462). Active transport of bile acids (accompanied by an equivalent number of cations) into the canalicular lumen may provide the osmotic driving force for movement of water and diffusible solute into the bile. The secretion pressure of bile is sometimes much greater than that of blood perfusing the liver, thus excluding ordinary hydrostatic filtration as the mechanism of bile formation. Bile salts given by mouth cause a marked choleresis (flow of bile). In animals, bile flow rates and excretion of chloride and bicarbonate are directly proportional to the excretion of the bile salt taurocholate. The osmotic activity and choleretic potency of several actively secreted compounds can be correlated.

Other substances such as sodium, potassium, chloride and calcium are present in approximately the same concentration as in blood. Active transport of the inorganic ions sodium and potassium almost certainly occurs, and accounts at least in part for their appearance in bile. Marked elevations of bicarbonate concentration in bile follow release of the hormone secretin from the duodenum (see Chapter 11). Secretin increases the volume of bile secreted, but is less choleretic than bile acids. It also stimulates active secretion of inorganic ions into the bile. The site of action is probably the bile ductules and ducts themselves. Bile flow may also be subject to nervous control.

Cholesterol is present in bile in lower concentrations than in the blood as are phospholipids, phosphate and glucose. Other substances found in small amounts include vitamin B_{12}, nucleoprotein, mucin, alkaline phosphatase, triglycerides and free fatty acids. Plasma proteins are present in very low concentrations because of the relative impermeability of canalicular membranes for large molecules.

Bile is stored in the gall-bladder where it is concentrated 5–10 times. This is the major site of reabsorption of water and electrolytes. Water reabsorption is coupled with active solute transport, and is inhibited by cyanide. The gall-bladder does not function unless sodium is present. Active reabsorptive processes probably also occur in the main bile ducts. Bile salts and pigments and cholesterol are not reabsorbed to any appreciable extent. The viscosity of bile increases in the gall-bladder which secretes a thick mucinous material.

Passage of bile into the duodenum results from simultaneous contraction of the gall-bladder and relaxation of the sphincter of Oddi and second part of the duodenum. Stimulation for this is release of the hormone cholecystokinin from the intestine upon the entry of food. The role of nervous control of gall-bladder and biliary function is not clear. The vagus may affect gall-bladder tone and is probably the mediator of contractions following emotional stimuli. Emptying of the gall-bladder in man is, however, unaffected by section of the vagi. Peristaltic waves occur in the common bile-duct which contains a varying amount of smooth muscle.

Physiology of bile constituents

Bile pigments. About 300 mg of *bilirubin* is produced daily in the adult. The majority is formed from the protoporphyrin moiety of haemoglobin released from effete red cells, but as much as 20 per cent may arise from other sources. The bone marrow and the liver itself produce this pigment which has been called 'early' bilirubin.

Bilirubin is transported in the plasma tightly bound to albumin. It is taken up by liver cells where 80 per cent is conjugated in microsomes under the action of the enzyme glucuronyl transferase to yield the diglucuronide. Bilirubin monoglucuronide and sulphate are also formed in animals but are of unproven importance in man. Conjugated bilirubin is actively secreted by the liver cell into the bile canaliculi. Uptake and excretion of bilirubin by the liver cell involve separate mechanisms.

Bacterial action in the lower bowel converts bilirubin to urobilinogen. This is largely reabsorbed into portal blood and returned to the liver for re-excretion. This process is called enterohepatic circulation. A small amount of pigment (1–2 mg daily) enters the systemic circulation and appears in the urine as urobilinogen and that remaining in the gut is converted to stercobilin which colours the faeces brown.

Bile acids are sterols formed by metabolism of cholesterol in the liver. Approximately 700 mg is formed daily. The two main compounds are cholic and chenodeoxycholic acids. Cholic acid, the most important compound, is conjugated in liver cells to form glycocholic and taurocholic acids which appear in the bile as sodium or potassium salts. Approximately 90 per cent of bile acids excreted in the bile undergo enterohepatic circulation with a cycle time of 8–16 hr. The remainder is lost in the faeces. Hepatic synthesis rate is closely regulated to the amount lost and the total amount circulating is virtually constant.

Cholesterol is a steroid alcohol found in many different tissue cells. Approximately 140 g is present in man. It is produced largely in the liver and to a lesser extent in kidneys and adrenals. 1–2 g is formed daily. The rate of synthesis is governed by a negative feed-back system. A cholesterol-lipoprotein complex acts upon cell microsomes and inhibits synthesis of cholesterol. In malignant hepatomas this feed-back system is absent. Administration of cholate suppresses the rate of synthesis and drainage of bile by way of a fistula increases it.

Ingested cholesterol, which is normally very much less in amount than that synthesized daily, is absorbed from the intestine along with other lipids. Fat and bile acids in the gut enhance absorption and plant sterols decrease it. Polyunsaturated fats given by mouth lower plasma cholesterol levels but the dietary intake of cholesterol has little effect upon plasma concentrations.

The chief route of excretion is into the gut by way of the bile or through mucosal cells. 1–2 g of cholesterol appears in the bile every 24 hr. The chief route of catabolism is oxidation to cholic acids (mainly in the liver), but a small amount is used for the synthesis of hormones in the gonads and adrenals (see Chapter 15). Two per cent of total body cholesterol is replaced in 24 hr. In the plasma, 75 per cent of cholesterol is combined with fatty acids as esters and is maintained in solution by phospholipids.

METABOLISM OF PROTEIN, CARBOHYDRATE AND FAT
Protein
The liver cell is the site of production of most plasma proteins except the immunoglobulins (p. 272). Proteins are formed in ribosomes on the rough endoplasmic reticulum which forms parallel tubes in contact with extracellular fluid. The proteins may leave the liver cell either by way of these structures or by reversal of the process of pinocytosis.

Albumin is the protein found in highest concentration in the plasma.

15

The total body pool is 250 g of which 40 per cent is intra-vascular and is responsible for approximately 70 per cent of plasma colloidal osmotic pressure (see Chapter 1). Each day 10 per cent of this fraction undergoes catabolism. The liver produces 10–12 g of albumin daily and approximately one-sixth of the dietary intake of nitrogen is utilized in this way. Factors controlling the rate of albumin synthesis are unknown. The plasma concentration alone is not responsible. An artificially induced fall in the plasma level following intravenous dextran infusion does not lead to an increased rate of synthesis and may even lower it. The rate of synthesis may be regulated by some function of colloidal osmotic pressure.

A number of plasma globulins are produced in the liver. The hepatic parenchymal cell is the site of formation of α_2-, β-, and some α_1-globulins. γ-globulins are made in the reticulo-endothelial system outside the liver (p. 272). Liver cells produce proteins important in the binding of hormones such as cortisol and oestrogen in the plasma. Others bind inorganic ions. Thus the β-globulin transferrin is involved in iron transport (Chapter 6) while the α_2-globulin caeruloplasmin plays an important role in the transport of copper in the plasma. The α_2- and β-globulins contain the lipoproteins.

The liver is probably also the sole site of production of other important plasma proteins including prothrombin, fibrinogen and other blood coagulation factors (see Chapter 6).

Degradation of amino-acids occurs mainly in the liver, where α-keto-acids and ammonia are formed. An alternative pathway is the transfer of amino-groups from amino-acids to α-keto-acids (transamination: see Chapter 13). Ammonia is converted to urea in the liver by the Krebs urea cycle (see Chapter 13). It may also be removed by the peripheral tissues, where it is converted to glutamic acid and glutamine, and by the kidney where its excretion is by non-ionic diffusion as it is a weak base.

Carbohydrate

Most of the galactose and about half the glucose absorbed from the intestine are metabolized in the liver. D-glucose undergoes phosphorylation to glucose-6-phosphate and this may be followed by conversion to uridine diphosphate glucose (UDP-glucose). This compound is involved in glucose-galactose interconversion and the synthesis of glycogen. It is also the precursor of UDP-glucuronic acid which is important in the conjugation of bilirubin and other substances (434 and 457). Glucose-6-phosphate in the liver may also be metabolized by way of the Krebs citric acid cycle and alternative pathways more fully discussed elsewhere (see Chapter 13). Glucose may also be formed in the liver from amino-, fatty and lactic acids as well as from other sugars. Fructose is phosphorylated by fructokinase.

The polymer glycogen is formed in the liver from glucose and other monosaccharides. Breakdown of this substance (glycogenolysis) by several different enzymes makes glucose available. The two processes are of importance in regulation of the blood sugar level (see Chapter 13).

Fat

The liver oxidizes a proportion of absorbed triglyceride, releasing energy in the form of ATP (see Chapter 13). It also converts unused free fatty acids (FFA), released from fat depots to meet energy requirements, to triglyceride and other lipids. The enzyme liver lipase hydrolyses neutral fat to glycerol and FFA. Glycerol is then utilized via the pathways of carbohydrate metabolism (see Chapter 13). FFA are oxidized to acetyl-Co-A units which undergo complete oxidation or recombine to form acetoacetic acid. The liver itself is unable to further metabolize this compound which is one of the 'ketone bodies'. When carbohydrate intake is deficient, metabolism of fat in the liver is increased. A small proportion is converted into glucose or glycogen.

The liver is a fat depot (see Chapter 13). Neutral fat accounts for 5 per cent of its bulk by weight. This proportion is increased when the diet is rich in fat but deficient in so-called lipotropic factors such as choline and methionine essential for its mobilization from the liver. It is also increased in starvation and in diabetes mellitus.

Fat-soluble vitamins A, D and K are stored in the liver.

METABOLISM AND DETOXICATION OF HORMONES AND DRUGS

The liver is the site of degradation of steroid hormones. Synthesis of cortisol, controlled through the hypothalamo-pituitary axis (see Chapter 14), is balanced by breakdown in the liver. Testosterone is also removed from the blood by the liver where rapid conjugation occurs. The metabolism of oestrogens is similarly primarily hepatic. Conjugated, partially-metabolized substances are excreted in the bile and undergo enterohepatic circulation (p. 434). Following absorption, the compounds are largely re-excreted in the bile, but some enter the systemic circulation and undergo renal excretion. About 80 per cent of oestradiol and oestrone eventually appears in the urine as conjugates or degradation products. Approximately one-fifth is present as oestradiol-17β, oestrone and oestriol. Antidiuretic hormone (vasopressin) is probably also removed from the circulation by the liver. Its subsequent metabolic pathway is not clear.

Some naturally occurring compounds, such as phenols and skatols, and many drugs cannot be excreted by the kidney until they are rendered more polar, i.e. water-soluble. This process takes place in liver cells under the influence of a number of enzymes including those producing conjugation and hydroxylation. Enzymes are bound to hepatic microsomes and are in life present in the endoplasmic reticulum. In the newly-born child microsomal enzymes are not fully developed. This explains the sensitivity of the very young to certain drugs, e.g. chloramphenicol, which are detoxicated by a conjugating enzyme system. Diminished oxidation of drugs by the endoplasmic reticulum occurs during gluco-corticoid deficiency and in the presence of thyroxine excess. Competition by two drugs for microsomal enzymes may also occur.

The enzymatic degradation of drugs may be stimulated by the prior administration of a different agent. Induction of the non-specific microsomal enzymes is then said to have occurred. The drug pheno-barbitone, for example, increases the rate of hepatic detoxication of steroidal compounds and anticoagulant drugs. This is of practical importance as the person receiving these compounds may become tolerant to them.

IRON METABOLISM
The liver is the major site of storage of body iron. This is fully discussed elsewhere (see Chapter 6).

Disordered function

DISORDERS OF THE HEPATIC AND PORTAL
VENOUS CIRCULATION
Occlusion of the hepatic artery causes deepening jaundice and death in liver failure (p. 444). Obstruction of the main hepatic veins causes hepatocellular dysfunction and occasionally failure. Portal hypertension (p. 439) may develop. Hepatic venous obstruction is usually due to malignant disease but less severe obstruction results from raised inferior vena caval pressure as in congestive heart failure or constrictive disease of the pericardium (see Chapter 2).

Haemodynamic changes in cirrhosis
Nodular regeneration of the liver parenchyma and extensive fibrosis are hallmarks of cirrhosis. Sinusoids are encroached upon or destroyed

and short communicating vessels develop between portal and central hepatic veins. One quarter of the blood perfusing the liver may pass through such channels and by-pass the nodules. These receive almost all of their blood from the hepatic artery.

Portal hypertension

Presinusoidal. This form of portal hypertension exists when the pressure in the portal venous system and spleen is raised but sinusoidal pressure is normal. It may result from thrombosis or obstruction of the splenic or main portal veins (extrahepatic obstruction) or from intrahepatic obstruction in portal areas.

Postsinusoidal. Obstruction to flow above the sinusoids is largely responsible for the portal hypertension of cirrhosis. Regenerating nodules exert pressure in these areas and on sinusoids themselves so that a sinusoidal element also exists. Anastomoses between hepatic arterioles and abnormal intrahepatic venous channels (p. 440) contribute to the hypertension. Sometimes hepatic arterial blood passes retrogradely down the portal vein by way of these channels. Hepatic venous obstruction also causes postsinusoidal portal hypertension.

Primary portal hypertension. This is said to exist when portal pressure is elevated in the absence of demonstrable obstruction. In the ill-understood condition idiopathic tropical splenomegaly, portal hypertension is associated with high splenic and hepatic arterial flow. Postsinusoidal resistance is normal. Presinusoidal resistance is elevated in half of the patients. The reason for the two groups is obscure. In those patients where presinusoidal resistance is normal the portal hypertension is cured by splenectomy. Increased arterial inflow may be of greater importance in the pathophysiology of portal hypertension than previously believed.

Effects of portal hypertension

Raised portal pressure causes splenic enlargement. Collateral venous channels, by-passing the liver, appear around the lower end of the oesophagus and on the anterior abdominal wall where peri-umbilical veins (or a patent umbilical vein remnant) communicate with systemic venous channels. Communicating vessels penetrate the capsules of the spleen and liver and run to the diaphragm while others join renal and lumbar veins. The extent of the collateral circulation cannot be correlated with the degree of elevation of portal pressure. Extensive collateral veins may reduce portal pressure to normal, while hypertension of short duration can exist without a demonstrable collateral circulation.

Long-standing deprivation of portal blood supply, consequent upon venous obstruction or diversion of flow through collateral channels, renders the liver more dependent upon hepatic arterial oxygen. Although it diminishes in size, however, its ability to regenerate following partial hepatectomy is unimpaired. A small liver is often associated with extensive collateral venous channels.

Portal hypertension contributes to the formation of ascites (p. 449). Collateral channels form a means whereby substances absorbed from the intestine, including those believed to be responsible for portal-systemic encephalopathy (p. 446), can by-pass the liver. Prolonged engorgement of the spleen results in hyperactivity of its reticulo-endothelial cells and pancytopenia may develop (see Chapter 6). The low platelet count in portal hypertension is due in part to increased splenic removal but impaired release from the bone marrow is more important. Purpura is, however, rare in uncomplicated portal hypertension and usually signifies concurrent hepatic dysfunction with impaired synthesis of coagulation factors (p. 255). The most important clinical manifestation of portal hypertension is bleeding from oesophageal or gastric varices. The tendency to haemorrhage correlates roughly with the height of portal pressure; the mere presence of collateral vessels does not usually result in bleeding. They may persist for years following surgical relief of portal hypertension without haemorrhage occurring. Rapid increase in portal pressure caused, for example, by intravenous infusion of blood or fluid may precipitate haemorrhage. Coagulation defects aggravate bleeding from these vessels but are rarely the sole cause.

Effects of portacaval anastomosis

There are two main forms of operation. In end-to-side anastomosis the portal vein is completely divided and joined to the inferior vena cava. The hepatic end of the vein is ligated. The liver is then entirely dependent upon the hepatic artery for its blood supply. Total hepatic blood-flow is reduced but oxygen supply to the liver is maintained by increased extraction. Arterial-hepatic venous oxygen content differences are increased. Postsinusoidal resistance, calculated from the ratio of postsinusoidal pressure (p. 460) to blood flow, is unchanged and postsinusoidal obstruction is unrelieved by this operation. In side-to-side anastomosis the normal anatomy of the portal vein itself is preserved. Total hepatic bloodflow again falls. As blood can leave the liver through the patent portal vein, post-sinusoidal resistance is relieved. This would clearly be advantageous but diversion of hepatic arterial blood in this way may have a deleterious effect upon the nodules it supplies.

The incidence of mental changes (p. 446) in cirrhosis is much greater in patients who have undergone surgical portacaval anastomosis. Permanent neurological damage occurs most commonly in these patients. (p.446). There may be heavy deposition of iron in the liver (p. 449). An increased incidence of peptic ulceration may be related to the by-passing of hepatic histaminase by portal blood containing histamine, with resulting hyperchlorhydria. The explanation for the increased haemolysis and jaundice which may follow portacaval surgery is obscure. Most of these phenomena associated with man-made portacaval anastomosis may occur equally well when large naturally-occurring venous 'shunts' are present.

DISORDERS OF BILIRUBIN METABOLISM: JAUNDICE

When the bilirubin concentration in the plasma is elevated, yellow staining of the tissues occurs. This coloration, or jaundice, is most easily seen in the sclerae and is first detectable clinically when the plasma concentration exceeds about 2 mg/100 ml.

There are three main ways in which elevations of plasma bilirubin can occur:

1. The rate of production may be increased because of haemolysis (see Chapter 6) or when increased amounts of haem or other haemoglobin precursors are converted directly to bilirubin.

2. Transit of bilirubin through the liver cells may be impaired. This occurs when the cells themselves are damaged, as in parenchymatous jaundice, or because of specific defects in the mechanisms of uptake, transport or conjugation.

3. The rate of excretion of bilirubin by the liver cells may be hindered either by changes up to the level of bile canaliculi (intrahepatic cholestasis) or when the large bile ducts are blocked (obstructive jaundice).

A combination of these factors is often present. For example, in jaundice due to obstruction of main bile ducts, secondary changes in liver cells soon occur and red cell survival (see Chapter 6) is usually reduced.

Haemolytic jaundice

The excess bilirubin in the plasma is unconjugated. It is protein bound and does not appear in the urine. The hepatic output of bile pigment is increased which predisposes to gallstone formation. Unconjugated bilirubin has great affinity for lipids and is taken up by the brain where it may cause severe damage (kernicterus) if plasma levels exceed 20 mg/100 ml. This occurs in haemolytic disease of the newborn (see Chapter 6). The jaundice is accentuated by impaired conjugation in the immature liver. In the presence of drugs such as salicylates and sulphonamides which displace unconjugated bilirubin from binding sites on albumin, kernicterus may develop in the presence of relatively low plasma bilirubin levels. Other drugs such as novobiocin intensify jaundice in the newborn by competing for glucuronyl transferase. Yet others, such as water-soluble vitamin K, if given in large doses to infants make jaundice more severe in an unknown way.

In the absence of haemolysis, the bone marrow may produce bilirubin too rapidly. This occurs in certain families and is responsible for so-called primary 'shunt' hyperbilirubinaemia. In this condition, haem in the marrow is converted directly to bilirubin without being incorporated in red cells. The term 'shunt' is used to imply this short-circuiting of the usual metabolic processes. When erythropoiesis is ineffective, as in pernicious anaemia (see Chapter 6), increased amounts of bilirubin are produced from haemoglobin in the marrow.

When jaundice is due to an increased rate of bilirubin production, the output of urobilinogen and stercobilinogen is increased.

Parenchymatous jaundice

Parenchymatous jaundice can best be considered in relation to the various metabolic processes occurring during passage of bilirubin through the liver cell.

Decreased uptake of bilirubin is responsible for the unconjugated hyperbilirubinaemia of the familial Gilbert's disease. Conjugation of test substances such as salicylamide is unimpaired. Liver cells appear normal and the patients are healthy. The plasma bilirubin level rarely exceeds 3 mg/100 ml. Decreased hepatic uptake of bilirubin may also occur when male-fern is used to treat tape-worm infestation.

Failure of conjugation of bilirubin in liver cells is responsible for the so-called 'physiological' jaundice appearing soon after birth. It is due to deficiency of glucuronyl transferase in the immature liver. Progesta-tional steroids in human milk may cause prolonged hyperbilirubinaemia in newborn babies These substances inhibit conjugation. Jaundice also occurs when they are administered in purified form. Congenital absence of glucuronyl transferase causes severe unconjugated hyperbilirubinaemia in the familial Crigler–Najjar syndrome. Kernicterus is common. The drug novobiocin may also cause jaundice by inhibition of conjugation.

In the commonest forms of parenchymatous jaundice such as virus hepatitis, and cirrhiasis, hyperbilirubinaemia is due to a combination of disorders. Transport of bilirubin across the liver cell is reduced, conjugation is probably impaired and intrahepatic cholestasis may be severe. In addition, a mild degree of haemolysis is almost invariably present. If the ability to form bilirubin conjugates is maintained, excess 'direct' reacting pigment (p. 451) is detected in blood and urine. Conjugated bilirubin in the plasma is largely bound to albumin. The quantity of bile pigments reaching the intestine is often reduced so that the stools are pale. Failure of liver cells to excrete absorbed urobilinogen leads to its appearance in excess in the urine.

'Obstructive' jaundice

Intrahepatic cholestasis describes interference with bile flow anywhere along the pathway from the liver microsomes, where conjugation occurs (p. 433), to the main bile ducts. It does not include organic obstruction of these major channels. The major causes of this condition may be classified anatomically as shown in Table 14.

TABLE 14

Level of obstruction	Condition	Comment
Hepatocellular	Virus hepatitis Alcoholic hepatitis Cirrhosis	Mechanism unknown. Plasma bilirubin level lowered by corticosteroid drugs (p. 459).
Canalicular and pericanalicular	Steroid induced Methyltestosterone	(and many other ^{17}C substituted compounds of testosterone)
	Pregnancy Hodgkin's disease	Probably due to a naturally-occurring hormone.
Ductular	Sensitivity-type jaundice Chlorpromazine Idiopathic recurrent cholestasis	
Larger ductules, interlobular and septal ducts	Primary biliary cirrhosis Intrahepatic biliary atresia	

Defective excretion of conjugated bilirubin is responsible for the familial Dubin-Johnson and Rotor syndromes. Other substances which undergo conjugation such as bromsulphthalein and cholecystographic

15*

media are also retained. Classical cholestasis with pruritus and hyper-cholesterolaemia does not, however, occur (p. 456). The congenital defect is probably within the liver cell and occurs before bile is presented for canalicular excretion.

Obstruction of main bile ducts, usually due to gallstones, fibrous stricture or growth, results in similar changes to those seen in intrahepatic cholestasis.

Jaundice appears in the majority of cases. The bilirubin in the plasma is chiefly in the conjugated form. Accumulation of bile salts in the circulation causes pruritus. In the absence of complete biliary obstruc-tion this may be relieved by oral administration of cholestyramine resin which absorbs bile salts entering the bowel, thus preventing their entero-hepatic circulation.

The urine contains bile pigments; its urobilinogen content is reduced in proportion to the degree of obstruction. If this is complete, sterco-bilinogen is not produced in the bowel and urobilinogen disappears from the urine. The faeces become pale and bulky due to decreased excretion of bile pigments and salts. In chronic obstruction steatorrhoea is proportional to the depth of jaundice. Secondary effects arise from malabsorption of fat soluble vitamins A, D and K and calcium from the intestine. A combination of osteomalacia and osteoporosis (see Chapter 8) is produced if the obstruction is prolonged. There may be marked hypercholesterolaemia (p. 456), resulting in cutaneous xan-thomata.

When main bile-ducts are obstructed, bile of normal composition and volume continues to be secreted until pressure in the biliary tree is greater than about 25 mm Hg. The time required for this level to be reached depends upon the presence and condition of the gall-bladder. If this is absent or functionless, biliary pressure rises rapidly. The function of liver cells is affected after as little as 24 hr. complete obstruc-tion. Bile formed after this time is normal in volume but contains very little of its normal constituents (p. 433) and is virtually colourless. Obstruction of main ducts causes dilatation of the biliary tree. The gall-bladder becomes distended if the obstruction is below the junction of cystic and common hepatic ducts.

DISORDERED LIVER CELL FUNCTION AND HEPATIC FAILURE

In view of the many metabolic processes occurring in the liver it might be assumed that hepatic disease would lead to widespread disturbances and serious ill-health. Such is not necessarily the case. This is due chiefly to the great reserve capacity and regenerative powers of the liver. In addition, other tissues and organs may take over some of the liver's functions. For example, despite the extensive part played by the liver in carbohydrate metabolism (p. 436), significant alterations in blood glucose levels are rare in hepatic disorders.

When particular parameters of liver function are abnormal it is best to speak of 'disordered liver function'. The terms 'hepatic failure' and 'hepatic decompensation' are reserved for the more serious clinical manifestations of impaired hepatocellular function in the form of jaundice, ascites, haemorrhagic phenomena and neuropsychiatric changes. These features may result from a variety of disease processes affecting the liver. They may be acute or chronic and are in no way specific for any one cause.

Disordered bilirubin metabolism
See p. 441.

Disordered protein metabolism
Decreased albumin synthesis results in lowered plasma levels in severe hepatocellular disease. Changes in plasma concentration occur relatively slowly and do not at once reflect acute functional impairment of the liver. A complete halt in albumin synthesis would result in a fall of only 25 per cent in the plasma level by the end of a week. The rate of catabolism of albumin is reduced in proportion to the plasma concentration. Hypo-albuminaemia is a factor in the production of fluid retention (p. 449). If hepatic dysfunction is marked the nails become white due to opacity of the nail-bed. The severity of the changes correlates with the depression of the plasma albumin level.

Disordered protein metabolism in chronic liver disease is also manifested in the form of muscle wasting. Haemorrhagic phenomena result from impaired synthesis of coagulation factors (p. 255). The metabolism of certain amino-acids, particularly methionine, tyrosine and cystine is impaired. These substances appear in increased amounts in blood and urine. When liver cell damage is massive, as in acute yellow atrophy, these and other amino-acids are found in high concentration.

Severe liver dysfunction results in impaired conversion of ammonia to urea. Following oral administration of ammonium chloride, arterial blood ammonia levels (p. 462) become elevated. The magnitude of these changes correlates roughly with the severity of liver cell disease as estimated by the plasma albumin level.

Neuropsychiatric changes. Hepatic coma

The exact nature of the biochemical defects causing reversible mental changes in acute and chronic liver disease is unknown. A number of processes, possibly interacting, may be responsible for the same end result. The most consistent abnormality is elevation of the arterial blood ammonia level. A high intake of dietary protein and the oral administration of ammonium salts or urea all result in 'flapping' hand tremor, hyper-reflexia and ultimate coma. Blood ammonia values become further elevated. The importance of degradation of nitrogenous substances in the bowel is shown by the clinical improvement in mental condition which follows restriction of dietary nitrogen intake, administration of antibiotics which reduce the gut flora, purgation and surgical 'exclusion' of the colon.

Portal-systemic encephalopathy implies that diversion of portal blood to the systemic circulation is the cause of the cerebral disturbance. In all patients with mental changes there is such a pathway. In acute liver disease the 'shunt' is functional. Hepatic cells are unable to deal adequately with portal venous blood. In cirrhosis, portal blood may by-pass the liver cells by way of collateral venous channels (p. 439) or anatomical 'internal shunts' in the liver itself (p. 439). Some degree of liver cell dysfunction must always exist before mental changes occur. If the liver is normal, even the most gross collateral venous channels may be present without evidence of any cerebral disturbance.

Hepatic foetor—a characteristic musty smell on the breath—is frequently detected in patients with severe liver disease. It is abolished by measures which also produce mental improvement (see above) suggesting a common origin for the two disorders.

Arterial blood ammonia levels are usually raised in hepatic coma. Apart from decreased conversion in the liver (p. 462) elevation may also result from impaired renal excretion consequent upon the use of diuretic drugs such as thiazides which produce elevated renal vein ammonia concentrations and this effect is also produced by potassium loss. A high dietary protein intake and 'shunting' past the liver cells are also contributory factors (p. 439). Impaired conversion to glutamic acid and glutamine in peripheral tissues may also play a part. Ammonia may have a deleterious effect on the brain by depleting it of glutamic acid or α-ketoglutarate which is an essential link in the Krebs citric acid cycle (see Chapter 13). There is, however, no proof that this is responsible for the cerebral disturbance in man. A direct 'toxic' effect is also unlikely as the brain in hepatic coma does not always take up ammonia and sometimes may release it. Ammonia has no *in vitro* effect upon cerebral oxygen utilization in animals. There is no absolute correlation between the degree of elevation of blood ammonia and the clinical state (p. 462).

Amines of different types, e.g. dimethylamine and ethanolamine have sometimes been isolated from the urine in patients with hepatic coma. Satisfactory qualitative or quantitative correlation with clinical findings has not been achieved. Serotonin deficiency has also been suggested as a cause of hepatic coma but there is no proof that this occurs in man.

Prolonged exposure of the central nervous system to the agents responsible for hepatic coma results eventually in organic change manifested as dementia, paraplegia and other disorders.

Disordered carbohydrate metabolism

Massive damage to liver cells resulting in acute hepatic failure causes hypoglycaemia. This is probably due to failure of the liver to split phosphate from glucose-6-phosphate. Severe hypoglycaemia does not occur in chronic hepatic disease, but the liver may incompletely metabolize glucose in portal blood. Reduced fasting blood levels may occur while hyperglycaemia and glycosuria may follow meals (see Chapter 13). Oral glucose tolerance tests in cirrhosis may show the same changes as in diabetes mellitus.

Absence of the enzyme glucose-1-phosphate uridyl transferase, essential for interconversion of galactose and glucose (see Chapter 13), from the liver results in the disease galactosaemia. Muscle wasting, cataracts, mental damage, renal tubular defects and sometimes cirrhosis may result.

Severe accumulation of glycogen in the liver may result from several different genetically-determined enzyme deficiencies. Absence of phosphorylase in muscle or liver is the cause of two types of glycogen storage disorder (McArdle's and Her's diseases). Absence of glucose-6-phosphatase which splits phosphate from glucose-6-phosphate (in turn formed from glycogen) gives rise to the better known von Gierke's disease. Absence of amyloglucidase is responsible for another variant (Pompe's disease) which also occurs when enzymes responsible for the 'debranching' of glycogen are lacking.

Disordered fat metabolism

Lipoprotein-lipase activity is depressed in chronic liver disease and may result in failure of transport of fat which then accumulates in the liver. Serum lipids may also be abnormal in the presence of liver cell dysfunction. Plasma concentrations of phospholipid as well as cholesterol and its esters (p. 456) may be reduced. Increased mobilization of fat causes elevation of plasma levels of free fatty acids.

Disordered metabolism of hormones and drugs

In the presence of liver cell dysfunction, cortisol activity in the body is normal or slightly increased. Decreased hepatic metabolism is balanced by reduced production by the adrenals. Urinary excretion rates of cortisol metabolites are low and do not adequately reflect the degree of activity of the hormone in the body or its pool size. The presence of acne, hirsutism, skin striae and mooning of the face sometimes seen in chronic liver disease cannot, however, be correlated with the relatively minor changes in cortisol metabolism.

Increased urinary excretion of oestrogens and their degradation products, determined by bio-assay methods, occurs in many instances in severe liver disease. These urinary 'oestrogens' may, however, consist chiefly of metabolites that have leaked into the general circulation, and hence the urine, from the enterohepatic cycle because of liver dysfunction. Their presence alone does not imply increased production or activity of these steroids in the body. Accurate urinary studies based on direct chemical analysis suggest, however, that conversion of oestrone to 16α-hydroxyoestrone (a step in the degradation of 17β-oestradiol to oestriol) is abnormal in severe liver disease. Nevertheless, no direct correlation exists between the clinical manifestations of hyperoestrogenism in the form of gynaecomastia, testicular atrophy, changes in body hair distribution and arterial spider naevi and the biochemical findings. Sensitivity of individual persons to slight increases in oestrogen activity may be of significance. Urinary androgen excretion measured by bioassay is reduced in patients with cirrhosis. This is probably due to these compounds being metabolized by alternative pathways.

Disordered liver cell function may result in delayed disappearance from the plasma of drugs excreted mainly by the liver. This is not, however, true in all cases. In many instances drug metabolism is only slightly impaired even in the presence of severe hepatocellular damage. Induction of hepatic microsomes (p. 438) by previously administered compounds is not significantly affected. Abnormal responses to therapeutic agents in patients with liver disease may be due not so much to impaired metabolism of the drug as to increased sensitivity of other organs in the presence of hepatic dysfunction. Thus the brain in patients with cirrhosis is unduly sensitive to exogenous intoxication (p. 446).

Disordered iron metabolism

Deposition of iron in the liver occurs in some patients with cirrhosis. This is particularly true in chronic alcoholism, where increased intestinal absorption is probably the cause, and following portacaval anastomosis (p. 440). Serum iron values may be elevated but full saturation of the total iron binding capacity (see Chapter 6) does not occur. The reason for increased iron deposition following operation is obscure. It may be related in some way to failing liver cell function. Increased absorption of iron from the bowel is probably the cause of haemochromatosis where it may be determined on a genetic basis. Elevation of the serum iron concentration and of the iron content of the liver is frequently seen in relatives of patients with this disease. In haemochromatosis the serum iron concentration is usually elevated and the iron binding capacity fully saturated.

Circulatory dysfunction

Patients with chronic liver disease frequently have an increased cardiac output and diminished systemic vascular resistance. Cutaneous vasodilatation results in warm extremities and capillary pulsation. The coronary and renal blood-flow, however, is diminished. There is, therefore, a redistribution of the circulation. Pulmonary vasodilatation is universal, at least in severe hepatic failure. Arterial oxygen desaturation may occur due to pulmonary arterio-venous fistulae. The mechanism of the circulatory changes is obscure. A vasodilator substance released from or not detoxified by the failing liver may be responsible. In terminal hepatic failure systemic hypotension becomes severe.

Fluid and electrolyte disturbances: ascites

Retention of fluid, as ascites or oedema, is a common manifestation of chronic hepatic disease. It may also occur in severe acute liver damage. A variety of factors may be responsible. Decreased production of albumin (p. 435) with lowering of plasma colloid osmotic pressure occurs and there is increased production of renin and aldosterone (see Chapter 15). Portal hypertension (p. 439) explains the predilection of the fluid for the abdominal cavity but the degree of elevation of pressure cannot be correlated with the presence or amount of ascites. Raised portal venous pressure alone does not cause ascites formation in the absence of liver dysfunction. Lymphatic obstruction in the liver and increased hepatic lymph formation may be important contributory factors in the formation of ascites. Plasma concentrations of antidiuretic hormone are increased in patients with cirrhosis (see Chapter 14).

Ascites may be massive. The fluid is nevertheless in equilibrium with the plasma. As much as 80 per cent of the water in the abdomen is exchanged each hour. Interchanges of albumin also occur.

Abnormalities of water and electrolyte metabolism are common in liver failure: water retention; sodium retention; potassium depletion. The results depend upon the relative importance of these and upon shifts between body fluid compartments. The usual findings are oedema and ascites, with an increased plasma volume, low plasma sodium and potassium concentrations, and an increased total exchangeable sodium and low total exchangeable potassium. The impaired water excretion results chiefly from proximal tubular reabsorption of sodium in the kidney which means that little passes to a distal site to allow free water to be generated (see Chapter 4). The sodium retention and potassium depletion are largely due to secondary hyperaldosteronism (see Chapter (15 but other factors are operative in governing plasma levels. Low plasma sodium concentrations result from expansion of the extracellular space and redistribution of sodium between intracellular and extra-cellular body fluids compartments. Low plasma potassium concentrations may result from poor dietary intake, vomiting and the use of diuretic drugs in addition to hyperaldosteronism.

In acute massive liver cell injury, low blood urea levels are due to decreased hepatic synthesis (p. 436) and expansion of the extra-cellular space. Values of less than 10 mg/100 ml may occur. Less marked reduction in blood urea levels may also occur in chronic liver disease. In terminal liver failure, blood urea levels are almost invariably elevated due to renal insufficiency. Oliguria becomes profound. The plasma potassium is elevated and hyponatraemia becomes more severe. The mechanisms underlying these changes are not clear. Impaired renal perfusion is the most likely explanation available at the present time. These changes are reversible only in the presence of improving liver function.

In hepatic coma there is a respiratory alkalosis, possibly because intracellular (H^+) is raised (see Chapter 5).

Principles of tests and measurements

Many clinical observations and numerous 'liver function tests' may help in the diagnosis of hepatic disease. Only a limited number in fact give quantitative information about the functional activity of the liver.

BIOCHEMICAL TESTS

TESTS OF BILIRUBIN METABOLISM

Bilirubin metabolism and its disorders have been discussed on pages 433 and 441.

Plasma bilirubin. There are three main ways in which the concentration of bilirubin in the plasma may become elevated. The rate of production may be increased, uptake and passage through the liver cell may be abnormal, and biliary excretion may be impaired.

Bilirubin glucuronides are water soluble (p. 433) and combine with Ehrlich's diazo-reagent to produce a violet colour in the Van den Bergh test. This is the 'direct' reaction. Unconjugated bilirubin is much less water soluble but is soluble in alcohol. It is estimated with the diazo-reaction. In routine practice, measurements of direct and indirect reacting bilirubin are used to estimate conjugated and unconjugated pigment. Results correlate closely with chromatographic separation methods which are too complicated for general use. Normal plasma contains up to 0·2 mg/100 ml of conjugated pigment. Its total bilirubin content is less than 1·0 mg/100 ml. In jaundice due to liver cell injury or bile-duct obstruction, the predominant pigment in the plasma is conjugated. Precise knowledge of the proportions of conjugated and unconjugated bilirubin is seldom useful but in congenital hyperbilirubinaemia (p. 442) it is essential to know if conjugated pigment is present and its exact amount. The same is true of haemolytic jaundice.

Urinary bilirubin. Glucuronides of bilirubin appear in the urine to which they may impart an orange-green hue. The froth obtained on shaking the specimen is coloured yellow. This is a useful preliminary clinical test. Qualitative estimation may be performed with the use of Fouchet's reagent. Bile pigments adsorbed on to a barium chloride precipitate of the urine produce a blue-green colour. As little as 0·2 mg/100 ml of bilirubin can be detected. The use of tablets containing a diazo-dye producing a purple colour with bile pigments is more popular. This test is specific, easy to perform, and will detect as little as 0·1 mg/100 ml of bilirubin in the urine. Accurate quantitation of urinary bilirubin is difficult because of interfering pigments and has little practical value.

Conjugated bilirubin enters the urine principally by glomerular filtration. Its excretion is influenced by substances affecting protein-binding of the pigment in plasma. A small amount of this is dialyzable and probably accounts for urinary excretion of conjugated bilirubin. Bile salts increase this dialyzability and may explain the greater renal clearance of bilirubin in obstructive than in parenchymatous jaundice. Tubular secretion is unimportant. Urinary excretion of bilirubin is pH dependent. The controlling factor is the pH of blood, the proportion of bilirubin which is dialyzable being greater at higher values. Urinary pH is unimportant and non-ionic diffusion is not involved.

Urinary urobilinogen. Urobilinogen is colourless but becomes oxidized to urobilin on standing which makes the urine turn orange. It is a weak, divalent organic acid and is predominantly lipid-soluble in the unionized form. The pK of urobilinogen is 5·4. It is excreted in the urine in a manner typical of many similar compounds. This involves glomerular filtration of the unbound plasma fraction (which is less than 20 per cent) and proximal tubular secretion of that which is ionized. pH-dependent back-diffusion of the unionized fraction occurs in distal tubules (non-ionic diffusion). Urinary urobilinogen excretion is greater in alkaline urine. There is also a diurnal variation in urobilinogen output. Maximal excretion occurs in the early afternoon, and very little is excreted at night. This rhythm is independent of pH changes, but is intensified by diurnal variation of urinary pH.

Urobilinogen produces a red colour with Ehrlich's aldehyde reagent. Both the urine and the reagent must be fresh. Increased amounts of urobilinogen appear in the urine when the liver cells are unable to re-excrete the pigment following intestinal absorption. The test is a sensitive index of liver function. It may be positive when other biochemical tests are normal. Mild hepatic dysfunction secondary to circulatory failure or pyrexia may produce a positive test when plasma bilirubin levels are normal. Elevated urinary concentrations also occur when bilirubin production is increased (p. 441) and when transit of bowel contents is abnormally slow permitting increased intestinal absorption (p. 391). Bacterial colonization of the small intestine has a similar effect.

The urinary content of urobilinogen is abnormally low in biliary obstruction (p. 443). It is also decreased when transit through the bowel is rapid or when antibiotic drugs have reduced intestinal bacterial flora. Impaired renal function and reduced proximal tubular secretion of the pigment, e.g. as produced by the drug probenecid, as well as extreme acidity of the urine all lead to reduction in urinary urobilinogen content.

Intravenous bilirubin tolerance tests. Bilirubin may be administered intravenously in alkaline solution either as a single injection, followed by analysis of plasma disappearance curves, or by constant infusion when maximum hepatic clearance is assessed. The technique is used in research to study the hepatic handling and site of action of drugs which affect the liver. Tolerance tests are available in the study of congenital disorders of bilirubin metabolism (p. 457).

Studies with radio-active labelled bilirubin. Much of the detailed knowledge concerning normal and abnormal bilirubin metabolism (pp. 433 441) has resulted from the ability to label this substance and related pigments with radio-active ^{14}C. Use of this material is confined to research.

ENZYMATIC TESTS
Plasma alkaline phosphatase and 5′-nucleotidase. Plasma alkaline phosphatase is derived from those of bone, intestine and liver. The normal range in adults is 3–13 King–Armstrong units/100 ml. The enzyme is excreted in the bile. In patients with liver disease, values greater than 35 usually indicate some form of biliary obstruction (p. 441). Less marked elevation of plasma levels is seen in acute liver cell necrosis due to increased permeability of cellular membranes. Moderate to marked elevations also occur in conditions characterized by proliferation of bile ducts in the absence of obstruction, as seen in cirrhosis. The enzyme is then probably derived from the proliferating cells themselves.

The problem of differentiating elevations of plasma alkaline phosphatase due to osteoblastic activity (see Chapter 8) from those associated with liver disease may occur. It is of greatest significance in young adults when a physiological increase in plasma alkaline phosphatase results from bone growth. Experimentally, the isoenzymes derived from extracts of these two tissues may be distinguished by starch-gel electrophoresis, but in plasma difficulties arise. Estimation of the related enzyme 5′-nucleotidase may be of value. It is present in normal plasma, the range of values being 2–15 international units/l. Plasma levels are increased in the same liver disorders which cause elevation of alkaline phosphatase but are normal in diseases of bone. Phosphatase derived from osteoblasts is inactive against a nucleotide phosphate substrate.

Plasma transaminases. Many enzymes involved in different metabolic processes are released into the plasma due to increased permeability or destruction of tissue cells, including those of the liver. Those usually assayed are *aspartate transaminase* (serum glutamic oxaloacetic transaminase, SGOT), and *alanine transaminase* (serum glutamic pyruvic transaminase, SGPT). Aspartate transaminase is present in both mitochondria and cytoplasm. In liver disease only the cytoplasmic enzyme is usually released. Severe cell damage must occur before the mitochondrial enzyme appears in the plasma. The normal range of values is 5–15 international units/l. Alanine transaminase is wholly cytoplasmic in origin. Greater plasma elevations of this enzyme than of aspartate transaminase are produced by acute liver cell injury not involving mitochondria. They are also more specific for the liver.

Isocitrate dehydrogenase. This enzyme is chiefly cytoplasmic. Elevated plasma levels occur following hepatocellular damage. The test is sensitive and is often positive in the absence of elevation of plasma bilirubin, e.g. following administration of hepatotoxic drugs.

These enzyme determinations provide a means of following the degree of activity of acute or chronic liver injury. They do not reflect cellular function. Biliary obstruction also causes mild elevation of plasma enzyme levels as the cells become damaged.

Plasma cholinesterase is synthesized by liver cells. The range of normal values is 2–5 international units/l. Increased levels occur in hepatocellular disease, e.g. cirrhosis. The estimation yields no more information than that of the plasma albumin and is less reliable. Its use is confined to research.

PLASMA PROTEIN DETERMINATIONS
The plasma albumin concentration may be determined by electrophoresis following estimation of total proteins or by the more standard salt fractionation procedure which gives somewhat higher values. Immunological techniques are being developed. The normal range is 3·5–4·5 g/100 ml. Of all the routine tests employed, the plasma albumin level provides the most adequate overall indication of liver cell function. Changes in concentration occur relatively slowly (p. 436). The plasma albumin level in protracted viral hepatitis or cirrhosis correlates closely with the clinical condition and may provide information regarding the efficiency of treatment as well as having prognostic value. Normal levels in cirrhosis merely reflect the great functional reserve of the liver. In assessing the significance of plasma albumin determinations, extrahepatic factors must be taken into account. Malnutrition, infection and fever lower the concentration as may expansion of the plasma volume in the absence of a change in synthesis.

Globulins are usually estimated by electrophoresis of serum when five distinct boundaries are noted. Electrophotometric scanning yields quantitative information regarding the different fractions but the method is inaccurate. The fractions, in order of decreasing mobility, are:—albumin, α_1-, α_2-, β- and γ-globulins. The fractions themselves are not homogeneous. Gamma globulin contains the immunoglobulins and is formed in the reticulo-endothelial system. The normal liver does not produce γ-globulin (p. 436), but in cirrhosis the liver contains γ-globulin producing cells, while plasma levels are elevated. The reasons underlying this enhanced production of γ-globulin are unknown. 'Auto-immunization' to liver tissue has been suggested but not proven. Hyper-reactivity of the immunological apparatus may be the cause. Increased production of antibodies to bacterial antigens in patients with chronic liver disease supports this hypothesis. Most of the γ-globulin elevation in cirrhosis can be accounted for by an increase in one or more of the known types of immunoglobulin (IgA, IgG or IgM). The significance of variations in the ratios between these immunoglobulins in various liver diseases is unknown.

Changes in the plasma concentration of α_1 globulin, manufactured by the liver cell, parallel those in plasma albumin. Elevated values may be associated with neoplastic disease of the liver, but the reason for this is not known. In biliary obstruction the degree of elevation of α_2- and β-globulins in the plasma correlates with the rise in serum lipids. These combine with peptides and appear in the β-globulins.

The time-honoured practice of calculating serum albumin–globulin ratios should be abandoned. The two protein fractions are formed at different sites, and their concentrations are affected by different factors. Their ratio as such is meaningless.

FLOCCULATION AND SEROLOGICAL TESTS
Serum flocculation reactions
These depend upon changes in the plasma proteins in liver disorders. Two types of mechanism are involved. Firstly, certain stabilizing factors normally present in the plasma disappear immediately following liver cell injury. Their absence may result, for example, in a positive cephalin flocculation reaction. There is no demonstrable quantitative change in plasma γ-globulin level. Secondly, a number of positive tests are due to increases in plasma γ-globulin concentration (whatever its cause). These include the cephalin flocculation, ammonium sulphate, zinc sulphate and thymol turbidity tests. Correlation between positive

reactions and the total globulin concentration is, however, poor. The thymol turbidity test depends upon changes in other stabilizing factors in the α- and β-globulins and upon albumin as well as γ-globulin alterations.

These tests are empirical and depend upon protein changes in no way specific for liver disease. They are of very limited value in assessment of liver function.

Serological studies

The Latex-FII agglutination test is frequently positive in patients with liver disease and is probably due to production of macroglobulins. Serum antinuclear factors are usually found only in chronic hepatic disorders where their occurrence is unexplained. Their presence in diseases of other organs and in the general population reduces their practical value. Antibodies to the mitochondria of various tissue cells of different animal species have recently been isolated. Their high incidence in primary biliary cirrhosis assists in the differentiation of this condition from cirrhosis secondary to main bile-duct obstruction and from other forms of cholestasis. They are present in a few cases of cirrhosis due to other causes but are rarely found in alcoholic liver disease. Mitochondrial antibodies occur in approximately 1 per cent of people with normal liver function. Although usually associated with a marked elevation of the plasma IgM level, this is not invariably the case. Other antibodies reacting with the cells of bile ductules, with smooth muscle and with bile canaliculi have recently been described. Their significance is obscure.

PLASMA CHOLESTEROL ESTIMATION

The total plasma cholesterol level is 150–300 mg/100 ml. Increased levels in obstructive jaundice (p. 443) are not due to bile retention but to overproduction by the liver. This may result from decreased utilization of cholesterol for bile acid formation. Increased plasma levels in acute obstructive liver disease are slight compared with those which occur when the condition is chronic. Low values in chronic obstructive jaundice carry a grave prognosis, indicating that hepatic decompensation is severe. They may be accompanied by disappearance of cutaneous xanthomata. In other forms of chronic liver disease plasma levels are usually normal. Decompensation or concurrent malnutrition, however, produce low values. In acute and chronic hepatocellular dysfunction esterification of cholesterol is depressed.

CLEARANCE AND TOLERANCE TESTS

A number of tests depend upon the ability of the liver to metabolize or excrete an administered substance. The rate of disappearance from the circulation is then an index of hepatic function. The validity of such tests depends upon the compound being removed entirely by the liver. Three mechanisms of hepatic 'clearance' are:

(1) by metabolism. Such substances as galactose, laevulose and ammonia are metabolized in liver cells.

(2) by biliary excretion. Such substances as bromsulphthalein, Rose Bengal and bilirubin itself are cleared in this way.

(3) by phagocytosis. Particulate matter such as colloidal gold is taken up by Küpffer cells.

Many tests relying on hepatic metabolism have been abandoned for various reasons. The oral galactose tolerance test has the disadvantage of being dependent upon intestinal absorption and adequate renal function. It is also affected by thyroid activity. The intravenous galactose tolerance test overcomes these snags but severe liver cell damage must be present before impairment is obvious. Other compounds such as ammonia are no longer used because of technical disadvantages or because of poor correlation with clinical findings. Yet other substances such as sodium benzoate have the disadvantage of being metabolized outside the liver.

The most satisfactory compound is one which is metabolized or excreted almost entirely by the liver and which can be given intravenously following which serial blood determinations are made. This obviates the difficulties introduced by variable intestinal absorption and impaired renal function. The substance which fills these criteria most satisfactorily is the tricarbocyanine dye indocyanine green. It becomes firmly bound to albumin in the plasma and renal excretion does not occur. It can be recovered almost totally from the bile but does not undergo enterohepatic circulation and extraction outside the liver does not occur. It is, however, expensive and minor technical disadvantages exist in estimating plasma levels. Its chief use is in the estimation of liver bloodflow (p. 462) .

The most satisfactory substance for routine use in assessing overall liver cell function is the dye *bromsulphthalein* (BSP). This is rapidly excreted by the liver but some extrahepatic removal does occur, being greatest in the presence of jaundice and at high plasma bromsulphthalein levels. Over 80 per cent of administered BSP can be recovered from the bile inside 2 hr. Here it is present both unchanged and in the form of various derivatives. These are chiefly conjugates with glycine, glutamic acid and cysteine. An enterohepatic circulation exists. The standard test is performed by intravenous administration of 5 mg/kg body weight of the dye as a 5 per cent solution. Forty-five minutes later a blood sample is obtained from a different site. The dye is simply estimated in separated plasma by comparison of the colour obtained when alkali is added with a standard curve. A 10 mg/100 ml solution is taken as 100 per cent retention. Normal people retain less than 5 per cent of the dye at 45 min.

The test finds its chief use in assessing liver cell dysfunction in the absence of jaundice. In experimental animals the excess dye retained correlated inversely with functioning liver tissue available after hepatectomy. The test is, however, not helpful in the presence of jaundice. It may be normal in well-compensated cirrhosis due to the reserve capacity of the liver. Since the test is dependent upon liver bloodflow it may be disproportionately abnormal in the presence of circulatory failure or portal venous obstruction. It is of special use in the diagnosis of Dubin–Johnson hyperbilirubinaemia (p. 443). A blood sample obtained 2 hr. after a standard intravenous test dose shows a higher concentration of dye than the 45 min specimen. This is due to release of conjugated BSP into the blood after normal initial uptake by hepatic cells.

The use of BSP for measurement of liver bloodflow should be abandoned in favour of indocyanine green (p. 462).

Estimation of storage capacity and secretory transport maximum for BSP. Hepatic excretion of BSP has been found to result from two independent processes: uptake and storage (S) in the liver cell and active secretion into the bile. A secretory transport maximum (Tm) has been defined for this process. Values for (S) and (Tm) can be derived indirectly from comparison of the disappearance rates of BSP from the plasma during two different constant infusions of dye. The amount stored is proportional to the plasma concentration. (Tm) is measured in mg/min. This test is a much more sensitive index of liver cell function than the simple routine procedure. Its chief use is in the detection of minor functional impairment of the liver and in research. A selective reduction of (S) occurs with advancing age.

The uptake of colloidal particles by Küpffer cells is the basis of several methods of measuring liver bloodflow (p. 462). It provides no information regarding hepatocellular function or reserve.

SPECIAL TESTS USED IN EVALUATION OF JAUNDICE

Prednisolone test. If prednisolone, given in high dosage, produces a definite fall in the plasma bilirubin level in a jaundiced patient this indicates hepatocellular dysfunction. Little change occurs in patients with other forms of cholestasis or main bile-duct obstruction. The test may not make a clear distinction in all instances. A fall of at least 40 per cent is necessary for a conclusive result. The fate of the bile pigment leaving the blood under these circumstances is unknown. Changes in faecal and urinary urobilinogen or in urinary bilirubin do not occur. It appears likely that bilirubin follows an alternative metabolic pathway. The drug probably acts upon the liver cells themselves in that a marked increase in the storage capacity (S) for BSP is observed (p. 458).

Percutaneous trans-hepatic cholangiography. If the plasma bilirubin level is elevated due to obstruction of main bile ducts, dilatation of the intrahepatic biliary tree occurs. Its magnitude is related to the degree and duration of obstruction. It is usually possible to enter a dilated biliary radicle by percutaneous puncture of the liver substance with a needle. If bile is aspirated, X-ray films are obtained following injection of contrast medium. Dilatation of ducts does not occur when intra-hepatic cholestasis is present (e.g. chlorpromazine jaundice). Failure of an experienced operator to enter a dilated radicle may be taken as good presumptive evidence of an intrahepatic origin for cholestasis.

TESTS OF GALL BLADDER AND BILIARY FUNCTION

Cholecystography utilizes orally administered compounds which are excreted by the liver and concentrated in the gall-bladder. This organ can then be visualized with the use of X-rays. A poorly functioning or diseased gall-bladder fails to concentrate the contrast material and cannot be seen. The contractile powers of the gall-bladder are assessed by observation of its shape following ingestion of a fatty meal. Its response to injected cholecystokinin may also be studied.

Intravenous cholangiography. Following intravenous injection of an iodine compound, the bile ducts become outlined at an early stage of excretion by the liver.

Cineradiography. When this technique is coupled with the above investigations, information about the contraction of the biliary tree as a whole as well as the gall-bladder may be obtained. These tests are impracticable in the presence of all but the mildest jaundice due to failure of hepatic excretion of the contrast medium in sufficient amount or concentration.

INVESTIGATION OF HEPATIC AND PORTAL
CIRCULATORY DYSFUNCTION

PORTAL VENOUS MANOMETRY

Intrasplenic pressure. Pressure recordings obtained from a needle inserted into the splenic pulp, which is in contact with portal venules, bear a close relation to portal venous pressure. The measurement is unaffected by splenic size and varies little in different parts of the organ. It provides a measure of presinusoidal pressure and is slightly higher than the true portal venous pressure. The investigation is carried out in practice by percutaneous puncture of the spleen. It is used diagnostically, for following changes during treatment, and in research.

Direct estimation of the portal pressure can also be made by introducing a fine catheter into a portal venous radicle under direct vision at operation or by insertion of a needle into varices on oesophagoscopy. The left main portal vein may be catheterized percutaneously by way of the falciform ligament.

Intrahepatic sinusoidal pressure measurement

This is performed by direct, percutaneous introduction of a fine needle into the liver substance. Blood drips back down the needle when it is satisfactorily placed. The mean of pressure obtained in several different areas is taken. The technique is used chiefly as a means of checking portal pressure measurements obtained by other techniques.

Portal venography

Percutaneous trans-splenic venography. Following percutaneous puncture of the spleen (above), radiopaque dye is rapidly injected. With the use of rapid serial films it is possible to assess flow in splenic and portal veins. Portal collateral venous channels are demonstrated and the pattern of intrahepatic venous radicles may also be studied. This information is essential if surgical portacaval anastomosis is considered.

Arteriovenography. When splenic puncture is impracticable, the portal venous system can be studied by injection of contrast medium into the superior mesenteric or splenic arteries following selective catheterization of these vessels. This can be easily carried out with modern radiological equipment and may provide haemodynamic information obtainable by no other means.

Determination of free and wedged hepatic venous pressure
The pressure recorded from a semi-stiff catheter with a single end-hole lying free in a main hepatic vein is termed the *free hepatic venous pressure*. It is normally the same as inferior vena caval pressure. It is raised when intra-abdominal pressure is elevated, as in the presence of tense ascites, or when flow in the vena cava is impeded by cardiac failure or constriction of the pericardium (p. 60). If the catheter is further advanced into the hepatic venous system until further progress is impossible, *the wedged hepatic venous pressure* is recorded. If contrast medium is injected down the catheter in this position it fills hepatic sinusoids and does not reflux into the inferior vena cava. Transmitted arterial pulsations are seen in recorded pressure tracings. Readings should be obtained from several different hepatic venous radicles and the mean pressure calculated. When the catheter is in the wedged position it produces stasis in a column of blood extending from the catheter tip deep into the vascular system of the liver. There is no pressure fall along this column because there is no flow and therefore no resistance. The catheter is in effect 'extended' further into the hepatic vasculature as far as the sinusoids. The normal wedged pressure is 6–8 mmHg. Elevation in liver disease means that the column of blood is traversing an area of abnormally high vascular resistance. Portal hypertension in the absence of wedged pressure elevation usually results from vascular abnormalities in the main portal vein or portal venules. This is presinusoidal portal hypertension. When wedged hepatic vein pressure is markedly raised it is usually the result of diseases affecting hepatic venules, central veins or channels connecting sinusoids and central veins. This is post-sinusoidal portal hypertension and results almost always from cirrhosis. Mild or moderate elevations may be caused by changes in the sinusoids themselves or in the sinusoids and hepatic outflow tracts together.

The measurement is of value in distinguishing between the different causes of portal hypertension and can be used when splenic puncture is impractical. It is also used in pre- and post-operative study of the portal circulation. Hepatic vein catheterization is essential for several of the methods of estimating liver bloodflow (p. 462).

Wedged hepatic venography is carried out with a forceful injection of contrast medium down the hepatic venous catheter in the wedged position. The medium fills hepatic sinusoids and retrograde filling of the portal vein may occur. This procedure coupled with cine-radiography yields valuable haemodynamic data particularly following the various types of surgical portacaval anastomosis (p. 440).

ESTIMATION OF HEPATIC BLOODFLOW

The constant infusion method utilizes the Fick principle. Ideally the infused substance must be removed only by the liver and at a steady rate. Arterial levels must remain constant and significant enterohepatic circulation should not occur. The dye indocyanine green (p. 433) fulfils these criteria most satisfactorily and has now replaced the hitherto popular BSP (p. 457). Radio-active gold may be used. It is taken up by Küpffer cells. A similar principle underlies the use of heat-denatured colloidal albumin labelled with radio-active [131]I. In the absence of liver disease, analysis of peripheral blood disappearance curves following a single injection suffices. When extraction by the liver may be impaired, hepatic vein catheterization is essential. Total bloodflow may also be estimated by external scintillation counting over the liver following intravenous injection of a gamma-emitter. The method is unreliable, however, if extraction by the liver is impaired.

A more direct method makes use of the indicator dilution technique. Following hepatic venous catheterization, an indicator substance is injected forcefully in retrograde fashion. Sampling is simultaneously carried out at some distance proximally in the same vessel.

The relative contributions of hepatic artery and portal vein may be estimated directly at operation with an electromagnetic or other flow meter.

SPECIAL TESTS USED IN EVALUATION OF
HEPATIC ENCEPHALOPATHY

Arterial blood ammonia. Methods of determination usually depend upon the release of ammonia gas from the blood upon the addition of alkali. They are technically difficult in unskilled hands and the range of normal values varies in different laboratories. The upper limit of normal is 0·8 to 1 μg ammonia nitrogen per ml blood. Arterial values are of greater significance than venous determinations because of possible uptake of ammonia by peripheral tissues. Blood samples should be taken at a time of fasting and rest. Although a little ammonia may be synthesized in lungs, kidneys and brain, its chief source is exogenous nitrogenous material in the form of dietary protein. It is produced by bacterial and non-bacterial enzymatic action in the bowel. Defective hepatic conversion of ammonia in portal venous blood results in elevated concentrations in the general circulation. Arterial levels correlate to some extent with the severity of the mental changes in patients with liver disease, but normal values are obtained in about 10 per cent of cases of frank coma. Estimations in terminal hepatic failure fluctuate widely and show little relation to the neurological state. Patients who have undergone surgical portacaval anastomosis may have arterial ammonia levels twice the normal value without apparent mental impairment. A number of facts (p. 446) suggest that neuropsychiatric changes and ammonia intoxication cannot be completely equated.

Electro-encephalography. EEG changes consist of slowing of the frequency from the normal α-rate right down to the δ-range of less than 4 cycles/sec. Changes can be graded. They are not specific for liver disease and may precede neuropsychiatric symptoms. EEG studies are useful in the early diagnosis of mental change and in following the effects of treatment (including portacaval surgery). The mechanism of the EEG changes is unknown. Borderline abnormalities may be clarified by high protein feeding or the administration of a small dose of morphine. The brain in patients with liver disease is unusually sensitive to exogenous intoxication and electrolyte disturbances, particularly potassium depletion. The reason for this is unknown.

OTHER TESTS

Radio-scanning of the liver. The use of radio-active substances such as iodinated-Rose Bengal allows photoscanning of the liver. Its chief use is in diagnosis of space occupying lesions. However, methods of study of uptake patterns and subsequent excretion of such substances may be developed in the future to provide data about liver cell function in a way analogous to the renogram in kidney diseases.

Serum B_{12} estimation. Vitamin B_{12} is stored chiefly in the liver (see Chapter 6). Elevated serum levels occur in acute liver necrosis but less constantly in chronic hepatocellular disease where they may even be low. Increased serum concentrations probably result from direct release of the substance from damaged cells. In cirrhosis, the total Vitamin B_{12} content of the liver is reduced to about a third, indicating that a storage defect also exists. Elevated serum concentrations often occur with space occupying lesions of the liver such as tumour or abscess. The reason for this is unknown.

SPIDER NAEVI

These occur in skin drained by the superior vena cava and more rarely in the mucosae of the nose, mouth and pharynx. They consist of a central arteriole from which numerous small vessels radiate. Pressure on the central area causes blanching of the whole lesion. If hepatocellular function deteriorates, spider naevi may become more obvious and new ones appear. Pulsation is seen to occur in association with other circulatory changes (p. 449). If liver function improves the naevi may disappear. In association with these lesions small scattered vessels may give the appearance of *paper money skin* while *white spots* on the arms and buttocks may be seen. At the centre of such spots are the beginnings of a vascular spider.

Arterial spider naevi may occur in acute as well as chronic hepatocellular disease and in some normal people. In pregnancy they may be marked between the second and seventh months. Although usually attributed to oestrogen excess, this association is unproven (p. 449). The uneven distribution of the lesions requires an alternative explanation. The presence of a local vascular predisposition in exposed areas as well as a humoral factor may be responsible. Children sometimes develop spider naevi on the lower limbs.

Practical assessment

HEPATIC AND PORTAL CIRCULATION
Portal hypertension and collateral circulation.
Clinical observation: gastro-oesophageal bleeding; splenic enlargement; abdominal wall collateral veins; venous hum; ascites. A soft liver suggests extrahepatic portal venous obstruction.

Routine methods: barium swallow and meal, oesophagoscopy, for varices.

Special techniques: intrasplenic pressure; trans-splenic venography; hepatic vein catheterization (wedge pressure); direct measurement. To study flow patterns: cine-radiography coupled with splenic venography, arteriovenography, wedged hepatic venography.

Hepatic bloodflow
Clinical observation and routine methods: a small liver implies a low total bloodflow. No other observations or routine methods available.

Special techniques: hepatic venous catherization and use of Fick principle or indicator dilution techniques; radio-active particle uptake by the liver and scanning; direct estimation at operation.

Portal-systemic shunting
Clinical observation: mental changes; flapping tremor; hepatic foetor. Portal hypertension and venous collateral circulation. Hepatocellular dysfunction.
Routine tests: Assessment of portal venous collateral circulation. Assessment of hepatocellular function.
Special tests: EEG; arterial blood ammonia; protein, ammonia and rarely morphine provocation.

HEPATO-CELLULAR FUNCTION
Clinical observation: general nutrition; protein depletion (muscle wasting, fluid retention, white nails, haemorrhagic phenomena); anaemia. Mental changes; flapping tremor; hepatic foetor. Jaundice. Other empirically established but poorly-understood signs: spider naevi, paper-money skin, white spots; gynaecomastia, testicular atrophy, body hair changes; acne, hirsutism, striae, mooning of the face; red palms, Cardiovascular changes. Hypotension and oliguria.

Routine methods: plasma proteins and bilirubin. Bromsulphthalein retention. Prothrombin time. Plasma cholesterol. Other routine 'liver function tests' occasionally helpful in diagnosis but not in assessing hepatocellular function. If oedematous: plasma electrolytes. Blood urea.

Special techniques: 'Tm and S' determination for BSP in borderline cases. Blood sugar and urinary amino-acids in acute hepatic failure. Serum iron and total iron-binding capacity. Serum B_{12} and cholinesterase.

BILE PIGMENT METABOLISM: JAUNDICE
Clinical observations: colour of skin: pale lemon in prehepatic jaundice; orange-yellow in hepatocellular jaundice; green-yellow in obstructive aundice.
Colour of urine: dark in all forms of jaundice, least dark in prehepatic; yellow froth in hepatocellular and obstructive jaundice.
Colour of stools: dark in prehepatic jaundice; pale in other forms. Pruritus in presence of cholestasis or biliary obstruction.

Routine methods: urinary urobilinogen and bilirubin. Plasma bilirubin, conjugated and total. Assessment of haemolysis (see Chapter 6). Plasma alkaline phosphatase and aspartate transaminase. Plasma proteins and cholesterol.

Special techniques: Serological tests. Prednisolone test. Percutaneous cholangiography. Intravenous bilirubin tolerance tests. Prolonged BSP test (p. 457).

References

KEELE C.A. & NEIL E. (eds.) (1965). *Samson Wright's Applied Physiology* (11th edn). pp. 370–6. London: Oxford University Press.

BRAUER R.W. (1936) Liver circulation and function. *Physiol Rev.*, **43**, 115–213.

SHERLOCK S. (1963) *Diseases of the Liver and Biliary System* (3rd edn). Oxford: Blackwell.

POPPER S. & SCHAFFNER F. (eds.) (1965). *Progress in Liver Diseases*. vol II. New York: Grune & Stratton.

GAMBLE J.R. & WILBUR D.L. (eds.) (1965). *Current Concepts of Clinical Gastroentrology*. Boston: Little, Brown and Company.

McCONNELL R.B. (1966) *The Genetics of Gastro-intestinal Disorders*. London: Oxford University Press.

TAYLOR E. (ed.) (1965). *The Biliary System*. Oxford: Blackwell.

SHERLOCK S. (1965). *Jaundice*. In *Recent Advances in Gastroenterology* (eds. BADENOCH J. & BROOKE B.N.). London: J. and A. Churchill Ltd.

READ A.E.A. *Biochemistry of cirrhosis and liver failure. Ibid.*

SHERLOCK S. (1966) Biliary secretory failure in man. The problem of cholestasis. *Ann. int. Med.*, **65**, 397–408.

BOUCHER I.A.D. & BILLING, B.H. (eds.) (1967) *Bilirubin Metabolism*. Oxford: Blackwell.

ZIEVE L. (1966) Pathogenesis of Hepatic Coma. *Arch. int. Med.*, **118**, 211–23.

WALKER J.G., DONIACH D., ROITT I.M. & SHERLOCK S. (1965) Serological tests in diagnosis of primary biliary cirrhosis. *Lancet*, i, 827–31.

BARON D.N. (1966) The clinical significance of serum enzyme estimations. *Abstr. World Med.*, **40**, 377–87.

13

Energy Sources Utilization

Normal function

Energy liberated by the oxidation of food and body reserves is converted to a basic biologically useful form (mainly adenosine triphosphate) and thence to other forms such as mechanical, osmotic and electrical energy. The efficiency of fuel utilization by the body is impaired by the loss of a little energy at each of the many steps involved in biological oxidations. When glucose is completely oxidized to CO_2 and water, only 40 per cent of its energy is recovered in a potentially useful form; the remainder is liberated as heat, which is not entirely wasted as it serves to maintain body temperature at a level at which metabolic processes proceed most efficiently.

ENERGY SOURCES

Carbohydrate, fat and protein, whether endogenous or of dietary origin, can all be oxidized with the liberation of biologically useful energy.

Carbohydrate

Glucose, fructose and galactose are obtained from the diet, usually as digestion products of larger carbohydrate molecules, e.g. glucose from starches and maltose, glucose and fructose from sucrose, and glucose and galactose from lactose. In the fasting state, glucose may be produced directly from liver glycogen and indirectly by the deamination and further metabolism of glucogenic amino-acids.

The extracellular glucose pool of a normal adult is approximately 15 g. Although turnover is rapid and variable, numerous independent and opposing mechanisms are integrated to maintain a constant concentration of glucose in the extracellular fluid.

Carbohydrate is stored, chiefly in liver and muscle, in the form of glycogen, a branched-chain polysaccharide formed by the condensation of glucose molecules. The liver of a well-nourished adult contains

16

approximately 100 g of glycogen, whilst the muscle mass contains approximately 250 g. Glycogen is degraded to glucose-6-phosphate which may be metabolized *in situ*: but only liver glycogen contributes to the available free glucose pool since muscle contains no glucose-6-phosphatase. This enzyme hydrolyses glucose-6-phosphate to free glucose, which then enters the blood. The glucose-6-phosphate derived from muscle glycogen can contribute indirectly to the glucose pool because the lactate produced by its oxidation may be released into the circulation, carried to the liver, and used for the resynthesis of glucose. The kidneys share the ability of the liver to synthesize glucose from the intermediates of glycolysis and glucogenic amino-acids, and are able to liberate free glucose into the blood, but it is unlikely that they play a significant part in carbohydrate metabolism except by preventing the loss of glucose in the urine.

Fat

Neutral fats (triglycerides) are formed by the combination of 1 molecule of glycerol with 3 molecules of fatty acid. Fatty acids are derived either from the hydrolysis of dietary triglyceride or by synthesis from acetyl CoA (p. 470) produced by the metabolism of glucose or amino-acids. Glycerol is formed from glyceraldehyde (one of the breakdown products of glucose).

Fatty acids can be metabolized by all tissues except those of the central nervous system. In the fasting state there is a very high rate of turnover of these acids which are the chief source of energy of the liver and muscles. Fatty acids diffuse freely into cells and their utilization is partly dependent upon their plasma concentration. Factors which inhibit the oxidation of fatty acids (e.g. an increased concentration of glucose and insulin in the blood) also inhibit the breakdown of stored triglycerides to glycerol and fatty acids (lipolysis).

Free fatty acids (FFA)—also known as non-esterified (NEFA) or unesterified fatty acids (uFA)—are released from fat depots following lipolysis or absorbed from the gut (p. 418). They circulate in the plasma loosely bound to albumin from which they are detached before entering cells for oxidation or incorporation into fat stores. There appears to be a continuous cycle in which FFA, released from adipose tissue in amounts in excess of the energy requirements of the body, pass to the liver where they are used for the resynthesis of triglycerides. The triglycerides formed in the liver are complexed with proteins to form lipoproteins which are released to the fat depots. Here the lipoproteins are split and the triglycerides are taken up. The accumulation of fat within hepatic parenchymal cells in some forms of liver disease is due to the failure of lipo-protein formation.

Fat is the most compact way of storing energy sources. The complete combustion of 1 g of fat produces 9·3 Cal whereas 1 g of carbohydrate yields 4·2 Cal. Fat storage does not require the retention of water as does storage of glycogen.

Although the amount of depot fat is variable, it represents a very large energy store even in lean people. The body of a normal (non-obese) 70 kg man contains approximately 10 kg of depot fat, which would be sufficient to maintain the basal metabolic processes for two months. In addition to storing energy, subcutaneous fat conserves energy by insulating the body against heat loss. Adipose tissue by its metabolic activity contributes to heat production and is one of the most active tissues biochemically.

There are two kinds of adipose tissue—white and brown. Adult humans have very little brown fat, but newborn infants and many small mammals have relatively large quantities. These are concentrated in the interscapular and cervical regions. Brown fat is metabolically very active. The fat in deposits of brown fat is not made generally available as a source of energy. Most of the fat is metabolized in the tissue and its energy dissipated as heat. The heat production by brown fat is regulated centrally through the autonomic nervous system and plays a considerable part in temperature control.

Protein

Amino acids derived from dietary proteins and not required for protein synthesis during growth and tissue replacement are metabolized to products formed during glucose oxidation, or to acetoacetate. Their energy is released by immediate oxidation or conserved by the synthesis of glycogen and depot fat triglyceride.

Although energy is released by the catabolism of endogenous protein during starvation, in uncontrolled diabetes and after injury, excess energy is not stored in the form of protein, and body protein acts as an emergency reserve.

Transport forms

The principal transport forms of fuels are glucose and FFA. These substances are oxidized to CO_2 and water with the liberation of energy. The factors which determine their relative rates of utilization are discussed below.

OXIDATION OF ENERGY SOURCES (Fig. 46, p. 472)
Fat, protein and carbohydrate are ultimately degraded to acetate which combines with co-enzyme A, forming acetyl CoA. This key substance is oxidized to CO_2 and water in the Krebs (citric acid, or tricarboxylic acid) cycle, where most of the energy of the original fuel substances is liberated. Oxidation and energy release are severely limited by lack of oxygen.

Glucose is phosphorylated by ATP in the presence of the ubiquitous enzyme hexokinase, forming glucose-6-phosphate. This is oxidized either anaerobically to two molecules of pyruvate or aerobically via the direct oxidative pathway (pentose cycle; hexose monophosphate shunt). In the presence of oxygen, pyruvate is converted into acetyl CoA by oxidative decarboxylation, and under optimal circumstances each molecule of glucose yields 6 molecules ATP. The direct oxidative pathway is an important alternative route for the metabolism of glucose-6-phosphate which operates in adipose tissue and liver, but not in muscle. This system, which involves the intermediate formation of various 5- and 7-carbon sugars, is involved in the synthesis of fatty acids and adrenocortical steroids by producing nicotinamide adenine dinucleotide phosphate (NADP, also known as triphosphopyridine nucleotide) necessary for their synthesis from acetyl CoA. However, it is likely that the supply of glycerophosphate and not NADP is the rate-limiting factor in fat synthesis. The direct oxidative pathway is not a significant source of energy.

Fatty acids are degraded step by step. Each stage frees a 2 carbon unit which yields one molecule of acetyl CoA. Acetyl CoA may be oxidized or, in the liver, 2 molecules may condense to form acetoacetyl CoA. Acetoacetyl CoA is used particularly for the synthesis of the cholesterol ring. It is also hydrolyzed in the liver to yield acetoacetic acid, most of which is then reduced to β-hydroxybutyric acid. A smaller amount is decarboxylated to acetone. These 'ketones' are usually oxidized but if they are produced in excessive amounts they are excreted by the lungs and kidneys.

Amino acids derived from protein are converted in the liver to keto-acids. Glucogenic amino acids are converted to pyruvate. Ketogenic amino-acids are degraded to acetyl CoA either directly or via acetoacetate.

Oxidation of acetyl-CoA by the Krebs cycle

Acetyl CoA reacts with oxaloacetate forming citrate, which undergoes a series of reactions resulting in the reformation of oxaloacetate. As a result, acetate is oxidized to CO_2 and water, and 12 molecules of ATP are formed for each molecule of acetate oxidized. The Krebs cycle requires oxygen, operates in all tissues and is the final common pathway for the oxidation of all energy sources. Oxalo-acetate and other intermediate compounds are themselves metabolized to some extent by pathways unrelated to the Krebs cycle, but losses are made good, chiefly from pyruvate.

Under optimal conditions and in the presence of oxygen, 1 molecule of glucose when completely oxidized via pyruvate yields 38 molecules of ATP. This compares with a yield of 35 molecules of ATP when oxidation follows the direct oxidative pathway and with only 2 molecules of ATP in the absence of oxygen.

ENERGY REQUIREMENTS

Energy is needed both to maintain basal metabolism and to carry out the many extra activities of the body. Basal metabolic activities consist mainly of cardiac contraction, breathing, secretion of urine, hormones and digestive juices, and maintenance of body temperature. Other energy requirements are created by the activity of muscles in addition to that present in the basal state, by the maintenance of body temperature on exposure to cold (largely by increased skeletal muscle activity, manifest by shivering), and by growth of tissues, requiring the synthesis of chemical compounds. In addition, some energy is necessarily dissipated in the form of heat during the metabolic processes involved in the storage of food as glycogen and fat, a process referred to as specific dynamic action. It consumes between 5 and 8 per cent of the calorific value of a mixed diet.

The basal energy requirements in health depend on age, being reduced in old age. Body mass, in proportion to surface area, is 6–10 per cent lower in women than in men of equal body weight. A healthy man weighing 70 kg, aged 20–30 years, requires approximately 40 Cal/m²/hr or 1700 Cal/day.

Muscular activity requires relatively large amounts of energy and variations in total energy expenditure depend very largely on differences in muscular work. Energy requirements (above basal requirements) for a 70 kg man are of the order of 70 Cal/hr for typing, 240 Cal/hr for walking at 3 mph on level ground, and 1000 Cal/hr for climbing stairs. A man who has a sedentary job and takes little exercise requires approximately 2500 Cal/day, while the same man would need 3000–4000 Cal/day if he did moderate to strenuous physical work.

Inter-relationships between metabolism of carbohydrate, fat and protein
Carbohydrate is converted to fat in the form of triglyceride for energy storage, while protein is converted to carbohydrate (or its oxidation

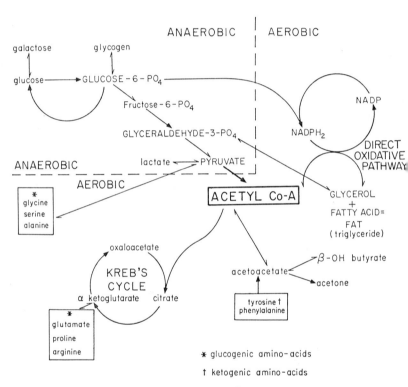

FIGURE 46.
Metabolic inter-relationships between carbohydrate, fat and protein

products) and aceto-acetate for energy release. Glycerol liberated during the hydrolysis of fat may be converted to glucose. The interconnecting pathways linking the metabolism of carbohydrates, fats and proteins are shown in Fig. 46. The principal linkages are through glyceraldehyde-3-phosphate, pyruvate and acetyl-CoA.

HORMONES INFLUENCING ENERGY LIBERATION
AND UTILIZATION

The complex, inter-related processes by which energy is liberated from food and endogenous reserves are adjusted to meet the energy requirements of the body which vary from moment to moment. The secretions of the pancreatic islet cells, adenohypophysis, thyroid and adrenal cortex, and the catecholamines released by the adrenal medulla and liberated at sympathetic nerve endings, influence and in some instances control these processes.

Pancreatic hormones
Insulin is a polypeptide consisting of 2 chains of 30 and 21 amino-acids joined by 2 disulphide bridges. There are small species differences in the amino-acid composition of the molecule. These differences do not modify the biochemical performance of the hormone, but account for the development of antibodies in animals injected with insulin derived from a different species.

Insulin is formed in the β-cells of the islets of Langerhans where it is stored in granules until released. This hormone causes a fall in the blood glucose concentration, both by increasing the rate of uptake of glucose in the periphery, and by reducing the output of glucose from the liver. This peripheral action of insulin, which mainly affects adipose tissue and muscle, is probably achieved by accelerating the carrier-mediated glucose transport system of the cell surface. Insulin also increases the rate of passage of potassium and some amino-acids across cell membranes. The direct inhibitory effect of insulin upon the glucose output by the liver is not well understood but it is not the result of any change in glucose transfer at the cell surface. Hepatic parenchymal cells, like pancreatic β-cells, are freely permeable to glucose at all times. Glucose transport in brain is also little affected by insulin. The breakdown of fat to fatty acids and glycerol is inhibited by insulin, an action which seems to be partially independent of any effect of the hormone upon carbohydrate metabolism. Other consequences of the presence of insulin are the stimulation of fat and glycogen synthesis (lipogenesis and glycogenesis), the suppression of glycogen breakdown (glycogenolysis), the enhancement of protein synthesis and the inhibition of glucose formation from amino-acids (gluconeogenesis) by the liver.

The release of insulin from the pancreas depends largely upon the concentration of glucose in the pancreatic arterial blood. The ' ketones ' acetoacetate and β-hydroxybutyrate are also capable of causing an increase in the rate of insulin secretion. No ' trophic ' hormone has been discovered, but glucose appears to be a more efficient stimulus for insulin release when given orally than parenterally so that there may be an intestinal factor involved. Certain drugs (e.g. the sulphonylureas) and amino-acids can also stimulate the output of insulin. Adrenaline can inhibit the secretion of the hormone *in vitro* and *in vivo* even in the presence of a high concentration of glucose.

Insulin is released into the portal venous blood and carried to the liver where approximately 50 per cent is removed at each passage. Insulin in the blood is associated with the α_2-globulin and may be neutralized with anti-insulin serum. This insulin can be measured by immuno-assay methods (p. 492). In addition there exists in plasma a fraction with insulin-like activity in biological assay systems which cannot be inhibited by insulin anti-serum. This fraction of plasma insulin-like activity (variously called ' atypical ' or ' non-suppressible ' insulin) does not disappear after pancreatectomy. It appears that the plasma immuno-reactive insulin (IRI) represents the hormonally active insulin *in vivo*. Insulin is inactivated by the enzyme insulinase which is found in liver, kidney and to a lesser extent in other tissues.

Glucagon, a straight chain polypeptide containing 29 amino-acid residues, is secreted by the α-cells of the islets of Langerhans. It stimulates glycogenolysis in liver and causes a temporary rise of blood glucose concentration. This hyperglycaemia in turn leads to a fall in plasma FFA. Unlike adrenaline, glucagon does not stimulate glycogenolysis in muscle. Glucagon causes an increase in the rate of secretion of insulin. These effects are observed after the administration of large doses and it is not known whether the hormone plays any part in the physiological regulation of carbohydrate metabolism.

Adenohypophysial hormones

Growth hormone stimulates lipolysis which causes a rise in plasma FFA concentration and an increase in the rate of ketone body formation by the liver. Carbohydrate oxidation is reduced; a change which is probably secondary to the alteration in fat metabolism. The transport of amino-acids across cell membranes is facilitated and the rate of incorporation of amino-acids into protein is increased. The effects of growth hormone upon lipolysis are reduced in the presence of an excess of glucose. Growth hormone secretion varies inversely with the blood glucose concentration and is increased by exercise, stress and the ingestion of protein.

Corticotrophin (p. 525) causes lipolysis *in vitro*. Its major effects on energy metabolism are, however, mediated through its action in stimulating the secretion of the adrenocortical hormones. During even moderate hypoglycaemia, there is an immediate rise of corticotrophic secretion which is independent of any release of adrenaline.

Adrenocortical hormones (also see Chapter 15)
Cortisol (hydrocortisone) and other 11-oxy adrenocortical steroids cause a diminution in the peripheral utilization of glucose and an equivalent reduction in the hepatic glucose output. They stimulate gluconeogenesis from protein, inhibit protein anabolism and increase the rate of glycogenesis by the liver. They increase the rate of turnover of FFA.

Withdrawal of gluco-corticoid hormones by hypophysectomy or by adrenalectomy also reduces the rate of insulin breakdown. The fasting blood glucose is low and the degree and duration of hypoglycaemia produced by insulin is greater than in normal subjects. The hyperglycaemic activity of both adrenaline and glucagon is reduced in the absence of glucocorticoids.

Catecholamines (also see Chapter 15)
Adrenaline stimulates the breakdown of glycogen in liver and muscle and causes a rise in the blood glucose concentration by increasing the glucose output of the liver. Noradrenaline has about one-twentieth the hyperglycaemic potential of adrenaline. Both catecholamines in physiological amounts increase the rate of lipolysis of depot fat, so causing a rise of plasma FFA concentration. Tissues which are able to use either energy source use more FFA and less glucose.

Only adrenaline is released from the adrenal medulla during hypoglycaemia. The rate of secretion is probably controlled by the hypothalamus, and is mediated by the splanchnic nerves. Sympathetic denervation of adipose tissue reduces the rate of lipolysis in the denervated region, presumably by stopping the liberation of noradrenaline at post-ganglionic nerve endings.

Thyroid hormones (also see Chapter 16)
Thyroxine and *tri-iodothyronine* decrease the efficiency of the oxidative energy-yielding processes. Increased amounts of glucose and FFA are oxidized and there is a rise in oxygen consumption. Synthesis of glycogen in the liver is diminished. More rapid lipolysis causes depletion of depot fat and faster gluconeogenesis leads to an increase in protein catabolism.

16*

The rate of absorption of glucose from the gut is accelerated. This causes an excessive rise in the blood glucose during the first half-hour after meals.

REGULATION OF BLOOD GLUCOSE AND PLASMA FREE FATTY ACID CONCENTRATIONS

The organization of metabolism requires that the basic energy needs of the body should be met at all times, that rapid increases in energy expenditure should be possible, and that the load of raw material resulting from an intermittent feeding pattern should be quickly and efficiently stored in a form which will allow easy metabolism and utilization. These basic organizational requirements are still further modified by the characteristics of individual cells. The brain can metabolize only glucose. In the fasting state, 70 per cent of the glucose output of the liver is used by the brain which constitutes less than 3 per cent of the total body weight: this distribution of glucose comes about because its access to all other tissues is restricted. This restriction is achieved by a low rate of insulin secretion and a low blood glucose concentration. It is also encouraged by the presence of FFA which provide an alternative source of energy. During the absorption of carbohydrate from the gut this pattern is completely changed. The blood glucose rises. As a direct consequence of this rise, there is an increased secretion of insulin and a diminished release of growth hormone from the pituitary. These factors combine to limit the degree and duration of hyperglycaemia by increasing glycogenesis, the synthesis of fat and the use of glucose instead of FFA as a source of energy by adipose tissue, muscle and the liver. The hepatic glucose output is suppressed by the raised blood glucose. Lipolysis is inhibited, and there is an elevated plasma insulin with a consequent rapid decline in plasma FFA concentration. (Resistance to the inhibitory effect of insulin upon lipolysis may be an important factor in the development of human diabetes mellitus; p. 479).

In the post-absorptive state as the blood glucose falls the plasma insulin concentration declines and rather later the rate of secretion of growth hormone rises. All 3 circumstances lead to an increase in the breakdown of fat with the liberation of glycerol and FFA. The declining plasma insulin concentration gradually restricts the access of glucose to muscle and adipose tissue and this restriction is reinforced by the rising levels of plasma FFA and 'ketones' which both affect the permeability of certain cells to glucose. FFA becomes the major source of energy. Glycogen synthesis ceases. The production of glucose by the liver is resumed. The concentration of glucose in the blood tends to stabilize at a fasting level which still provokes a small resting secretion of insulin. This continuing secretion of insulin in the basal metabolic period probably helps to limit the rate of lipolysis in the periphery and to prevent the development of severe keto-acidosis during prolonged fasting.

During the first day of life the fasting blood glucose is of the order of 50 mg/100 ml. Within a few weeks it reaches the level maintained during the remainder of life, 70–100 mg/100 ml for arterial and capillary blood and 5–10 mg/100 ml lower for mixed venous blood. The concentration in the plasma of free fatty acids in a normal adult after an overnight fast is 0·3–0·6 m-equiv/l. The blood glucose concentration represents at any time the balance between the rate of addition of glucose to the blood and the rate at which it is removed.

APPETITE AND HUNGER

Appetite is an agreeable sensation experienced in anticipation of food which has previously caused pleasure. It is an acquired, conscious, psychological process, probably mediated by the cerebral cortex and modified by psychological influences such as anxiety.

Hunger is an innate, involuntary, physiological effect which becomes active within a few hours of birth. Its symptoms are unpleasant and signal a physiological need for food. It may, however, be modified to some extent by psychological factors and suppression of hunger is seen in some forms of mental illness.

Experiments in animals in which different parts of the brain were stimulated electrically or destroyed by electro-coagulation and observations in patients with brain tumours, head injuries and encephalitic lesions show the existence of hypothalamic hunger regulating centres. Stimulation of the medial satiety centre in animals abolishes hunger, while destruction of the centre causes persistent hunger and over-eating. The lateral feeding centre is normally dominated by the satiety centre, but stimulation and destruction of the centre cause effects opposite to those seen after stimulation and destruction of the satiety centre.

Hunger is a complex physiological phenomenon and depends upon many factors. Numerous hypotheses have been put forward to explain it, none of which is satisfactory. The 'glucostatic' hypothesis of hunger regulation depends upon the observed association of satiety with increased peripheral glucose arterio-venous (a–v) difference after meals. It cannot explain why a carbohydrate-free meal can abolish hunger even though there is no change in the peripheral a–v glucose difference. Hyperglycaemia *per se* (as in diabetes) does not suppress hunger. The 'thermogenic' hypothesis suggests that hunger is abolished by the rise of body temperature which occurs after meals, due to the specific dynamic action of food. It cannot explain why fat, which has the lowest specific dynamic action, is the most satisfying of all foods.

The presence of the stomach is not essential for the perception of hunger which may be experienced after gastrectomy. Hunger is only partially relieved by distension of the stomach by nutritionally inert material.

Disordered function

DIABETES MELLITUS

The syndrome of diabetes mellitus is the result of a deficiency of physiologically effective insulin. Although the characteristic and most easily measured disorder of function is in the handling of carbohydrate by the body, there are also profound alterations in the organization of energy metabolism, especially in relation to fat metabolism.

Types of diabetes
Two main types of diabetes mellitus are recognized clinically.

1. *Insulin-dependent* diabetes sometimes known as juvenile or severe diabetes. This type appears chiefly in children and young adults. The interval between the onset of symptoms, weight loss and polyuria, and diagnosis is short. Unless treatment with insulin is started there is a rapid progression to ketosis and coma.

2. *Adult-type* diabetes, also known as maturity-onset or non-insulin dependent diabetes. Symptoms are mild, insidious in onset, often unnoticed by the patient and appear characteristically in later life. Patients are often obese and do not become ketotic if not treated with insulin.

These 2 types of diabetes represent the extremes and there is some overlap of features in individual patients. It is not uncommon for patients with 'adult-type' diabetes to become insulin dependent. It is very exceptional for a diabetic with a history of episodes of ketosis to cease to be dependent upon exogenous insulin.

Causes of diabetes

Insulin production may fail because of damage to the β-cells of the pancreatic islets. Islet cells may be damaged by acute inflammation of the pancreas, by chronic fibrosis, as in chronic pancreatitis and haemochromatosis, and occasionally by pancreatic neoplasms.

Spontaneous diabetes mellitus is an inherited condition. Population studies suggest that the disease is a recessive trait and it has been estimated that approximately 6 per cent of the population are homozygous for the gene. There is no evidence that the 2 types of diabetes are genetically distinct. They rather seem to represent 2 facets of the same condition. Although diabetes mellitus is an inherited disorder other factors affect its expression. Of these factors age, repeated pregnancy, obesity and diet are among the most important in the development of adult type diabetes. The incidence of this type of the disease fell sharply during the war in all countries where rationing was enforced—a clear example of the effect of environment upon the expression of an inborn error of metabolism. The factors which precipitate the development of insulin-dependent diabetes are probably associated with the hormonal changes of growth and puberty and with the degenerative changes of old age. Insulin-dependent diabetes occurs most commonly in childhood, adolescence and old age whereas adult-type diabetes has a maximum incidence during the fifth and sixth decades. The gene may also have a variable penetration and the overt disorder of carbohydrate metabolism may represent the last phase in the development of the disease. There is increasing evidence that the premature development of arteriosclerosis may be associated with a hidden diabetic trait.

The cause of diabetes mellitus is unknown. In the early stages of the disease the effectiveness of insulin is decreased. Two explanations have been put forward to account for this diminished effectiveness. It has been suggested that fatty acids in high concentration in blood and tissues compete with glucose for utilization by muscle and that under such circumstances muscle is relatively insensitive to the action of insulin (p. 473). Alternatively, it has been proposed that there is a circulating antagonist to insulin. An antagonist to the action of insulin on muscle has been found to be present both in normal people and, in a higher concentration, in diabetics. The antagonist is associated with the serum albumin and is dependent upon the pituitary and adrenal glands. A proportion of the normal relatives of diabetics has been found to have an increased amount of this antagonist. The pattern of inheritance suggests a Mendelian dominant character and therefore differs from that of diabetes mellitus.

Metabolic changes in diabetes mellitus

Patients with adult-type diabetes have an increased concentration of immuno-reactive insulin in the blood. In the earliest detectable phase of the disease, both the fasting blood glucose and plasma insulin are normal. However, there is a greater than normal rise in the blood glucose and plasma insulin concentration after a glucose load (p. 489). In the next phase the fasting glucose and insulin levels are also raised. Finally, a state may be reached when the pancreatic secretion of insulin is maximal even when the patient is fasting and under such conditions there is no increase in the plasma insulin concentration when the blood glucose rises after the administration of carbohydrate. Obesity has a special relationship with this form of diabetes; it is uncertain whether the diabetic trait plus obesity causes the abnormal glucose tolerance curve or whether the diabetic trait predisposes to obesity first and diabetes second. The biochemical disturbances present may disappear after weight loss.

Adult-type diabetes is characteristically associated with a high plasma FFA concentration which falls only slowly after oral glucose. It has been suggested that in patients with this type of the disease there is a metabolic abnormality which leads to a greater release of fatty acids, and that the combination of a high blood glucose and an increased plasma insulin concentration is a less effective inhibitor of lipolysis in such patients. In the post-prandial state the action of insulin on muscle would be antagonized by the high plasma FFA concentration and the uptake of glucose by this tissue would therefore be restricted. The oxidation of fatty acids by muscle would therefore continue until the inhibition, by glucose and insulin, of lipolysis in adipose tissue had led to a fall in plasma FFA concentration. This fall would in turn permit the uptake and utilization of glucose by muscle in the presence of insulin. This explanation accounts for the delayed response to insulin seen in patients with adult-type diabetes and in normal people on a low carbohydrate diet. It might also account, in part, for the development of obesity before the onset of hyperglycaemia, for the glucose excluded from muscle can only be laid down as fat. This theory does not explain the raised fasting blood glucose.

Patients with insulin-dependent diabetes have little or no circulating insulin, the insulin content of the pancreas is negligible, and irreversible degenerative changes may be seen in the β-cells of the pancreatic islets. These are, however, secondary developments. There is increasing evidence that such patients pass briefly through all the phases described in the adult form of the disease before the pancreatic secretion of insulin fails completely. The factors which cause the pancreatic exhaustion are not known, but obesity rarely precedes the onset of this form of the disease.

Diabetes due to an excess of a physiological insulin antagonist is sometimes seen in acromegaly (growth hormone excess), in Cushing's syndrome (adrenocortical glucocorticoid excess) and in patients treated with corticotrophin or corticosteroids. Patients with phaeochromocytoma (p. 546) often have glycosuria or a diabetic form of glucose tolerance curve. In each instance, antagonism to the activity of insulin may lead to hyperglycaemia and glycosuria. The situation may be aggravated by an hereditary predisposition to diabetes. The elimination of the hormonal excess usually results in the disappearance of the diabetes but it is possible to cause irreversible β-cell degeneration and permanent diabetes in dogs by the injections of growth hormone given over a short period (metahypophysial diabetes).

Diabetes mellitus has been produced in cats by the prolonged infusion of large amounts of glucose intravenously. It is not known if persistent post-prandial hyperglycaemia is a subsidiary factor in the development of diabetes in man. Patients who have been burnt and given intravenous glucose over a period of days occasionally develop acute diabetes.

Metabolic disturbances in uncontrolled diabetes

The magnitude and to some extent the nature of the metabolic disturbances depend on the degree of deficiency of physiologically effective insulin. The abnormal glucose tolerance curve (p. 489) is due to defective removal of glucose from the blood by peripheral tissues. Fasting hyperglycaemia results from a failure of the inhibition of the glucose output by the liver by blood glucose concentrations higher than normal.

Hyperglycaemia has 2 main consequences. First, glycosuria occurs when the amount of glucose in the glomerular filtrate exceeds the amount which can be reabsorbed by the renal tubules (p. 155). The presence of glucose in the renal tubules causes an osmotic diuresis (p. 166). Second, rapid and marked alterations in blood glucose concentration alter the refractive index of the media of the eye, causing changes in accommodation.

Protein loss, manifest by general muscular wasting, is seen in un-controlled insulin-dependent diabetes and is due to excessive catabolism and defective anabolism, the former resulting in increased rates of gluconeogenesis and acetoacetate synthesis.

Patients with uncontrolled insulin-dependent diabetes lose depot fat because of increased fat catabolism and defective fat synthesis due to the very low level of plasma insulin. Increased rate of lipolysis results in an increased plasma FFA concentration and production of acetoacetate by the liver in excess of the quantity that can be metabolized.

The accumulation of acetoacetic and other organic acids in the blood and tissues in patients with uncontrolled juvenile-type diabetes causes a metabolic acidosis (p. 210 and p. 486). Pulmonary ventilation is increased and the P_{CO_2} of blood and tissues is reduced. The great increase in the amount of organic anions excreted by the kidneys, and the osmotic diuresis due to glycosuria cause sodium and potassium depletion. Electrolyte depletion is aggravated by reduced intake and by extrarenal loss due to vomiting. Polyuria, decreased fluid intake and loss by vomiting cause dehydration. Studies in which the amount of cations, water and nitrogen required to replenish body stores were measured indicate losses in patients in severe diabetic keto-acidosis of the order of 500 m-equiv sodium and 350 m-equiv potassium (approximately 17 per cent and 10 per cent of the total exchangeable pools respectively), 2 l. of intracellular and 3 l. of extracellular fluid (approximately 7 per cent and 20 per cent of the normal volumes of these respective compart-ments), and 40 g nitrogen (equivalent to approximately 250 g protein).

Despite considerable body depletion, the plasma sodium and potas-sium concentrations are usually normal in untreated patients with diabetic ketoacidosis because of the concomitant reduction of the extracellular fluid volume. Treatment with potassium free fluids expands the extracellular space. The plasma potassium concentration may fall, and if sufficiently low (less than 2·0 m-equiv/l.) may cause muscular weakness and cardiac arrest. Hypokalaemia is aggravated by insulin treatment as increased uptake of glucose by tissues is accompanied by movement of potassium from the extracellular into the intracellular fluid compartment.

Hyperosmolar non-ketotic diabetic coma occurs usually in 'adult-type' elderly diabetes. It is characterized by severe dehydration and may be associated with focal or generalized seizures. The blood glucose concentration is very high, often exceeding 1000 mg/100 ml, and the plasma sodium is usually greater than 155 m-equiv/l. There is no excess of ketones in the blood and the plasma bicarbonate is normal, although occasionally it is reduced when the condition is accompanied by a lactic acidosis. The coma is probably due to the extracellular hyperosmolarity. The factors which lead to the development of this condition are unknown.

Complications of diabetes mellitus
It is not yet possible to explain the origin of the complications of long-standing diabetes (angiopathy, nephropathy, retinopathy, neuropathy, etc.) in terms of disordered metabolism. There is some evidence that the onset of these complications may be delayed if the blood glucose is kept, as nearly as possible, within normal limits. Regression of early retinal changes has been reported to have resulted from improved control of the disease.

Prediabetes
If diabetes mellitus is a recessive inherited disorder all persons homozygous for the gene but with normal glucose tolerance curves must be considered to be 'prediabetic'. Such individuals cannot be identified except during episodes of temporary impairment of carbohydrate tolerance. These episodes may be precipitated by the administration of steroids or ACTH or by an increase in adrenocortical secretion in response to stress.

An abnormal glucose tolerance curve develops only in the last and most easily defined phase of a progressive metabolic disorganization. It is preceded by an elevation of the concentrations of circulating FFA and insulin and by alterations in other factors at a cellular level which cannot yet be assessed. It is not therefore surprising that certain changes considered typical of diabetes may antedate frank hyperglycaemia (e.g. the skin changes of necrobiosis lipoidica diabeticorum and the large birth weights of infants born to 'prediabetic' mothers) nor that pathological changes in the basement membrane of the renal glomeruli may be present at the time that a raised blood glucose concentration is first discovered.

HYPOGLYCAEMIA

Causes
Hypoglycaemia occurs when the rate of removal of glucose from the blood exceeds the rate at which it enters the circulation. It most commonly results from insulin overdosage in the treatment of diabetes, but can also arise from excessive insulin secretion, deficiency of the

physiological antagonists to the action of insulin, defective glycogenolysis in the liver or, rarely, in association with extrapancreatic neoplasms.

Excessive insulin secretion may be from an insulinoma (β-cell islet tumour), or due to a therapeutically excessive dose of sulphonylureas (usually chlorpropamide), or to certain 'functional' hypoglycaemic states. The amino-acid *l*-leucine causes hypoglycaemia in man by the release of insulin. The mechanism of this release is not known, but children with so-called idiopathic hypoglycaemia of childhood and patients with insulinoma are especially sensitive to this effect of leucine.

Deficiency of insulin antagonists. Patients with untreated hypopituitarism and adrenal cortical insufficiency (Addison's disease) are unusually sensitive to the hypoglycaemic action of insulin and recover from hypoglycaemia very slowly. This is partly due to impairment of insulin degradation. Absence of gluconeogenesis and deficiency of liver glycogen contribute to the mild fasting hypoglycaemia observed in these conditions.

Defective glycogenolysis. Hypoglycaemia during fasting is seen in patients who are unable to break down liver glycogen. In some forms of glycogen storage disease the liver contains an excess of glycogen, but degradation to free glucose is blocked by the absence of a necessary enzyme (glucose-6-phosphatase, debranching enzyme or hepatic phosphorylase). Hypoglycaemia in chronic hepatic disease is rare and cause is not understood for its occurrence correlates poorly with the severity of structural liver damage and impairment of other liver function.

Effects

The manifestations of hypoglycaemia are due to deprivation of the brain of its major source of energy and to activation of the sympathetic nervous system, including increased secretion of adrenaline from the adrenal medulla.

The nature and severity of the symptoms depend on the degree of hypoglycaemia and on individual susceptibility. Symptoms usually appear when the blood glucose concentration is less than 40 mg/100 ml for this is the threshold for the stimulation of the autonomic nervous system by hypoglycaemia. All subjective symptoms of hypoglycaemia are due to the activity of the sympathetic nervous system. The patient is not aware of the symptoms of brain dysfunction which include confusion, abnormal behaviour and eventually coma and convulsions.

Increased secretion of adrenaline stimulates glycogenolysis in liver and muscle and mobilization of FFA from depot fat, thus increasing the blood glucose and the availability of an alternative source of energy. Sympathetic activation also causes tachycardia, sweating, pupillary dilatation and cutaneous vasoconstriction with pallor.

OBESITY

Causes

Obesity can only result from the intake of food in excess of energy requirements. Excess food is converted to fat and stored in adipose tissue.

Excessive food intake may be due to abnormal eating habits, a pathological craving for food as a means of obtaining psychological gratification, and occasionally to pathological hunger produced by hypothalamic lesions. In each instance carbohydrate consumption is characteristically excessive and lipogenesis is stimulated by increased secretion of insulin in the presence of large amounts of glucose substrate.

Efficient lipogenesis is necessary for the development of obesity. There is evidence from animal experiments of adaptive changes occurring in enzyme systems, especially those of the direct oxidative pathway, with alteration in feeding patterns. Rats trained to take all their food in 1 hr. lay down more fat than similar animals with free access throughout the day to food of the same calorific value. Lipogenesis in the former group is stimulated by the relatively greater release of insulin provoked by a single, large, daily meal. The ability to make fat from excess carbohydrate has an obvious survival value to animals with inconstant food supplies. Some species of desert rodents when kept under laboratory conditions with free access to food, develop first obesity and then diabetes. These animals are an exact experimental model of adult-type diabetes.

Obese subjects have elevated plasma FFA concentrations and their low respiratory exchange ratio (p. 489) suggests that they metabolize fat as their chief source of energy. There is some evidence that obesity is associated with an impaired capacity to oxidize glucose.

Obesity is usually attributed to increased fat synthesis. Defective lipolysis may also be important. Adrenaline has a relatively poor lipolytic action in obese persons. Similarly fasting causes a smaller rise in plasma FFA than in normal subjects. Starvation causes a less severe ketosis in obese than in normal persons.

Effects of obesity
Total metabolism is increased, because of the increased mechanical work required in physical activity and the metabolic activity of the increased amount of adipose tissue. The probability that diabetes will develop increases with the duration of obesity. Evidence described above indicates, however, that obesity may be the first evidence of metabolic abnormality in individuals who subsequently become diabetic.

KETOSIS

The term ketosis describes the accumulation of 'ketones' (acetoacetate, β-hydroxybutyrate and acetone) in the blood and tissues. The conditions in which ketosis occurs are uncontrolled insulin-dependent diabetes, fasting, glycogen storage disease and the consumption of calorically adequate but carbohydrate deficient diets. Ketosis occurs when lipolysis is excessive and the rate of production of 'ketones' exceeds the rate at which they can be metabolized. In diabetic ketoacidosis the production of 'ketones' is not only excessive but there is also evidence that the rate of utilization of acetoacetate and β-hydroxybutyrate is diminished. The increase in insulin secretion provoked by ketone bodies (p. 474) in normal subjects may serve as a feedback mechanism which, by slowing the rate of lipolysis, prevents the development of severe ketoacidosis during fasting.

Ketosis causes ketonuria, i.e., the excretion of 'ketones' in the urine. Acetoacetic and β-hydroxybutyric acids are both almost completely ionized in body fluids. In uncontrolled insulin-dependent diabetes they are present in sufficient concentrations to cause acidosis. Increased availability of acetyl-CoA results in increased cholesterol synthesis and is associated with an increase of plasma cholesterol. The elevated plasma lipoprotein concentration that accompanies ketosis is probably a reflection of excessive lipolysis.

FASTING

The metabolic changes associated with complete abstinence from food for a short period (fasting) are different from those resulting from a prolonged consumption of a calorically inadequate diet (starvation).

During fasting the blood glucose concentration is maintained initially by breakdown of the limited amount of glycogen in the liver (approximately 100 g in a previously well nourished adult) and subsequently by increased gluco-neogenesis from amino acids and decreased removal of glucose from the blood associated with increased utilization of FFA by many tissues.

Breakdown of depot fat glycerides results in an increased plasma FFA concentration and over production of acetoacetate which results in a moderate ketosis and ketonuria.

Urinary nitrogen excretion in adults is of the order of 10–15 g/day, representing the catabolism of approximately 60–90 g protein (equivalent to 240–360 Cal energy). Cortical secretion is increased and stimulates gluconeogenesis from amino acids.

Energy metabolism in fasting is inefficient. Excessive breakdown of fat causes ketosis (except in the obese). Energy is required to convert acetoacetate to acetoacetyl-CoA before it can be oxidized by tissues; and potential sources of energy (acetoacetate, β-hydroxybutyrate and acetone) are lost in the urine. The high rate of tissue protein breakdown is wasteful. The fundamental difference between short term fasting and prolonged undernutrition (starvation) is the better use which is made of available energy supplies in the latter condition.

STARVATION

The term 'starvation' is used here to describe the prolonged intake of insufficient food to balance energy expenditure. Its effects in man have been studied in volunteers, famine victims and patients with anorexia nervosa and disorders of intestinal absorption. Leaving aside the manifestations of associated vitamin deficiencies the most important metabolic changes are utilization of depot fat and some body protein as sources of energy, and reduction of overall energy expenditure.

Increased lipolysis of depot fat is associated initially with an increase in the plasma FFA concentration and mild ketosis and ketonuria. These changes disappear within a few days despite continued caloric deficiency. Persons dying of starvation show almost complete absence of depot fat, but the amount of lipid in certain tissues, notably brain, is unaffected. Catabolism of protein is shown by wasting and weakness of skeletal muscles and later by atrophy of viscera and skin, and sometimes hypoproteinaemia and oedema. The protein content of bone, however, is little affected. The fasting blood sugar falls by 10–20 mg/100 ml, and thereafter remains relatively constant.

Basal energy expenditure is reduced within a few days. Contributing factors include reduction of 'active' tissue mass, decreased cardiac work (shown by a reduced cardiac output which is associated with a minor fall of blood pressure and a decrease of heart size), reduction of skin temperature (due to cutaneous vasoconstriction, permitting better conservation of body heat), and suppression of growth. The secretion of hormones by the adenohypophysis, thyroid, adrenal cortex and gonads is decreased. Reduced thyroid activity is of particular importance in decreasing basal energy expenditure but, except during exposure to cold, body temperature is well maintained until just before death. Starving people are lethargic and decreased voluntary muscular activity contributes to the overall reduction of energy expenditure.

The fall in the serum cholesterol concentration is probably due to depression of hepatic cholesterol synthesis.

Changes in body fluid distribution in starvation include contraction of intracellular fluid space and maintenance of, or a slight increase, in the size of the extracellular fluid pool. The ratio of extracellular to intracellular fluid volumes is therefore increased. Plasma sodium concentration is reduced and that of potassium increased slightly. This may reflect a partial breakdown of the energy-requiring mechanism which maintains the concentration gradient of these cations across cell membranes.

Deprivation of dietary fat produces effects only because caloric intake is reduced. However, deficiency of essential fatty acids in infancy may cause skin lesions. Protein deprivation, however, causes very definite effects unrelated to reduction of dietary caloric intake. These are most striking in childhood and include failure of growth and wasting of certain tissues, particularly skeletal muscle, impairment of plasma protein synthesis with oedema and defective synthesis of digestive enzymes. The latter aggravates the existing nutritional deficiency by interfering with digestion and thus absorption of food from the gut.

Principles of tests and measurements

MEASUREMENT OF ENERGY EXPENDITURE

Direct calorimetry
The energy expenditure of a subject placed in a small, sealed insulated chamber is determined from measurements of heat lost by the subject to the chamber and its water cooling system. The principal use of this method has been in the validation of the simpler techniques.

Indirect calorimetry

This requires the measurement of rates of O_2 consumption, CO_2 production and urinary nitrogen excretion. The rate of protein metabolism is calculated from the urinary nitrogen excretion, assuming that each gram of nitrogen represents the catabolism of 6·25 g protein. The amounts of O_2 consumed and CO_2 liberated during the metabolism of protein is calculated on the basis of 0·97 l. O_2 and 0·78 l. CO_2/g. The non-protein respiratory exchange ratio (RQ) is calculated as the ratio of CO_2 produced to O_2 consumed after allowing for the contribution of protein metabolism to each factor. The proportion of carbohydrate (RQ 1·0) and fat (RQ 0·7) metabolized is calculated from the non-protein RQ and the actual amounts from the observed O_2 consumption, less the amount required for the oxidation of protein. Total energy output is calculated as the sum of the energy liberated by the oxidation of protein, carbohydrate and fat, on the bases of 4, 4 and 9 Cal/g respectively.

Basal metabolic rate

This is usually measured by a simplified form of indirect calorimetry. Oxygen consumption is measured, usually with a simple recording spirometer, after an overnight fast with the subject recumbent and mentally and physically relaxed. It is assumed that under these conditions the RQ is 0·85 and that the consumption of 1 l. of oxygen corresponds to the liberation of 4·83 Calories. The rate of energy output is thus calculated from the oxygen consumption. Results are expressed in terms of Calories/m² of body surface area per hour, or more usually in clinical practice as the percentage difference between the estimated value and a standard value for persons of the same age, sex and surface area.

The basal metabolic rate has been used chiefly as an index of thyroid function but as it is greatly affected by other factors, especially anxiety and unfamiliarity with the apparatus, it is now being superseded for this purpose by other tests (p. 562). Increased values are obtained in patients with hyperthyroidism and fever, severe anaemia, cardiovascular disease, and with certain types of malignant disease, including leukaemia. Low results are seen in patients with hypothyroidism, whether primary or secondary to hypopituitarism, and during starvation and hypothermia.

CARBOHYDRATE METABOLISM

The glucose tolerance test (GTT)

The rise and fall of the concentration of glucose in the blood after the administration of a glucose load, reflects the difference between the rate of absorption of glucose and the rate at which it is dispersed into the tissues. It is normally controlled, both in degree and duration, by the secretion of insulin which increases in response to the raised blood glucose.

The oral GTT is widely used. Glucose is given in solution after an overnight fast. The amount is not critical but should be of the order of 1 g/kg ideal body weight. Arbitrary amounts of 50 g or 100 g are often used in adults. The oral GTT is affected by numerous factors unrelated to carbohydrate metabolism. The rate of absorption of glucose may be reduced by delay in the rate of gastric emptying when concentrated solutions of glucose are given and also by a diminished rate of absorption by the small intestine. Glucose absorption is accelerated in thyrotoxicosis and by surgical procedures resulting in the rapid entry of stomach contents into the small intestine. The rate at which a glucose load may be handled is reduced by a previous low carbohydrate intake (p. 480). A diet containing about 300 g a day should be given for at least 3 days before performing a GTT.

The upper limits of the normal response to an oral GTT have been determined using venous blood. Although the fasting capillary blood glucose is only very slightly higher than the fasting venous blood glucose, the capillary-venous blood glucose difference increases during the test. At the time of the blood glucose peak this difference is about 40 mg/100 ml in normal individuals but may be as great as 100 mg/100 ml. This difference between the capillary and the venous blood glucose concentration is determined by the amount of insulin secreted in response to the test hyperglycaemia and the effectiveness of this insulin in accelerating the transfer of glucose into the peripheral tissues.

When the oral GTT is performed the blood glucose concentration is estimated immediately before and at intervals after glucose ingestion. Blood samples are usually taken at $\frac{1}{2}$, 1 and 2 hr. If the absorption of glucose is very rapid the peak concentration in the blood may be reached at $\frac{1}{4}$ hr, and reactive hypoglycaemia may not occur until 3 hr, after glucose is taken; therefore many laboratories take samples at these times. Particular attention is paid to the following points when interpreting the results. (All values quoted are for venous blood glucose estimated by a method specific for glucose).

Fasting blood glucose is normally 65 to 95 mg/100 ml. This value is increased in most but not all diabetics.

Peak value is normally less than 160 mg/100 ml and usually occurs at $\frac{1}{2}$ hr. In diabetes the value is greater than normal and usually occurs late.

The peak value may be delayed and only slightly above the fasting blood glucose in diseases of the small intestine causing malabsorption of glucose. In such conditions the rate of absorption of glucose barely exceeds the rate at which a glucose load may be handled by the liver and peripheral tissues.

Two hour value. This is normally less than 120 mg/100 ml. It is increased in diabetes and this is the single most important value on the glucose tolerance curve.

Steroid-augmented GTT. The GTT in 'prediabetes' is by definition normal. An underlying diabetic trait may be unmasked if the test is performed after the administration of either cortisone or prednisone.

Intravenous GTT. This test excludes variations in the rate of intestinal absorption of glucose, which affects the oral GTT. Several techniques have been proposed. Usually glucose (0·3 g/kg body weight or 25 g) is given intravenously within three minutes. The nearly exponential fall in the blood glucose which follows the injection is plotted semi-logarithmically against time. The slope of the resulting straight line is calculated and multiplied by 100 for convenience of expression. This constant (K) which is the conventional turnover constant × 100 for a first order reaction, is normally between 1·1 and 2·4 but in diabetes is less than 1·0.

Intravenous tolbutamide test

Tolbutamide stimulates the secretion of insulin by β-cells of the pancreas and also by the cells of insulin-secreting tumours (insulinomas). The intravenous tolbutamide test is chiefly used to distinguish between causes of spontaneous hypoglycaemia. Patients with insulinomas show a profound and abnormally prolonged fall in blood glucose whereas patients with functional hyperinsulinism have a normal or near normal response. The results of the test are unpredictable in patients with other kinds of hypoglycaemic episodes.

Adult-type diabetics respond to intravenous tolbutamide by a fall in blood glucose that is slower than normal and the return to the initial level is delayed. The blood glucose is unaffected by tolbutamide in established diabetes of the insulin dependent variety, except in cases of very recent onset when the pancreatic β-cells may still contain some insulin.

In normal subjects the intravenous administration of 1 g sodium tolbutamide in the fasting state causes a fall in the blood glucose concentration to a minimum of 40 mg/100 ml after 25–45 min. Three hours after the start of the test the blood glucose exceeds 70 per cent of the fasting value. Patients with insulinomas may develop symptoms of hypoglycaemia or even coma and usually the blood glucose is less than 40 mg/ml after 3 hr.

Glucagon test

Glucagon stimulates hepatic glycogenolysis and when injected into normal subjects causes a rise of blood glucose maximal at $\frac{1}{2}$–1 hr and over by 3 hr. This response does not usually occur in patients with glycogen storage disease or severe liver damage or in normal people who have fasted for a long time. The rise of blood glucose following glucagon is normal in the presence of an insulinoma but is rapidly succeeded by a fall to a level at which symptoms of hypoglycaemia develop. This effect, which does not occur in subjects with functional hyperinsulinism, is due to the liberation of insulin from the tumour by glucagon (p. 474). It is not a sequel to the modest hyperglycaemia produced by the latter hormone.

Plasma insulin concentration

The measurement of the plasma insulin concentration is likely to become a routine laboratory procedure. Assay methods are either biological or immunological. Most biological methods depend upon the biochemical action of insulin on either muscle or adipose tissue *in vitro*. Immunological assay of plasma insulin depends upon the competition of insulin in the sample to be assayed with isotopically labelled insulin for combination with a specific antibody. The amount of radioactivity associated with the insulin antibody complex is inversely related to the concentration of insulin in the sample. This technique measures the immunoreactive insulin (IRI) which is associated with the plasma α-globulins (p. 273). This determination is not dependent on the physiological activity of the insulin which is measured. The greatest difficulty with all the methods for the assay of insulin in the blood is to relate the values obtained to the physiological effectiveness of the hormone in any particular set of circumstances. When discussing plasma insulin levels in the preceding sections all references are to insulin concentration as determined by immuno-assay.

OBESITY AND STARVATION

Depot fat accounts for 15–17 per cent of the body weight of normal young subjects. The proportion of fat may increase in old age, even in the absence of weight gain, as muscle is replaced by adipose tissue.

Excess or deficiency of depot fat is obvious on inspection. The degree of abnormality is most easily determined by comparison with the standard weight of individuals of the same age, sex, height and somatotype.

The actual amount of body fat may be determined for research purposes in a number of ways. *Body weight,* and the difference between the *specific gravity,* determined by weighing in air and under water, and the standard specific gravity of non-fat body constituents can be measured. *Intracellular and extracellular* fluid volumes can be estimated. 'Active cell mass' is calculated on the assumption that cells contain 67 per cent water. The weight of depot fat is calculated by subtracting from the observed body weight the sum of the weights of 'active cell mass', extracellular fluid and an allowance for skeletal minerals.

An approximate assessment of the amount of depot fat may be made by measuring the thickness of the subcutaneous fat by soft tissue radiography or more simply with calipers.

Practical assessment

DIABETES MELLITUS

Clinical observations
Symptoms of hyperglycaemia: polyuria and temporary visual disturbance.

Symptoms of water and electrolyte loss: thirst and eventually dehydration with low plasma volume (p. 481).

Increased gluconeogenesis: weakness and wasting of muscles (protein depletion).

Increased lipolysis: loss of depot (including subcutaneous) fat and ketosis.

Recognition of known complications: retinopathy, nephropathy and neuropathy, and a high incidence of mature cataracts and peripheral vascular disease.

Evidence of causative disease: acromegaly, Cushing's syndrome, phaeochromocytoma, chronic pancreatitis, haemochromatosis.

Routine urine tests
Glucose oxidase tests (Clinistix and Testape), for detection of glucosuria and *copper reduction tests* (Clinitest and Benedict's test) for measurement of glycosuria.

For ketonuria, see below.

Routine laboratory methods
Fasting blood glucose: > 100 mg/100 ml, except in mild adult-type patients.

One to two-hour post prandial blood glucose: > 150 mg/100 ml.

Glucose tolerance test: peak value > 160 mg/100 ml, usually occurs later than ½ hr. 2 hr value > 120 mg/100 ml.

Tests for diagnosis of primary causative disease: acromegaly (p. 513), Cushing's syndrome (p. 531), phaeochromocytoma (p. 546), chronic pancreatitis, haemochromatosis.

KETOSIS

Clinical observations
Increased depth and rate of breathing when severe and associated with acidosis. Odour of acetone in expired air.

Routine methods
Urine tests: Rothera test and Acetest for acetone. Ferric chloride test: less sensitive test for acetoacetate. The latter test must always be performed if Acetest is strongly positive, to determine the severity of ketonuria. The larger part of urinary 'ketones' is β-hydroxybutyrate (for which there is no simple test). There is five to ten times as much acetoacetate as acetone in the urine of ketotic patients. The normal urinary secretion of 'ketones' is less than 100 mg/day; in diabetic ketoacidosis the urinary loss may exceed 100 g/day.

Plasma (HCO_3^-), pH and P_{CO_2} measurements (p. 213). Plasma 'ketones' (normal 1–2 mg/100 ml) are difficult to measure. A rough estimate, however, may be obtained by using Acetest and serial dilution of plasma with water; in mild ketosis the test is positive at a dilution of 1 : 2.

'PREDIABETES'

Clinical observations
Obesity; family history of diabetes; hyperglycaemia during stress of pregnancy, severe infection or injury; in women, birth of large babies.

Routine urine tests: glycosuria when present is due to low renal threshold (renal glycosuria). In the last trimester of pregnancy lactose (a reducing sugar) is often present in the urine.

Routine laboratory tests
Glucose tolerance test: normal.

Steroid-augmented glucose tolerance test: higher blood sugar curve than in GTT. The administration of steroids often causes glycosuria.

OBESITY AND STARVATION

Clinical observations: body size, contour and weight.

Special techniques: measurement of depot fat (p. 493) and assessment of amount of subcutaneous fat (p. 493).

HYPOGLYCAEMIA

Clinical observations:
Episodes of weakness, palpitation, tremor, sweating, abnormal behaviour. Coma and convulsions occur chiefly after fasting with insulinomas. In functional hyperinsulinism symptoms develop 2–5 hr after meals. Symptoms relieved by glucose administration.

Signs of causative disease: hypopituitarism, Addison's disease, history of gastric operation, glycogen storage disease, severe liver damage.

Routine methods:
Blood glucose: usually < 40 mg/100 ml during episode.

Intravenous tolbutamide test: blood glucose < 40 mg/100 ml after 3 hr, with insulinoma but not with functional hyperinsulinism.

Tests for causative disease: hypopituitarism (p. 506), Addison's disease (p. 526), glycogen storage disease.

References

LEVINE R. (1964) Carbohydrate metabolism. In *Disease of Metabolism* (5th edn). (Ed. DUNCAN G.G.) Philadelphia: Saunders. pp. 105–90.

CANTAROW A. & SCHEPARTZ B. (1967) *Biochemistry* (4th edn). Philadelphia: Saunders.

RANDLE P.J. (1964) Insulin. In *The Hormones IV* (Ed. PINCUS G., THIMANN K.V. & ASTWOOD E.B.). New York: Academic Press, pp. 481–530.

RENOLD A.E., CROFFORD O.B., STAUFFACHER W. & JEANRENAUD B. (1965) Hormonal control of adipose tissue metabolism with special reference to the effects of insulin. *Diabetologia* 1, 4–12.

BERSON S.A. & YALLOW R.S. (1966) Insulin in blood and insulin antibodies. *Amer. J. Med.*, **40**, 676–690.

MAYER J. (1966) Some aspects of the problem of regulation of food intake and obesity. *New Engl. J. Med.*, **274**, 610–616; 662–673; 722–731.

STRANG J.M. (1964) Obesity. In *Diseases of Metabolism* (5th edn). (Ed. DUNCAN G.G.). Philadelphia: Saunders. pp. 693–804.

KEYS A., BROZEK J., HENSCHEL A., MICKELSEN O. & TAYLOR H.L. (1950) *Biology of human starvation*. Minneapolis: Univ. of Minnesota Press.

RENOLD A.E. & CAHILL G.F. (1966) Diabetes mellitus. In *The Metabolic Basis of Inherited Disease* (2nd edn). (Ed. STANBURY J.B., WYNGAARDEN J.B. & FREDRICKSON D.S.). New York: McGraw-Hill. pp. 69–108.

RANDLE P.J., GARLAND P.B., HALES C.N. & NEWSHOLME E.A. (1964) The glucose fatty acid cycle and diabetes mellitus. In *Ciba Colloquia on Endocrinology*. vol. 15. London: Churchill. pp. 192–210.

VALLANCE-OWEN J. (1964) Synalbumin insulin antagonism and diabetes. In *Ciba Colloquia on Endocrinology*. vol. 15. London: Churchill. pp. 217–234.

NUTTALL F.Q. (1965) Metabolic acidoses—diabetic. *Arch. Intern. med.*, **116**, 709–716.

WILLIAMS R.H. (ed.) (1960) *Diabetes with a chapter on hypoglycaemia*. New York: Hoeber–Harper.

MARKS V. & ROSE F.C. (1965) *Hypoglycaemia*. Oxford: Blackwell.

14

The Pituitary Gland

STRUCTURAL ORGANIZATION

The mammalian pituitary gland originates from 2 independent anlages which coalesce during foetal life and then occupy a common site in the sella turcica of the sphenoid bone. One portion of the pituitary is typically glandular in structure: the other resembles nervous tissue. The glandular elements (adenohypophysis) develop from the somatic ectoderm of the posterior nasopharynx (Rathke's pouch); the nervous elements (neurohypophysis) develop as a downward evagination of the neural ectoderm from the floor of the diencephalon.

The adenohypophysis consists of the pars distalis (anterior lobe), the pars intermedia (intermediate lobe) and the pars tuberalis. The neurohypophysis consists of the infundibular process (posterior lobe), the infundibular stem and the median eminence of the tuber cinereum. The pars tuberalis surrounds the infundibular stem to form the pituitary stalk.

There are structural connections between the hypothalamus and both divisions of the pituitary. The connection between the hypothalamus and the adenohypophysis is believed to be exclusively vascular. It consists of a group of venules, the hypophysial portal vessels, which arise from the capillaries of the median eminence and terminate in a secondary capillary plexus in the pars distalis. The neurohypophysis is connected to the supra-optic and paraventricular nuclei of the anterior hypothalamus by the hypothalamo-hypophysial tract.

THE ADENOHYPOPHYSIS

Normal function

THE ADENOHYPOPHYSIAL HORMONES

At least 6 hormones are secreted by the cells of the anterior pituitary gland, and these hormones account for most of the physiological effects attributed to extracts of this gland. The 6 hormones are: (1) growth or somatotrophic hormone (GH), (2) prolactin or lactogenic hormone, (3) thyrotrophin or thyroid-stimulating hormone (TSH), (4) follicle-stimulating hormone (FSH), (5) luteinizing or interstitial-cell stimulating hormone (LH, ICSH), and (6) corticotrophin or adrenocortico-trophic hormone (ACTH).

In some species, including man, which lack a distinct intermediate lobe, the cells which produce melanocyte-stimulating hormone (MSH) are intermingled with those of the adenohypophysis. Some other species, such as the rat, have a distinct intermediate lobe from which MSH is elaborated.

Pituitary cell types
The use of histochemical and cytochemical staining procedures in conjunction with altered physiological states due to castration, thyroid-ectomy, adrenalectomy, hormone injections and different stages of the reproductive cycle have made it possible to associate individual hormones with specific cell types. Knowledge of the fine structure of the gland has been advanced by the use of newer and more refined techniques including electron microscopy, autoradiography and fluorescent anti-body microscopy. By fractionation of homogenates of rat anterior pituitary glands it has been possible to isolate secretory granules and to confirm that each hormone, with the possible exception of ACTH, is incorporated into secretory granules of a specific size. A summary of current views of rat anterior pituitary cell types and their secretions is shown in Table 15.

Chemical properties
Hundreds of proteins and peptides may now be characterized in pituitary extracts by the use of zone electrophoresis in gel media (Ferguson, 1965). Undoubtedly, many of these have intracellular functions in the pituitary gland, and many may be the result of enzymatic hydrolysis during extraction. However, the possibility that a number of these proteins are hormones with as yet unknown functions cannot be excluded. Meanwhile it is important to note that none of the protein hormones has yet been unequivocally identified in its secreted form. Growth hormone from human pituitary glands has been isolated in highly purified form and consists of a single polypeptide chain containing 188 amino acids, with a molecular weight of 21,500.

'Plasma growth hormone' as determined by radioimmunoassay ranges from less than 5 ng/ml in normal people to more than 50 ng/ml in acromegalics: biological assay of plasma, however, may give higher

TABLE 15. A summary of current views of rat anterior pituitary cell types and their secretions (modified from McShan & Hartley, 1965).

Hormones	Cell type		Staining reactions			Electron micro-scopic description
	General	Specific	AF	PAS	Acid stains	
Growth hormone	Acidophil	Somatotrope	—	—	+	350 mμ granules, cells columnar and arranged in groups on sinusoids.
Prolactin	Acidophil	Mammo-trope	—	—	+	600 mμ elliptical granules, cells located individually in interior of cell cords.
TSH	Basophil	Thyrotrope	+	+	—	140 mμ granules, cells angular and not usually located on sinusoids.
FSH	Basophil	FSH gonadotrope	—	+	—	200 mμ granules, cells located on sinusoids and are usually rounded.
LH	Basophil	LH gonadotrope	—	+	—	200 mμ granules, cells usually located on sinusoids, rounded and contain bizarre cytoplasmic formations.
ACTH	Chromophobe (identification still uncertain)	Corticotrope	—	—	—	100–150 mμ acido-philic granules. Large cells best seen after adrenalectomy.
No specific hormone	Chromophobe	Acidophilic chromophobe. Basophilic chromophobe.	—	—	—	Few characteristic granules

AF=aldehyde-fuchsin. PAS=periodic acid-Schiff stain.

values. A number of growth responses *in vitro*, such as ^{35}S uptake by the cartilage of hypophysectomized rats, are not given by pituitary growth hormone, but are given by serum. This activity is low in the serum of pituitary dwarfs and increased by the administration of human growth hormone (HGH) or in acromegalic serum. The substance responsible has been called the sulphation factor. It has a biological half-life of about 12 hr compared with 20 to 40 min for injected HGH.

17

Growth hormone preparations from different species differ considerably in some of their chemical properties and in biological specificity. All mammalian growth hormone preparations are active in the rat but man responds only to primate growth hormone. Attempts to modify the more readily available bovine and porcine growth hormones to make them effective in man have not yet been successful, but some growth hormone-like effects in man have been obtained with ovine prolactin. In human pituitary extracts growth hormone and prolactin are not clearly separate hormones as they are in most other species. During pregnancy the placenta secretes large amounts of material with weak growth hormone- and prolactin-like activities, usually referred to as chorionic growth-hormone-prolactin or placental lactogen.

Highly purified forms of TSH, LH and FSH have also been prepared, permitting the development of immunoassay methods for their determination in plasma.

ACTH appears to occur in the pituitary in both low (peptide) and high molecular weight forms. The peptide contains 39 amino acids in a single chain and has a molecular weight of 4500. The results of immunoassay suggest that it is the circulating form of the hormone. However, it is important to note that the immunoreactive groups reside in the terminal 15 amino acids, while only the first 24 amino acid portion of the molecule is necessary for full biological activity. Melanophore-stimulating hormone occurs in 2 peptide forms, designated α- and β-MSH. The structure of α-MSH is identical in all species examined and its amino acid sequence is the same as that of the last 13 amino acids of ACTH. β-MSH shows minor differences between species, the human peptide containing 22 amino acids compared with 18 for other species. A 7-amino acid sequence of β-MSH is common to both α-MSH and ACTH. The sequence of peptide I, a fat-mobilizing peptide of molecular weight 5000 isolated from pig pituitaries, is reported to contain the sequence for β-MSH.

Physiological effects

Growth hormone increases the transport of amino acids into cells and their incorporation into protein. It inhibits fat synthesis and causes release of fatty acids from adipose tissue. The uptake of glucose into cells is inhibited, perhaps as a consequence of the increased uptake of fatty acids (p. 476), and there is decreased sensitivity to the hypoglycaemic effect of insulin.

In man the administration of human growth hormone (HGH) leads to retention of nitrogen, phosphorus, sodium, potassium and chloride, and to a slight increase in plasma phosphate. Plasma concentrations of glucose, fatty acids, glycerol and ketone bodies are increased. There is persistent hypercalciuria, which appears to be parathyroid-dependent. The secretion of aldosterone may be increased. In pituitary dwarfs 5 mg HGH 3 times a week promotes a rate of growth equal to, or even greater than, normal. Since the half-life of HGH itself is only 23 min it appears likely, as has already been pointed out, that the circulating form of growth hormone differs from that present in pituitary extracts.

Despite the diverse sites of action of growth hormone and its apparent importance in regulatory metabolism (p. 474) it is interesting that in the adult hypopituitary patient, given replacement therapy with adreno-cortical steroids, thyroid hormone and the appropriate sex hormone, it is difficult to detect any signs of growth hormone deficiency.

Prolactin. Details of the hormonal regulation of lactation have been worked out most fully in the rat, in which it appears that mammary duct growth requires the combined action of adrenal corticoids, growth hormone and oestrogens, whereas progesterone and prolactin are needed in addition to bring about the growth of the alveolar lobules. Milk secretion is initiated when progesterone and oestrogen are simul-taneously withdrawn, but only in the continued presence of prolactin and adrenal corticoids. In certain animals, including human beings, the stimulus of suckling maintains milk production. This is due to a reflex effect of breast stimulation on prolactin secretion.

In primates prolactin closely resembles growth hormone in its meta-bolic effects and may have regulatory functions in addition to its role in lactation: it does not, however, function as a luteotrophic hormone as in the rat.

The gonadotrophic hormones. In primates ovulation divides the female reproductive cycle into two phases. In the first phase secretion of FSH leads to maturation of the graafian follicle and the small amount of LH released stimulates the secretion of oestrogen. After ovulation is induced by a sudden discharge of LH, the newly formed corpus luteum begins to secrete progesterone which is reflected by an increased urinary excretion of pregnanediol. Maintenance of the corpus luteum depends on LH.

In the male, FSH acts on the spermatogenic cells in the testis and promotes growth of the seminiferous tubules. Secretion of LH is more or less constant after puberty and promotes secretion of androgens by the Leydig cells of the testis. For further discussion of pituitary-gonadal relationships see p. 503 and Chapter 18.

The trophic functions of *thyrotrophin* are discussed in chapter 16 and those of *corticotrophin* in chapter 15. Both these substances may exert direct effects, e.g., on fat mobilization, not mediated through their respective target organs. The hormonal regulation of adipose tissue is discussed in chapter 13.

REGULATION OF ADENOHYPOPHYSIAL FUNCTION

Present concepts of anterior pituitary regulation are dominated by the portal-vessel-chemotransmitter hypothesis which states that the secretory activity of the adenohypophysial cells is controlled by humoral substances known as 'releasing factors' or, in the case of prolactin, 'inhibiting factor'. These substances are thought to be liberated by hypothalamic nerves ending close to the capillaries of the median eminence, and to be carried to the pars distalis in the hypophysial portal vessels. The hypothesis is supported by several different lines of evidence. If the pituitary is transplanted to a site remote from the median eminence, secretion of all the anterior lobe hormones declines to a low level, with the exception of that of prolactin. If the transplanted pituitary is then reimplanted beneath the median eminence normal function is restored. Section of the pituitary stalk, which includes the portal vessels, also leads to a marked decline in pituitary hormone secretion. Destruction or stimulation of discrete areas of the hypothalamus has helped to localize the sites of control for each pituitary hormone. Finally, separate releasing factors for each of the anterior pituitary hormones have been identified in extracts of the median eminence and in hypophysial portal blood.

The activity of the hypothalamus is modified by neural influences arriving from other parts of the brain, particularly the reticular activating system and the limbic area. The hypothalamus also contains centres for the regulation of food intake and for water seeking and water conservation (via the neurohypophysis) and responds to changes in the temperature, glucose concentration and osmolarity of the perfusing blood.

In the case of the trophic hormones there is a further important mechanism of regulation which serves to stabilize the plasma level of the target hormones. This is usually described as a 'negative feedback' control. An increase in the plasma cortisol level, for example, inhibits the secretion of ACTH, whereas a fall in plasma cortisol leads to an increased secretion of ACTH. The major sites of inhibitory control are believed to be hypothalamic in the case of ACTH and the gonadotrophic hormones, but in the pituitary itself in the case of TSH. Because the response is relatively slow and long-lasting, it has been suggested that the feedback regulatory system controls synthesis rather than release of trophic hormones.

Regulation of sexual function

In the pre-pubertal animal the hypothalamus exerts a tonic inhibitory control over gonadotrophin secretion. The infantile hypothalamus appears to be more sensitive to oestrogens than the adult, and therefore maintains the low oestrogen levels characteristic of the prepubertal state. Hypothalamic lesions, by reducing the size of the area from which pituitary-inhibiting stimuli arise, may initiate precocious puberty.

The pituitary gland itself is potentially bisexual. Grafts of pituitary glands from newborn male rats placed under the median eminence of hypophysectomized females quickly restore cyclic gonadal activity and can support pregnancy. A single injection of testosterone, administered before the fifth day of life to female mice and rats causes lifelong sterility. These animals manifest chronic FSH secretion without cyclic LH release. When the glands of such androgen-sterilized females are transplanted to the median eminence region of uninjected hypophysectomized female hosts normal reproductive function is restored. Moreover, the pituitary glands of androgen-sterilized rats will release LH if the hypothalamus is stimulated electrically. The inference is, therefore, that the neural signal and not the pituitary LH-synthesizing-releasing mechanism is at fault in androgen-induced sterility. It thus appears that, in the rat, the adult pattern of gonadotrophic activity depends upon hormone-controlled brain function. The brain centres involved in sexual regulation have a well defined period of maturation, the direction of which must depend upon a specific hormonal milieu during this critical phase.

In the human subject the onset of reproductive cycles appears to be due to intrinsic maturation processes of the brain. Cyclic pituitary-ovarian function is clearly under neural control as shown for example by the effects of emotional disturbances and psychotropic drugs. Neural regulation in other species is even more strikingly illustrated by the phenomena of environment-influenced breeding and reflex ovulation.

Regulation of TSH secretion

As noted above the TSH secretion of the pituitary gland is directly regulated by plasma free thyroxine concentration. Neural influences maintain a tonic control of pituitary-thyroid function over which responses to elevated and depressed blood levels of thyroid hormone are superimposed. The thyroid response to cold exposure involves thermo-sensitive structures in the preoptic area of the hypothalamus close to those concerned with autonomic heat-regulatory responses. This region for temperature and thyroid regulation is in turn anatomically close to the ventromedial nucleus which, together with the lateral hypothalamic area, comprises a system for the control of feeding and satiety. Inter-action between feeding and temperature control regions can be demonstrated in goats: local hypothalamic cooling induces eating even in food-satiated animals.

Regulation of ACTH secretion

After corticoid administration the adrenal glands atrophy and pituitary ACTH concentration falls; after adrenalectomy pituitary and blood ACTH concentrations rise. These observations illustrate feedback regulation of ACTH secretion by adrenal steroids. The locus of action appears to be in the hypothalamus rather than the pituitary itself. It should be remembered that the feedback inhibition depends upon the effective level of cortisol which is determined not only by the cortisol secretion rate but also by the extent of protein binding and rate of degradation of the hormone. The 'set-point' of the negative feedback device seems to undergo rhythmic diurnal variations under normal circumstances so that the secretion of ACTH is highest in the mornings and lowest in the evenings.

Secretion of ACTH can be evoked by 'stress'—a general term comprising a variety of physiological disturbances, e.g., acute hypoglycaemia, acute pyrogenic reactions, severe burns, severe gastroenteritis, electroconvulsive therapy and major surgery as well as 'stressful' emotions such as fear, anger or frustration. There is much evidence to suggest that stress-induced ACTH discharge is mediated through the anterior ventral hypothalamus. Moreover, this region is highly sensitive to the local inhibitory action of cortisol. A number of 'corticotropin releasing factors' (CRF) have been found in the ventral median eminence. The most potent, β-CRF, resembles vasopressin but contains 4 additional amino acids. Vasopressin itself is a potent stimulator of the pituitary-adrenal system, but its locus of action in the release mechanism of ACTH is unknown.

There are therefore 2 primary and opposing forces that determine ACTH secretion: the degree of hypothalamic activation, and the extent to which ACTH secretion is checked by the circulating corticoid level. They appear to be integrated within the ventral median eminence. Under conditions of stress the threshold for cortisol inhibition is raised so as to allow increased secretion of ACTH. Very severe stress, however, will completely over-ride the feedback control.

Regulation of growth hormone secretion
The mechanism for the control of growth hormone secretion also involves a hypothalamic centre responding to both chemical and neural influences, and regulating the activity of the pituitary somatotroph cells by means of a growth hormone-releasing factor. Plasma growth hormone levels as determined by radioimmunoassay have been found to change rapidly in response to changes in the availability of glucose. It appears that growth hormone secretion is stimulated by fasting and by insulin-induced hypoglycaemia. Feeding or glucose administration causes a prompt fall in plasma growth hormone which is succeeded by a late rise at about 3 hr. It has been suggested that the secretion of growth hormone serves to mobilize fatty acids as an alternative source of energy at times when glucose is not available: but the lipolytic response evoked by growth hormone seems to be too slow for short-term needs (see Chapter 13). It has also been found that plasma growth hormone is increased after intravenous administration of certain amino acids, including phenylalanine and the basic amino acids arginine, histidine and lysine, or oral beefsteak; plasma insulin also rises but there is little change in plasma glucose. During prolonged exercise in the fasting state plasma growth hormone shows large fluctuations which have not been satisfactorily explained.

It has been established that growth hormone levels in childhood are in general higher than in adults: and it seems likely that the pacing of somatic growth under the influence of growth hormone will prove to be a neurally timed phenomenon like the development of gonadotrophic activity at puberty.

Regulation of prolactin secretion
The secretion of prolactin is also under neural control via the hypothalamus, but in this case the control is inhibitory. Removal of hypothalamic control by the placing of lesions in the median eminence or transplantation of the pituitary to another site leads to a greatly increased secretion of prolactin. Mammary carcinoma is not infrequent in rats with heterotopic pituitary transplants. In women galactorrhoea may occur following section of the pituitary stalk for metastatic breast carcinoma or as an occasional accompaniment of tumours or inflammatory lesions in the hypothalamo-pituitary region.

Disordered function

UNDERSECRETION

In adults undersecretion usually involves all the adenohypophysial functions to some extent. Isolated loss of gonadotrophic function may occur; in some cases it is the earliest manifestation of a pituitary tumour, and later corticotrophin and thyrotrophin deficiencies appear. Isolated deficiencies of thyrotrophin or corticotrophin are very rare. Among children with idiopathic pituitary dwarfism about half are found to have isolated growth hormone deficiency, which is sometimes familial; the others have multiple deficiencies.

OVERSECRETION

Pituitary gigantism is due to an excessive secretion of growth hormone from an eosinophilic adenoma of the pituitary, arising before the age of epiphysial closure. Such an excess of growth hormone acting on the adult body causes overgrowth of the skeleton and soft tissues without increase in length; that is, *acromegaly*. During the active phase of the disease, which usually continues for several years, gonadotrophic activity may be diminished. Goitre due to increased secretion of thyrotrophin is occasionally seen. Diabetes occurs in about one-third of all cases and may be permanent. Panhypopituitarism is not infrequently the last stage of the disorder.

In *Cushing's syndrome* (p. 531) associated with bilateral adrenal hyperplasia plasma ACTH concentration is normal or high despite an increased cortisol production, indicating an abnormality in feedback control of pituitary ACTH; in addition, the normal circadian rhythm of plasma ACTH concentration is lost. Sometimes the source of increased corticotrophin production is a pituitary tumour which may escape detection until after the adrenals have been removed. Such tumours are usually composed mainly of chromophobe cells and they may produce MSH as well as ACTH, thus leading to intense skin pigmentation with melanin. In the 'ectopic ACTH syndrome' an ACTH-like peptide (possibly ACTH) is produced by a tumour of non-endocrine tissue most commonly a bronchial carcinoma. The relations between plasma ACTH and plasma cortisol are shown in Fig. 47.

Interference with the normal hypothalamic control of pituitary function leading to excessive secretion of prolactin and impaired secretion of gonadotrophins is believed to be responsible for the syndrome of galactorrhoea with amenorrhoea. It occurs more commonly in puerperal women, but a non-puerperal form is also recognized and some of these patients prove to have pituitary tumours.

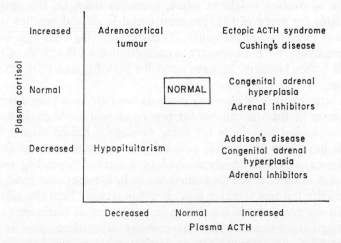

FIGURE 47. Relationships between plasma ACTH and plasma cortisol (after Liddle).

Principles of tests and measurements

DETERMINATION OF ANTERIOR PITUITARY HORMONES IN BLOOD AND URINE

The only method which is commonly available in routine laboratories is that for determination of human pituitary *gonadotrophins* (HPG) in urine using the mouse uterus test. The effect of injections of urine extracts on uterine weight is compared with that of a standard human menopausal gonadotrophin (HMG), one HMG unit being the amount of activity in 1 mg of HMG. Mean HPG excretion in normal males is 11 HMG units/24 hr (range 5 to 23). In normally menstruating females the average excretion throughout the cycle is 10 HMG units/24 hr (range 3 to 34), low values being found in the follicular and luteal phases with a peak at mid-cycle (due to LH). In ambulant post-menopausal women the mean excretion is 76 HMG units/24 hr (range 35 to 158): in women in hospital somewhat lower values are found. Plasma HPG can also be measured using the mouse uterus test and the mean level in post-menopausal women is 32 HMG units/100 ml (range

17*

17 to 59): normal men and normally menstruating women have less than 5 HMG units/100 ml. The mouse uterus test gives a measure of total gonadotrophic activity. Specific biological assays for FSH require further development: the best available method depends on the augmentation of ovarian weight in intact, immature mice. Of the methods available for assay of LH, the most useful in clinical practice is the ovarian cholesterol-depletion (OCD) test since, owing to its high degree of sensitivity, it is not necessary to concentrate the LH activity of body fluids before bioassay. Immunoassays for both LH and FSH are now in use.

A large number of bio-assay methods for *TSH* have been described but none of them is suitable for routine clinical application. Radio-immunological techniques are being developed. Raised plasma TSH levels have been reported in patients with untreated hypothyroidism.

Plasma *ACTH* is usually assayed by a method depending on the increase in adrenal venous corticosterone in hypophysectomized rats. A simpler but less sensitive procedure has recently been described in which the end point is the change in mixed venous corticosterone in dexamethasone-treated rats. Immunoassay of corticotrophin is also being developed. Normal plasma corticotrophin ranges from 0·09 to 0·4 m-units/100 ml with a diurnal variation, being highest in the morning and lowest in the evening.

Bio-assay methods for *prolactin* are not yet sufficiently sensitive for clinical use. The hormone can be determined in pituitary extracts by measurement of crop weight in pigeons or milk formation in rabbit mammary glands.

The standard biological assay for *growth hormone* activity is the tibia test, which depends on the increase in width of the proximal epiphysial cartilage of the tibia in hypophysectomized rats. Unfortunately the tibia test is not sensitive enough to detect growth hormone in plasma. The immunoassay of growth hormone, like that of insulin, is now a standard procedure and should become more widely available. It gives values for fasting plasma growth hormone ranging from below 5 ng/ml in normal adults to more than 50 ng/ml in acromegalics. Experience has confirmed the clinical usefulness of this measurement, despite the reservations already expressed (p. 488).

The method of disc electrophoresis has proved to be a rapid, sensitive and accurate procedure for detecting changes in concentration of growth hormone in pituitary homogenates, and it may be possible to develop chemical procedures of this sort for the rapid determination of protein hormones in plasma.

INSULIN TEST

Insulin (0·1 or 0·15 units/kg intravenously) causes a fall in plasma glucose and free fatty acid (FFA) levels which is normally greatest 20–30 min after injection. In hypothalamo-pituitary deficiency the rate of return towards control values is abnormally slow, particularly in the case of FFA. This is associated with deficient production of growth hormone, and sometimes ACTH, in response to hypoglycaemia. Plasma cortisol and plasma growth hormone concentrations may be measured before and 20, 30, 60, 90 and 120 min after injection.

ARGININE TEST

Rapid infusion of arginine causes large increases in plasma insulin and plasma growth hormone with little change in plasma glucose (p. 474). The response is inconstant in adult males. Standard conditions for a test of hypothalamo-pituitary function based on this phenomenon are now being worked out.

GLUCOSE TEST

Plasma growth hormone is measured 3 hr after oral glucose. A normal 'late rise' excludes growth hormone deficiency.

PLASMA INORGANIC PHOSPHORUS

Administration of growth hormone tends to raise the plasma phosphate concentration. The mechanism is unknown. High values are sometimes found in acromegaly, particularly in the active stage of the disease.

STIMULATION AND SUPPRESSION OF
ACTH SECRETION

Metyrapone test

Metyrapone (Metopirone, SU-4885) inhibits the activity of the adrenal enzyme responsible for hydroxylation at C-11 in the steroid nucleus (p. 531). Synthesis of cortisol is blocked, thus leading to increased secretion of ACTH, which in turn stimulates the adrenal production of steroids lacking the 11-hydroxyl group, particularly 11-deoxycortisol (compound S). These precursors contribute to the urinary 17-oxogenic steroids, the excretion of which rises by more than 10 mg/24 hr in those with normal pituitary and adrenal function. The precision of the test can be improved by measuring the urinary excretion of tetrahydro S, the main metabolite of 11-deoxycortisol. The biological half-life of metyrapone is very short, about 30 min. To ensure complete inhibition of 11-β-hydroxylase the drug must be given every 2 hr, or incorporated in a resin base to prolong its duration of action. As the response is rather slow the test should be continued for at least 2, and preferably 3 days. If the response is abnormal an ACTH stimulation test of adrenal function (p. 538) should be performed to establish whether the defect is at the adrenal or the pituitary level.

Pyrogen test

Intravenous injection of bacterial pyrogen is followed by increased corticotrophin secretion, leading to a rise in plasma cortisol. The locus of action of pyrogen is unknown but there is some evidence that it acts directly on the pituitary cells. The response is obtained whether or not fever is suppressed.

Lysine-Vasopressin test

Vasopressin can stimulate the pituitary-adrenal system (p. 502) and can be used to test its integrity. The test measures the rise in plasma cortisol during infusion of lysine-vasopressin. Growth hormone may also be increased but this effect is not found in all normal people. There is a risk of coronary vasoconstriction.

Dexamethasone suppression test

Dexamethasone, a potent synthetic glucocorticoid, can suppress ACTH secretion without contributing significantly to urinary 17-oxogenic steroid excretion. The 24 hr urinary excretion of 17-oxogenic steroids on the third day of treatment is compared with a control value obtained on the day before administration of dexamethasone. Normally, the 24 hr excretion is reduced to less than 3 mg when the daily dose of dexamethasone is 2 mg (0·5 mg every 6 hr). In Cushing's syndrome with adrenocortical hyperplasia suppression is incomplete with 2 mg, but may be achieved with higher doses of dexamethasone. Failure of suppression with higher doses may indicate the presence of an adrenal cortical tumour or of a corticotrophin-secreting tumour, usually a carcinoma of the bronchus.

The physiology of tests of target organ function is discussed under the individual organs: thyroid p. 558, gonads p. 622, adrenals p. 535.

Practical assessment

UNDERSECRETION

CHILDREN

Clinical methods

Hypopituitarism is a relatively uncommon cause of retarded growth. Hypopituitary dwarfs are of normal size at birth, and slowing of growth is not apparent before the age of 2–4 years. They do not show cranio-facial anomalies nor other congenital defects. Bony development is delayed, and sexual maturation does not usually occur. In most cases gross clinical evidence of thyroid and adrenal deficiency is absent, and in some, pituitary deficiency is entirely confined to growth hormone.

A pituitary tumour (usually a craniopharyngioma) is present in a third of all cases, and may produce pressure symptoms, including headache, vomiting and visual failure.

It may be impossible clinically to distinguish between hypopituitarism and primary gonadal dysgenesis with dwarfism (p. 585) unless some of the congenital abnormalities associated with gonadal dysgenesis are present; for example, webbing of the neck and coarctation of the aorta.

Most children in whom growth and sexual development are delayed eventually mature normally.

Routine methods

The insulin test gives valuable information, particularly if FFA, GH and cortisol can be measured as well as glucose, but may be dangerous. Essential precautions are the continuous presence of the physician and immediate availability of intravenous glucose. Arginine and glucose tests have the advantage of avoiding hypoglycaemia, but normal responses have not been so clearly defined.

Although gross clinical evidence is not apparent, thyroid and adrenal hypofunction can sometimes be revealed by appropriate tests. The plasma protein-bound iodine concentration is the most useful index of depressed thyroid function (p. 562). The metyrapone test (p. 509) is unreliable in children and may provoke acute adrenal insufficiency. A clear distinction can be made between hypopituitarism and primary hypogonadism by the urinary gonadotrophin output (p. 507) since excretion is abnormally high in primary hypogonadism and low in hypopituitarism. A 'negative' sex chromatin pattern in an apparently female child confirms gonadal dysgenesis and precise diagnosis may be made by chromosome examination (p. 594).

Radiography of the skull and delineation of the visual fields may reveal a pituitary tumour.

ADULTS
Clinical methods
By contrast with children, adults usually show evidence of multiple endocrine deficiencies and the symptoms may include those of thyroid, adrenal and gonadal insufficiency (see p. 540). The skin is very pale, fine and soft; body hair is sparse or absent; the genitals are atrophic, though the breasts in women may appear normal.

A pituitary space-occupying lesion may be suggested, as in children, by headache, vomiting, visual failure and optic atrophy. Weight gain and polyuria suggest hypothalamic involvement. Ischaemic necrosis of the pituitary is suggested by the absence of evidence of tumour, and by the history of a post-partum haemorrhage followed by failure of lactation (Sheehan's syndrome). Pituitary infarction may complicate severe head injuries.

Routine methods
The insulin test rarely produces alarming reactions in adults but the precautions mentioned on p. 511 should be observed. Its value is greatly increased by FFA, GH and cortisol measurements. It may be superseded by an arginine test. Urinary gonadotrophins should be measured and metyrapone and ACTH tests performed. Thyrotrophic function is assessed by radio-iodine uptake before and after TSH. The lysine-vasopressin and pyrogen tests have not been fully evaluated.

Skull X-ray and visual field examination may provide evidence of a tumour.

OVERSECRETION

Gigantism
Pituitary gigantism (i.e. pituitary hyperfunction present from an early age) should be distinguished from constitutional tall stature by the family history. It has also to be distinguished from precocious sexual development accompanied by a growth spurt, and from eunuchoidal gigantism in adults.

X-ray of the pituitary fossa will often show expansion of the sella turcica, and the presence of acromegalic features provides additional proof. Plasma growth hormone concentration is increased.

Acromegaly

Acromegaly is diagnosed clinically, and the problem usually lies in assessing the activity of the tumour. Activity may be presumed if there is a history of changing features and enlarging extremities up to the time of examination. In doubtful cases careful photography of the face and X-ray of the skull repeated after a few months are of great value. Diabetes may be revealed by a glucose tolerance test. Fasting plasma GH is usually markedly raised and is usually unchanged after glucose or insulin. (Additional tests are, however, unnecessary if the fasting value is unequivocally high.) A high plasma phosphate suggests activity but a normal value does not exclude it.

*Special methods of assessment in disorders of
the adenohypophysis*

LH, TSH and ACTH can be measured in body fluids by the methods outlined on p. 507.

THE NEUROHYPOPHYSIS

Normal function

THE NEUROHYPOPHYSIAL HORMONES

The typical mammalian neurohypophysis contains two active principles. One is oxytocin. The other is usually either arginine or lysine vasopressin: in man it is the arginine form.

Arginine vasopressin

CyS. Tyr. Phe. Glu (NH$_2$). Asp (NH$_2$). CyS. Pro. Arg. Gly (NH$_2$)

Lysine vasopressin

CyS......Phe......................CyS......Lys..........

Oxytocin

CyS......Ileu......................CyS......Leu..........

Both vasopressins contain basic amino acids in the 8-position. This is associated with strong vasopressor and antidiuretic activities. The antidiuretic function of the neurohypophysis appears to have evolved as an adaptation to terrestrial life, effects on sodium metabolism preceding those on water in phylogenetic terms.

Within the gland the octapeptides are reversibly bound to a specific protein, termed neurohypophysin. It is not yet certain whether the free peptides are secreted or whether the protein-peptide complex is released from the neural lobe. The latest evidence suggests that in the dog plasma antidiuretic activity is completely dialyzable.

The main function of *vasopressin* in man is to permit increased reabsorption of water by the kidney probably through an effect on the permeability of the distal tubular epithelium (p. 162). It is therefore often referred to as the antidiuretic hormone or ADH. Continued administration of the hormone to animals or to man can cause a progressive retention of water with hypotonicity of body fluids. After 2 or 3 days an increase in urinary excretion of sodium occurs, continuing as long as water is taken freely, and body weight levels off at a new steady state. The rise in sodium excretion is not due to a direct effect of vasopressin on the kidney, but is probably related to an increase in glomerular filtration rate and to a decrease in aldosterone secretion. The possible role of vasopressin in corticotrophin release is mentioned on p. 504.

Oxytocin causes contraction of the parturient uterus. Its other major function in mammals is to cause ejection of milk from the breasts. The stimulus of suckling excites a reflex discharge of oxytocin which in turn causes contraction of myoepithelial fibres surrounding the mammary ducts. Animals in whom neurohypophysial function has been destroyed can no longer rear their young. In some species, including the rat, oxytocin has a powerful natriuretic action; but in man this effect appears to be insignificant. In rats low doses of oxytocin can inhibit the antidiuretic response to vasopressin, while higher doses are themselves strongly antidiuretic. The possibility that oxytocin is implicated in the regulation of prolactin release is now largely discounted.

Regulation of neurohypophysial hormone release

The posterior pituitary hormones are formed in the hypothalamus by the cells of the supraoptic and paraventricular nuclei, transported in the form of neurosecretory granules along the hollow axons of the hypothalamo-hypophysial tract and stored in dilated nerve endings within the posterior lobe. These endings are closely applied to capillaries into which the hormones can be rapidly released in response to impulses propagated by the supraoptic nerve fibres.

Vasopressin release can be elicited (1) by an increase in plasma osmolality—probably detected by the supraoptic cells, since intracarotid injections of hypertonic saline increase the firing rate of the supraoptic but not the paraventricular neurones (p. 502); (2) by a reduction in circulating blood volume—possibly detected by stretch receptors in the atria and great veins; (3) by sensory or emotional stimuli—pain, fear, rage, etc.; (4) by muscular exercise; (5) by fainting; (6) by surgical trauma (p. 26); (7) by suckling (see below); (8) by certain drugs—acetylcholine, nicotine, morphine, barbiturates and some anaesthetic agents. Release of vasopressin can be inhibited (1) by a decrease in plasma osmolality; (2) by expansion of the circulating blood volume, manipulations which increase the intrathoracic blood volume being particularly effective; (3) occasionally by emotional stimuli; (4) by ethanol.

Oxytocin secretion is increased during parturition (p. 610), suckling (p. 611), coitus (p. 608) and by certain stimuli which excite vasopressin release—e.g. hypertonic saline infusion. Indeed most stimuli appear to provoke release of both hormones, although some degree of independent control probably exists.

Disordered Function

UNDERSECRETION

Lack of oxytocin has not been described as an isolated defect. The manifestations of neurohypophysial insufficiency are essentially those of lack of antidiuretic hormone; that is, diabetes insipidus. As a result of diminished reabsorption of water by the renal tubules the urine becomes copious and very dilute. Plasma osmolality rises and intense thirst develops.

A genetic defect in the synthesis of vasopressin with normal synthesis of oxytocin has been shown in rats with hereditary diabetes insipidus. Whether this situation obtains in human hereditary hypothalamic diabetes insipidus remains to be established.

Lesions of the hypothalamo-hypophysial system must be fairly complete (i.e. more than 85 per cent) to cause permanent diabetes insipidus. Thus surgical division of the pituitary stalk usually causes only transient polyuria since it leaves the median eminence intact. When adenohypophysial as well as neurohypophysial secretion is deficient, polyuria is slight or absent, but frank diabetes insipidus may appear during cortisone administration. (The influence of cortico-steroids on renal function is considered on p. 522.)

Oxytocin lack does not seem to affect parturition in human diabetes insipidus: the effect on suckling is not clear. Difficulties with both functions have been observed in animals with diabetes insipidus.

HYPERSECRETION

(1) Primary hypersecretion of oxytocin has not been definitely recognized. A sustained and inappropriate secretion of ADH is held responsible for the hyponatraemia and renal 'sodium-wasting' which occur in some patients with malignant disease (especially carcinoma of the bronchus), cerebrovascular disorders or acute porphyria. In certain patients with malignant disease the source of the antidiuretic activity may be the tumour tissue itself. (2) Secondary hypersecretion of ADH occurs in oedematous states and may occur in adrenocortical deficiency. In oedematous states increased secretion is for the most part simply an appropriate response to increased sodium retention. In some cases, however, where water is retained in excess of sodium, the neurohypophysis may be responding to a volume stimulus as well as to an osmotic one. In cirrhosis of the liver decreased hepatic inactivation of ADH may contribute to water retention (p. 449). The cause of the impaired diuretic response to water in adrenocortical insufficiency is considered on p. 538: the evidence for hypersecretion of ADH is unconvincing.

Principles of tests and measurements

DETERMINATION OF NEUROHYPOPHYSIAL
HORMONES IN BLOOD AND URINE

Vasopressin in urine or plasma can be assayed by preparing extracts which are injected intravenously into hydrated rats. The changes in urine volume and electrical conductivity are compared with those produced by arginine vasopressin. Non-specific antidiuretic activity is excluded by establishing that the activity is destroyed by thioglycollate, that the response is identical with that to arginine vasopressin and that the extract is ineffective in rats during a mannitol diuresis. Normally no activity is detectable in mixed venous blood and urinary excretion is less than 15 m-units/24 hr. Oxytocin can be assayed in blood using the contraction of the isolated guinea-pig uterus or milk ejection in the cannulated rabbit mammary duct.

PLASMA OSMOLALITY

Methods for determining plasma osmolality are now widely available. The normal range is 280–300 m-osmole/l. Values in diabetes insipidus tend to be above normal, because replenishment of water loss may be delayed or incomplete. By contrast, in compulsive water-drinking (primary polydipsia) some degree of overhydration is usual, and plasma osmolarity is decreased.

WATER DEPRIVATION
If a normal subject is deprived of water the plasma osmolarity tends to rise. ADH is secreted and causes increased tubular reabsorption of water. A urine specific gravity greater than 1·020 is found after 12–18 hr. The retention of water prevents dehydration and thirst. In a subject with diabetes insipidus little or no ADH is released. The urine specific gravity does not exceed 1·014. Water loss continues and severe thirst and dehydration develop with rapid loss of body weight. To minimize discomfort a standardized water deprivation test is now used which is terminated when body weight has fallen by 3 per cent. Urine osmolality then normally exceeds 700 m-osmole/l.

HYPERTONIC SALINE INFUSION
A hypertonic solution of sodium chloride is infused intravenously in the hydrated subject. If the neurohypophysial function is normal the increased plasma osmolality elicits a release of ADH and a fall in urine volume. A definite antidiuretic effect is thought to exclude diabetes insipidus. Patients having a partial deficiency of ADH may, however, respond normally. The procedure is dangerous in patients with heart disease.

ADMINISTRATION OF NICOTINE
The patient should be well hydrated. He rapidly inhales the smoke of 1–3 cigarettes until definite nausea and dizziness appear. Alternatively nicotine may be injected intravenously. The duration of any antidiuretic effect is compared with that produced by graded intravenous doses of Pitressin. Patients with severe diabetes insipidus invariably give responses equivalent to less than 10 m-units of Pitressin. In normal subjects the response is equivalent to more than 100 m-units. Nicotine should not be given parenterally to patients with coronary artery disease.

Practical assessment

Clinical
Polyuria and thirst may occur in diabetes mellitus, chronic renal failure (p. 171), potassium deficiency, hypercalcaemic states (p. 536), and with

excessive corticosteroid administration. In the following discussion it is assumed that these conditions have been excluded.

In infants with diabetes insipidus, thirst and polyuria often go unnoticed, and fever, dehydration or simply failure to thrive may be the presenting symptoms. In adults the main difficulty lies in distinguishing between true diabetes insipidus and compulsive water-drinking. Expert psychiatric assessment can be most helpful. An abrupt onset may favour diabetes insipidus. About one-third of cases result from intracranial tumours, which can be sought by the usual methods, including skull X-ray and visual field examination. A search should also be made for evidence of primary malignancy elsewhere in the body, and for granulomatous conditions and lipoidoses.

Routine methods
Response to vasopressin. In diabetes insipidus injection of 1 unit (0·2 ml) of Pitressin tannate intramuscularly is followed by prompt reduction in thirst and polyuria: placebo injections are ineffective. In compulsive water-drinking the patient may continue to drink large quantities of water despite reduction in urine volume; or he may respond to both hormone and placebo injections by a reduction in thirst and in urine volume. A true resistance to vasopressin occurs in the rare hereditary 'nephrogenic' form of diabetes insipidus.

Plasma osmolality measurements have the virtue of freedom from risk or discomfort, and will clearly differentiate diabetes insipidus from primary polydipsia.

Stimulation of ADH release provides a quantitative assessment of neurohypophysial function. The standardized water deprivation test with measurement of urinary osmolality has now largely superseded the nicotine and hypertonic saline tests on grounds of simplicity, freedom from risk and ease of interpretation.

Special procedures
The assay of vasopressin and oxytocin has been discussed on p. 516.

References

General
The Pituitary Gland (3 vols.) ed. Harris G.W. & Donovan B.T. London: Butterworths, 1966.
Neuroendocrinology (2 vols.) ed. Martini L. & Ganong W.F. New York and London: Academic Press, 1966–7.

McSHAN W.H. & HARTLEY M.W. (1965) Production, storage and release of anterior pituitary hormones. *Ergebn. Physiol.* **56**, 264–96. (In English).

DIXON H.B.F. (1964) Chemistry of pituitary hormones. *In 'The Hormones'*, Vol. 5, ed. Pincus, Thimann & Astwood. New York and London: Academic Press.

Recent studies on the hypothalamus. *Brit. med. Bull.*, **22**, 3. (Sept., 1966).

REICHLIN S. (1963) Neuroendocrinology. *New Eng. J. Med.* **269**, 1182–91, 1246–50, 1296–303.

FERGUSON K.A. (1965) Human pituitary hormones. *Med. J. Aust.* **1**, 329–34.

FRIESEN H. & ASTWOOD E.B. (1965) Hormones of the anterior pituitary body. *New Eng. J. Med.* **272**, 1216–23, 1272–7, 1328–35.

DAUGHADAY W.H. & KIPNIS D.M. (1966) The growth-promoting and anti-insulin actions of somatotropin. *Rec. Progr. Hormone Res.* **22**, 49–99.

LORAINE J.A. & BELL E.T. (1966) Hormone assays and their clinical application. 2nd Ed. Edinburgh and London: Livingstone.

SAWYER W.H. (1964) Vertebrate neurohypophysial principles. *Endocrinology* **75**, 981–90.

Other selected references

MERIMEE T.J., LILLICRAP D.A. & RABINOWITZ D. (1965) Effect of arginine on serum levels of human growth hormone. *Lancet* ii, 668–70.

GREENWOOD F.C., LANDON J., STAMP T.C.B. & WYNN V. (1966) The plasma sugar, FFA, cortisol and growth hormone response to insulin. *J. clin. Invest.*, **45**, 429–36 and 437–49.

LANDON J., JAMES V.H.T. & STOKER D.J. (1965) Plasma cortisol response to lysine-vasopressin. *Lancet* ii, 1156–9.

The investigation of hypothalamic-pituitary-adrenal function. *Memoirs of the Society for Endocrinology*. In press.

ROSS E.J. (1966) Cancer and the adrenal cortex. *Proc. Roy. Soc. Med.* **59**, 335–8.

LEE J., JONES J.T. & BARRACLOUGH M.A. (1964) Inappropriate secretion of vasopressin. *Lancet* ii, 792–3.

Proceedings of the International Symposium on Growth Hormone, Milan, 11–13 September, 1967. Amsterdam: Excerpta Medica Foundation, 1968 (in press).

15

The Adrenal Glands

ADRENAL CORTEX

Normal function

The cortex of the adrenal glands is the source of all the known steroid hormones elaborated in the body except for those derived from the gonads and placenta. Adrenocortical steroid hormones play an important role in the regulation of the body's metabolic processes and without them life is hazardous. In particular, they appear to be responsible for the normal regulation of salt and water metabolism, normal renal function, normal carbohydrate and protein metabolism and for the normal response of the body to such noxious stimuli as severe injury, surgical operations and infections (the so-called 'resistance to stress').

THE ADRENOCORTICAL STEROID HORMONES

Adrenocortical steroids are synthesized from cholesterol which is particularly abundant in adrenal cortical tissue. The high fat content is responsible for the vivid yellow colour of the adrenal glands. The chemical basis of all steroid molecules is the reduced cyclopenteno-phenanthrene ring (Carbon atoms 1 to 17 of Fig. 48 (i)). In contrast to other steroids such as oestrogens and androgens, which have 18 and 19 carbon atoms respectively, the characteristic features of the adrenocortical steroids are that they have: (1) 21-carbon atoms; (2) an unsaturated ketone group in the A ring—the Δ^4, 3-ketone grouping Fig. 48 (ii)); and (3) a 2-carbon side-chain at carbon 17 (that is, carbon atoms 20 and 21)—the α-ketol side-chain (Fig. 48 (iii)). This α-ketol side-chain has strong reducing properties and is the basis of many chemical tests.

The important chemical differences between the various adrenocortical steroids consist mainly of varying substitutions with OH or O in the C-17 or C-11 positions, but aldosterone is unique in having an aldehyde grouping at C-18. Of the many C-21 steroids with this type of basic chemical structure that have been isolated from adrenal tissue, probably only cortisol, corticosterone and aldosterone are important physiologically. It is only these three which have been identified in the adrenal venous blood in sufficient amounts likely to have a significant biological effect. The proportions of each of these steroids varies considerably from species to species, but in man cortisol predominates.

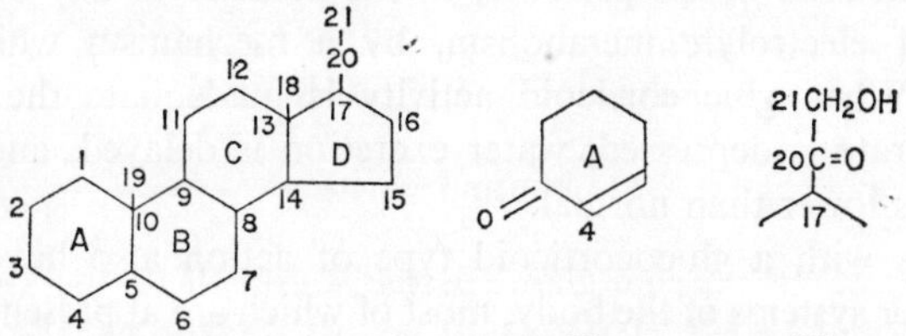

FIGURE 48.—*Steroid configurations*

Cortisone and desoxycorticosterone have also been identified in adrenal venous blood but only in amounts which are most unlikely to be important physiologically.

BIOLOGICAL ACTIVITIES OF THE
ADRENOCORTICAL STEROID HORMONES
Although all adrenocortical steroid hormones share many biological activities when assessed pharmacologically, they are conventionally classified on the basis of what appears to be the predominant physiological effect or effects of the steroid in question. That is, an attempt is made to classify them according to their likely role in the normal function of the body. In the present state of our knowledge this classification can only be approximate because the biological activities of adrenocortical steroids overlap considerably. With this proviso the adrenocortical 21-carbon atom steroid hormones can be considered as being either glucocorticoids (i.e. affecting carbohydrate metabolism principally) or mineralocorticoids (i.e. having a predominant effect on sodium and potassium metabolism).

Glucocorticoids influence carbohydrate metabolism by promoting the conversion of protein to glucose (gluconeogenesis), by inhibiting the peripheral utilization of glucose (possibly because they antagonize insulin) and by increasing glycogen deposition in the liver. Deficiency of glucocorticoids causes a lowered fasting blood sugar which is probably largely the result of depressed gluconeogenesis.

Apart from the qualifications mentioned above, the term 'glucocorticoid' is additionally deceptive because these steroids have other very important physiological actions which are unrelated to carbohydrate metabolism.

Glucocorticoids help to maintain normal renal function: they increase the glomerular filtration rate and promote water excretion. They also raise the arterial blood pressure, in the absence of any demonstrable change of electrolyte metabolism, by a mechanism which remains obscure. When glucocorticoid activity is inadequate the glomerular filtration rate is depressed, water excretion is delayed, and the blood pressure is lower than normal.

Steroids with a glucocorticoid type of action also have effects on many other systems of the body, most of which are at present ill-defined, but which may be of profound physiological importance and are certainly very useful therapeutically. The resistance to the 'stress' caused by non-specific harmful influences such as mechanical or thermal injuries, severe infections, or the harmful effects of antibody-antigen reactions is lowered in the absence of adequate glucocorticoid activity. An increased concentration of glucocorticoids in the blood gives rise to a fall of eosinophils and lymphocytes and an increase of neutrophil granulocytes: erythropoiesis is also enhanced. The inflammatory response to tissue irritants is suppressed when pharmacological doses of glucocorticoids are given and wound healing may be delayed. Large amounts of glucocorticoids also reduce the rate of antibody formation; infections spread easily, and the survival of autologous tissue transplants is prolonged. Mental changes are frequent. The type of psychiatric manifestation depends largely upon the basic type of personality of the individual patient, but euphoria is especially common. More specific actions include stimulation of acid and pepsin secretion from the gastric mucosa and also suppression of normal pituitary activity, particularly, of course, the secretion of corticotrophin.

Mineralocorticoids primarily influence the rate of sodium and potassium transport across cell membranes, promoting entry of sodium into cells, and extrusion of potassium from them. This is most easily seen in the case of the renal tubule because the characteristic changes are quickly reflected in the urine. With increased mineralocorticoid activity the rate of sodium excretion falls and that of potassium rises. Conversely, lack of mineralocorticoids leads to sodium loss and potassium retention.

Similar effects can be demonstrated on the ratio of sodium to potassium concentration in saliva and faeces and on the concentration of sodium in the sweat. Probably many other tissue cells (if not all of them) respond to mineralocorticoid activity in a similar fashion.

In man the principal adrenocortical steroid hormones are cortisol, corticosterone and aldosterone. Cortisol is the principal 'glucocorticoid' but it also has a considerable 'mineralocorticoid' type of action even in physiological amounts. Aldosterone, however, is more important physiologically as a mineralocorticoid type of hormone despite its low concentration in the adrenal venous blood (of the order of $\frac{1}{100} \mu g/ml$), although in pharmacological doses it has also some glucocorticoid activity. Corticosterone has both mineralocorticoid and glucocorticoid activity in quantities which are likely to be physiological, but its exact role is not yet fully understood.

Sex hormones of the adrenal cortex. Apart from the C-21 or so-called adrenocortical steroid hormones described above, androgens (C-19 steroids) and oestrogens (C-18 steroids) have also been detected in extracts of adrenal tissue. It is uncertain, however, whether the elaboration of androgens and oestrogens is a specific function of the normal adrenal cortex or whether their presence merely reflects the production of C-21 steroids. The adrenals probably contribute very little to normal sex hormone activity, but the over-production of androgens (and very rarely of oestrogens) by the adrenal is important in pathological conditions. Adrenal androgens appear to be necessary for the growth of body hair in women but they cannot maintain secondary sexual characteristics of castrated male animals even if the gland is under the influence of prolonged maximal ACTH stimulation. However, although they are unable to prevent the effects of loss of ovarian function, the adrenals may produce enough oestrogen to stimulate the growth of 'oestrogen-dependent' breast carcinoma after the main source of oestrogen has been removed by oophorectomy.

THE METABOLISM OF CORTISOL,
CORTICOSTERONE AND ALDOSTERONE

Biologically active adrenocortical steroid hormones are almost insoluble in water, but protein solutions (e.g. albumin) increase their solubility by some sort of binding process. In plasma, corticosteroids are loosely bound to albumin, but cortisol and possibly other adrenal steroids are also more strongly bound to an α-globulin (the corticosteroid-binding globulin or transcortin). At the temperature and hydrogen-ion concentration of the extracellular fluid about 90 per cent of cortisol is protein-bound. This is considerably weaker than the binding of thyroxine to its specific binding globulin (p. 530).

Radio-isotopic studies show that cortisol and aldosterone are rapidly degraded in the body. Cortisol has a biological half-life of about $1\frac{1}{2}$ hr but aldosterone has one of only about 20 min, which is probably a reflection of the fact that corticosteroid-binding globulin has little affinity for aldosterone.

The liver is largely responsible for the degradation of cortisol, corticosterone and aldosterone into biologically inactive metabolites, mainly the tetrahydro derivatives. Both these and the unchanged steroids are then conjugated with glucuronic acid and sulphate. This makes them easily soluble in water and the conjugates are excreted into the urine. The urinary steroids consist largely of conjugated steroids of adrenal origin, although in adult males about half of the total 17-oxosteroids (the metabolites of androgen metabolism) come from the testes. The rate of urinary corticosteroid excretion can be considerably influenced by alterations of hepatic metabolism, renal function and plasma protein steroid-binding capacity.

This relatively simple view of steroid metabolism may have to be modified because there is now good evidence that in the metabolism of C-18 and C-19 steroids, their metabolites may not only possess special biological activities of their own, but may also act as substrates for hormone production in other glands. For example dehydroisoandrosterone sulphate, which is partly secreted as such from the adrenal gland, may be an important substrate for the production of oestrogens by the placenta.

RATE OF HORMONE PRODUCTION

Using refined radio-active techniques it is now possible to measure indirectly the actual rate of cortisol and aldosterone production by the adrenals (p. 535). Under normal conditions the adrenals of an adult man or woman produce about 16 mg of cortisol daily. This can normally be increased by endogenous or injected corticotrophin up to a secretion rate of about 100 mg per day. In patients with partial adrenocortical failure the basal secretion rate of cortisol may be normal but the response to corticotrophin may be impaired. On a diet containing the usual amount of salt (150–250 m-equiv daily) the secretion rate of aldosterone is about 100 μg daily. Severe sodium depletion will increase this four- or five-fold. The secretion of adrenocortical steroids is subject to a diurnal rhythm. Both the blood glucocorticoid levels and the rates of urinary excretion of corticosteroids, androgens and their respective metabolites reflect this. Secretion is usually greatest between 4 a.m. and midday and falls to the lowest level at about midnight. An absence of this diurnal variation is an early sign of adrenocortical overactivity. Aldosterone excretion usually parallels that of cortisol but is additionally increased during the day when the patient is up, and decreased during rest in bed at night.

CONTROL OF ADRENOCORTICAL HORMONE PRODUCTION

The rate of cortisol and corticosterone secretion is almost exclusively controlled by the level of circulating corticotrophin. Without the pituitary hormone adrenal production of these two steroids falls to vanishingly small levels. In turn the rate of corticotrophin (ACTH) production by the pituitary is influenced by the level of cortisol in the extracellular fluids so providing a 'feed-back' mechanism to maintain a constant cortisol level in the peripheral blood. However, a more important influence is the hypothalamus which appears to stimulate ACTH release by means of a neuro-hormone (the corticotrophin-releasing factor), which is carried to the anterior pituitary gland from the median eminence of the hypothalamus via the hypothalamo-hypophysial portal vessels. This hypothalamic system is stimulated by many factors, both nervous and humoral (p. 504). It is responsible for the increased ACTH secretion which results from stressful stimuli such as fear, pain, or severe injuries, and it also provides the mechanism by which adrenaline causes ACTH release.

In contrast to cortisol, aldosterone production is only slightly affected by ACTH and it continues largely unchanged following removal of the pituitary. It is an old observation that in experimental animals hypophysectomy is followed by atrophy of the two inner zones of the adrenal cortex (the zona fasciculata and the zona reticularis) but aldosterone is produced almost exclusively by the outer zona glomerulosa. Clinically the independence of aldosterone from pituitary control is well illustrated by the contrast between patients with panhypopituitarism and those with Addison's disease. Patients without adrenal glands may die within a few days from sodium depletion and potassium intoxication, whereas those without pituitary function linger on for much longer before finally succumbing not to any electrolyte disturbance but rather to an ill-defined failure to respond to some stressful influence.

The rate of aldosterone secretion depends on the blood volume and on the potassium concentration in the plasma. Aldosterone secretion is increased by reduction of the circulating blood volume as, for example, in sodium depletion and also by an increase of plasma potassium concentration. It is decreased by expansion of the blood volume, as, for example, in sodium loading and also by potassium depletion. These changes occur in the absence of the pituitary except that they may be somewhat sluggish. Another system, therefore, must be responsible and there is now good evidence that some hormone is involved. A neuro-humour from the hypothalamus or the region of the pineal has been suggested, but the evidence is compelling that the renin-angiotensin system of the kidney is involved. Angiotensin, in small amounts, selectively increases the rate of aldosterone production from the adrenal glomerulosa and, in dogs, haemorrhage does not increase the rate of aldosterone production in the absence of the kidneys. A raised plasma renin concentration has been observed in many situations associated with hypovolaemia, such as sodium depletion, and a low one has been observed in situations associated with hypervolaemia, such as sodium loading. The way that changes of blood volume influence renin output is still conjectural. In some situations, changes of mean pressure in the renal artery are likely to be relevant but alterations of activity of sympathetic nerves to the kidney are probably more important (p. 44).

Disordered function

Functional disorders of the adrenal glands usually show themselves in one of two ways. Either there is a defect in the amount (too much, or too little) of a physiologically important steroid hormone which is produced normally (e.g. cortisol or aldosterone) or, alternatively, there is a qualitative defect so that steroids which are normally produced in physiologically unimportant amounts are secreted into the blood stream in excess.

HYPOFUNCTION OF THE ADRENAL CORTEX

Since the adrenal cortex is neither functionally nor anatomically homogeneous, it is difficult to describe under a single heading the effects of 'hypofunction' of the gland. A pathological process which diffusely and slowly destroys the adrenal cortex without respect for functional zones (e.g. Addison's disease) will understandably produce a different clinical picture from one which causes differential atrophy of the inner two zones (e.g. anterior pituitary failure). Similarly, a failure of synthesis of physiologically important hormones such as cortisol, due to enzymic defects in the biosynthetic pathway (e.g. adrenogenital virilism) will impair cortisol secretion (and hence produce the signs of cortisol deficiency) but may also cause hyperplasia of the gland and the over-production of other steroids.

Clinically two important and interdependent syndromes are recognized. One is due, primarily, to an acute failure of cortisol secretion and the other to a more chronic failure of both cortisol and aldosterone secretion. The first can be completely reversed by adequate glucocorticoid therapy but the second requires the replacement of salt and water as well. Once the initial sodium depletion is made good, an adequate body content of sodium can then be maintained by treatment with mineralocorticoids.

Acute failure of cortisol secretion (acute adrenal insufficiency) usually occurs when patients whose adrenals are incapable of secreting more than basal amounts of glucocorticoids, are exposed to a relatively sudden stress. The adrenal cortex is incapable of increasing the secretion of glucocorticoid in response to a greater demand. This unresponsiveness may be the result of primary disease in the adrenal cortex itself, as in Addison's disease and congenital adrenal hyperplasia, or it may develop as a result of a secondary atrophy due to chronic failure of corticotrophin secretion. This occurs, of course, in panhypopituitarism; but it most commonly develops as a result of prolonged treatment with suppressive doses of some glucocorticoid type of preparation such as cortisone, prednisone or dexamethasone. Sometimes, especially in children, the disease responsible for the 'stress' may also itself damage the adrenal cortex by causing adrenal haemorrhage. This is sometimes seen in severe meningococcal septicemia, in diphtheria and occasionally after severe abdominal injuries.

The clinical picture is usually one of profound shock (see p. 25). The blood pressure falls and severe oliguria or even anuria develops; there is urea retention and the plasma potassium concentration rises. The body temperature is often raised initially but becomes subnormal with severe shock. Vomiting is common and the patient may become dehydrated, but usually the external losses of sodium are modest. Nevertheless, the plasma sodium concentration often falls not because of overall sodium depletion but because the distribution of water and sodium between cells and the extracellular fluid is altered. Superficially, therefore, the clinical picture resembles that of severe water and salt loss, but treatment with saline solutions and/or mineralocorticoids is not enough. All the changes, including the hyponatraemia, can be reversed by giving cortisol, cortisone or one of their synthetic analogues. However, when acute adrenal insufficiency occurs in patients already the victims of prolonged mineralocorticoid deficiency, as in Addison's disease or when vomiting has been severe, then correction of the circulatory and electrolyte disturbance requires sodium repletion.

Chronic insufficiency of both glucocorticoid and mineralocorticoid secretion occurs in Addison's disease. This condition is the result of a diffusely destructive pathological process affecting the whole adrenal cortex. Tuberculosis, haemochromatosis or carcinomatosis may all be responsible but usually no cause can be found. Some patients also suffer from Hashimoto's thyroiditis (p. 290), which suggests that an auto-immune process may be responsible for at least some of the cases of Addison's disease due to an 'idiopathic' atrophy of the adrenal cortex. Clinically the condition is characterized by progressive weakness and loss of weight, thirst and polyuria, and pigmentation of the skin and mucosae. The pigmentation tends to accumulate in areas exposed to friction such as flexor surfaces (e.g. palmar creases) and the buccal mucosa.

Lack of mineralocorticoid activity leads to characteristic changes in the plasma concentrations of sodium, potassium and urea in severe cases. The kidneys fail to conserve sodium adequately and tubular secretion of potassium is impaired so that the plasma level of sodium tends to fall and that of potassium to rise. In mild cases the urinary sodium loss is at least partially counterbalanced by increased salt consumption, because many patients with Addison's disease have an excessive taste for it. Obvious hyponatraemia is therefore a late sign but an elevation of the plasma potassium level occurs relatively early. When sodium depletion does supervene it causes a reduction of the plasma volume with haemoconcentration, a fall in the systemic blood pressure, and urea retention as a result of impaired renal blood flow.

Lack of 'glucocorticoid' activity, however, is primarily responsible for most of the other manifestations of chronic adrenal insufficiency. Although, in moderate or severe cases, progressive weakness may be partially due to sodium loss, only treatment with glucocorticoids will relieve it completely. The impairment of renal function and particularly the impairment of water excretion as a result of glucocorticoid deficiency (see above) leads to delayed water excretion, nocturia and urea retention. Since gluconeogenesis from protein is impaired, glucocorticoid deficiency tends to cause a fasting hypoglycaemia and the hypoglycaemic effects of insulin are potentiated. Patients with acute adrenal insufficiency should always be given glucose.

The fall of plasma cortisol concentration abolishes the normal suppressive effect of cortisol on the release of pituitary corticotrophin. Corticotrophin secretion becomes excessive and can relatively easily be detected in peripheral blood. In the absence of the usual target organ one would not expect this to have any particular biological effect, but corticotrophin, which is a simple polypeptide containing 39 amino-acids, shares many chemical features with the melanocyte-stimulating hormone (p. 500). For example, they both share an identical sequence of 7 amino-acids and even the purest corticotrophin preparations have slight melanocyte-stimulating activity. Moreover, suppression of the pituitary by treatment with glucocorticoids will slowly clear Addisonian pigmentation. It is therefore probable that an excessive secretion of the melanocyte-stimulating hormone is a secondary result of cortisol deficiency and that this causes the excessive pigmentation seen in chronic adrenal insufficiency.

ADRENAL INSUFFICIENCY IN PITUITARY FAILURE

As mentioned above, corticotrophin lack causes failure of cortisol secretion from the zona fasciculata and the zona reticularis, both of which eventually atrophy. Mineralocorticoid function, on the other hand, is preserved because aldosterone is produced by the zona glomerulosa which remains relatively unaffected.

Therefore, patients with adrenal insufficiency secondary to a pituitary lesion differ clinically from those with a primary lesion of the adrenal gland itself by having (1) normal electrolyte balance, (2) reduced skin pigmentation and (3) evidence of hypofunction of the other endocrine glands controlled by pituitary trophic hormones, e.g. the gonads and the thyroid. Otherwise they suffer from the effects of cortisol lack as described above, particularly an inability to respond adequately to infections and other stressful stimuli.

The cause of the pituitary lesion may be a tumour or some other more obscure lesion but it is most commonly due to postpartum necrosis (Sheehan's syndrome).

CONGENITAL ADRENAL HYPERPLASIA (VIRILISM)

Congenital adrenal virilism is caused by an inborn deficiency of one or more of the enzymes responsible for adequate hydroxylation of the steroid nucleus; the production of cortisol is therefore defective. In the most common form hydroxylation at the C-21 position is impaired so that 17-hydroxyprogesterone accumulates and its urinary metabolite, pregnanetriol, appears in excessive amount in the urine. The low level *(feedback)* of circulating cortisol stimulates ACTH release from the pituitary which then in turn causes hyperplasia of the adrenal glands and stimulates them to over-produce other steroids, particularly androgens. The clinical result of this is virilism and excessive growth. Boys show precocious sexual development and the girls are masculinized. If the defect is severe, genetic female children are born with male-looking external genitalia (pseudo-hermaphroditism) and they are often mistakenly reared as boys. Clinically most of these children suffer from a relative lack of cortisol. In boys the endocrine disorder may be first suspected only because of a failure to respond normally to the stress of a minor infection or injury.

About one-third of the cases also show evidence of mineralocorticoid deficiency. Vomiting is common and sodium depletion occurs rapidly unless treated. In boys the condition is often unsuspected until the correct diagnosis is made by finding severe hyperkalaemia. A number of different mechanisms have been suggested to explain this salt-wasting syndrome in some children with congenital adrenal hyperplasia. Cortisol deficiency is rather more pronounced than in children without salt-wasting but lack of the weak mineralocorticoid action of cortisol seems hardly sufficient to explain it. Aldosterone production is superficially adequate but these children cannot increase aldosterone production when deprived of salt. This may be an adequate explanation but the sodium depletion can be so profound that oversecretion of another, as yet undiscovered, steroid hormone with a predominantly salt-losing action may be responsible. It is relevant that critical sodium depletion may follow the administration of ACTH. Alternatively, the biological effect of aldosterone may be directly antagonized. We now know that a number of steroids with a chemical structure reminiscent of that of aldosterone will compete with aldosterone (and also other mineralocorticoids) for receptor sites on the renal tubule, so causing sodium loss and potassium retention. Synthetic steroids with a spirolactone grouping attached to C-17 have been prepared which do have this effect, and they are useful adjuncts to diuretic therapy because they do not cause potassium loss. It is quite possible that steroids which are potent aldosterone antagonists may be produced naturally in congenital adrenal hyperplasia. Rarely the salt-wasting syndrome may be associated with deficiency of 3β-steroid dehydrogenase.

More rarely, children with congenital adrenal virilism develop severe arterial hypertension and this may be associated with oversecretion of desoxycorticosterone, a mineralocorticoid which regularly produces hypertension experimentally. In these cases there is a predominant defect of 11β-hydroxylation as when 11β-hydroxylase is inhibited artificially. Compounds with this type of action can be produced synthetically and when administered to normal people the adrenal production of 11-deoxygenated steroids is increased, especially 17α-hydroxy-11-deoxycorticosterone (Reichstein's compound S), and 11-deoxycorticosterone. Since ACTH production rises as a result of the low circulating levels of cortisol the urinary excretion of 'glucocorticoids' is greatly elevated (p. 537). Rarely, a defect of 17-hydroxylase may lead to the adrenogenital syndrome and hypertension; the predominant steroids are related to corticosterone.

Administration of some form of glucocorticoid will reduce the adrenal androgen output to normal if given in amounts which produce a sustained suppression of the pituitary and yet do not give rise to signs of overdosage. All the manifestations of congenital adrenal hyperplasia can be controlled if adequate treatment is started early enough; girls can undergo a normal puberty and even become pregnant.

HYPERFUNCTION OF THE ADRENAL CORTEX

As with hypofunction of the adrenal the effects of adrenal overactivity depend upon which steroids are primarily affected.

CUSHING'S SYNDROME

Glucocorticoid over-production is essentially synonymous with cortisol over-production and it leads to Cushing's syndrome if sustained for long enough. Clinically most of the effects can be interpreted in terms of the known actions of cortisol. Carbohydrate metabolism is impaired largely because there is excessive glucose formation from protein so that diabetes mellitus is common; even those patients without overt glucosuria usually show a diabetic type of glucose tolerance curve. Whether or not there is a demonstrable abnormality of glucose handling is largely a function of the reserve of insulin within the pancreatic β-cells; but, characteristically, the diabetes when it occurs is of the non-ketotic adult type. Large doses of insulin are often required to control it. The excessive protein breakdown is responsible for the atrophied skin which bruises easily and readily cracks at stress points to form striae. It is also responsible for the wasted, weak muscles and contributes both to the classical picture of trunk (central) obesity with

18

match-stick limbs and to the development of osteoporosis. Excess cortisol leads to arterial hypertension by some unknown mechanism and also causes erythrocytosis by what appears to be a direct stimulating effect on the bone marrow. The cause of the striking central obesity of Cushing's syndrome is obscure. Women usually develop oligomenorrhea or amenorrhea and may become slightly hirsute as a result of excess androgen production. An abnormally high output of the androgen, dehydroepiandrosterone, is particularly characteristic of adrenal carcinomata.

Since cortisol does have some mineralocorticoid activity it might be expected that manifestations of this would appear in Cushing's syndrome even though aldosterone production is apparently not elevated. In mild cases, particularly those due to adrenal hyperplasia, no abnormality of electrolyte balance is usually demonstrable, but with adrenal or extra-adrenal carcinomata hypokalaemia and a raised plasma bicarbonate concentration are common. These may be useful differential diagnostic points.

Aetiology

Cushing's syndrome may be due to either a benign or malignant primary tumour of the adrenal or to bilateral hyperplasia of the adrenal cortex. Rarely Cushing's syndrome is caused by malignant tumours of other tissues, e.g. the bronchus. Most cases in children are due to a tumour whilst in adults hyperplasia is more common. Cortisol production by tumours is largely autonomous, whereas with hyperplasia, cortisol output may still be influenced by alterations of circulating corticotrophin. Clearly there is likely to be some extra-adrenal cause of the trouble in patients with Cushing's syndrome due to bilateral adrenal hyperplasia. *A priori* one would expect this to be an excessive production of corticotrophin by the pituitary, but in the past attempts to detect increased levels of circulating corticotrophin have usually met with failure. But now, with the development of more sensitive corticotrophin assay techniques, there is good evidence that, taking into consideration the elevated circulating cortisol levels, the concentration of corticotrophin in the peripheral blood is definitely excessive. Further evidence of a primary pituitary mechanism leading to sustained, inappropriate overproduction of corticotrophin is the fact that pituitary adenomas—either the small basophil ones or the larger, more serious chromophobe tumours—are common in Cushing's syndrome due to adrenal hyperplasia. These tend to show themselves particularly when the restraint of high circulating cortisol levels on pituitary activity has been removed by adrenalectomy. Furthermore, irradiation damage to the pituitary, whether supplied externally or internally (e.g. by implanting radio-active gold seeds), often causes remission of the disease.

HYPERALDOSTERONISM

Mineralocorticoid over-production is seen in fairly pure form without involvement of the production of other steroids in the syndrome of hyperaldosteronism. So-called primary hyperaldosteronism is almost always due to an adrenal adenoma. Secondary aldosteronism is seen in patients with cirrhosis of the liver, severe cardiac failure or the nephrotic syndrome who are actively forming oedema fluid.

The clinical manifestations of the primary and secondary form are very different.

In *primary aldosteronism* the dominating features are systemic hypertension (which is only rarely malignant) and potassium depletion with alkalosis. Muscle weakness and overt tetany are not uncommon and the kidneys may be damaged by potassium deficiency (see p. 20). In the absence of hypertensive cardiac failure oedema is rarely seen. The plasma renin concentration is low. These patients must be distinguished from the many patients with essential hypertension. The widespread use of the benzothiazide diuretics, which frequently induce potassium loss, has meant that hypokalaemic alkalosis is commonplace, and the diagnosis has now been made additionally difficult because accelerated or malignant essential hypertension may also be associated with raised aldosterone secretion rate; a hypokalaemic alkalosis is often present but, in contrast to patients with hypertension due to an adrenal adenoma, the plasma sodium concentration is often low and the hypertension is more severe. The cause of the hyperaldosteronism is almost certainly a raised plasma renin concentration. Although the clinical syndrome of *primary* hyperaldosteronism is superficially present, patients with severe essential hypertension represent another form of *secondary* hyperaldosteronism (see below). Apart from the clinical information, tests designed to test the autonomy of aldosterone production and measurements of the plasma renin concentration (particularly when the patient is sodium-depleted) help to distinguish. Another example of this variety of secondary hyperaldosteronism, characterized by hypokalaemic alkalosis without hypertension, is caused by hyperplasia of the juxta-glomerular apparatus of the kidney. Plasma renin concentrations are high and there is resistance to the cardiovascular effects of angiotensin infusions.

Although aldosterone has a potent sodium-retaining action in adrenalectomized animals and in Addison's disease, alterations of sodium metabolism are not prominent in primary hyperaldosteronism. However, intracellular sodium concentrations may be elevated, and the serum sodium tends towards the high side of normal. Possibly a continued expansion of the extracellular fluid volume raises the glomerular filtration rate sufficiently to allow sodium equilibrium although increased urinary potassium loss continues unabated.

By contrast *secondary aldosteronism* is dominated by oedema formation; potassium loss is modest and the serum levels of potassium are usually normal unless benzothiazide diuretics have been used. The blood pressure tends to be low and the plasma renin concentration high. The hypothesis that angiotensin is over-produced is attractive because angiotensin in suitable doses stimulates aldosterone production (p. 526), without changing the production of cortisol appreciably.

The ion-exchange mechanism in the distal tubules of the kidney probably explains why the syndrome of primary aldosteronism is characterized by hypokalaemia whilst that of secondary aldosteronism is not. The increased proximal tubular sodium reabsorption seen in oedematous states will reduce the amount of sodium delivered to the distal tubule and so reduce the potassium loss which would otherwise occur in exchange for sodium. The fact that the hypokalaemia of primary aldosteronism can be corrected by feeding a low sodium diet probably reflects this process.

ACQUIRED ADRENAL VIRILISM

Sex hormone over-production occurs in Cushing's syndrome but, in the presence of adrenal tumours in children and in some adult women the clinical manifestations are sometimes dominated by sexual virilism giving rise to the so-called adrenogenital syndrome, or, more simply, adrenal virilism. This syndrome when it occurs after the age of about one is almost always due to an adrenal tumour. In very young children sex hormone over-production occurs in congenital adrenal hyperplasia (as described on page 529); but in these cases there is an associated deficiency of cortisol secretion and it is for this reason that the syndrome has been discussed separately.

The over-production of androgens is chiefly responsible for the clinical manifestations but very occasionally a feminizing adrenal tumour may cause gynaecomastia in boys. Androgen excess in children of both sexes causes unusually rapid growth and their muscles become strong and well developed because androgens stimulate protein anabolism (producing the 'infant Hercules'). Their bony epiphyses fuse prematurely so that ultimately growth is stunted. Body hair appears prematurely and the skin may become greasy and develop acne. The voice is husky and boys show precocious secondary sexual development although the testes remain infantile because the excess androgen production suppresses the secretion of pituitary gonadotrophin. Girls show enlargement of the clitoris, a masculine body build and a male distribution of the pubic hair. They do not undergo puberty because of gonadotrophin suppression. In women similar changes occur, but in addition, ovarian activity is suppressed so that menstruation ceases and the breasts atrophy.

IDIOPATHIC HIRSUTISM IN WOMEN
This is a psychologically distressing condition which, since it is often associated with irregular or infrequent menstruation and reduced fertility, suggests that some endocrine abnormality is present rather than an abnormal sensitivity of the hair follicles to normal amounts of circulating androgen. The rate of urine excretion of the 17-ketosteroids is usually normal but the plasma testosterone concentration or the output of testosterone in the urine is increased in about half the patients. Some patients show an enhanced response to exogenous ACTH and it is probably these who show some response to adrenal suppressive therapy. Others respond to ovarian suppression, as, for example, when contraceptive steroids are administered (p. 619). The fundamental defect is therefore, either an enhanced sensitivity of the hair-follicles or overproduction of androgens, particularly testosterone, from the adrenal glands or from the ovaries.

Principles of tests and measurements

Procedures for the assessment of adrenal cortical function fall into three groups: firstly, tests designed to provide some measure of the basal secretion rate of specific steroid hormones; secondly, tests designed to measure the adrenal responsiveness to appropriate stimuli; and thirdly, indirect tests designed to assess changes in physiological functions which are influenced by the adrenal cortical steroid hormones.

ASSESSMENT OF THE BASAL RATE OF STEROID PRODUCTION
Secretion rate of specific steroids
By the application of elegant double isotope dilution-derivative assay procedures it is now theoretically possible to measure specifically the

actual secretion rate of many individual steroid hormones by the adrenal glands. Following a tracer dose of radio-active steroid, the specific activity of an exclusive urinary metabolite is measured in a 24 or 48-hr urine sample. The extent to which this has fallen as compared with the specific activity of the administered steroid is a measure of the endogenous steroid production. The details of the methods have now been carefully worked out for aldosterone, cortisol and testosterone. However, the measurements are time-consuming, and can only be undertaken in specialized laboratories.

For most general clinical purposes an attempt is made to assess the secretion rate of a given steroid or group of steroids indirectly. Usually the assessment is doubly indirect and certain assumptions are made which must be remembered. Not only is the plasma level or urine excretion rate of appropriate metabolites assumed to be an index of glandular secretion rate but also, in many instances, the steroid hormone concerned is not measured specifically. Thus, the *plasma level* of a particular steroid or group of steroids at any given time is the result of the balance struck between the amount of steroid entering the circulation from the adrenal gland and the rate of its disappearance. The latter, in turn, is determined by the degradation rate (chiefly a function of the liver) and the renal clearance of the steroid concerned. Furthermore, the adrenal glands have a diurnal rhythm of secretion which can cause considerable fluctuation of plasma level so that a plasma sample taken at any one time during the day may be quite unrepresentative of the mean daily glandular secretion rate. By the same type of reasoning the 24-*hr urinary excretion rate* of a steroid metabolite is a function not only of the integrated plasma level of free unbound steroid over a 24-hr period but also depends on the vagaries of renal and liver function. Finally, the chemical methods used routinely are only partially specific because the estimation of individual steroids is too tedious and rarely essential. But, despite these qualifications, it is surprising how much useful information can be gleaned from urinary and plasma 'steroid' levels, although the diagnosis of primary hyperaldosteronism is uncertain without an estimation of the rate of aldosterone secretion. The detection of abnormal amounts of dehydroepiandrosterone and of pregnanetriol in the urine is most useful in the diagnosis of adrenal carcinoma and congenital adrenal hyperplasia respectively.

Routine methods

Methods which are sufficiently simple for routine hospital laboratory use have been devised to estimate glucocorticoids and their metabolites and androgen metabolites in urine. Refinements of these methods are applied to plasma. Urinary estimations alone are commonly used in clinical practice.

Urine is treated with acid or enzymes to hydrolyse steroid conjugates and the freed steroids are extracted with organic solvents and measured by colour reactions given by all steroids with certain common structural features, e.g. the Porter–Silber reaction for 17,21-dihydroxy-20-keto-steroids, the blue tetrazolium reaction for α-ketols (20-oxo,21-hydroxy steroids) and the Zimmerman reaction for 17-oxosteroids. Results are expressed in terms of standard substances which usually do not have the same chromogenicity. Glucocorticoids and their metabolites (hereafter called 'glucocorticoids') are estimated as 17-hydroxycorticoids, 17-oxogenic steroids or total 17-hydroxycorticosteroids. The difference between these various ways of obtaining an index of 'glucocorticoid' secretion is usually unimportant clinically. Androgen metabolites are estimated as 17-oxosteroids. Routine steroid estimations are made on aliquots of 24-hr collections of urine. The interpretation of results obtained on random specimens is complicated by the normal diurnal rhythm of steroid excretion. Most methods for plasma steroids measure only the unmodified steroids and not their conjugates, but modifications are available which also measure steroids liberated from conjugates by enzymic hydrolysis.

The following points should be kept in mind when interpreting the results of steroid estimations: (1) The excretion of 17-oxosteroids is very low in children of both sexes until puberty, when it rapidly rises to adult levels. It is also low in old age and in many chronic illnesses without evidence of endocrine involvement. Approximately one half of the 17-oxosteroid excretion of men is derived from adrenal androgens and most of the remainder from testicular androgens. Very small amounts are derived from glucocorticoids but the actual amounts may become appreciable when glucocorticoid secretion is excessive. (2) Routine methods measure steroids which have common chemical properties, and they do not necessarily differentiate between biologically active and inactive substances and their metabolites. This is particularly important in the case of tumours, which often secrete large amounts of chemically reactive but biologically inert steroids. (3) The actual values obtained depend on the method used. The several methods for estimating 'gluco-corticoids', for example, measure slightly different groups of steroids and therefore give different results with the same sample of urine.

Normal values for specified methods are given in Table 16, p. 543.

INDIRECT TESTS

Most of the indirect methods of assessing adrenal function became obsolete when practicable methods were introduced for the estimation of 'glucocorticoids' and 17-oxosteroids. Tests which remain useful include: (1) estimation of the plasma concentrations of sodium, potassium and urea; (2) the water excretion test.

(1) The plasma concentrations of urea and potassium rise with chronic primary adrenal insufficiency, and later the plasma sodium and bicarbonate concentrations may fall. These changes do not occur in adrenal insufficiency secondary to hypopituitarism because aldosterone production is not diminished. Primary hyperaldosteronism is associated with hypokalaemia, a high normal sodium and an increased plasma bicarbonate concentration. The presence of considerable hypokalaemia in patients with Cushing's syndrome suggests the presence of a carcinoma of the adrenal.

(2) Delayed water excretion is caused by glucocorticoid deficiency as well as by several other conditions, the most important of which are: dehydration, small intestinal malabsorption states, myxoedema, renal disease and oedematous states. A normally hydrated, fasting, healthy adult excretes at least 80 per cent of a standard oral dose of water of 9 ml/lb or 20 ml/kg body weight within 4 hr. The administration of 100 mg cortisone acetate or an appropriate analogue by mouth, 2–4 hr before the water load, restores excretion to normal when delay is due to glucocorticoid deficiency, but only rarely does so in the other conditions mentioned. This test, although useful because it is so simple, is potentially dangerous in patients with severe glucocorticoid deficiency and should not be performed in patients suspected of Addison's disease unless the plasma electrolytes are normal. They may develop water intoxication, especially if they are already hyponatraemic. Excretion may be hastened in these circumstances by an intravenous injection of hydrocortisone.

Outmoded tests include random absolute eosinophil counts and insulin tolerance tests. The latter may cause severe, prolonged and dangerous hypoglycaemia in patients with adrenal insufficiency.

The Na/K ratio of saliva and sweat gives an indication of mineralocorticoid activity but depends to some extent on the rate of formation. The test is not widely used.

TESTS OF ADRENAL RESERVE
Hypofunction
The adrenal reserve of cortisol production is most easily determined by observing the response to maximal doses of corticotrophin and the

reserve of aldosterone production by the response to sodium deprivation and depletion.

To test cortisol reserve it is usually sufficient to estimate the urinary excretion of glucocorticoid metabolites by one of the methods described above, but it is sometimes useful to make simultaneous determinations of the plasma 17-hydroxycorticosteroid levels. The simplest procedure is to give intramuscular injections of corticotrophin for 3 days, or an intravenous infusion for 8 hours. A normal person will show a clear increase of corticosteroid and 17-oxosteroid excretion and a fall in the urinary sodium to potassium ratio. Since large doses of ACTH stimulate the production of mineralocorticoids such as 11-deoxycorticosterone and since cortisol has a considerable mineralocorticoid type of action in its own right, primary adrenal insufficiency can usually be excluded for practical purposes if there is a clear reduction of the urinary sodium/potassium ratio of more than 80 per cent. Patients with Addison's disease show little or no response. This is a useful test because it can be done while the patient is still receiving appropriate replacement therapy. It is particularly appropriate in recognizing mild cases of Addison's disease where there is only sufficient adrenal tissue to secrete normal amounts of steroids under basal conditions and additional ACTH from exogenous sources cannot increase steroid production any further. The test may also help to distinguish between chronic adrenal insufficiency of adrenal and pituitary origin. However the response is often considerably less than normal in pituitary disease. If doubt still exists the test can be repeated over a longer period of time to allow regeneration of the atrophied adrenal cortex. The Cutler salt deprivation test is now obsolete as a test for Addison's disease because it is dangerous, but the change of secretion rate or urinary excretion of aldosterone in response to sodium depletion determines the adrenal reserve of aldosterone production.

Hyperfunction

Stimulation. The hormone production of tumours is largely independent of pituitary control and is often unaffected by corticotrophin injections. Some increase of glucocorticoid and 17-oxosteroid excretion may be produced, however, by stimulation of normal adrenal tissue. In contrast, hyperfunctioning normal-sized or hyperplastic glands causing Cushing's and the adrenogenital syndromes usually show an unusually great secretory response. In Cushing's syndrome the 'glucocorticoid' response is greater than that of the 17-oxosteroids.

Suppression. Glucocorticoids inhibit secretion of corticotrophin and suppress the output of glucocorticoids and androgens by normal and

18*

(feedback)

normal-sized, or hyperplastic, hyperfunctioning glands but not usually of tumours. Metabolites of administered cortisone or hydrocortisone mask changes in the excretion of endogenous 'glucocorticoid', so that suppression is best detected when a powerful glucocorticoid such as dexamethasone is used. The metabolites of the small amounts required (2–8 mg daily) contribute little to the total urinary 'glucocorticoid' excretion. With a dose of 2 mg daily for 3–4 days all normal people show a fall of urinary corticoid excretion to very low levels, whereas patients with Cushing's syndrome fail to do so. When 8 mg daily for 3–4 days is used it is often possible to differentiate between adrenal hyperplasia and a tumour as the cause of Cushing's syndrome. Patients with hyperplasia suppress excretion of glucocorticoid metabolites at this dose level, but most patients with adrenal tumours do not.

Practical assessment

ADRENAL HYPOFUNCTION

PRIMARY—ADDISON'S DISEASE
Clinical observations:
> Tiredness, weakness, vomiting, nocturia, increased pigmentation, hypotension (particularly on standing) and poor response to stress.

Routine methods
> Water excretion—delayed, restored by cortisone.
> Plasma K^+ and blood urea increased; plasma Na^+ normal or low.
> X-rays for tuberculous adrenal calcification.

Special techniques:
> ① Basal steroid excretion—'glucocorticoids' low or in mild cases, low normal.
> 17-oxosteroids very low in women, about 5 mg daily in men.
> ② No significant response to corticotrophin test, as shown by failure of reduction of urinary Na/K ratio, or by lack of increase in 'glucocorticoid' and 17-oxosteroid excretion.

SECONDARY—HYPOPITUITARISM
Clinical observations:
> Tiredness, weakness, pallor, amenorrhoea, feeling cold, nocturia, absence of pubic and body hair, poor response to stress. There is

often a history of haemorrhage associated with childbirth with subsequent failure of lactation. There may be symptoms and signs of intracranial tumour.

Routine methods:
Water excretion—delayed, restored by cortisone.
Plasma potassium normal. Plasma sodium may be low.
Skull X-rays for evidence of tumour; assessment of visual fields.
Laboratory evidence of thyroid hypofunction (see p. 558).
Vaginal epithelium is 'basal', indicating oestrogen deficiency.

Special techniques:
Basal excretion of 'glucocorticoids' and 17-oxosteroids very low in both sexes.
Significant response to corticotrophin test (p. 539).
Very low or absent urinary excretion of follicle-stimulating hormone (p. 501).
Increased radioiodine uptake by the thyroid after administration of thyroid-stimulating hormone (TSH) (p. 559).

ADRENAL HYPERFUNCTION

GLUCOCORTICOID EXCESS—CUSHING'S SYNDROME
Clinical observations:
Central obesity, plethoric moon face, atrophic skin with bruises and purple straie, muscular weakness and wasting, backache, occasional psychosis, hypertension, polycythaemia, glycosuria; and in women, hirsutism and menstrual disturbances.

Routine methods:
Glucose tolerance test—often diabetic (p. 489).
Plasma K^+ may be decreased if a tumour is present.
X-rays of spine for osteoporosis.
Basal 'glucocorticoid' excretion increased. 17-oxosteroids may be increased, but less than 'glucocorticoids'.

Special techniques:
Estimation of cortisol secretion rate or urinary free cortisol excretion rate.
Plasma 11-hydroxycorticosteroid concentration fails to show the

normal diurnal rhythm.
Corticotrophin stimulation and dexamethasone suppression tests
may differentiate cases due to tumour (p. 539).
Presacral gas insufflation X-ray studies or aortography for detection
of tumour.

MINERALOCORTICOID EXCESS—PRIMARY HYPERALDOSTERONISM
(CONN'S SYNDROME)
Clinical observations:
Severe hypertension, muscular weakness, tetany.

Routine methods:
ECG changes of hypokalaemia. Plasma K^+ low, Na^+ high normal,
and bicarbonate high.

Special techniques:
Estimation of urinary aldosterone excretion or aldosterone secretion
rate.
Effect of Na^+ deprivation, and Na^+-loading on aldosterone
secretion or urinary excretion rates.
Effect of K^+-loading on plasma K^+ concentrations and on aldosterone production.

ANDROGEN EXCESS—ACQUIRED ADRENAL VIRILISM
Clinical observations:
In children: Precocious secondary sexual development in boys
with infantile testes, virilization in girls, accelerated somatic
growth in both sexes.
In women: Masculine body build and hair distribution, baldness,
coarse, greasy skin with acne, deep voice, menstrual disturbances
including amenorrhoea, enlarged clitoris.

Routine and special techniques:
Basal 17-oxosteroid excretion increased. 'Glucocorticoids' variable.
Corticotrophin stimulation and dexamethasone suppression tests
may differentiate cases due to tumour.
Presacral gas insufflation X-ray studies or aortography for detection
of tumour.

CONGENITAL ADRENAL VIRILISM

Clinical observations:
Precocious secondary sexual development in boys with infantile testes; pseudohermaphroditism in girls; accelerated somatic growth and poor resistance to stress in both sexes. Sometimes associated with sodium depletion and occasionally with hypertension.

Routine methods:
Determination of chromosomal sex by examination of buccal epithelial cells or leucocytes (p. 594).

Special techniques:
Basal 'glucocorticoid' excretion low. 17-oxosteroid and pregnenetriol excretion increased.

17-oxosteroid and pregnanetriol excretion reduced and excessive androgenic activity abolished by small doses of cortisone or one of its analogues.

TABLE 16.—Normal values for adrenal steroid estimations

Method	Men	Women
URINE (mg/24 hr)		
'Glucocorticoids'		
17-hydroxycorticoids	3–12	1–9
17-oxogenic steroids	5–22	4–18
total 17-hydroxycorticosteroids	8–22	5–17
17-oxosteroids	10–20	5–15
PLASMA (μg/100 ml)		9–10 a.m.: 6–26
11-hydroxycorticosteroids		Evening: <8

References

FORSHAM P.H. (1962) The Adrenal Cortex. In *Textbook of endocrinology* (3rd edn). (Ed. WILLIAMS R.H.). Philadelphia: Saunders. pp. 282–383.

Proceedings of a conference held at the University of Glasgow, July 1960. Ed. CURRIE A.R., SYMINGTON T. & GRANT J.K. (1962) Edinburgh: Livingstone.

The adrenal cortex. Ed. PRUNTY F.T.G. (1962). *Brit. med. Bull.*, **18**, 89–173.

Proceedings of a conference on aldosterone. Ed. BAULIEU E.E. & ROBEL P. (1964). Blackwell, Oxford.

WILKINS L. (1957) Adrenal Cortex: hyperadrenocorticism—adrenogenital syndrome and Cushing's syndrome. In *The diagnosis and treatment of endocrine disorders in childhood and adolescence* (2nd edn). Illinois: Thomas. pp. 330–78.

JAILER J.W. & HOLUB D.A. (1960) Congenital adrenal hyperplasia. In *Clinical endocrinology* 1. Ed. ASTWOOD E.B. New York: Grune & Stratton. pp. 354–62.

PRUNTY F.T.G. (1967) Current techniques for the assessment of adrenocortical function and their interpretation. In *Recent advances in Endocrinology*. Ed. GARDINER-HILL. London: Butterworths. pp. 169–92.

Proceedings of the second international conference on hormonal steroids, May 1966. Ed. MARTINI L., FRASCHINI F. & MOTTA N. Excerpta Medica, London.

ADRENAL MEDULLA

Normal function

The adrenal medulla is a specialized part of the sympathetic nervous system. It represents the postganglionic neurones and, like them, secretes sympathetic amines in response to stimulation by preganglionic sympathetic neurones. The adrenal medulla differs from postganglionic sympathetic neurones, however, in two ways; firstly, in adults but not in children, adrenaline as well as noradrenaline is liberated, and secondly, the amines are discharged into the blood stream (thus making the adrenal medulla an endocrine or ductless gland) so that they act indirectly rather than directly on the effector organs. In contrast to other endocrine glands, abolition of adrenal medullary function does not apparently interfere with the body's metabolic processes and medullary secretion only seems to have physiological significance in response to specific stimulation by the hypothalamus. In fact the gland provides many of the immediate reactions to a sudden potentially harmful stimulus as, for example, in preparing the organism for 'fight or flight'. This underlines the fact that, in contrast to other hormones, those of the adrenal medulla act very swiftly.

Biological activities of noradrenaline and adrenaline (see also p. 46)
Adrenaline causes excitatory responses in some regions and inhibitory ones in others. It excites constriction of the blood vessels of the skin, it stimulates pilo-erection and dilatation of the pupil and in very large quantities may cause sweating. Adrenaline also increases the excitability of the myocardium and induces tachycardia. The cardiac output rises and there is an elevation of the systolic blood pressure. The diastolic pressure does not increase, however; in fact, the peripheral resistance falls. This is because adrenaline has important inhibitory effects on the

smooth muscle of all arterioles except those of the skin. It also relaxes the smooth muscle of the uterus (in man but not in all species), the bronchioles, the intestine and the bladder. (The subject of α- and β-adrenergic receptors is fully discussed in Chapter 2.)

Adrenaline also has metabolic effects. It produces a rise of the blood sugar concentration by stimulating the breakdown of liver glycogen to glucose and it increases the metabolic rate.

In contrast *noradrenaline* has predominately excitatory effects on the arteriolar musculature. There is a generalized vasoconstriction so that both systolic and diastolic blood pressures rise sharply and the peripheral resistance is greatly increased. Bradycardia occurs and the cardiac output remains unchanged. Sweating, pilo-erection and pupillary dilatation are minimal in doses which cause hypertension and noradrenaline is approximately eight times weaker than adrenaline in causing hepatic glycogen breakdown.

Biosynthesis and metabolism of the adrenal medullary hormones

Noradrenaline and adrenaline are synthesized from tyrosine by a series of enzymic steps. The benzene ring is hydroxylated to form 3,4-dihydroxyphenylalanine (DOPA) which is decarboxylated by a dopa decarboxylase to form dopamine. A hydroxyl radical is then added to the side-chain to form noradrenaline, which is methylated by N-methyl transferase to form adrenaline. The decarboxylation of dopa to dopamine can be specifically inhibited by alpha-methyl dopa, a hypotensive drug.

Hydroxylation of tyrosine, the initial step, is controlled by a specific enzyme, tyrosine hydroxylase. Its activity is probably the main factor governing the rate of synthesis of noradrenaline. Noradrenaline inhibits tyrosine hydroxylase (an example of end-product inhibition) and it now seems clear that the rate of noradrenaline formation is controlled by the rate of noradrenaline secretion. The rate of secretion and the hormone content of the gland vary directly and not inversely, in contrast to other endocrine glands such as the pancreas.

Both hormones are stored in the chromaffin granules of the medullary cells and they are responsible for the characteristic staining reaction with potassium dichromate. The store of catechol amines is greatly depleted by hypotensive drugs such as reserpine and guanethidine both in the adrenal medulla and the postganglionic neurones.

In contrast to other endocrine glands the secretion of noradrenaline and adrenaline into the blood stream seems to occur only in response to some specific stimulus; there is little or no secretion under basal conditions. The hypothalamus discharges impulses down the pre-ganglionic neurones to the adrenal medulla in response to severe injury, emotion (particularly fear), hypoglycaemia and severe cold. The immediate stimulus to the medullary cells is, of course, the chemical transmitter substance of the sympathetic ganglia, acetylcholine; and the synapses between the preganglionic nerve endings and the medullary cells, like those in the sympathetic ganglia, respond to drugs in the same way. For example, hexamethonium blocks catechol amine release whereas parasympatheticomimetic drugs stimulate it.

Noradrenaline and adrenaline are metabolized into biologically inactive derivatives at a remarkably rapid rate in comparison with other hormones. Within a very few minutes of stopping an infusion of nor-adrenaline its cardiovascular effects have worn off although the effects of adrenaline may persist for a little longer. Both amines are excreted in the urine largely as o-methylated, deaminated metabolites, produced by the action of o-methyl transferase and monoamine oxidase respectively. The main metabolite is 3-methoxy-4-hydroxy mandelic acid (vanillyl mandelic acid or VMA) but smaller amounts of the o-methylated metabolites, normet- and metadrenaline are also excreted, either free or as glucuronides. Only about 5 per cent of the catechol amines are excreted in the urine as such, i.e. in biologically active form. Whereas there is normally about 4 times as much adrenaline as noradrenaline in the adrenal medulla the reverse is true in the urine. Total adrenalec-tomy barely affects noradrenaline excretion although adrenaline excretion virtually vanishes. It is clear, therefore, that extra-adrenal tissues (probably the postganglionic sympathetic nerves) are normally responsible for most of the noradrenaline found in the urine.

Disordered function

The only known abnormality of the adrenal medulla is oversecretion. This is nearly always the result of a phaeochromocytoma, a tumour of the chromaffin cells which is usually benign.

The clinical manifestations depend firstly on the relative amounts of noradrenaline and adrenaline oversecreted, and secondly on whether the oversecretion is continuous or intermittent. Since all phaeochromo-cytomata produce an absolute excess of noradrenaline the dominating feature is nearly always systemic hypertension. This is sustained in most patients and paroxysmal in a minority (25 per cent). Episodes of severe symptoms are not invariable, but when they occur they usually consist of headache, sweating and apprehension, and they are often precipitated by cold, fasting, exercise or palpating the region of the tumour.

Overt diabetes develops in about 10 per cent and many patients with phaeochromocytoma show an impaired glucose tolerance, but whether or not carbohydrate metabolism is affected will depend on the absolute quantity of adrenaline secreted. For example, disordered carbohydrate metabolism has not been a feature of the few cases reported in children presumably because their adrenal glands contain only noradrenaline. Increase of the metabolic rate and nervousness sometimes mimics thyrotoxicosis. In patients who continuously oversecrete noradrenaline alone hypertension is sustained and carbohydrate metabolism is not detectably disordered, so that differentiation from essential hypertension can be difficult.

Practical assessment

Adrenal medullary function may be assessed by measurement of the urinary excretion of hormones and by observing the effects of drugs which influence hormone secretion or activity. With the development of rapid and reasonably specific methods of chemical assay, the use of pharmacological tests is becoming less frequent.

Urine tests
Medullary hormones are estimated biologically by comparing the effect on the blood pressure of an anaesthetized cat with that of standard amounts of adrenaline and noradrenaline, and chemically by several fluorimetric methods. Normal urine contains less than 0·1 μg/ml or 100 μg/day of adrenaline or noradrenaline. Relatively simple screening tests are available to detect the presence of greater amounts of hormones. Although large amounts of catecholamines may be present in the urine in quiescent phases, it is best to collect the urine of patients with intermittent hypertension during a paroxysm. The biological test may give false positive results in patients who are taking antihistamines and sympathomimetic drugs. Conversely, cases of phaeochromocytoma have been described in which no excess of catechol amines could be detected in the urine when measured by bio-assay. Many drugs interfere with the fluorimetric tests.

The urine output of vanillyl mandelic acid provides a convenient chemical method for the detection of patients with phaeochromocytoma.

Normally, and in essential hypertension, less than 7 mg/day is found in the urine. Eating bananas (which contain noradrenaline), and foods containing tyramine (such as strong cheeses) or vanilla may give falsely positive results, among other foods and drugs.

Pharmacological tests
Provocative tests are useful in patients with intermittent hypertension. The intravenous injection of 0·01–0·025 mg of histamine causes a fall, or occasionally a slight rise in the blood pressure of normal subjects and patients with hypertension not due to a phaeochromocytoma. If a phaeochromocytoma is present, histamine stimulates the secretion of noradrenaline and precipitates a hypertensive paroxysm. The blood pressure may rise by as much as 200 mm systolic and 100 mm diastolic and, once the effect has been observed, should be reduced by an adrenolytic drug. The test should not be performed in patients with sustained hypertension. The use of tyramine as the provocative agent may be more reliable diagnostically.

Blocking tests are performed with adrenolytic drugs which antagonize the peripheral activity of noradrenaline. The intravenous injection of phentolamine ('Regitine', 'Rogitine') causes the prompt fall of at least 40 mm systolic and 25 mm diastolic in the blood pressure of patients with a phaeochromocytoma but not in those with sustained hypertension due to other causes. False positive results are common particularly in patients who have poor renal function or who are sedated with barbiturates. The test is only useful in patients with sustained hypertension. Other drugs, including benzodioxane, have been used as diagnostic blocking agents, but are inferior to phentolamine because they give more frequent false positive results or unpleasant side effects.

References

FORSHAM P.H. & THORN G.W. (1962) Adrenal medulla. In *Textbook of Endocrinology* (3rd edn). (Ed. WILLIAMS R.H.). Philadelphia: Saunders. pp. 383–91.
HAGEN P. (1960) Adrenal medulla and its secretions. In *Clinical Endocrinology* I. Ed. ASTWOOD E.B. New York: Grune & Stratton. pp. 397–406.
VON EULER U.S. & HELLNER S. (1951) Excretion of noradrenaline, adrenaline and hydroxytyramine in the urine. *Acta. physiol. scand.*, 22, 161–7.
Second symposium on catecholamines. *Pharmacol. Rev.*, 18, No. 1 (1966).

16

The Thyroid Gland

Normal function

Thyroid function is closely related to iodine metabolism because the hormones made by the thyroid gland—thyroxine and tri-iodothyronine—contain a high proportion of iodine and are the only compounds of physiological importance known to contain this element. The effects of these 2 hormones are qualitatively very similar but differ dramatically in their time-course of action in man.

This chapter is limited to consideration of these 2 hormones but the recent discovery of a new hormone, calcitonin, must be mentioned. Calcitonin may be of importance in human calcium metabolism and has been extracted from the thyroid of man. It is discussed further on p. 316.

In mammals, thyroid hormones play an important role in the regulation of growth and heat production but in lower orders they also influence metamorphosis. Although the function of many different tissues can be affected by thyroid hormones no single key site of physiological action has yet been defined.

Thus, the assessment of thyroid function in patients may be made either by measurement of the basal metabolic rate which depends on the peripheral utilization of thyroid hormones or by studying some aspect of iodine metabolism in the thyroid itself which reflects the rate at which thyroxine and tri-iodothyronine are synthesized.

The availability of suitable radioactive iodine isotopes and sensitive chemical techniques for the measurement of stable iodine in body fluids enables both approaches to be used to determine with great precision whether the hormones are being produced in smaller or larger amounts than normal.

THE THYROID HORMONES

Chemically these hormones are iodinated forms of thyronine, the formula of which is shown below.

$$HO - \langle \rangle - \langle \rangle - CH_2 - CH(NH_2)COOH$$

3' 3

5' 5

Thyroxine has 4 iodine atoms, attached to the 3:5 and 3':5' positions. Tri-iodothyronine has 3 iodine atoms, attached to the 3:5 and 3' positions.

Synthetic analogues have been prepared by substitution of other halogens for iodine in these 2 molecules; they possess some physiological activity but are much less potent than the naturally occurring compounds. In common with many other physiologically active compounds the naturally occurring forms of thyroxine and tri-iodothyronine are both laevorotatory.

Within the thyroid gland the greater part of its store of iodinated compounds is in the colloid as mono- and di-iodotyrosine which are precursors of the fully formed hormones made from them by oxidative coupling. Thyroxine, tri-iodothyronine and the iodinated tyrosines are all bound to thyroglobulin by peptide bonds which are broken by the action of thyroidal-protease. In the circulating blood thyroxine is present in 9 times greater concentration than tri-iodothyronine and is mostly bound to a specific carrier protein known as thyroxine-binding globulin. This carrier protein migrates in the inter-α-region on electrophoresis and is only partially saturated in health (about 20 per cent); the metabolically active free-thyroxine fraction is minute compared with the protein bound hormone. A stable equilibrium exists between the free and bound thyroxine, and the concentration of thyroxine binding globulin does not vary greatly in thyroid diseases. Because of this the level of protein bound iodine may be used as a measure of the level of thyroid hormones.

Production of thyroid hormones

The outstanding physiological property of thyroid cells is their ability to concentrate iodide by an active transport system which normally results in the gland concentration being 25 times greater than in serum. In states of iodine deficiency, or when the thyroid is stimulated, this gradient becomes even greater, thus conserving body iodine.

Dietary iodine intake is mainly derived from some species of fish, iodized salt and cow's milk which may contain substantial quantities if the cattle are fed on artificial cake to which supplemental iodine has been added. In urban communities without evidence of iodine deficiency most measurements show an intake of the order of 100 μg/day.

In health the concentration of plasma free inorganic iodide is quite low (less than 1 $\mu g/100$ ml) and its clearance is by the thyroid or kidneys. Other tissues such as salivary or mammary glands also actively transport iodide from the blood but only the thyroid is capable of synthesizing its hormones.

Certain anions—notably perchlorate and thiocyanate—inhibit the transport of iodide by the thyroid and may be used as antithyroid drugs in some circumstances.

The iodide in the thyroid is oxidized and becomes incorporated into tyrosine radicals to form mono- and di-iodotyrosine. This step is controlled by an enzyme system not yet identified. The tyrosine radicals which are thus iodinated are already part of the protein molecule which is to become thyroglobulin.

The formation of thyroxine is accomplished by the coupling together of the di-iodotyrosine radicals:

$$HO-\underset{I}{\overset{I}{\bigcirc}}-CH_2-CH(NH_2)COOH$$

with the extrusion of alanine. This step is also an oxidative process. The formation of tri-iodothyronine is probably by coupling 1 mono-iodotyrosine radical and 1 di-iodotyrosine radical.

Both the iodination of tyrosines and the coupling of iodotyrosines can be prevented by small quantities of antithyroid substances of the thiourea series. Thus, it is possible to do a 'pharmacological dissection' of thyroid hormone synthesis; perchlorate prevents iodide concentration whereas thiourea prevents the iodination of protein without affecting the iodide concentrating mechanism.

Thyroglobulin is stored within the colloid of the thyroid acini. When hormone is required, thyroglobulin is broken down by a protease to release thyroxine and tri-iodothyronine which pass out into the blood. The same proteolytic process also releases mono- and di-iodotyrosine, which are then acted upon by a di-iodinase which releases the iodide they contain. This iodide is mostly used again within the thyroid. After thyroxine and tri-iodothyronine are broken down in the peripheral tissues part of their iodine is also reutilized by the thyroid. Thus, both these methods are employed by the body to conserve its store of iodine.

CONTROL OF THYROID FUNCTION

The anterior pituitary gland secretes a thyroid stimulating hormone (TSH or thyrotrophin) which stimulates all known aspects of thyroid function: iodide concentration, iodination of protein, proteolysis of thyroglobulin and release of hormone into the blood. Thyroid function persists after complete hypophysectomy albeit at a greatly diminished level compared with intact animals. Thus, there is no single metabolic step which is dependent upon TSH.

The release of TSH from the pituitary is controlled by the level of thyroid hormones in the circulating blood through a 'negative feed back' mechanism. The release of TSH is stimulated when blood thyroid hormone level falls and vice versa so that, in health, the output of hormonal iodine from the thyroid is approximately 70 μg/day, of which most is contained in thyroxine. The level at which this system operates is itself probably under hypothalamic control through the influence of a thyrotrophin releasing factor (TRF).

In experimental animals, thyroid function responds to changes in environmental temperature, increasing when it is cold and declining when it is higher than normal. It is not clear whether these adjustments depend chiefly upon hypothalamic influences or upon changes in the rate of peripheral utilization of thyroid hormones.

Thyroid function may be depressed by stresses such as surgical operations and by the administration of adrenal steroids. Whether or not emotional stresses, acting through the hypothalamus, influence thyroid function is still uncertain.

The operation of the pituitary-thyroid 'servo' (p. 503) mechanism is seen clearly in experiments which interfere with hormone synthesis either by depriving an animal of its dietary iodine, or by inhibiting thyroidal transport of iodide with potassium perchlorate or by preventing the iodination of protein by one of the drugs of the thiouracil group. All of these situations result in a decline in circulating thyroid hormone which stimulates the pituitary to release more TSH, which, in turn, increases thyroid function and will, in time, lead to thyroid enlargement. This thyroid enlargement can be prevented by the simultaneous administration of any substance having thyroid hormone-like activity. This is the basis of the goitre prevention test, used for the assessment of the thyroid hormone-like activity of substances chemically related to thyroxine.

The thyroid is able to compensate for low blood iodide levels by increasing the efficiency of the iodide transporting mechanism; the ability to transport iodide is preserved although in a greatly enfeebled way after hypophysectomy and there is some evidence from hypophysectomized animals that there is also an internal regulating mechanism in thyroid follicles which limits the accumulation of iodide when colloid stores are adequate.

In spite of these observations there is no doubt that, in health, thyroid function is controlled by TSH which reaches the gland in the circulating blood. The influence of the long-acting thyroid stimulator (LATS) in the overactive thyroid glands of patients with thyrotoxicosis is discussed below.

PHYSIOLOGICAL EFFECTS OF THYROID HORMONES

The precise primary mechanism and sites of action of thyroid hormones are not yet known. There is a latent period of many hours between the administration of thyroid hormones and any measurable effect even when very large doses are given. The 'uncoupling' of oxidative phosphorylation which can be demonstrated under the influence of high concentrations of thyroxine is most likely to be related to a general demand for readily available energy consequent upon stimulation of synthetic functions of the cell. Most of the experiments upon which the older hypothesis depended involved doses far above the physiological range.

In physiological concentrations the thyroid hormones are anabolic and failure of growth is one of the most striking effects of removal or destruction of the thyroid in young animals. In some amphibia metamorphosis cannot occur in the absence of thyroid hormones.

In adult animals thyroidectomy is followed by a dramatic fall in heat production. Approximately 40 per cent of an animal's heat production is under thyroid control and its caloric output, therefore, falls by this amount after thyroidectomy. Accompanying this decline in heat production there is a parallel decrease in oxygen consumption and carbon dioxide output.

The changes induced by thyroidectomy can all be reversed by thyroxine or tri-iodothyronine. If these hormones are given in greater than physiological doses the metabolic rate of all tissues is increased and with this goes a parallel increase in general activity and respiration and pulse rate. The increased caloric output is partially compensated for by an increased food intake, but if the dose is sufficiently high this compensation is inadequate and weight loss results. The qualitative effects of thyroxine and tri-iodothyronine are indistinguishable; the latter compound acts much more rapidly because it is less firmly bound to plasma proteins, in mammals, and when compared on a weight for weight basis is 3–5 times more potent. In birds, which lack a specific thyroxine-binding plasma protein, thyroxine and tri-iodothyronine are equally potent.

Disordered function

HYPOTHYROIDISM

Clinically hypothyroidism is seen either as a consequence of a pituitary lesion or, more commonly, because of defective function of the thyroid itself. The thyroid lesion may be of various types: *congenital* deficiency of enzymes (sporadic goitrous cretinism); *embryological* failure of thyroid development; *biochemical* (as a result of iodine deficiency or ingestion of anti-thyroid substances); *immunological* (associated with formation of auto-antibodies against thyroglobulin or some other constituent of the thyroid—see p. 290); *surgical* (removal of an excessive amount of thyroid tissue at partial thyroidectomy); *post irradiation* thyroid failure (after treatment with X-rays or radioiodine). If the pituitary is functioning normally, it reacts to hypothyroidism by secreting abnormally large quantities of TSH which will cause thyroid enlargement if the gland is capable of growth. This occurs in genetically determined goitrous cretinism and in goitre due to iodine deficiency or the ingestion of anti-thyroid substances. Thyroid enlargement is also a feature of some cases of lymphadenoid goitre associated with auto-immunization (Hashimoto's disease). In the remaining groups the lesion is destructive so that the thyroid cannot respond by enlargement.

Hypothyroidism also results when the pituitary fails to produce TSH. If the other trophic hormones are also absent the clinical picture is complicated by hypogonadism and hypoadrenalism. In the absence of TSH the thyroid shrinks but does not atrophy completely. Residual function persists at a very low level and the amounts of thyroid hormones produced are insufficient for normal requirements.

Compensated hypothyroidism

Any thyroid lesion capable of causing complete failure may also occur in an incomplete form. Under these circumstances, if there is enough thyroid tissue capable of increased function under the influence of TSH, the compensatory process operated through the 'feed back' mechanism will sometimes be completely successful in restoring the deficiency. In that event there are no signs of thyroid deficiency but the thyroid is enlarged so that a goitre is said to be present. This occurs in areas of iodine deficiency where most of the inhabitants may be euthyroid but many have goitres as the price they pay for normal levels of thyroid hormone production.

EFFECTS OF HYPOTHYROIDISM

In the adult

The physiological changes are considered here: the clinical manifestations, some of which cannot be fully explained, are listed on page 566.

General metabolic effects. There is a reduction in the basal metabolic rate of up to 40 per cent. Associated with this there is a general slowing down of many body processes and a tendency to gain weight which may be partly due to retention of fluid.

Cardiovascular effects. The heart rate is slowed and the cardiac output is decreased. The heart is often said to be enlarged; but this may be due to a pericardial effusion whose cause is unknown. The electrocardiogram characteristically shows low voltages and flattened or inverted T-waves.

Skin changes. The skin is thickened, dry and shows a tendency to scale. The cutaneous thickening is due to a mucinous infiltration which has histological staining characteristics due to an increased content of mucopolysaccharides; this change in its fully developed state is called 'myxoedema' and gives its name to the syndrome of severe thyroid deficiency in adults.

Neurological effects. Apart from the general slowing down of mental processes which almost invariably accompanies thyroid deficiency there may be a psychosis. The severe mental disturbances in myxoedema are not necessarily depressive or apathetic in nature and manic states are also seen.

Paraesthesiae and aches and pains which cannot be accounted for may occur anywhere and myxoedematous tissue may cause a 'carpal tunnel' syndrome. Muscle tone is increased (myxoedematous myotonia —p. 348) and is associated with delayed relaxation of tendon reflexes which can be elicited during routine physical examination. Patients with thyroid deficiency may suffer from deafness.

Hypothyroid coma. Severe untreated hypothyroidism may proceed to coma with hypothermia—a very low metabolic rate and CO_2 retention (respiratory acidosis).

In the child

'Cretinism' refers to hypothyroidism present from birth; 'juvenile myxoedema' describes hypothyroidism developing in a previously healthy child. The chief effects are retardation of growth and mental development; there are certain other characteristics (p. 566) whose physiological explanation is uncertain.

HYPERTHYROIDISM

In most cases of hyperthyroidism, the thyroid is diffusely hyperplastic. The underlying cause of this condition is unknown. In recent years there has accumulated a convincing body of evidence which suggests that the increased thyroid activity is associated with the presence of an abnormal thyroid stimulator in the circulating blood. Because of its prolonged time course of action in assay animals this material is known as the 'long-acting thyroid stimulator', abbreviated as LATS.

LATS is recovered with gamma-globulins and has not been separated from this fraction of serum proteins by techniques originally developed in the study of antibody structure. Chemical fractionation shows that the thyroid stimulating activity of LATS resides within the same region of the gamma-globulin molecule as antigen binding sites in antibodies. There is thus much speculation at the present time about the possibility that LATS is a thyroid auto-antibody. There can now be little doubt that LATS is the ultimate cause for the increased thyroid activity of thyrotoxicosis but its site of origin and the mechanism of its formation remain uncertain. Furthermore, there is no convincing precedent for stimulation of any tissue by an antibody.

Exophthalmos

Patients with hyperthyroidism often (but not invariably) show a number of eye signs of which the best known is exophthalmos, or protrusion of the eye from the orbit. This may be associated with weakness of the muscles which move the eyeball (ophthalmoplegia) and spasm of the levator palpabrae superioris muscle (lid retraction and lid lag). The periorbital tissues may be greatly swollen and oedematous.

The cause of the eye signs associated with thyrotoxicosis is not known but it is clearly not a direct result of the increased production of thyroid hormones.

Although most commonly the eye signs and hyperthyroidism develop concomitantly this is not invariably so. Thus, the eye changes may present in euthyroid subjects who never subsequently develop hyperthyroidism; more commonly thyroid overactivity will occur subsequently. Sometimes the episode of thyroid overactivity has responded satisfactorily to treatment and thereafter eye signs develop or they may appear during the recovery phase. These latter two sequences have led some physicians to consider that treatment of thyroid overactivity will invariably be followed by deterioration in any associated eye signs. This is not necessarily so; indeed, control of thyroid overactivity probably offers the best chance of amelioration of the associated eye involvement.

There is no clear and consistent relationship between the serum level of LATS and the severity of the associated eye signs in thyrotoxicosis. The blood of patients with these eye signs has been shown to contain a factor which causes exophthalmos in fish. A similar effect in fish can be seen after the injection of certain pituitary extracts. The relationship between this factor and pituitary TSH is not clear but it cannot be the same as LATS which is not found in pituitary extracts.

'Solitary toxic adenoma'
Hyperthyroidism may sometimes result from overactivity of a localized part of the thyroid seen pathologically as a discrete encapsulated nodule in a gland which is otherwise inactive. Exophthalmos does not occur in such cases and the lesion is usually regarded as a benign new growth.

Thyroid addiction
Finally hyperthyroidism can be produced by an excessive intake of thyroid hormones. There are a few individuals who appear to relish the sensation of hyperthyroidism and become 'thyroid addicts'. In such cases (which are very rare) the thyroid is not enlarged and there are no abnormal changes in the eyes.

EFFECTS OF HYPERTHYROIDISM
Specifically clinical manifestations are summarized on p. 566.

General metabolic effects. There is an increase in the metabolic rate which may be as great as 80 per cent. Associated with this there is an increase in rate of many body processes and weight loss is very common. Severe cases, particularly following exposure to the stress of an acute infection or surgical operation, may develop a 'thyrotoxic crisis', with extreme tachycardia, hyperpyrexia and collapse. The condition may be fatal unless rapidly treated.

Cardiovascular effects. There is an increase in heart rate and cardiac output. Thyroid hormones may induce atrial fibrillation, or occasionally flutter, especially in older patients. Heart failure may ensue in severe cases. These symptoms are related to increased sensitivity to sympathetic nervous activity and to circulating adrenaline and can be largely reversed by treatment with adrenergic blocking agents.

Neurological effects. Normal variations in mood are exaggerated and many patients confess to increased nervousness and irritability. In a severe case there may be mania. Tremor is frequently present and is best demonstrated by observing the outstretched fingers. The mechanism for tremor is not understood.

Thyrotoxic myopathy is discussed on p. 346. Lid retraction is at least partly caused by the direct action of thyroid hormones on the levator palpebrae superioris.

SIMPLE GOITRE

In this condition the thyroid is enlarged, but the output of thyroid hormones is normal. There are, therefore, no other consequences remote from the thyroid although when the enlargement is very great mechanical effects such as tracheal obstruction or displacement may cause respiratory distress.

IMMUNOLOGICAL REACTIONS OF THE THYROID

It is now well established that auto-antibodies can be formed against normal constituents of the thyroid both in man and in rabbits deliberately immunized against extracts of their own thyroids. Such antibodies occur in certain thyroid diseases and high titres of antibody to thyroglobulin, for example, are frequently encountered in Hashimoto's disease. Thyroglobulin, however, is not the only intrathyroidal component which may be antigenic as auto-antibodies also exist to an antigenic component within thyroidal microsomes.

The mechanism whereby these antigens are 'exposed' and whether auto-antibodies are the direct cause of thyroid diseases or merely an accompaniment remains uncertain. There is a relationship between the presence of thyroid auto-antibodies and the extent to which the thyroid shows infiltration with plasma cells and lymphocytes.

Principles of tests and measurements

There are several different methods of assessing the functional state of the thyroid gland. Radioactive isotopes of iodine are now readily available everywhere and afford a simple means of making direct observations on the state of thyroidal iodine turnover. Such tests, however, may be difficult to interpret in iodine deficiency or after the prolonged administration of excess iodine or certain antithyroid drugs.

Alternatively, chemical techniques enable the stable iodine in blood to be determined with precision and the protein bound fraction is usually a valid measure of the level of thyroid hormone in the circulation (see p. 562).

Finally, estimations of the basal metabolic rate reflect the effects of thyroid hormones on tissues generally.

Although these widely differing methods for assessing thyroid function usually give concordant results there are occasionally apparent discrepancies which require experienced interpretation. For example, in iodine deficiency states or after removal of the greater part of the thyroid the turnover rate of a dose of radioactive tracer iodine may be very rapid but the absolute production of thyroid hormones lies within the normal range.

RADIOIODINE TRACER TESTS

As in other similar tracer studies, the principle upon which these tests depend is that radioactive isotopes of iodine are handled by the body in exactly the same manner as the stable, naturally occurring isotope ^{127}I; but their radioactivity enables us to follow their movement without difficulty and to measure the concentrations in the thyroid and various body fluids.

Although a number of radioactive isotopes of iodine have been produced the only ones of clinical interest are ^{131}I, with a half-life of 8 days and ^{132}I, with a half-life of 2·3 hr. In most centres conducting tracer tests these isotopes are administered orally to fasting subjects.

Because of the short physical half-life of ^{132}I, the radiation received by the thyroid is only about 1/50 that from a similar dose of ^{131}I. With tracer doses of ^{132}I (5–40 μc) the radiation hazards are negligible so that ^{132}I is preferred for tracer studies in young patients. However, the much shorter half-life limits the duration of thyroid uptake studies with ^{132}I to approximately 2 hr. Useful serum measurements of the rate at which the isotope becomes protein bound are not possible. For this reason, many still prefer a longer period of study with ^{131}I with which studies of urinary excretion and thyroidal uptake may be combined with protein bound ^{131}I measurements to give a much more complete record of the way in which the thyroid gland utilizes iodine. Tracer doses of ^{131}I are not given in pregnancy.

Factors influencing radioiodine distribution

The most fundamental measurement that may be made with radioactive iodine is the thyroid clearance rate; that is, the volume of blood cleared of iodide by the thyroid in unit time. This may be measured by timed serial records of the counting rate over the thyroid to calculate what proportion of the dose administered has entered the thyroid per minute; this figure is then divided by the mean concentration of radioiodine/ml of plasma over the same period. This gives the thyroid clearance in ml of plasma cleared per minute; the average normal value is 17 ml/min. By similar means the renal clearance rate for iodide can be obtained; normal values are about 34 ml/min or twice the normal thyroid clearance rate. For practical purposes a dose of labelled iodide is removed from the circulation by thyroidal uptake or renal excretion; losses through skin, lungs or alimentary tract are all negligible.

Thus, in complete anuria the thyroid eventually accumulates 100 per cent of administered radioiodine; in complete hypothyroidism 100 per cent of the dose is excreted in the urine. In practice when patients suspected of thyroid disease are investigated, the assumption is made that they have a normal renal clearance for iodide.

Uptake measurement

In normal subjects the curve of thyroidal uptake of radioiodine rises steeply at first and gradually flattens out to a plateau after about 24 hr. Thereafter the concentration of radioiodine in the thyroid declines very slowly because a substantial proportion of the radioactive isotope, released from the gland after incorporation into fully formed hormones, is re-utilized following the peripheral breakdown of thyroxine and tri-iodothyronine.

In hyperthyroidism both the rate of rise and the rate of fall of this curve are greater so that there is typically a clear peak on the thyroid uptake curve which may be very sharp and occur as early as 4–6 hr. These changes reflect the more rapid uptake of iodide by the thyroid and the greatly increased output of hormonal iodine.

Serum protein-bound [131]I

Measurements of thyroid uptake may be combined with another type of procedure which measures the rate at which labelled iodine passes through the thyroid and emerges in the hormones. This is usually done by measuring the proportion of the plasma radioactivity which is bound to protein in a blood sample within 48 hr after an oral dose of [131]I. The result is expressed as protein bound ^{131}I per cent of administered dose per litre (PB[131]I per cent dose/l.) and gives excellent discrimination between normal and thyrotoxic subjects. It is not satisfactory in detecting thyroid deficiency and may be abnormally high when the metabolic pool of iodine is diminished (see p. 559). With modern counting equipment measurements of PB[131]I may be combined with thyroid uptake studies using doses as low as 10 μc.

It is obvious that ^{131}I tracer tests which include uptake measurements in the first few hours after giving radioiodine as well as at later times up to 48 hr and PB[131]I levels will give more complete, and clinically more useful, information than single early observations of radioiodine uptake. Nevertheless, using the isotope [132]I in this way reasonably satisfactory differentiation between patients with thyrotoxicosis and normal subjects can be achieved and some centres use this method exclusively.

Factors influencing radioiodine studies
It is generally agreed, however, that there may be great difficulties in interpreting tests solely based on uptake measurements in simple goitre in which uptake in the thyroid is increased but the PB[131]I is usually not elevated to the range found in thyrotoxicosis.

In interpreting tracer studies care must be exercised to make sure the patient has not been taking drugs which may modify the results. The list of drugs which may do this is long; apart from obvious culprits like excess iodides (present in many cough medicines), antithyroid drugs and thyroxine, it also includes agents such as phenylbutazone, iodopyrine, resorcinol and para-amino salicylic acid which all possess weak antithyroid effects. Iodine containing opaque media used for radiology can also seriously interfere with these tests which should not be performed within 3 months of cholecystography and up to 2 years after bronchography. The tests are permanently invalidated by myelography.

Neither abnormally low levels of uptake nor abnormally low PB[131]I levels are easily measured with precision. For the diagnosis of thyroid deficiency the pattern of radioiodine excretion by the kidneys is more useful; by appropriate timing of urine collections it is possible to detect the characteristically high excretion rates especially in the early period after the administration of radioiodine which reflects the failure of normal thyroidal uptake. This type of study is liable to great errors as a result of incomplete urine collections or imperfect timing. Not all patients may be able to comprehend the importance of following instructions regarding urine collections carefully and supervision in hospital may be necessary to obtain satisfactory results.

'Scintiscanning' of the thyroid
In addition to its use in determining the state of thyroid function, ^{131}I is also useful in localizing the site of iodine concentration anatomically. Studies of this type require a highly collimated scintillation counter and are made 48 hr after a dose of [131]I. Lingual or intra-thoracic thyroid tissue may be located and nodules of hyper-functioning tissue detected

within a normally placed thyroid. This technique may also be used to establish that areas of the thyroid are not functioning and, in highly differentiated malignant thyroid tumours, may show function in remote secondary deposits.

^{131}I-labelled tri-iodothyronine ('T3') 'uptake' tests

Thyroxine and tri-iodothyronine can both be bound to specific sites on thyroxine binding protein but the affinity for thyroxine is much greater. Thus, the ability of serum to bind ^{131}I-labelled tri-iodothyronine reflects the number of unoccupied binding sites on the carrier protein. Serum, ^{131}I-tri-iodothyronine and resin (capable of taking up ^{131}I-tri-iodothyronine not bound to serum) are incubated under rigidly controlled conditions. The resin, which may be incorporated into a sponge, is then separated and the distribution of ^{131}I-tri-iodothyronine between it and the serum is measured. In hyperthyroidism the number of unoccupied serum binding sites is low so that resin uptake is high. Conversely, in hypothyroidism the uptake by the resin is diminished.

This test has the great advantage of being carried out solely on serum. No exposure of the patient to radioactive materials is involved and the sample can be sent by post to suitably equipped laboratories. Further experience will be required before its final role in the diagnosis of thyroid disorders is established.

CHEMICAL MEASUREMENT OF CIRCULATING THYROID
HORMONES

Although direct chemical estimation of thyroxine and tri-iodothyronine in blood is not practicable except as a research procedure, it is possible to measure the amount of protein bound iodine which comes to much the same thing. Very sensitive methods are available for the estimation of iodine by its catalytic effect on the reduction of ceric sulphate by arsenite. The difficulties encountered are mostly in eliminating contamination of reagents and glassware with extraneous iodine.

An essential preliminary is the separation of iodides from the organic iodine of plasma, which is assumed to be thyroxine and tri-iodothyronine, bound to carrier proteins. This is usually effected by precipitation of the proteins followed by an ashing procedure under carefully controlled conditions. An alternative is to extract thyroxine and tri-iodothyronine with butanol, which is afterwards washed with alkali to remove iodides. This procedure adds to the time and labour of the estimation, but effects a more complete separation of hormonal iodine in the presence of high plasma iodide levels.

Radiological contrast media interfere with measurements of protein bound or butanol extractable plasma iodine just as they do in radio-iodine tracer tests. There are also certain diseases, for example the nephrotic syndrome, in which the protein bound iodine is lowered because of a lack of thyroxine binding globulin. Conversely, in pregnancy and in women taking oestrogens, e.g. in the form of contraceptive pills, the protein bound iodine rises into the range otherwise diagnostic of thyrotoxicosis because of an increase in the available protein binding sites for thyroxine. There may also be corresponding paradoxical changes in the ^{131}I-labelled tri-iodothyronine uptake tests so that complete knowledge of a patient is needed to interpret the results of thyroid investigations which may be outside the normal ranges for reasons other than disturbed thyroid function.

In most laboratories the normal range of serum or plasma protein bound iodine is 3·5–8·0 μg/100 ml. Butanol-extractable iodine is approximately 0·5 μg/100 ml less.

BASAL METABOLIC RATE (BMR)

This old-established method of assessing thyroid function has not been entirely displaced by more recent techniques. The BMR remains the only means of measuring the effects of thyroid hormones upon the body as a whole. Essentially, this is a measurement of the heat output of a fasting subject at complete rest (p. 489). In practice, what is measured is the oxygen consumption or carbon-dioxide output, or both together. Theoretically, both these measurements should be made, so that the subject's respiratory quotient can be calculated. However, it is so much simpler to measure oxygen consumption alone in a closed circuit machine with a carbon-dioxide absorber, that this is what is done in routine practice. The test is done after an overnight fast and at least 1 hour's complete rest. An airtight connection is made between the patient's mouth and the bell of the spirometer which contains oxygen, the subject's nose being occluded by a clip. The rate of descent of the spirometer bell is recorded directly, and is a measure of the rate at which oxygen is being consumed. After correction for temperature and barometric pressure this figure is divided by the oxygen consumption to be expected from the average normal subject of the same age, sex, height and weight. These average normal figures are obtained from tables; in this country those prepared by Robertson & Reid (1952) should be used. The result is conventionally expressed as a percentage of average normal.

There are so many potential sources of error in this procedure that it

19

is remarkable that it works as well as it does. The main ones are: incomplete absorption of CO_2 (soda-lime used up); leaks in the connections between subject and apparatus; inapplicability of the normal standards because of gross deviations of the subject's body proportions; apprehension on the part of the subject, resulting in tense muscles, so that he is not in a truly 'basal' state. The last is probably the most frequent source of error, but can be overcome by the tact of the operator and by repetition of the test on successive days until a stable result is obtained. In some clinics the test is done with the patient asleep after administration of a barbiturate, in order to eliminate nervous tension.

In normal subjects the results usually fall within ± 15 per cent of those expected from the tables. Results greater than + 15 per cent can be taken as indicating hyperthyroidism provided certain other disease states can be excluded (e.g. fever, heart failure, leukaemia, polycythaemia). Results below— 15 per cent indicate hypothyroidism in the absence of gross malnutrition or adrenal cortical deficiency. The theoretical basis of the test is discussed more fully on p. 489.

'DELAYED-RELAXATION' OF TENDON REFLEXES

Thyroid deficiency has a characteristic effect on the time course of muscular relaxation after the induction of a stretch reflex. This is manifested by a delay in the relaxation phase and is not the consequence of any change in the conduction of nervous impulses.

There are several relatively simple devices which record the duration of the contraction and relaxation phases of the ankle jerk which may be conveniently followed in the movement of the foot. The most usual measurement for differentiating patients with thyroid disturbances from normal subjects is the 'time to half relaxation' which is prolonged in thyroid deficiency and shortened in hyperthyroidism. The test is simple to perform, gives an immediate result and the patient is not subjected to any inconvenience or discomfort. The relaxation time is, of course, also altered in primary muscular disorders and many other diseases so that it cannot be used as the sole basis for confirming the diagnosis of a thyroid disorder. It may, however, be a most useful screening procedure as the changes in thyroid disorders are remarkably consistent and revert to normal after appropriate treatment.

BLOOD CHOLESTEROL

In hypothyroid animals the production and excretion of cholesterol are both decreased, but since the latter is reduced to a greater extent than the former the net result is an increase in blood cholesterol level. In hyperthyroid animals the reverse occurs and blood cholesterol falls. Similar changes occur in patients with hypo- and hyperthyroidism. The elevation of plasma cholesterol in hypothyroidism is usually above the upper limit of normal (approximately 300 mg/100 ml) and is a fairly constant phenomenon. Exceptions occur when the disease is exceptionally advanced (myxoedema coma) probably because malnutrition is also present, and in young children the increase may not be found. In hypothyroidism secondary to a pituitary lesion the rise in blood cholesterol, though it may occur, is less constant. Hypercholesterolaemia is also encountered in other diseases, such as obstructive jaundice, diabetes mellitus and nephrotic syndrome; it also occurs as an inherited trait associated with premature excessive atheroma.

In a group of hyperthyroid patients it is easy to demonstrate that the mean blood cholesterol concentration is less than normal. Most of the values, however, lie in the lower part of the normal range so that the estimation of serum cholesterol has little practical value in supporting a diagnosis of hyperthyroidism.

OTHER TESTS

The output of creatine in the urine is decreased in hypothyroidism and increased in hyperthyroidism. Many other conditions (e.g. muscular dystrophies) also cause excessive creatinuria (see p. 349) so that this cannot be used as a test for hyperthyroidism.

Radiology is useful in assessing the mechanical effects of goitres. For example X-ray pictures of the thoracic inlet will show the extent to which the trachea is deviated from its normal course and compressed by thyroid enlargement. Similar information for the oesophagus can be obtained on barium swallow.

Estimation of skeletal age by X-ray pictures of appropriate joints provides a good index of the state of thyroid function in childhood in that 'bone age' lags behind chronological age when hypothyroidism is present during childhood.

The diagnostic use of drugs

Drugs can usefully be employed in combination with radioiodine tests. TSH preparations of bovine origin are principally of use in distinguishing between diminished thyroid function due to primary disease of the thyroid and thyroid failure secondary to pituitary disease. Both conditions are associated with a low uptake of radioiodine. In the first case uptake will not be increased by an injection of TSH; in the second the uptake will increase. In some cases of hypopituitarism a single injection of 10 units of TSH will restore uptake to normal although others require up to 4 repeated doses to achieve this.

Thyroxine and tri-iodothyronine are also useful in differentiating cases of simple goitre, which frequently have a high uptake of radio-iodine, from true cases of hyperthyroidism. A brief course of treatment with either hormone (e.g. 120 μg of tri-iodothyronine for 8 days) is sufficient to suppress the uptake of radioiodine by a person with normal thyroid function or with a simple goitre. In hyperthyroidism uptake is virtually unaffected by this treatment. The distinction is almost certainly related to the failure of the normal feed back control of the thyroid which occurs in hyperthyroidism where LATS is probably responsible for the excessive thyroid function (see p. 556).

Practical assessment

Clinical observations
Hypothyroidism in adults. Main difficulties are insidious onset and lack of specific manifestations. Question relatives and ask for old photographs.

Slowing down mentally and physically; dislike of cold; gain in weight; constipation; vague aches and pains; paraesthesiae; puffiness of face; localized swellings around eyes and lips; loss of hair; hoarseness of voice; dry, coarse and cold skin particularly in older subjects; slow heart rate; heart sounds quiet; deafness; tendon jerks relax slowly; psychosis of no characteristic type; coma with hypothermia.

Presence of goitre suggests drugs (phenylbutazone, para-amino salicylic acid, resorcinol) or Hashimoto's thyroiditis (p. 554).

Hypogonadism or hypoadrenalism suggest pituitary failure.

Hypothyroidism in children. Failure of mental and physical development; large tongue; distended abdomen with umbilical hernia; retarded bone age. Goitrous cretinism may indicate congenital enzyme deficiency (p. 554).

Hyperthyroidism. Goitre usually diffuse, may be nodular; occasionally inconspicuous; very rarely solitary hyperactive nodule.

General metabolic effects; loss of weight; increased appetite especially in younger subjects; feels hot and sweaty; warm moist skin.

Other local manifestations probably due to general metabolic effects; tremor; weakness and wasting; diarrhoea; emotional lability; psychosis without characteristic features.

Circulatory effects, often predominant in older patients; palpitations; tachycardia; elevated sleeping pulse rate; atrial fibrillation; wide pulse pressure; heart failure; rarely oedema without heart failure.

Eye manifestations; lid retraction; exophthalmos; ophthalmoplegia (diplopia or squint); periorbital oedema; oedema of conjunctivae.

Routine methods

Laboratory confirmation always advisable lest diagnosis later doubted and treatment interrupted.

Hypothyroidism: PBI (p. 562); Cholesterol (p. 564); BMR (p. 563); relaxation time of tendon jerks (p. 564); ECG; Urinary excretion pattern of ^{131}I; immunological evidence; ESR; serum floculation tests and electrophoresis; specific antibodies (p. 290); radiological estimation of 'bone age'.

Hyperthyroidism: PBI; radioiodine uptake; PB^{131}I; BMR; scintiscan for local nodule (p. 561).

Special techniques

Needle biopsy for histology in lymphadenoid change or for chromatography after radioiodine.

Perchlorate after radioiodine to test for protein binding (p. 551); labelled 'T$_3$' resin uptake tests; TSH or LATS assay; measurement of circulating thyroxine by saturation analysis.

References

General

The Thyroid: a Fundamental and Clinical Text: 2nd Edition. Ed. WERNER S.C. (1962). London: Cassell.

PITT-RIVERS R. & TATA J.R. (1959) *The Thyroid Hormones.* London: Pergamon.

WAYNE E.J., KOUTRAS D.A. & ALEXANDER W.D. (1964) *Clinical Aspects of Iodine Metabolism.* Oxford: Blackwell.

The Thyroid Gland, Vol. 1 and 2. Ed. PITT-RIVERS R. & TROTTER W.R. (1964). London: Butterworths.

MEANS J.H., DeGROOT L.J. & STANBURY J.B. (1963) *The Thyroid and its Diseases.* New York. McGraw-Hill Book Company.

TROTTER W.R. (1962) *Disease of the Thyroid.* Oxford: Blackwell.

Other selected references

RIGGS D.S. (1952) Quantitative aspects of iodine metabolism in man. *Pharmacol. Rev.,* 4, 284–370.

ROBERTSON J.D. & REID D.D. (1952) Standards for the basal metabolism of normal people in Britain. *Lancet* i, 940–3.

MALOOF F. & SOODAK M. (1963) Intermediary metabolism of thyroid tissue and the action of drugs. *Pharmacol. Rev.* 15, 43–97.

17

Genetics

Normal function

UNITS OF INHERITANCE

The transmission of discrete traits from each parent is termed *segregation*. Each discrete unit of transmission is termed a *gene* and each inherited character is determined by the actions of two genes, one from each parent.

The genes are located on the chromosomes in the nucleus of the cell. In man there are 46 chromosomes, comprising two sex chromosomes (XX in the female and XY in the male) and 22 pairs of like chromosomes known as *autosomes* (Fig. 48).

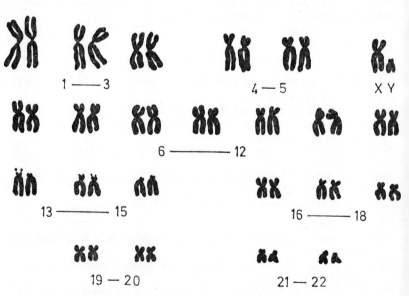

FIGURE 48. *Chromosomes from a normal male.*

The 22 autosomal pairs can be considered in groups according to size and position of the *centromere* joining the two arms. The acrocentric chromosome pairs numbered 13, 14, 15 and 21, 22 have the centromere near one end and carry small *satellites* on fine stalks on their short arms, which are involved in the organization of the nucleolus. Those with the centromere at the middle of the chromosome or off-centred are termed metacentric or submetacentric. Normal variations in arm length, centromere position and size of satellite are commonly seen for several of the chromosomes, especially the acrocentrics, the Y and number 16.

Between cell divisions the individual chromosomes are very thin and long and cannot be distinguished microscopically. With the onset of somatic cell division or *mitosis* each chromosome contracts, becomes thicker, and splits along its length to form a pair of *chromatids*, joined only at the centromere (Fig. 53 (a)). When the spindle is formed the chromosomes line up on the metaphase plate and then split through the centromere and the two daughter chromatids of each chromosome separate and migrate to opposite poles of the spindle. Each daughter cell is left with exactly the same number of chromosomes as the parent cell and each carries exactly the same genes.

In the gonads the spermatogonia and oogonia undergo a different type of division, known as *meiosis* to form the germ cells. This consists of two divisions, a first or *reduction division* in which the total number of chromosomes is halved and a second division similar to a somatic mitosis. The reduction division differs from mitosis in that when the chromosomes line up on the metaphase plate the like, or *homologous*, chromosomes come together in pairs and exchange segments of their material, crossing-over, and then instead of splitting at the centromere the whole chromosomes of each pair migrate in opposite directions. As a result the daughter cells contain only 23 chromosomes each instead of the somatic number of 46. These 23 in the case of ova will consist of 22 different autosomes and one X-chromosome and in the case of spermatozoa of 22 different autosomes and either an X or a Y chromosome. The genes determining a particular trait and carried at corresponding positions or *loci* on the two chromosomes of each homologous pair are not necessarily identical and each pair of chromosomes can exchange genes at crossing-over. Hence the possible variations in the precise genetic constitution of the germ cells of a single individual are enormous.

Knowledge of the mechanisms of cell division derives from cytological studies. The genes carried on individual chromosomes and their linear sequence have been determined in certain plants and animals, such as the fruit fly Drosophila, by observations on the way in which the characters determined by the genes segregate during breeding experiments. These classical observations can now be fitted into the more recent knowledge of the biochemical nature of this genetic material. According to the Watson-Crick model the nuclear protein *deoxyribonucleic acid* (DNA) consists of a double spiral each helix of which consists of a backbone of repeating deoxyribose-phosphate molecules. Attached to each sugar moiety is one of four nucleic acid bases: adenine, guanine, cytosine or thymine. The two helices of the spiral are held together by hydrogen bonds linking their bases. Since adenine is always linked to thymine, and vice versa, and guanine to cytosine, and vice versa, the two helices are complementary. Before cell division the two DNA strands separate and a fresh complementary strand is synthesized on each of the two original strands. This provides a mechanism for the replication of the DNA with an exact reproduction of the original sequence of nucleic acid bases and is the biochemical counterpart of the chromosomal division that follows it.

The replication of DNA can be studied by growing cells in a medium containing tritiated thymidine, which is incorporated into thymine. It is found that replication of the DNA of any one chromosome starts at different points at slightly staggered time intervals and that different chromosomes replicate at different times within the whole synthetic period. In particular in cells from normal female subjects one of the two X-chromosomes always replicates much later than all the other chromosomes. It is this late replicating X-chromosome that subsequently

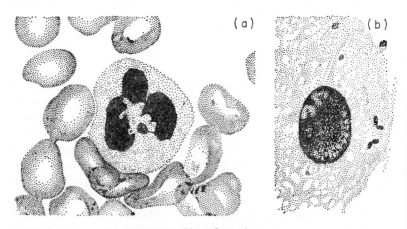

FIGURE 49. *Normal sex chromatin:*
(a) Drumstick in neutrophil, (b) Sex chromatin in buccal epethelial cell.

chain of DNA coiled back on itself to give a basic strand of 60 Å width and this strand is itself probably rather irregularly coiled or folded to give the 200 Å wide resting chromosome. Even if this interpretation is correct it still remains to be seen precisely how DNA replication and chromosome splitting take place within this structure. Autoradiographic studies suggest that replication starts at several different points along the DNA chain rather than at one end.

MODES OF INHERITANCE

The two genes at the same locus on homologous chromosomes are termed alleles. If they are identical the individual is *homozygous* for the gene concerned but if they differ he is *heterozygous*. If a gene is present on the X chromosome in the male but not on the Y he is said to be *hemizygous*.

For most known loci in man there are from one to three or four alleles of relatively frequent occurrence and a larger number of rare alleles. Two genes present at a given locus constitute the *genotype* for that locus and the number of possible genotypes depends on the number of alleles (N). It is given by the formula $(N+N^2)/2$, which for two alleles gives three genotypes, for three gives six, and for four gives ten genotypes.

Alleles and genotypes in man have been most extensively studied for the genes determining blood groups and those for certain serum or red cell enzymes and proteins. For a high proportion of such systems studied multiple alleles have been found, a phenomenon known as *genetic polymorphism*. Obviously this phenomenon provides the basis for extensive variation of genetic origin. The major alleles within a polymorphic system arise by mutation and their frequencies in any community are determined by natural selection. Selection, acting differently from one part of the world to another, accounts for the finding of differing gene frequencies among human communities. Much research in human genetics is devoted to determining the number of allelic genes for particular traits and their frequencies in different populations.

Some characters such as stature, birth weight and intelligence do not segregate because they are the composite result of a number of different factors, each determined by independent pairs of genes whose collective effect is additive. As a result these characters show continuous variation. The inheritance of such continuously varying traits is termed *multifactorial*.

The effect of a major gene may be apparent whether it is present in single or double dose, i.e. in heterozygous or homozygous state, or it may only be apparent when it is present in the homozygous state. This difference accounts for the two common modes of inheritance of characters determined by a single gene pair, *dominant* and *recessive* inheritance. Both modes of inheritance may be illustrated by the ABO blood group system.

In this system there are three genes, A, B and O. The A and B genes determine the blood group whenever they are present, that is they are *co-dominant*. Their expression is dominant over that of the O gene which is not expressed in their presence. Individuals who have the genotypes AA or AO are group "A", those who have the genotypes BB or BO are group 'B' and those who have the genotype AB are group 'AB'. It is evident from Fig. 51 that in dominant inheritance the trait inherited, in this case the A antigen, is passed to half the offspring of a parent carrying the gene in single dose, is present equally in the two sexes and is expressed in each individual carrying the gene in each generation.

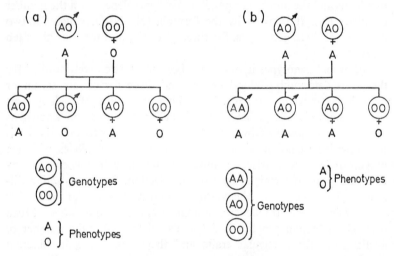

FIGURE 51. *Autosomal dominance and recessivity in the inheritance of a normal character, the ABO blood group.*

(a) Dominant inheritance of Group A, (b) Recessive inheritance of Group O.

On the other hand the inheritance of the O antigen is recessive to the A and B antigens. In recessive inheritance the trait is expressed in only 1 in 4 of the children of two heterozygous parents neither of whom shows the trait. The trait is only present in individuals inheriting the gene from both parents but one in two of the offspring will carry the gene without showing the trait but will pass it on. As with dominant inheritance the sexes are equally affected.

With a common recessive trait, like blood group O, one or even both parents may also be homozygous for the gene and show the trait, but with rare traits both parents are usually heterozygous. With rare recessive traits it is common for the parents to be related, usually as first cousins. This is because any individual has half his genes in common with his first degree relatives, a quarter in common with second degree relatives (uncles, aunts, nieces and nephews) and one eighth in common with first cousins. Thus if a man carries a rare gene and he marries his first cousin there is one chance in eight that she will also carry the gene concerned.

Dominance and recessivity are qualities not of the gene itself but of its expression. They depend on the method of observation used and are subjective rather than objective. For example, if the O antigen stimulated the production of antibody or if it were possible to recognize the actual protein determined by the ABO genes it would be possible to detect the O antigen in AO or BO individuals. The O gene would then in this sense be expressed in a dominant manner.

Sometimes the expression of a gene is influenced by environmental factors or other genes so that it is manifest in some people carrying the gene but not in others. In this situation it is said to show *incomplete penetrance*. Whether penetrance is complete or incomplete, the degree to which the gene is expressed may vary from maximal expression to a degree that is only just detectable. This sort of modified dominant inheritance merges into incomplete recessive inheritance. Another modification of the typical pattern is that in which the gene is expressed in a marked form in the homozygote and in a weak form in the heterozygote. This is called *intermediate inheritance*.

The pattern of inheritance is also modified when the locus is on a sex chromosome. Apart from genes directly involved in sex differentiation there are no known genes on the Y chromosome of man, with one possible trivial exception. Hence for practical purposes sex-linked inheritance in man is X-linked. In recessive X-linked inheritance the gene is expressed only in the hemizygous male whereas in dominant X-linked inheritance it is expressed also in the heterozygous female. A great many normal and abnormal traits are known to be X-linked (p. 592).

The expression of many characters determined by genes on autosomes is modified by the sex of the individual, or may be manifested in only one sex. These are termed *sex-influenced* or *sex-limited* conditions and are not to be confused with sex-linkage. An example of a sex-limited character is the normal baldness that develops in many men with age. Sex influence on autosomal genes has always to be taken into account in interpreting the sex ratio of any character studied.

SEX DETERMINATION (Table 17).
Sex in man is initially determined by the sex chromosomal constitution with the Y-chromosome having a strongly masculinizing effect. Since the ovum normally always has an X-chromosome it is the sperm that determines the sex of the zygote. In the absence of the Y-chromosome, differentiation is in the female direction but the presence of an extra X-chromosome does not override the male differentiation induced by a Y-chromosome. This masculinizing effect induces the medulla of the primitive gonad to develop into a testis with atrophy of the cortex. In the absence of the Y-chromosome the medulla atrophies and the cortex of the gonad develops into an ovary. If the gonad, for any reason, fails to develop, subsequent development is female regardless of genetic sex. The embryonic gonad and adrenal gland secrete sex hormones and defects of these may interfere with sexual differentiation (p. 583).

The genital duct system develops from the paramesonephric and mesonephric ducts. In the presence of a normal ovary the paramesonephric duct persists and develops into the Mullerian duct and normal female genital tract. In the absence of gonads the Mullerian duct still persists but development of the female genital tract is incomplete. If the gonads are testes the mesonephric duct persists and becomes the Wolffian duct from which the male genital tract develops. Errors can occur at any stage in the development of the Mullerian or Wolffian ducts giving rise to congenital malformations of the genital tract and are of course closely associated with urinary tract abnormalities.

TABLE 17. Determinants of sex

Sex chromosome constitution	} Genetic sex
Sex chromatin	
Gonadal sex—ovarian, testicular or both	
Hormonal sex	
Genital ducts—Mullerian or Wolffian	} Anatomical sex
Genitalia and Secondary Sex Characters	
Social and Psychological Sex—Gender role	

EVOLUTION
Although genetic aspects of evolution have been widely studied in other organisms comparatively little is known in man. There are, however, a

number of observations that can be regarded as the first few pieces of the jig-saw.

Firstly, a comparison of man and other primates such as the gorilla show a remarkable degree of overall similarity of their chromosomes but a number of differences in points of detail, which suggest that there may have been a reduction in the total chromosome number during the course of human evolution.

Secondly, differences in the amino-acid sequences of the polypeptide chains of certain protein variants such as the haemoglobins and the haptoglobins suggest that the different alleles of polymorphic systems may arise through structural rearrangements of the chromosome at the site of the locus concerned, as well as by single point mutations.

Once a new variant of a gene has arisen it would soon be eliminated by selection if its effects were entirely harmful. One way in which a gene which is deleterious in the homozygote achieves a stable frequency in a population is by conferring advantage on the heterozygote. For example, heterozygotes for sickle haemoglobin are more resistant to malaria than homozygotes for normal adult haemoglobin.

LINKAGE

In organisms with a short life span, such as the fruit fly, Drosophila, it is relatively easy to establish by planned breeding experiments which gene loci lie on a particular chromosome pair and the linear relationship of the loci to one another. In man this can only be done by studying the offspring of individuals who carry both of the genes in question.

Linkage of genes implies not that the characters determined by them are inherited in association with one another, but that the loci in question are carried on the same chromosome pair, either on the same chromosome or else one on each of the homologous pair of chromosomes. In practice, owing to the assortment arising from crossing-over, widely separated loci on the same chromosome behave like loci on different chromosome pairs and linkage can only be demonstrated when the loci are close together.

Evidence of linkage may be obtainable when families are studied in which one parent happens to carry the two genes under consideration. One of three situations may be found. The genes may be alleles in which case they must be at the same locus on two homologous chromosomes in the parent and will *segregate* in the children. They may be at different loci and either on different chromosomes or too far apart on the same chromosome to show evidence of linkage in which case they will show *independent assortment* in the children. By this is meant that any child will have equal chances of inheriting both genes, neither gene, one gene or the other gene. Thirdly the genes may be close together on either the same chromosome or on homologous chromosomes, that is to say *linked*. If the genes were on the same chromosome then they will tend to remain together, the children either inheriting both genes or neither. This situation is termed *linkage in coupling*. However owing to separation of the genes by crossing-over there will be some offspring in whom only one of the genes is inherited, termed *recombinants*. The closer the two loci are the fewer will be the number of recombinants, whereas with independent assortment the proportion of recombinants equals that of non-recombinants. If the genes were on opposite chromosomes of a pair they will tend to be inherited separately only one or other going to each child, this is *linkage in repulsion*. In this case crossing-over results in recombinants carrying either both or neither of the genes concerned, the opposite of the situation in coupling (Fig. 52).

The proportion of recombinants in either coupling or repulsion gives a quantitative estimate of the closeness of the loci concerned.

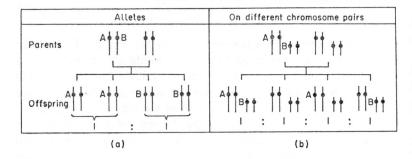

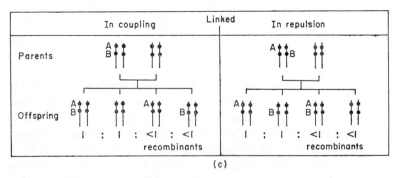

FIGURE 52. *Segration (a), independent assortment (b) and linkage (c) in gene transmission.*

By determining this estimate, the *recombination fraction*, for different pairs of loci it is possible to build up a chromosome map of loci. A start has been made on this process in man for the X-chromosome but only a few isolated instances of linkage of autosomal loci have so far been established.

Abnormal function

CHROMOSOMAL DISORDERS

Chromosome abnormalities may involve loss or increase in the number of chromosomes or alteration in the morphology of individual chromosomes. All the cells of the body may be abnormal or only a proportion of them or only the cells of a particular tissue. Abnormalities may be inherited, they may arise during gametogenesis, they may occur in the first few divisions of the zygote or they may be induced during later foetal or post-natal life.

The last mentioned group include chromosomal damage induced by radiation, chemicals, viruses or mycoplasma and aberrations observed in neoplastic tissues. They are clearly not genetic. The other classes are either clearly genetic or are possibly due to environmental influence on the very early embryo and give rise to recognizable syndromes of developmental abnormality.

Variation in total chromosome number is due to *non-disjunction* at cell division (Fig. 53 (b)). If during meiosis one pair of chromosomes fail to separate and both migrate to the same pole the resultant gametes will have either one too many, that is 24, or one too few chromosomes, that is 22. The effect is that in the subsequent zygote one chromosome pair is represented by three homologous chromosomes, *trisomy* or by only one, *monosomy*.

A similar abnormal migration can involve one of the chromatids of a chromosome following splitting of the centromere in mitosis. In this case the daughter chromatids may migrate to the same pole with a similar effect to non-disjunction in gametogenesis or one chromatid may fail to migrate and become lost to the cell.

Apart from monosomy for one of the X-chromosomes it appears that monosomic zygotes are not viable. Trisomy is occasionally due to inheritance of an extra chromosome from a trisomic parent, a phenomenon known as *secondary non-disjunction*.

Mitotic non-disjunction is associated with *mosaicism*, that is the presence of more than one cell line in the zygote. Non-disjunction at the first mitotic division in the zygote results in two cell lines, one with 47

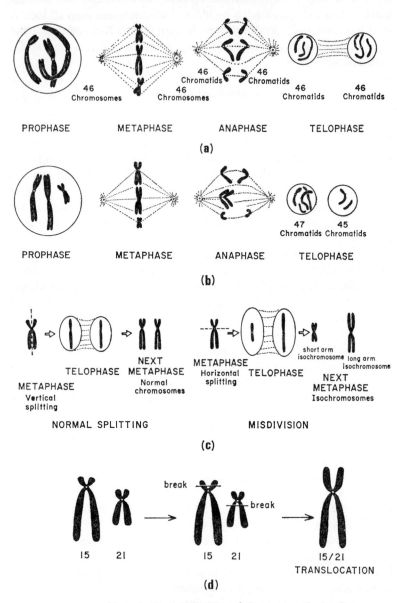

FIGURE 53. *Normal mitosis and origins of chromosome abnormality.*

(a) Normal mitosis, (b) Mitotic non-disjunction, (c) Formation of isochromosomes, (d) Formation of a translocation.

and one with 45 chromosomes. At the second division three cell lines result with 46 chromosomes in half the cells and 45 or 47 chromosomes in a quarter each. Non-disjunction at later divisions results in abnormal cell lines representing progressively smaller proportions of the total cell population so that by about the sixth or seventh division they would no longer be readily detectable.

Abnormalities of morphology arise in several ways. Breaks occurring simultaneously in two chromosomes with rejoining of part of each chromosome to a part of the other, translocation, results in two abnormal chromosomes (Fig. 53 (d)). In the commonest stable type of translocation in man, *centric fusion*, two acrocentric chromosomes are involved with the loss of one centromere and the small arms of both chromosomes.

Such a translocation is balanced in that there is no significant alteration in the total amount of chromosomal material and no clinical abnormality. If however such a translocated chromosome is transmitted to a child it may not be balanced but result in effective trisomy producing corresponding clinical abnormalities.

Horizontal splitting of the centromeres at metaphase instead of the normal vertical splitting is known as *misdivision* and results in two *isochromosomes*, one consisting of two long and the other of two short arms for the chromosomes concerned (Fig. 53 (c)).

Another fairly common abnormality is a *deletion*, loss of part of an arm of a chromosome following a break with failure to rejoin. Deletions are not infrequently associated with non-disjunctional errors. Small deletions are not detectable by cytological methods and if associated with a gene deficiency could be transmitted as an apparently dominant condition.

Inversions, especially involving the centromere, and ring chromosomes are also rarely associated with clinical abnormality. Ring chromosomes arise from breaks close to each end of the chromosome with joining of the two ends.

AUTOSOMAL ANOMALIES

The major autosomal anomalies have certain clinical features in common. In contrast to single gene defects all the tissues of the body tend to show abnormalities and these are mostly developmental defects rather than metabolic errors. Despite the fact that most of these syndromes are trisomic states with triplication of the genes of the trisomic chromosome there is no evidence that any of the clinical features are due to gene dosage effects. This may be because the genes controlling development are largely unknown or it may be that the developmental errors are due to some gross effect of the total amount of chromatin present unconnected with any specific genes. The total incidence of autosomal anomalies is about 2·5 per 1000 live births, but in addition they are found together with sex anomalies in about one fifth of all spontaneous abortions.

Down's syndrome
The commonest autosomal anomaly is Down's syndrome or mongolism which is present in about 1 in 600–700 live births. In the majority of cases there are 47 chromosomes, the extra chromosome being a small acrocentric, number 21. This is due to non-disjunction during oogenesis in the mother. In a minority of instances maternal non-disjunction may result from a predisposing gene or from a specific environmental factor but in most instances the cause is unknown although it shows a marked association with the age of the mother. The overall incidence of Down's syndrome in children born to 18 year old mothers is about 1 in 2300 while at a maternal age of 46 it is about 1 in 46.

Occasionally the mother herself is a mosaic of normal and trisomic cells. When the ovum is trisomic the fertilized zygote is also trisomic, an example of secondary non-disjunction. In about 3 per cent of cases of Down's syndrome there is the normal number of chromosomes, 46, but an abnormal translocated chromosome is present. The translocation arises by centric fusion of a number 21 with one of the group 13 to 15 with loss of the short arms of each chromosome (see Fig. 53). Alternatively there is a centric fusion of a number 21 with a 22 or another 21. Such translocations arise either *de novo* in the affected child or they may be inherited from a clinically normal parent who carries the translocation in a balanced form.

The presence of the extra chromosome 21, whether as an independent chromosome or as part of a translocated chromosome results in the familiar defects of development of the face and limbs of the mongol child and in mental retardation. There may also be developmental abnormality of the heart or of the alimentary tract. Characteristic alterations of the dermatoglyphic patterns, a distally placed axial triradius in the palm and an absence of pattern in the hallucal area of the sole, provide further examples of developmental effects.

Other autosomal trisomic syndromes
Another syndrome, with an incidence of about 1 in 1500 live births, is is characterized by a different spectrum of congenital anomalies, and by

frequent arches on the finger tips. It is associated with early death. Chromosomal analysis again shows 47 chromosomes with in this case the extra chromosome in the group 17-18. Familial translocated cases have also been described.

A third syndrome, with an incidence of less than 1 in 2000, shows yet a further set of developmental defects and a persistence of foetal haemoglobin and at birth even of embryonic haemoglobin. Most affected infants die within a few months but a few have survived several years. The dermal ridges show an even more distally placed triradius than that seen in Down's syndrome and a tendency to marked thenar patterns. Chromosomal analysis once again shows 47 chromosomes, the trisomic chromosome belonging to group 13-15. As with 21-trisomy and 17-18-trisomy, translocated cases have been reported. The persistence of foetal and embryonic haemoglobins in this syndrome is more likely to be a gene dosage effect than are the other anomalies.

Among the chromosomal abnormalities found in aborted foetuses is triplication of each chromosome pair, *triploidy*, giving 69 chromosomes. Partial triploidy in mosaic form has been reported in living subjects. Partial deletion of the short arms of a chromosome in the 4 to 5 group is found in the 'cri-du-chat' syndrome. Many other autosomal anomalies have been reported in isolated cases including other deletions and trisomies, ring chromosomes and multiple trisomies.

SEX CHROMOSOMAL ANOMALIES

Genetically determined sexual disorders can be classified into disorders of sex chromosome number and inter-sex states due to a variety of causes (see Table 18). Most, but not all, of these conditions are associated with sterility or severe infertility and account for a major proportion of all infertility, especially in the male.

Klinefelter's syndrome

This is a disorder of men characterized by small atrophic testes, azoospermia, low 17-oxosteroid excretion and raised urinary gonadotrophin. Other variable features include eunuchoidal stature, gynaecomastia and mild mental retardation. Histologically the testes show 'ghost' tubules devoid of elastic tissue. However, the Leydig cells, which secrete androgen, persist so that the secondary sexual characters are normal. There is no gross distortion of the dermal ridge patterns.

The majority of cases are chromatin positive, i.e. their cells show the presence of sex chromatin. This technique provides the only means of diagnosis at birth. The incidence of chromatin positive males is about one in 800 live births.

TABLE 18.

Genetically determined disorders of sexual development.

I Abnormalities of sex chromosome number

1 Klinefelter's Syndrome
2 Turner's Syndrome
3 Triple-X Syndrome
4 XYY Syndrome

II Inter-sex states

1 Pure Gonadal Dysgenesis
2 Testicular intersex
  a Testicular feminization
  b Other forms of testicular intersex
3 Ovarian Intersex
  a Congenital adrenal hyperplasia
  b Other forms of ovarian intersex
4 Ovo-testicular intersex

Chromatin positive cases of Klinefelter's syndrome have been found to possess 47 chromosomes with an XXY sex-chromosome constitution. It is not usually possible to tell whether the non-disjunction leading to the XXY constitution is paternal or maternal but in some instances this can be determined from the Xg blood groups of the patient's family. Such studies have revealed a maternal age effect in cases due to maternal non-disjunction, similar to that in Down's syndrome but less marked. There is also inconclusive evidence implicating parental auto-immune disease in the aetiology of sex-chromosomal non-disjunction. A minority of chromatin positive cases has been found to have a complex chromosomal constitution with more than two X-chromosomes or more than one Y-chromosome. They include XXXY and XXXXY, with cells containing two or three sex chromatin bodies respectively and showing more severe mental defects than the XXY cases; and XXYY. Others include mosaics XY/XXY, XX/XXY, XXY/XXXXY and XXY/XXXY.

There are also patients with the clinical picture of Klinefelter's syndrome who are chromatin negative and prove to have a normal male chromosomal constitution. In these cases the testicular tubules are of uniform size and are rich in elastic tissue but are devoid of germ cells. The aetiology of this group is unknown.

Turner's syndrome

This is a disorder of women; the features are primary amenorrhoea, sterility and short stature. There is an increased excretion of pituitary gonadotrophin and biopsy shows the gonads to consist of fibrous streaks lacking ovarian follicles. Included in the syndrome as originally described by Turner was neck webbing but this is not an invariable finding. Other features that may be present are an increased carrying angle at the elbow, dyplasia of nails, cardiac defects especially coarctation of the aorta and pulmonary stenosis, a low hair line on the neck, renal malformations and lymphoedema at birth. The finger tips show well developed ridge patterns and the palm a distally placed axial triradius. The subjects are of normal intelligence.

The incidence at birth is about 1 in 2500. This low incidence is at least in part, if not entirely, due to the fact that a high proportion of cases are non-viable and are lost through spontaneous abortion.

They lack sex chromatin in their cells and chromosomal analysis shows only 45 chromosomes with only one sex chromosome, an X and no Y, designated as XO. Mosaic forms are fairly common and include XO/XX, XO/XY, XO/XYY, XO/XXY and XO/XX/XXX. The XO/XY or XO/XYY cases may show masculinization and in extreme cases present as males with low stature and other stigmata of Turner's syndrome.

In a minority of cases the clinical syndrome is associated with chromatin positive cells. Some of these are XO/XX or XO/XXX mosaics. Others have one normal X-chromosome and one isochromosome for the long arms of the X, when large drumsticks are found on the neutrophils. Yet others have a deletion of the short arms of one X-chromosome with small drumsticks.

Other sex chromosomal anomalies

Another sex chromosomal anomaly is the finding of three X-chromosomes in women who may be clinically normal. In some cases there is secondary amenorrhoea or mild mental retardation. They are chromatin postive with a high total sex chromatin count and have two sex chromatin bodies in some of their cells. Patients with four X-chromosomes are infertile and severely mentally retarded. Mosaics such as XX/XXX, XO/XXX and XO/XX/XXX are also encountered.

The triple-X syndrome has a similar incidence to Klinefelter's syndrome at birth (1 in 800).

In males a double-Y syndrome has recently been described. Males who are XYY may be fertile and do not necessarily show any abnormalities. However, their average height is greater than that of the general male population. A high proportion of the taller inmates of criminal mental hospitals, especially among those patients sentenced for aggressive or violent crimes have been found to have an XYY constitution. Males who are XXYY usually present as tall Klinefelter's but may occasionally be fertile. There have not been any surveys of incidence of the YY syndrome.

A few women have been described with primary amenorrhoea, normal stature but eunuchoidal proportions and an infantile uterus. When laparotomy has been performed small fibrous ovaries with primordial follicles have been found. The cells have either no sex chromatin or small sex chromatin bodies, and chromosomal analysis reveals one normal X chromosome and one X chromosome from which the long arms have been deleted. The clinical picture is identical to that seen in 'pure gonadal dysgenesis', described below.

INTERSEX STATES

Patients with intersex states can be classified according to the type of gonad present. Patients in the first group have only fibrous streaks for gonads similar to those in Turner's syndrome, and include so called *'pure' gonadal dysgenesis*; the group of testicular intersex or male pseudohermaphroditism is a heterogeneous one having in common testes, chromatin negative cells and ambiguous external genitalia; ovarian intersex or female pseudohermaphroditism forms another mixed group in which the gonads are ovaries, chromatin is positive and the sex chromosomal constitution is XX; in the final group ovo-testicular intersex or true hermaphroditism both an ovary and a testis or else ovo-testes are found. Where gonads are present in intersex states they are liable to neoplastic change.

The aetiology of such states is very variable, some are due to chromosomal mosaicism; some to a single major gene; some to congenital malformation and others to a hormone secreting tumour in the mother or the foetus. The administration of hormone preparations to the mother can also affect the genital development of the foetus.

'Pure' gonadal dysgenesis

Patients with 'pure' gonadal dysgenesis are women with primary amenorrhoea, chromatin negative cells and streak gonads but having normal stature and no other features of Turner's syndrome. They tend to have eunuchoidal proportions and a normal vagina, with or without clitoral enlargement, and an infantile uterus and fallopian tubes. Their breasts do not enlarge normally. Urinary gonadotrophin excretion may be raised. The majority of cases have an XY sex-chromosome constitution. Another variant shows an XX chromosome constitution with chromatin positive cells. The cause of the failure of gonadal development is unknown.

Testicular intersex
The commonest form of testicular intersex is *testicular feminization*. Such patients typically have female external genitalia with a short vagina, absent or rudimentary uterus, normal breasts and little or no sexual hair. They have XY sex chromosomes. The defect is a failure of the tissues to respond to normal testicular hormones. Inheritance is probably X-linked but as the individuals do not reproduce it is not possible to exclude sex-limitation of an autosomal dominant inheritance. Some degree of masculinization is seen in incomplete forms of the disorder.

A number of chromosomal mosaics involving XY, XO and XXY cell lines may be associated with testicular intersex. Steroids received either via the placenta or post-natally by XY males may induce ambiguity of the genitalia.

Ovarian intersex
The great majority of cases of ovarian intersex are due to *congenital adrenal hyperplasia* (p. 529). This condition is due to a defect in one of several enzymes involved in the synthesis of cortisol. Lack of cortisol leads to increased secretion of pituitary corticotrophin with consequent adrenal hyperplasia and raised androgen secretion and urinary 17-oxosteroid excretion, which in the female foetus causes ambiguous development of the genitalia. Other clinical features depend on the enzyme involved, deficiency of 21-hydroxylase causes marked virilization and deficiency of 11-β hydroxylase is associated with hypertension. 3β,Δ^4 dehydrogenase is concerned in the earlier stage of conversion of Δ^5 pregnenolone to progesterone; deficiency of this enzyme produces a vary rare fatal form with severe salt depletion and adrenal hyperplasia with infiltration of the gland by cholesterol. All forms are inherited in an autosomal recessive manner.

Tumours of the adrenal cortex also produce an increase in 17-oxosteroid excretion and give rise to intersex states in the female. They may develop antenatally or postnatally. On the other hand 17-oxosteroid excretion is normal in arrhenoblastoma which, if occurring either in the infant or in the mother during pregnancy, can cause an intersex state. Both genito-urinary tract malformations and androgen administration in the female can produce ambiguity of the genitalia.

Ovo-testicular intersex
The majority of patients with ovo-testicular intersex have an XX-chromosome constitution and normal 17-oxosteroid excretion. Cases have been reported with XX/XY or XX/XXY/XXXXX mosaicism and chromatin negative cases with XO/XY and XY, the latter possibly an undetected mosaic.

GENE ABNORMALITIES
A gene producing some abnormality of structure or function may be present in an individual because it has been inherited by one of the normal mechanisms of inheritance already discussed or it may arise by fresh mutation. A gene mutation is the sudden appearance of a new and usually harmful gene and represents a change in the nucleic acid base sequence in the DNA, a 'point' mutation being a substitution of a single nucleic acid base by another base. Such a substitution in a structural gene may alter a single amino-acid in the polypeptide chain controlled by the gene and thus lead to the synthesis of an abnormal enzyme or other protein, as for example the replacement of glutamic acid by valine in the β-chain of haemoglobin S. If occurring in a regulating gene substitution may lead to a failure of protein synthesis or even to excessive synthesis.

Mutation
Harmful mutations tend to be selected against and an equilibrium between mutation rate and elimination produces a stable frequency. Genes that are wholly lethal depend entirely on mutation for their frequency, as illustrated by the gene for retinoblastoma. This condition was formerly never inherited as it was fatal before reproductive age and therefore depended entirely on fresh mutation for its occurrence. Recent advances in treatment have led to a number of affected patients giving birth to affected children. Mutation rates can be determined by direct observation in the rare circumstances of a gene regularly expressed in the heterozygote. Otherwise the mutation rate of deleterious genes has to be estimated indirectly. For this it is necessary to know the mode of inheritance, the frequency of the condition due to the gene and the relative fitness of affected persons. For recessive disorders, lethal before

reproductive age, the mutation rate per gene per generation is equal to the frequency of the disorder.

Inborn errors of metabolism

Inborn errors of metabolism are due to an abnormal gene causing a deficiency of a specific enzyme or the synthesis of an inactive enzyme with metabolic block at the step concerned:

$$A \longrightarrow B \longrightarrow C \overset{\vdots}{\longrightarrow} D$$

$$\downarrow \qquad \text{block}$$

$$\text{minor}$$

$$\text{pathway}$$

There are several possible consequences of a block. There may be effects arising from the failure to produce the final metabolite D, as in the failure to synthesize cortisol in congenital adrenal hyperplasia discussed earlier. Accumulation of the immediate precursor C may produce toxic effects, as does unconjugated bilirubin from lack of glucuronyl transferase in Crigler-Najjar syndrome (p. 442). The more remote precursors A or B may be harmful factors, as in glucose-6-phosphatase deficiency (von Gierke's disease) in which glycogen accumulates in liver cells. This illustrates another point, that the harmful effects of a metabolite are not necessarily toxic to cells other than those producing them but may arise from accumulation of the substance within the cell of origin. Finally the block may lead to increased metabolism along a normally minor pathway with accumulation of a toxic metabolite, as in phenylketonuria. There are many metabolic disorders, such as fibrocystic disease of the pancreas in which the specific enzyme defect is not known although the mode of inheritance is understood.

Most inborn errors of metabolism are inherited as autosomal recessive conditions and are due to homozygosity for a rare harmful gene. A few are sex-linked, for example, glucose-6-phosphate dehydrogenase deficiency. Probably everyone carries several harmful genes in single dose. This surprising fact becomes less surprising if one considers the application of the Hardy-Weinberg equation to rare recessive disorders. The equation states that if two alleles a and b have gene frequencies in a population of p and q respectively then, with random mating, the homozygotes *aa* will have a frequency of p^2, the homozygotes *bb* a frequency of q^2 and the heterozygotes *ab* a frequency of $2pq$. This is expressed in the quadratic equation: $p^2 + 2pq + q^2 = 1$.

Suppose a severe disorder such as phenylketonuria, has an incidence of 1 in 40 000. In the equation:

$$p^2 + 2pq + q^2 = 1.$$
$$q^2 = 1/40\ 000$$
$$q = \sqrt{1/40\ 000} = 0.005$$
$$p = 1 - q = 0.995$$

The incidence of carriers (2pq) is given by

$$2pq = 2 \times 0.995 \times 0.005$$
$$= 0.00995$$
$$\text{or} \quad 10/1000$$
$$\text{and} \quad p^2 = 0.995^2 = 0.990$$

Thus in every 1000 of the population 990 are normal homozygotes, about 10 or 1 per cent are heterozygote carriers, and only 1 in every 40 000 is an affected homozygote. This high frequency of carriers, which applies to each of the many rare recessive disorders accounts for the probability that everyone carries several potentially harmful genes. It is a matter of chance as to whether both of two parents carry any harmful genes in common. It is obvious from this that eugenic measures directed towards the homozygote hardly affect the frequency of genes determining recessive disorders. Indeed, if the homozygote cannot reproduce eugenic measures directed towards preventing mating of heterozygotes are the only ones likely to be effective.

The elucidation of the biochemical lesion in recessive metabolic disorders is of assistance to an understanding of their genetics in several ways. First, a clinically single disorder may prove biochemically to arise from several different genes either at different loci as in the group of glycogen storage diseases or alleles forming part of a polymorphic system. Secondly, a knowledge of the metabolic error involved enables diagnostic screening tests, as for phenylketonuria, to be developed which can be used in surveys to determine the incidence of the disorder and hence the gene frequency. Thirdly in some cases it proves possible to distinguish the heterozygotes from normal homozygotes by biochemical tests. This has been done most successfully in the haemoglobinopathies.

Abnormal proteins

Gene mutation may be responsible for abnormalities of proteins other than enzymes. Several anaemias are due to defects of haemoglobin or of its synthesis (p. 235) and these serve particularly well to illustrate the kinds of genetic defect giving rise to protein abnormalities. The whole range of abnormal haemoglobins in the haemoglobinopathies due to variants of the α or β chains are examples of point mutations of structural genes leading to the synthesis of an abnormal protein (p. 235). Excess production of an enzyme has been demonstrated in two instances. Recently a family was described in which the type B variant of the sex-linked enzyme glucose-6-phosphate dehydrogenase was markedly increased in the red cells. Hemizygous males showed four times the normal activity whereas affected females showed a less marked increase. This apparent sex-linkage of the increased activity suggests that it is due to a mutation within the operon, either of the structural locus or of the operator gene. In acute intermittent porphyria the concentration of δ-amino-laevulic acid synthetase in the liver is raised as a result of enzyme induction and, since the disease is inherited as a dominant, is therefore probably due to a mutation of an operator gene with loss of the normal repression of the structural locus on one chromosome.

The majority of disorders due to gene mutations are clinical syndromes in which the biochemical lesion is either incompletely known or quite unknown. They are found affecting every physiological system of the body and also causing developmental malformations. They include clotting defects and congenital haemolytic anaemias; congenital hyperbilirubinaemias; cystic fibrosis of the pancreas and polyposis coli; muscular dystrophies and many other neurological diseases; hereditary nephritis, polycystic kidneys and renal tubular defects; genetic disorders of skin and the special sense organs and a number of specific forms of mental defect and of endocrine defects.

Congenital malformations
Most of the common major congenital malformations are not due to single gene defects but do show an increased incidence in the close relatives, especially in sibs of affected persons. This indicates that they are due to a complex of environmental and genetic factors. These have been at least in part identified in congenital dislocation of the hip. This condition is predisposed to by joint laxity, which is a dominant trait, by shallow acetabula, which is multifactorially determined, and by the intrauterine posture of flexed hips and extended knees commonly seen in breech presentation. Rarely a single gene is responsible as in sex-linked hydrocephalus. Other malformations are primarily environmental in causation as in the case of those following maternal rubella or thalidomide. Altogether probably some 2–3 per cent of all live born

children suffer from major malformations and many more from minor malformations such as those of the hand, some of which are inherited.

Research on the marine alga, *Acetabularia*, and on the eggs of sea-urchins and amphibia suggests that morphogenesis depends on protein synthesis and that this in turn depends on messenger RNA. It is probable that identification of the specific morphogenetic proteins will eventually lead to an understanding of developmental anomaly comparable to our present knowledge of metabolic errors.

GENETICS OF COMMON DISEASES

The difficulties in detecting genetic factors in common diseases are due to the fact that in most diseases multiple additive rather than single genes are involved. The effects of such genes on manifestation are greatly modified by environment and indeed in many cases they only determine susceptibility and not manifestation at all. A further difficulty is that a gene of very high frequency may be more rather than less difficult to detect. For example a gene determining susceptibility to a particular disease if universally present in man can only be surmised from the fact that other species do not develop the disease. Also the high incidence of cousin marriage of the parents of persons with rare recessive disorders is no longer seen when the condition reaches an incidence of 1 in 1000 or more. Furthermore a common recessive disorder will not be limited to one generation.

Common diseases are often heterogeneous in origin and refinement of diagnosis may reveal a proportion of cases due to a rare single gene. Examples are those cases of hydrocephalus due to a sex-linked gene, of carcinoma of the colon due to polyposis coli, of epilepsy due to Huntington's chorea and of nephritis due to Alport's syndrome.

Most common diseases show some familial tendency and this if very high, say ten times the population incidence, is strongly suggestive of genetic causation. Far more often the familial increase is of a lesser degree and reflects common genetic and environmental factors. Here a detailed analysis of incidence by age, sex, and degree of relationship may provide evidence for genetic factors. Such analyses suggest that gastric and duodenal ulcer, mammary carcinoma, epilepsy, congenital pyloric stenosis and a number of fairly common congenital malformations are in part genetic and probably multifactorial.

A comparison of incidence between identical and fraternal twins of affected individuals may also provide evidence for genetic causation. High concordance for monozygotic (identical) twins has been found for schizophrenia, susceptibility to tuberculosis and for *situs inversus* or isolated dextrocardia. However, such evidence does not exclude heterogeneity of causation.

Extensive studies have been made of the incidence of different blood groups in a number of common diseases and for a few, for example duodenal ulcer and group O, a significant but weak correlation with a specific gene has been demonstrated. This suggests that the gene concerned plays a minor role in predisposing the person carrying it to the disease with which it is associated.

In many rare recessive disorders a bimodal distribution, among relatives of affected individuals, of a continuously varying aspect of the disorder has been demonstrated. Attempts have been made to find evidence for a single specific gene in common disorders, as for example in essential hypertension (p. 67). However in no instance has the bimodality found been great enough to be conclusive.

The phenomenon of balanced polymorphism, discussed under normal inheritance, in which the heterozygote carriers of a gene that is harmful in the homozygous state have a selective advantage, can lead to a recessive disorder becoming common. In certain areas of Africa sickle cell disease reaches an incidence of 7–8 per cent of all births. In Britain the commonest recessive disorder, fibrocystic disease of the pancreas, has an incidence of about 1 in 2000 live births. Assuming a fitness of zero for homozygotes this would give a mutation rate of the order of 1 in 2000, a quite unacceptably high figure. It is, therefore, very likely that in this condition too carriers will be found to have some advantage.

Genetic incompatibility between a mother and her foetus can result in the haemolytic anaemia of erythroblastosis foetalis, described on p. 233.

PHARMACOGENETICS
Several instances of genetic variation in response to drugs are known. The administration of barbiturates to patients with acute intermittent porphyria provokes or exacerbates the acute attack. In this instance the drug aggravates the symptoms of an existing genetically determined disease. Haemolytic anaemia has also been described in some of the haemoglobinopathies following administration of certain drugs.

The drug isoniazid, used in the treatment of tuberculosis, is acetylated more slowly by some patients than by others, necessitating an adjustment of the dose if side-effects are to be avoided. This difference is recessively determined and is an example of a simple genetic difference in the break-down of a drug. A dominantly determined drug resistance has been reported in one family to the anticoagulant warfarin.

Other drugs have been found to provoke abnormal reactions in patients who lack a specific enzyme but are otherwise clinically normal. Hydrolysis of the muscle relaxant suxamethonium depends on the enzyme serum cholinesterase. About 1 in 2000 people develop prolonged apnoea when given suxamethonium and these individuals have been shown to be homozygous for a gene determining the synthesis of an atypical form of cholinesterase. Another instance of this type of reaction is that found in American Negroes who have a deficiency of the red cell enzyme glucose-6-phosphate dehydrogenase. Deficient subjects develop an acute haemolytic anaemia when given the anti-malarial drug primaquine or any one of a number of other drugs including sulphonamides, certain analgesics and quinine. Owing to the risk of such reactions it will become necessary in some cases to test for the genetic abnormality concerned before administering certain drugs.

Principles of tests and measurements

SEX CHROMATIN

The role of sex chromosomes in the determination of sex is described on p. 596 and normal sex chromatin on p. 571. In the investigation of sex chromosomal disorders sex chromatin determination has two uses. First it gives an indication of the number of X-chromosomes present. Secondly it may indicate the presence of a structurally abnormal X-chromosome. It gives no information as to the number of Y-chromosomes and, therefore, does not indicate the sex of the individual.

The buccal smear is a simple test to perform and in a normal female about 30–60 per cent of squamous cell nuclei contain a single sex chromatin body. Lower percentages may be obtained in mosaic individuals or from technically poor preparations and also from patients receiving steroid or antibiotic therapy. Subjects with one X-chromosome, that is XO, XY or XYY, have no sex chromatin while those with more than two X-chromosomes tend to have high counts and also show some nuclei with more than one sex chromatin body, up to one less than the number of X-chromosomes.

A count of the proportion of neutrophil leucocytes with drumsticks provides confirmation of the findings in the buccal smear and also may indicate the presence of a structurally abnormal X-chromosome. An isochromosome for the long-arms of the X-chromosome gives unusually large drumsticks and conversely small drumsticks may be seen when there is a partial deletion of one X-chromosome. This is because whenever one of a pair or more of X-chromosomes is structurally abnormal the abnormal chromosome always forms sex chromatin.

CHROMOSOME ANALYSIS

Apart from the cytological study of malignant conditions or of cell damage by chemical, radioactive or infective agents chromosomal analysis provides information of anomaly of chromosome number, of gross structural abnormality or of mosaicism. It will not reveal small deletions such as would mimic gene mutations nor will it show inversions unless they are large pericentric inversions. However, inversions not shown by analysis of mitotic metaphases may prevent the formation of normal bivalents in meiosis and be detectable in testicular biopsy. These principles have been described on pp. 568–573 and pp. 579–581.

The method most widely used is that of lymphocyte culture from peripheral blood and recently micro methods have been developed. When blood is not obtainable or for any reason this method fails cultures of fibroblasts from small skin biopsies or from connective tissue obtained at operation may be used. This technique is essential when it is important to detect mosaicism. In leukaemia or malignant neoplasia marrow, effusions, or teased out tumour tissue can be examined directly or after a short period of incubation. It is also possible to study meiotic chromosomes from testicular biopsy in males.

In exceptional cases additional information may be provided by the technique of autoradiography using tritiated thymidine labelling of the dividing cells. For example an extra or an abnormal chromosome can be identified as an X by the fact that it takes up the label relatively late.

DERMATOGLYPHICS

The dermal ridges of the palms and finger tips carry the openings of the sweat ducts which are just visible to the naked eye. Their function is still unknown, it may help to give better friction in grip or it may be to prevent obstruction of the sweat ducts on flexion of the skin. They form parallel lines covering the surface. Where three systems of parallel lines meet, provided each of the angles between them is at least 90°, they form a central point termed a *triradius*. There are three main types of pattern that may interrupt the parallel system on the finger tips. These are the simple *arch*, the *loop* in which a ridge turns back on itself through 180° and which is always associated with one triradius and the *whorl* associated with two triradii (Fig. 54).

The ridges are formed during the third and fourth months of foetal life and follow patterns that are retained for the rest of life. The departures from simple parallel ridges to more complex patterns reflect the shape at the time the ridges are laid down, and the patterns formed cover the surface in the most economical way possible following topological principles. Quantitative studies have shown that the ridge patterns are genetically determined in a multifactorial manner.

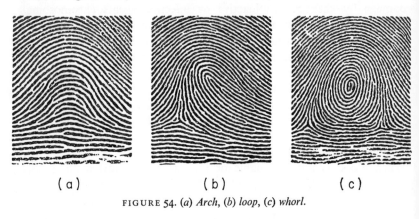

(a)　　　　　　　　(b)　　　　　　　　(c)

FIGURE 54. (*a*) *Arch*, (*b*) *loop*, (*c*) *whorl*.

The major practical application of these studies is obviously forensic but they do have clinical uses. The ridges can be observed by direct inspection in good light, with if necessary a magnifying lens. They are easily recorded by a clean method using a starch impregnated paper containing an iodide which is released by oxidizing agent wiped on the skin.

Characteristic patterns are seen in most of the established chromosomal disorders. Unusual patterns in children with retarded mental development, especially if unlike those of the parents, are suggestive of a developmental insult dating from the time the ridges are laid down. They are also of value in determining the zygosity of twins.

BIOCHEMICAL AND OTHER TESTS

Biochemical tests may be used to detect the presence of an abnormal enzyme or protein or the deficiency of a normal one ; to measure levels of metabolites that either accumulate or are deficient as a result of a metabolic block or to detect increased utilization of a minor pathway due to such a block. These principles are more fully discussed on pages 589–590. They have several applications in the assessment of genetic aspects of biochemical disorder.

On the other hand biochemical and other methods are sometimes developed in the attempt to identify clinically normal carriers of genes determining recessive disorders. For example, a phenylalanine tolerance test may reveal heterozygotes for the phenylketonuria gene and, less reliably antihaemophilic globulin assay may reveal low levels in female carriers of haemophilia.

There are also conditions in which for purposes of prognosis or genetic counselling it is necessary to carry investigation further than is needed for clinical diagnosis or management. This is well illustrated by the Hunter–Hurler syndrome in which the staining of fibroblasts, cultured from skin biopsies from the parents of affected patients, for mucopolysaccharides enables the sex-linked recessive form to be distinguished from the autosomal recessive form.

Mention has already been made of the use of tests to identify patients liable to react atypically to drugs owing to their genetic constitution (p. 593).

ASSESSMENT OF GENETIC RISK

There are three essential steps in assessing the risk of a genetic disorder recurring in a family. These are an accurate initial diagnosis; family history, and if necessary family investigation, including details of age, sex and medical history of relatives, miscarriages, consanguinity and the ante-natal and labour record of the index patient; and a knowledge either of the mode of inheritance or of the observed frequency of recurrence of the disorder in question. Such information is available in standard textbooks and original reports. Only a minority of diseases or malformations are determined by a single major gene with Mendelian inheritance. Most disorders for which genetic advice is sought are either chromosomal or due to a complex of environmental and genetic factors.

Recurrence of chromosomal disorder

Most forms of chromosomal disorder carry a low risk of recurrence. If a normal couple has one child with Down's syndrome due to standard trisomy-21 and if parental mosaicism is excluded the risk of recurrence will depend on the mother's age. However since some families have a predisposition to non-disjunction the risk is slightly higher than that usual for the mother's age, especially if any close relatives have had a child with Down's or any other chromosomal anomaly. If either parent has Down's syndrome or is mosaic for it then the risks of recurrence are very high, up to 1 in 2. Higher risks are also found in translocation cases. A fertile male of XYY sex constitution is liable to have a proportion of XYY and of XXY sons and similarly an XXX woman may have an XXY son or an XXX daughter. These possibilities should, therefore, be excluded if advice is sought as to the recurrence of the triple-X, XYY or Klinefelter anomalies.

A succession of children with multiple congenital anomalies, even if different, could be due to a structural chromosomal rearrangement in one of the parents and can be looked for in such cases. Although recurrent abortion is seldom due to genetic factors it is known that in a fifth of all spontaneous abortions the foetus has a demonstrable chromosomal abnormality. It is, therefore, to be expected that in occasional instances recurrent abortion will be due to a transmissible chromosomal anomaly in a parent.

Recurrence of single gene defects

In disorders due to a single major gene advice is easy to give and will usually be just a matter of quoting the Mendelian ratios of 1 in 2 in a dominant disorder or 1 in 4 for a recessive. However even here a number of complicating factors may be present. In a dominant disorder the expression of the gene may not always be complete and then the risk of recurrence will be less than 1 in 2, although the carrier rate will be unchanged. If the parent is not himself affected but some other member of his family is so an estimate may have to be made of the risk of the parent being a carrier who may manifest the disorder late in life. This may be a problem in Huntington's chorea, for example. A parent can also carry a harmful gene without manifesting any disease, as in dystrophia myotonica. If a dominant disorder has appeared in a child for the first time the relative probability of fresh mutation or of prior failure to manifest have to be estimated.

In recessive disorders advice may be sought on the risk of a potential carrier having affected children. Even in the absence of any method of directly detecting carriers it is always possible to calculate a probability based on the known gene frequency. In conditions with intermediate inheritance like thalassaemia carriers can always be directly detected.

In sex linked disorders it may be possible to detect carriers in all cases or only in some as by antihaemophilic globulin assay in haemophilia. Again the probability of being a carrier can also be calculated. Another complication with sex linked disorders is that the probability of a female being a carrier when a brother is affected is less than 1 in 2 if no earlier cases are known as the brother may represent a fresh mutation. This probability can be calculated when there is a reasonable known estimate of the mutation rate.

Occasionally clinically indistinguishable disorders may be inherited either in an autosomal recessive or in a sex-linked manner. This occurs in retinitis pigmentosa where only family history can help and in the Hunter–Hurler syndrome where as mentioned earlier tests can distinguish the two forms (p. 597).

Recurrence of genetically complex disorders
This problem of heterogeneity of aetiology also arises with conditions that are not determined by a single gene. Whatever the overall risk of recurrence, as determined from observations on many families, the individual family history may lead to modification of the empirical risk. Such empirical risks vary from one community to another and that for the community of the family concerned must be used. Reliable risks have been determined for common disorders like the major malformations of the central nervous system, the common cardiac defects, talipes, congenital dislocation of the hip and pyloric stenosis. For rarer congenital disorders the number of recorded instances of familial recurrence is too small for any reliable figure to be given. For all these conditions the likelihood of recurrence is greatly increased if there is already more than one affected child. For example the risk of recurrence of anencephaly rises from about 1 in 20 after a single anencephalic child to about 1 in 10 after two such children.

Cousin marriage
Occasionally advice is sought on the risk of a cousin marriage. Cousins have 1 in 8 of their genes in common and hence have a greater risk of having children homozygous for a recessive condition. If there is any evidence of recessive disorder on either side of the family the risk for the particular condition is obviously increased. Suppose the husband has a sister with retinitis pigmentosa. He has a 1 in 2 chance of being a carrier and the chance that both he and his first cousin are carriers is 1 in 16. If however, there is no evidence for the presence of any particular harmful gene in either partner then they only carry a risk about 3–4 times that of an unrelated couple of having a child with any recessive disorder, say of the order of 1 in 150 instead of about 1 in 500.

Practical assessment

CLINICAL OBSERVATIONS
(i) Family history; ante-natal and developmental history and menstrual history;
(ii) facial abnormalities, minor defects of the hand or feet and cardiac defects;

(iii) bone age and the height and proportions;

(iv) examination of the genitalia and secondary sexual features;

(v) measurement of the width and length of the head as well as its circumference. In some cases the height of the cranial vault obtained from lateral X-rays may also be of value. The ratio of width/length is termed the cephalic index and has been established for a number of disorders.

DERMATOGLYPHS

Dermatoglyphic studies are of value in new born infants in whom clinical features are less marked than at later ages. Dermatoglyphic patterns may assist in the diagnosis of Down's syndrome in which some at least of the palmar and finger-tip features are nearly always found. In the 50 per cent of cases with an open field on the hallucal area of the sole this is almost diagnostic. Characteristic patterns may also be of great help in the diagnosis of other trisomic states.

Parents who are clinically normal but who are mosaic for normal cells and for an abnormal line occasionally show dermatoglyphic patterns suggestive of the abnormal line. Such patterns in a parent of a child with Down's syndrome may suggest the possibility of parental mosaicism as the origin of the trisomy in the child. Unusual patterns may provide more general evidence of developmental defect originating in at least early foetal life, but will not distinguish intra-uterine environmental causes from genetic ones. The correlation of the total finger ridge count between twins can be used as an additional factor in the determination of zygosity.

ROUTINE METHODS

Sex chromatin determination is useful in new born infants with ambiguous genitalia or with neck-webbing or lymphoedema; in infertile men especially with azoospermia; in women with amenorrhoea and short stature; and in adults with any form of intersex.

SPECIAL TESTS

Chromosomal analysis is particularly valuable in cases of suspected autosomal or sex chromosomal anomaly at birth in which the diagnosis is in doubt. Analysis of more than one tissue is needed in diagnosis of patients who present a partial clinical picture suggestive of mosaicism.

Chromosomal analyses and sex chromatin determination, are also helpful in all cases of intersex and of infertility or amenorrhoea not clearly due to typical Klinefelter's or Turner's syndrome or to non-chromosomal causes.

Chromosomal analysis of the parents of a child with Down's syndrome, when there is a family history of the syndrome or the mother is under 30 years of age, will exclude or confirm the presence of a balanced translocation in either parent.

References

FRASER ROBERTS J.A. (1967) *An Introduction to Medical Genetics* (4th Ed.). London: Oxford University Press.

THOMPSON J.S. & THOMPSON M.W. (1966) *Genetics in Medicine*. Philadelphia and London: W.B. Saunders.

BRITISH MEDICAL BULLETIN (1961) *Human Genetics*. 17, No. 3.

Progress in medical genetics in STEINBERG A.G. & BEARN A.G. (eds.) Vols 1–4. (1961 etc.). New York and London: Grune and Stratton.

HARRIS H. (1959) *Human biochemical genetics*. London: Cambridge Univ. Press.

PENROSE L.S. (1964). *The biology of mental defect* (3rd Ed.). London: Sidgwick & Jackson Ltd.

The metabolic basis of inherited disease. (2nd Ed.) in STANBURY J.B., WYNGAARDEN J.B. & FREDRICKSON D.S. (eds.) (1966). New York: McGraw-Hill.

VALENTINE G.H. (1966) *The chromosome disorders*. London: William Heinemann Medical Books Ltd.

18

Sex and Reproduction

Normal function

Sexual function is controlled by a combination of genetic, endocrine and nervous mechanisms.

The gonads produce gametes (which enable the organism to reproduce itself) and secrete hormones (which help to determine the characteristic morphology and behaviour of the two sexes). The sex hormones also have actions on the tissues and metabolism of the body as a whole. The difference between male and female is not as sharp as it might appear. The embryo's gonad is sexually neutral at first and genetic and hormonal aberrations may affect the development of the reproductive system in such a way as to produce a wide variety of disorders. In both sexes the gonads produce both male and female hormones whose actions overlap, and, in both sexes, the pituitary secretes the same gonadotrophic hormones. For these reasons male and female functions will be discussed as far as possible side by side rather than separately.

GENETIC DETERMINATION OF SEX (p. 576)
The nucleus of the normal human cell contains 46 chromosomes, consisting of one pair of dissimilar sex chromosomes (X and Y) and 22 other pairs of similar chromosomes (autosomes). Chromosomes are numbered in descending order of length and are classified into seven groups according to their size and form. The X chromosome is the seventh largest and carries female genes. The Y chromosome is the fourth smallest and carries male genes.

In the formation of gametes the division of cells is associated with halving of the number of chromosomes (meiosis), so that the ovum contains only a single X chromosome and the sperm either one X or one Y chromosome. When the ovum is fertilized by the sperm the original number of chromosomes is restored. If the sperm carries an

X chromosome the offspring will be female (XX); if it carries a Y chromosome the sex will be male (XY).

Female chromosomal sex (XX) is manifested by a local condensation of chromatin in the nucleus of most cells, in close contact with the nuclear membrane (Barr bodies), and by accessory nuclear lobules in the leucocytes ('drumsticks'). The normal female is thus said to be 'chromatin-positive'. Male cells invariably contain no chromatin body, the chromatin being distributed throughout the nucleus, and the normal male is thus 'chromatin-negative'.

EMBRYOLOGY

The gonad is at first sexually undifferentiated. It contains a cortical (female) component, derived from the primordial germ cells of the yolk-sac and from the germinal epithelium of the coelomic genital ridge, and a medullary (male) component derived from the mesonephros. If the embryo is to develop as a female, the cortical component predominates and develops into the Müllerian duct and thence into the Fallopian tubes, uterus and vagina. If the embryo is to develop as a male, the medullary component predominates and develops into the Wolffian duct and thence into the epididymis, vas deferens and seminal vesicles.

Between the third and the fifth month of foetal life the external genitalia develop from the urogenital sinus. Masculinizing influences which arise at this time in genetic females impair the separation of the urethra and lower vagina, giving rise to female pseudohermaphroditism. This is usually the result of congenital adrenal hyperplasia (p. 529).

In animals the development of a male reproductive tract depends upon secretion of a male hormone by genetically male embryos, whereas no such hormone is produced by genetically female embryos. If castration is performed before the gonads are differentiated, so that the influence of this masculinizing hormone is absent, the reproductive tract develops along female lines, regardless of the genetic sex of the embryo. Castration at a later stage produces male pseudohermaphroditism in genetic males.

The foetal male hormone is probably produced by the interstitial cells of the foetal testes which are particularly abundant at the time that the genital tract is becoming differentiated. It is interesting that this coincides in time with the phase of maximal excretion of chorionic gonadotrophin in the maternal urine (p. 507). Apparently the foetal male hormone is not the same as testosterone because it suppresses the development of the Müllerian system, whereas injected testosterone

20*

does not do so even though it masculinizes the external genitalia.

The foetal male hormone is in some way influenced by the pituitary because hypophysectomy of a male embryo has the same effect as castration. Furthermore, basophil cells of the gonadotrophic type have been seen in the foetal pituitary gland during the second half of foetal life.

The action of the foetal hormone is apparently a local one, since unilateral castration of a male embryo is followed by the development of a female genital tract on the side of castration only. This may have a counterpart in human hermaphroditism (p. 586).

The neonatal hypothalamus

The close interrelationship between the gonads and the hypothalamus, which involves some sort of servomechanism (p. 503), is a delicate one. Recent work suggests, in rats, that the threshold and response to 'feed-back' from gonadal hormones (and hence sexual behaviour) can be permanently modified by changing the hormonal environment quite briefly in the first few days after birth. If neonatal females are exposed to testosterone, they are sterile as adults; their ovaries are large and polycystic like the changes in an ovary when it is transplanted into an adult male castrate. On the other hand, if neonatal males are castrated, they behave, as adults, like females; transplanted ovaries remain normal, they ovulate and undergo normal female cyclical changes. Thus, whether the hypothalamus behaves like a male or a female in adult life, depends, like the urogenital system in foetal life, not so much on genetic factors but on the presence or absence of male hormone at a specific stage of early development.

POST-NATAL DEVELOPMENT OF THE GONADS

THE TESTES

At birth the testes contain small closely-packed tubules without lumina, consisting mainly of undifferentiated cells. A few germ cells are present and the interstitial tissue consists of Leydig cells which disappear within a few weeks of birth. There is little further development in the first 10 years, but, at puberty, they grow abruptly and continue to grow for the next 5 or 6 years, owing to proliferation of the seminiferous tubules. The latter produce germ cells which become differentiated by stages into spermatozoa under the influence of follicle stimulating hormone (FSH) from the anterior lobe of the pituitary gland. Spermatogenesis begins at about the age of 14 years and is well established by the age of 15 years; but it does not start unless the testes are in the scrotum. The Sertoli cells become differentiated at puberty. Their function is not understood. The presence of lipoid material in them, as in the interstitial cells, suggests that they may secrete a hormone, which may be an oestrogen. Alternatively, they may be concerned with the nutrition and development of the spermatozoa. The interstitial (Leydig) cells lie between the tubules along with undifferentiated connective tissue cells. They reappear at puberty, when they secrete testosterone under the influence of interstitial cell-stimulating hormone (ICSH) secreted by the anterior pituitary (p. 498).

Control of testicular function
Hypophysectomy causes atrophy of the seminiferous tubules which can be prevented by the administration of follicle-stimulating hormone (FSH). It also causes atrophy of the assessory sexual organs but this can only be prevented by the administration of ICSH (LH) and not FSH. In addition ICSH is probably necessary for fully normal spermatogenesis. Large quantities of androgens can inhibit the release of FSH from the pituitary but oestrogen, secreted by the testis, is a more potent inhibitor of FSH release and this, rather than testosterone, probably provides the pituitary feed-back mechanism normally used. Androgens in large amounts can maintain spermatogenesis but this is probably not a physiological function.

Spermatogenesis can only take place at a temperature which is some degrees lower then the central body temperature. It does not occur in abdominal testes. *In vitro*, the rate of synthesis of testosterone is also maximal at the cooler temperature of the scrotum.

PUBERTY
In girls, puberty begins at 10–11 years of age with enlargement of the nipples, areolae and lacteal ducts as a result of an increased rate of oestrogen secretion. Oestrogens also control the subsequent development of the genitalia. The growth of body hair probably depends on the secretion of adrenal androgens, although oestrogens may also have some influence. The development of the labia majora (which are the counterpart of the scrotum) may also be controlled by adrenal androgens.

In boys puberty starts with enlargement of the testes at about 11 years of age. This is followed closely by the development of the secondary sexual characters.

Physiological variations in puberty
Nutrition, chronic illness and climate as well as genetic factors cause considerable physiological variation both in the timing and the pattern of puberty. In girls it may start any time from 9 to 17 years of age and in boys about a year later. Sexual hair may grow in quite early childhood without other signs of puberty. Transient breast development often occurs in the newborn due to placental oestrogens but the breasts may also develop in childhood without other signs of puberty. Adolescent boys may develop gynaecomastia, particularly when virilization is rapid. This is probably due to oestrogen production either from the testes or by conversion from testosterone (testosterone administration can also cause gynaecomastia). Similarly, adolescent girls sometimes develop signs of virilization (hirsutism, muscularity and acne) although they menstruate normally. Appreciation of these normal variations is important clinically.

The underlying mechanism of puberty is obscure but it is not due to a change in the responsiveness of the gonads or the pituitary. There may be a reduction in the sensitivity of the hypothalamus to the inhibitory effects of circulating gonadal hormones, but if so the mechanism is also obscure. It may be an inherent property of the ageing hypothalamus.

THE OVARY

At birth the ovary contains 40,000 to 400,000 primordial follicles, each consisting of an ovum surrounded by a layer of granulosa cells. From infancy onwards some of these show varying degrees of development into Graafian follicles, but they do not completely mature or discharge their ova. Only about 10,000 to 30,000 of the primordial follicles survive to puberty. Approximately 300 ova are liberated before the ovary atrophies at the menopause.

THE MENSTRUAL CYCLE

Follicular phase
Towards the end of each cycle and in the early part of the following cycle a number of primordial follicles develop into Graafian follicles. Initially this is an autonomous process but later development depends on the presence of anterior pituitary follicle-stimulating hormone (FSH), which is released as the level of oestrogen falls in the last week of the cycle. Only one of these follicles matures fully and releases an ovum. The earliest changes in the developing follicle are proliferation of the granulosa cells surrounding the ovum and hyperplasia of the stroma to form the theca interna. The granulosa cells form the follicular

liquor, into which the cells of the theca interna secrete oestradiol. This hormone enters the blood stream and brings about the *proliferative phase* of the endometrium, in which the endometrial glands enlarge and the vessels become elongated, both becoming increasingly tortuous.

Ovulation

Ovulation is preceded by a transient, sharp increase in the plasma concentration of luteinizing hormone (LH) from the anterior pituitary which depends on a rising concentration of oestradiol, secreted under the influence of FSH in the first half of the cycle. The ovum, surrounded by its radiating layers of granulosa cells (the corona radiata), is extruded into the abdominal cavity and is directed into the Fallopian tubes by their fimbriae. The precise mechanism of ovulation is unknown.

Secretory phase

Under the influence of LH the theca interna secretes progesterone and its 20-hydroxylated form and the ruptured follicle is converted into a *corpus luteum*. The evidence now suggests that, in humans, there is no corpus luteum-maintaining substance in the menstrual cycle. In all species luteal function is initiated by rupture of the follicle but the requirement for a luteotrophin (prolactin) varies greatly. The mechanim by which luteal function wanes towards the end of the cycle is unknown, but it may depend on the production of a 'luteolysin' from the uterus. The plasma concentration of progesterone increases tenfold, from about 0·1 to 1·0 μgm per 100 ml.

The epithelium of the endometrial glands becomes vacuolated and discharges mucus and glycogen into the lumen. This phase is established about 48 hours after ovulation. It is at this stage that implantation of a fertilized ovum can occur with the development of the true decidua of pregnancy. If pregnancy does not supervene the corpus luteum degenerates and becomes fibrotic, the secretion of oestradiol and progesterone declines and the endometrium regresses. As the endometrium becomes thinner the spiral arteries become increasingly coiled and constricted, and this results in ischaemic necrosis. The vessels then relax temporarily and bleeding ensues; the bleeding is checked by a further phase of vasoconstriction and by thrombosis. Desquamation of the endometrium then follows. The withdrawal of oestrogen allows FSH to be released once more and a new cycle is initiated.

Breast changes

When ovular cycles begin the breasts undergo cyclical changes. During the second week of the menstrual cycle oestrogens cause the ducts to dilate and secrete and the stroma becomes oedematous; the breast as a whole becomes enlarged and nodular. After ovulation progesterone stimulates the formation of alveoli, which become arranged into lobules. The action of progesterone on the breast, as on the endometrium, is dependent upon the previous action of oestrogen. When the concentrations of oestrogens and of progesterone fall off towards the end of the mentrual cycle the breast regresses.

During pregnancy the changes resulting from oestrogens and progesterone are intensified.

REPRODUCTION

Fertilization

Ovulation occurs almost constantly at about 14 days before the first day of the next menstrual period. This is the mid-point of the 28-day cycle; in shorter cycles the pre-ovulatory phase is shortened but the post-ovulatory phase is maintained at 14 days. The ovum remains susceptible to fertilization for only 1 to 3 days, so that fertilization usually occurs around the mid-point of the cycle. Occasionally ovulation occurs much earlier or much later, and this accounts for the occasional failure of the 'safe period' method of contraception.

The prostate adds calcium and fibrinolysin to the semen. Calcium increases its tendency to coagulate and thus helps to prevent its escape from the female genital tract. Fibrinolysin subsequently liquefies it and thus allows the sperms to penetrate further into the uterus. The sperm is thought to enter the ovum by penetration with its flagellum and with the aid of the hyaluronidase which it contains.

The fertilized ovum takes about 4 days to pass along the Fallopian tube into the uterus and a further 2 or 3 days to become implanted. A decidual reaction in the endometrium precedes implantation which, at least in animals, is a delicately-timed event under hypothalamic control.

Pregnancy

By the time the ovum has become implanted it has already divided and multiplied to form a blastocyst surrounded by a trophoblast. The latter erodes the endometrium and develops into the placenta.

At an early stage of pregnancy the trophoblast begins to secrete the polypeptide hormone, chorionic gonadotrophin. This is predominantly luteinizing in type and is thought to maintain the corpus luteum and its secretion of progesterone during the first 3 months. The output of the hormone reaches its maximum level in the second and third months and then rapidly falls to reach a steady level by the fifth month, at which level it persists until after parturition.

After the first 3 months the corpus luteum is no longer indispensable and the secretion of progesterone is taken over by the placenta. This is revealed by a steadily increasing output of pregnanediol in the urine, which is maintained for the remainder of the pregnancy. The excretion of oestrogens also increases from the fifth week onwards. The predominant oestrogen in the urine is oestriol. This is secreted by the placenta and also by the foetus. In fact, the placenta and foetus are now considered to form a biosynthetic unit which, although unable to synthesize oestrogens from the precursors used by other steroid-producing organs, produce oestrogens by aromatization of steroids such as dehydroepiandiosterone and its sulphate. These C-19 steroids may originate in the foetal adrenal gland because women bearing anencephalic foetuses with atrophied adrenals, excrete very little oestrogen. The excretion of oestriol increases abruptly at 32 weeks, at a time when the growth of the placenta and its production of pregnanediol is beginning to slow up. After this the curve of increasing excretion flattens out for the remainder of the pregnancy. The high concentrations of oestrogen and progesterone produced by the placenta suppress the output of pituitary gonadotrophins, so that the cyclical activity in the ovaries is abolished; they also prepare the breasts for lactation (p. 611). Oestrogen is thought to make the genital tract softer, more vascular and more easily stretched and to make the pelvic ligaments more elastic. A polypeptide named 'relaxin' has also been recovered from the blood during pregnancy which enhances these effects. It is found mainly in the corpus luteum but its physiological role remains undefined.

Apart from chorionic gonadotrophin the placenta also produces another polypeptide hormone, human placental lactogen (HPL), which appears to be formed by the foetal part of the placenta. It is luteotropic and stimulates the crop-sac of the pigeon. It cross-reacts immunologically with human growth hormone (p. 498) but is separable from it immunochemically. Given alone it does not stimulate growth but, in hypophysectomized rats, the effect of growth-hormone is enhanced. The physiological significance of HPL is unknown.

In pregnancy and also in people taking oestrogens or in women taking the contraceptive 'pill', the concentration of total cortisol in the plasma increases. The rate of removal of cortisol from the plasma is delayed. The rate of secretion of cortisol is normal or reduced in people taking oestrogens but increased in pregnancy. The concentration of the α-globulin which binds cortisol (corticosteroid-binding globulin or CBG) increases but, if anything, the concentration of free, unbound cortisol also increases, although the proportion of free to bound cortisol may fall. Despite this, clinical evidence of excessive cortisol action is lacking, so that there is, presumably, some mechanism which inhibits the action of cortisol on tissue cells.

The rate of aldosterone secretion is definitely and considerably increased during pregnancy, and the plasma level is elevated. In contrast to cortisol, there is no change of protein-binding, and the rate of removal of aldosterone from the plasma is normal. Gross alterations of mineral metabolism are not seen and this probably reflects on increased plasma concentration of steroids such as progesterone (p. 614) which attenuate the action of aldosterone on the renal tubules.

The concentration of protein-bound iodine in the plasma rises during pregnancy, and, as in the case of cortisol, this is due to an increased concentration of a specific binding-protein, TBG or thyroxin-binding globulin. Again it can be reproduced in the non-pregnant state by the administration of oestrogen. Removal of thyroid hormone from the plasma is also delayed and hyperthyroidism is exceptional.

Parturition

The mechanism is not fully understood but it is clear that the placental portion of the uterine muscle must remain largely inactive up to the time of birth. Local injections of progesterone into the uterus decrease its spontaneous activity and we know that the placenta secretes progesterone, so that a local inhibitory action of progesterone on the muscle cells near the placenta may be the mechanism. The non-placental part of the myometrium gradually enlarges as pregnancy progresses; its spontaneous activity increases and it becomes more and more sensitive to the action of oxytocins so that the amniotic pressure rises progressively. Finally the force of uterine contractions reaches consciousness and labour pains ensue.

Formerly the onset of labour was attributed to a sudden withdrawal of progesterone but it now seems that the total concentration of progesterone in the circulating blood is not very meaningful because we do not know how much of it is biologically effective. A change in the plasma-binding of progesterone without any change of the total content might well occur at the onset of labour, but has not so far been demonstrated.

The role of oxytocin has not been fully elucidated. This hormone can be measured in the plasma during pregnancy and the uterine activity can be increased by infusing it at any stage of pregnancy. The concentration in the plasma rises sharply during the second stage of labour and the main action of the hormone is probably to aid the expulsion of the foetus, rather than to initiate labour.

Lactation

The physiology of lactation is not completely understood and most of the evidence is derived from animals. Prolactin appears to initiate the process and there is some evidence that the release of prolactin is stimulated by oxytocin and by a decline in the inhibitory influence of progesterone at parturition with a relative dominance of the stimulating effect of oestrogen. Growth hormone and thyroid hormone apparently help to maintain lactation. Milk is secreted by the alveolar epithelium and is stored by the expanded ducts. It is ejected in response to suckling, by sensory stimuli relayed from the nipple to the hypothalamus which cause the neurohypophysis to secrete oxytocin. The latter causes the 'basket cells' of the alveoli to contract and expel the milk. The reflex is inhibited by sympathetic impulses and this may account for the failure of lactation which is liable to result from emotional disturbances.

THE CLIMACTERIC

The process usually starts between the ages of 45 and 50 years, but occasionally as early as 35 years or as late as 55 years of age. In general, the earlier the menarche, the later the menopause. The ovaries gradually become atrophic, the output of oestrogens falls and the output of pituitary gonadotrophins consequently rises. Hot flushes appear to result from a change in balance between oestrogens and gonadotrophins. They occur also after castration but only occasionally in hypopituitarism, in which both gonadotrophins and oestrogens are suppressed, and not at all in ovarian agenesis, in which a deficiency of oestrogens and an excess of gonadotrophins exist from the beginning.

The fall of oestrogen output also leads to atrophy of the breasts and of the labia minora and to atrophic changes in the vaginal mucosa, often associated with pruritus and sometimes progressing to kraurosis or leukoplakia. Ovulation fails to occur and menstruation ceases gradually or abruptly. If the secretion of oestrogens persists at an adequate level after ovulation has ceased, the endometrium develops an exaggeration of the histological pattern characteristic of the proliferative phase of the menstrual cycle; failure of progesterone secretion in the absence of the corpus luteum prevents the development of the secretory phase and the greatly proliferated and vascular endometrium may bleed heavily and for prolonged periods.

PITUITARY GONADOTROPHINS

The gonads are stimulated by two pituitary gonadotrophins, whose secretion is regulated by the hypothalamus. Hormones secreted by the gonads in turn inhibit the release of their respective trophic hormones when the former reach a certain concentration. This preserves homeostasis and represents a 'feed-back' mechanism (see Chapter 14).

The actions of FSH and LH in the menstrual cycle are described on p. 606. In the male FSH stimulates spermatogenesis and LH stimulates the interstitial cells of the testis to secrete testosterone (hence it is also known as interstitial-cell-stimulating hormone or ICSH).

Luteotrophin (LTH), which is identical with prolactin, is also produced by the pituitary and probably acts in synergism with ICSH and testosterone in maintaining the accessory sex glands.

GONADAL HORMONES

These are all steroid compounds. Oestrogens contain eighteen carbon atoms, androgens nineteen and progesterone twenty-one (like the adrenal corticosteroids) (see p. 521).

Androgens

Androgens are produced by the Leydig cells of the testes but also by the adrenals and the ovaries. The biosynthetic pathways are broadly similar in all three steroid-producing glands and it is differences of the local concentration of particular enzymes which determine the main steroid hormone actually produced. In the testes the predominance of enzymes which split the side-chain at $C17$ means that production of testosterone and Δ^4-androstene-3,17-dione is favoured. Recent studies show that a chemically different androgen, dehydroandrosterone (p. 523) is also an important secretion of the testis. It belongs to the Δ^5-pregnene series whereas testosterone belongs to the Δ^4-pregnene series. Therefore there are at least two different pathways for androgen synthesis which share points of crossover. Double isotope studies show that both pathways are used simultaneously.

Androgens are metabolized in the liver (and elsewhere) to other

17-oxosteroids and 17-oxosteroid conjugates. Some of these are themselves androgenic and some, like dehydroandrosterone sulphate, may act as precursors for steroid synthesis in other glands (p. 609). The chief urinary metabolities of androgens are the glucuronides of androsterone and aetiocholanolone.

Apart from the effects of androgens on the secondary sex characters testosterone increases the formation of protein, especially in the muscles and in the epiphyses, and stimulates growth. Consequently potassium, calcium, phosphorus and sulphur are retained. The β-lipoprotein fraction of plasma is increased and the α-lipoprotein fraction reduced. These changes are similar to those associated with coronary atherosclerosis, which is commoner in normal men than in women during the reproductive period and is relatively uncommon in eunuchs. Testosterone increases the vascularity and pigmentation of the skin and renal blood-flow is also increased. It plays some part in haemopoiesis and has been used in the treatment of aplastic anaemia. It stimulates libido and aggressiveness in both sexes.

Oestrogens

Oestrogens are so called because they induce oestrus in immature female or spayed adult animals. Chemically, oestrogens are C-18 steroids characterized by a phenolic ring A (p. 521). The ovary secretes oestradiol-17β and oestrone, which are readily interconvertible and which are, together, irreversibly converted to oestriol by pathways involving other oestrogens. The high concentration of aromatizing enzymes in the ovary favours the production of oestrogens but, in addition to the placenta and foetus, oestrogens are also produced by the adrenals and testes. About 80 per cent of the oestrogen excreted in the urine of normal men is derived from the testis, though a proportion of this is the result of conversion from testosterone.

The output of oestrogens in the urine reaches a peak at about the time of ovulation, and a second smaller peak occurs in the middle of the luteal phase. The output increases greatly during the second half of pregnancy. Low values during pregnancy suggest that pregnancy may not continue to full-term.

Oestrogens are largely inactivated in the liver by conjugation as sulphates and glucuronides. In this form they are soluble in water and are readily excreted in the urine. The three naturally occurring oestrogens are excreted in the urine in approximately the same proportions in both sexes.

Oestrogens promote the development of the female genitalia and breasts. The changes in the vaginal epithelium, particularly cornification, and in the uterine weight of immature animals, are frequently used for the bioassay of oestrogens. As with aldosterone, the biochemical basis of these effects probably depends upon the stimulation of enzyme synthesis.

Oestrogens are less potent than androgens in stimulating growth of the epiphyses but have a pronounced effect on their closure (p. 309). They have a stronger action in retaining sodium, chloride and water, but a relatively weak action in retaining nitrogen. Their effects on the concentration of cholesterol in β- and α-lipoproteins are the reverse of those exerted by androgens.

Progesterone

Progesterone is secreted by the corpus luteum, by the placenta, and also as an intermediary in the synthesis of corticosteroids from cholesterol in the adrenal cortex. Progesterone is excreted mainly in the form of pregnanediol in the urine, which increases during pregnancy and reflects placental function.

The effects on the female reproductive system are complex. After preliminary priming with oestrogen, progesterone causes the changes which occur during the luteal or secretory stage of the cycle. In castrates, progesterone has no effect alone but when combined with oestrogen, all the endometrial changes of the normal cycle can be reproduced. It inhibits further ovulation, delays menstruation and prevents the bleeding which normally occurs following oestrogen withdrawal but, paradoxically, it actually induces ovulation if given close to the time of expected, spontaneous ovulation. The mechanism by which progesterone inhibits ovulation is obscure; it does not affect the rate of growth of the follicle, the rate of oestrogen secretion or the responsiveness of the follicle to gonadotrophins. It may act by preventing the sudden, rapid rise of LH secretion that precedes ovulation (p. 607) but the tonic release of FSH or LH from the pituitary is unaffected.

Progesterone also has interesting extragenital effects. It antagonizes the action of aldosterone on the renal tubules, which may explain the high rate of aldosterone secretion and the relative ineffectiveness of aldosterone during pregnancy; it stimulates heat production, which may explain the changes in body temperature during the menstrual cycle; it depresses central nervous activity; and it induces maternal behaviour. It is also mildly catabolic.

Disordered function

MALDEVELOPMENT OF THE GONADS

Disorders of sex determination, such as Klinefelter's and Turner's syndrome, and disorders of sex differentiation such as hermaphroditism, are discussed on p. 583 to 588 in Chapter 17.

FUNCTIONAL DERANGEMENTS ARISING POST-NATALLY
HYPOFUNCTION IN MALES

HYPOGONADISM

This may arise either as a primary failure of testicular function or as a result of deficient secretion of pituitary gonadotrophic hormone with or without deficient secretion of other pituitary hormones.

Primary testicular failure

There may be a failure of development involving both the germinal epithelium and the interstitial cells, so that the individual is both sterile and deficient in androgenic development ('eunuchoidism' or 'functional prepubertal castration'; the same will result, of course, from artificial castration ('eunuchism')). Alternatively, the testis may atrophy as a result of cryptorchidism, trauma, infection with mumps or irradiation; in such cases the main brunt of the injury falls upon the germinal epithelium, the interstitial cells being relatively resistant, so that the individual becomes subfertile or sterile, but usually develops or maintains normal androgenic function. Klinefelter's syndrome (p. 583) falls in the same category. Both spermatogenesis and function of the interstitial cells may be impaired as a result of failure of a diseased liver to metabolize endogenous oestrogens or of the administration of exogenous oestrogens. Deposition of iron in the testes in haemochromatosis may have the same result. Occasionally the Leydig (interstitial) cells may by hypoplastic while spermatogenesis remains intact. The individual then shows evidence of androgenic deficiency but may be fertile, though fertility may be impaired as a result of deficient seminal fluid and consequent inability to transport the sperm.

Testicular failure secondary to hypopituitarism

Both seminiferous tubules and interstitial cells remain infantile, or, in acquired hypopituitarism, both atrophy.

MANIFESTATIONS OF ANDROGEN DEFICIENCY

Failure of the interstitial cells of the testis to develop and to secrete testosterone prevents the onset of puberty. The skeletal muscles develop poorly because protein anabolism is deficient and osteoporosis may occur in long-standing cases. The skin is pale and atrophic and the face becomes finely wrinkled. The normal aggressiveness of the male is absent. But sometimes the patient overcompensates and becomes unduly assertive. Libido may not be lacking and some untreated patients may achieve a form of coitus.

The effect of testosterone deficiency on body hair and bony growth depends on the presence or absence of other hormonal defects. If it is the sole lesion (as in primary testicular failure or *selective* pituitary gonadotrophin deficiency) then the body hair grows a little because adrenal androgens are still present, but the distribution of the pubic hair remains feminine. Fusion of the epiphyses is delayed and this allows the long bones to grow more than usual, so that the span of the out-stretched arms exceeds the height and the pubic symphysis is nearer the top of the head than the bottom of the feet. Normally the span equals the height and the height of the pubic symphysis is half the full height. By contrast, if testosterone deficiency is part of a *general* pituitary failure then the body hair remains infantile. The bones grow very slowly, so that, although the epiphyses may never fuse, the body proportions remain normal. All the manifestations described above can be corrected by early administration of testosterone with the exception of the bony changes, which can only be modified. A temporary acceleration in the rate of growth can be reproduced in cases of pituitary infantilism, but the long-standing deficiency of growth hormone cannot be compensated in this way.

Castration after puberty is followed by only partial impairment of the androgenic development which has already been achieved. The abrupt withdrawal of testosterone may cause hot flushes, like those occurring after castration or the menopause in the female. Physical strength and endurance may be impaired and nervous tension and emotional instability may result.

HYPOFUNCTION IN FEMALES

Ovarian failure, like testicular failure, may arise as a primary phenomenon or as a result of hypopituitarism. Primary ovarian failure may result from aplasia, as in Turner's syndrome, from surgical castration or from destruction of the pelvic organs by disease. Ovarian failure may also result from thyroid dysfunction, adrenal hyperplasia or from debilitating conditions, but often there is no discoverable cause. Secondary ovarian failure may result from hypopituitarism due to an organic lesion of the pituitary or hypothalamus, but more commonly it is due to interference with the hypothalamic control of gonadotrophin secretion, by emotional disturbances, or a change of environment. Either emaciation (as in anorexia nervosa) or obesity are common associated symptoms.

Before puberty ovarian failure causes primary amenorrhoea but the development of the breasts, genitalia and secondary sex characters is sometimes little affected. Lesions of the pituitary-hypothalamic region or of the ovaries arising after puberty result in secondary amenorrhoea and there may be some regression of secondary sex characters.

Patients with primary amenorrhoea due to ovarian failure must, of course, be distinguished from those in whom some mechanical obstruction (such as an imperforate hymen) prevents the menstrual flow from appearing externally and also from those patients whose endometrium is abnormally resistant to a normal pattern of hormone secretion.

Mild degrees of ovarian failure, usually without discoverable cause, are common and result either in secondary amenorrhoea or in 'dysfunctional' bleeding. Dysfunctional bleeding usually results from failure of ovulation. The endometrial pattern varies from hyperplasia with incompletely developed secretory changes to intense proliferative changes with no evidence of secretory activity (metropathia haemorrhagica); in extreme degrees the endometrium may become polypoidal and may even advance to the borders of malignancy.

The premenstrual syndrome

The retention of fluid resulting from the secretion of oestrogens during the first three weeks of the cycle may cause demonstrable oedema and increase in weight during the premenstrual phase, together with headache, tension, instability, depression, loss of efficiency and pain in the breasts. The threshold of sensitivity to these physiological changes varies from one individual to another, being particularly low in unstable persons.

STATES OF HYPERFUNCTION—SEXUAL PRECOCITY

Precocity is more than twice as common in the female as in the male. Most commonly it represents an extreme variation of the physiological norm and is then described as 'idiopathic' or 'constitutional', but it may result from disturbance of hypothalamic function by tumours, infections or congenital defects or from tumours of the gonads.

IDIOPATHIC AND HYPOTHALAMIC PRECOCITY
Idiopathic cases may have a genetic basis, a small percentage showing a familial tendency. These and the hypothalamic types show complete sexual maturation in all respects, including active spermatogenesis in the male and maturation of the Graafian follicles in the female. Puberty has been known to arise at as early an age as 4 to 6 weeks in idiopathic cases and not uncommonly occurs before the age of 2 years. Pregnancy has been reported at the age of 5 years, but lactation has never been recorded. As a result of the early onset of puberty there is at the same time an early spurt of growth, such as accompanies normal puberty; for the same reason the epiphyses ossify and close prematurely. This eventually results not only in permanent dwarfism but in disproportionate shortening of the limbs as compared with the trunk, so that the individual resembles a chondrodystrophic dwarf. Mental development and emotional maturation proceed less rapidly than physical development, though they gradually attain to the same level. The majority marry at the usual age, bear healthy children and die from natural causes. The menopause does not occur prematurely. Indeed, apart from their short stature they become essentially normal adults.

GONADAL HYPERFUNCTION
Ovarian tumours
These are all rare in childhood, the least uncommon being granulosa cell tumours, which are usually benign in children and are usually unilateral. The oestrogens which they secrete are entirely responsible for the precocious development of secondary sexual characteristics. The remaining normal ovarian tissue stays immature, with no evidence of ovulation. Uterine bleeding is almost invariable and the epiphyses close prematurely.

Testicular tumours
These are also extremely rare and include a number of cases of benign interstitial cell adenoma and one or two cases of teratoma. Since the neoplasia is confined to the interstitial cells, the individual develops precociously only so far as his secondary sex characters and skeletal changes are concerned. Spermatogenesis does not occur.

Congenital adrenal hyperplasia in the male results in precocious development of the secondary sex characters, though the testes remain infantile, presumably because the secretion of gonadotrophins is inhibited by the high concentration of androgens (p. 529).

STATES OF PERVERTED FUNCTION

VIRILISM IN FEMALES
Ovarian tumours
Certain rare types of ovarian tumour secrete excessive amounts of androgens. These include arrhenoblastoma and masculinovoblastoma (lipoid cell tumours). A third type of tumour arises from the hilus cells of the normal ovary, which resemble Leydig cells.

Stein–Leventhal syndrome
In this ill-defined condition the ovaries are usually enlarged and contain numerous follicular cysts. Their capsules are thickened, pale white, smooth and shiny. The follicles may or may not contain granulosa cells. The theca interna is often hyperplastic and luteinized but ovulation occurs infrequently and corpora lutea are seldom found. The endometrium usually shows proliferative changes and, because of the failure of ovulation, is seldom secretory in pattern. The cardinal clinical features are oligomenorrhoea or amenorrhoea and infertility. A proportion of patients are hirsute but other features of virilism are usually absent. Some are obese. The aetiology is obscure and its specificity has been questioned, but analysis of the steroids in the fluid obtained from the follicular cysts suggests that there may be a block in the synthesis of oestradiol from progesterone, with an accumulation of the intermediary metabolite androstenedione, which is weakly androgenic. The thecal hyperplasia may represent an attempt to overcome this metabolic block and the adrenal cortex may also produce an additional supply of androgens.

FEMINISM
This occurs in males as a result of excessive secretion of oestrogens, either by a carcinoma of the adrenal cortex or by a rare type of testicular tumour arising from the Sertoli cells. Atrophy of the remaining testicular tissue and gynaecomastia result. Testicular feminisation, where there is end organ resistance to androgens, is described on p. 587.

DISORDERS OF REPRODUCTION

COITUS

In men failure may occur at any stage of the sexual act. Disorders of the central nervous system may be responsible but psychogenic disturbances are far the commonest. Endocrine reasons are rare.

In women frigidity is nearly always psychogenic in origin. In any case libido tends to be less strong than in the male and a high proportion of women fail to achieve an orgasm during coitus.

INFERTILITY

In both sexes, no reason is usually discovered but disorders of sex determination or disorders of sex differentiation (p. 583–588) or hypogonadism for other reasons (p. 615) may be responsible. In men absent or scanty spermatozoa may account for about 25 per cent of infertile marriages. In women, infertility may be due to defective cervical mucous which is 'hostile' to spermatozoa, to pelvic inflammation or to emotional factors, which probably interfere with hypothalamic function.

DISORDERS OF PREGNANCY

Habitual abortion may be associated with a reduced rate of pregnanediol excretion, suggesting inadequate progesterone secretion at a time when the placenta takes over the secretion of this hormone from the corpus luteum. However, there is no conclusive evidence that the results of treatment with progesterone in this condition are any better than those which can be obtained with rest and reassurance. Low levels of oestriol and pregnanediol in the urine have been found in pre-eclamptic toxaemia, essential hypertension and placental insufficiency (discrepancy between observed and expected uterine size), but these are probably secondary changes, the output of oestriol reflecting the viability of the foetus and that of pregnanediol reflecting the state of the placenta.

DISORDERS OF THE BREAST AND OF LACTATION

Variations in breast development. Some women show little or no development of the breasts in spite of otherwise normal secondary sex characters and normal reproductive function. Selective failure of breast development must be regarded as a manifestation of end-organ resistance, probably determined by genetic factors. Even intensive administration of oestrogens is ineffective. Similarly, excessive development of the breasts is probably due to extreme sensitivity of the breast tissue to the action of oestrogens.

Failure of lactation. This is principally due to inadequate suckling or to emotional factors which inhibit the reflex secretion of oxytocin by increasing sympathetic activity (p. 515). Possibly it may result also from genetically unresponsive breast tissue or from deficient activity of the pituitary hormones, sex hormones and thyroid hormones which participate in lactation. Occasionally it results from hypopituitarism following post-partum haemorrhage (p. 512).

Persistent lactation. Lactation may persist for many years after a confinement, even until the menopause, and may be accompanied by amenorrhoea. The cause is obscure but it may be that some hypothalamic disturbance occurs which prevents the normal inhibition of lactogenic hormones from the anterior pituitary lobe. Persistent lactation may also occur without antecedent pregnancy and in association with amenorrhoea. This may be due to excessive production of growth hormone or prolactin, both of which are thought to be secreted by the eosinophil cells of the anterior pituitary lobe. Thus lactation is a comparatively common feature of acromegaly. It has also been reported in association with chromophobe adenomata, which, contrary to earlier beliefs, are capable of secreting excessive amounts of pituitary hormones.

Gynaecomastia. Hyperplasia of the glandular tissue of the male breast seems to result almost invariably from an excess of oestrogens and the histological features are similar to those in the female breast at normal puberty, consisting of proliferation of the ducts and stroma without the formation of alveoli. The excess of oestrogens may be due to various causes. (1) Maternal oestrogens may cause transient enlargement of the breasts with some secretion at birth. (2) Secretion of oestrogens by the interstitial cells of the testes, or the conversion of testosterone into oestrogens, commonly causes enlargement of the subareolar breast tissue at puberty (p. 606) and occasionally this leads to persistent and progressive gynaecomastia. The same phenomenon may be reproduced by the administration of chorionic gonadotrophin, which stimulates the interstitial cells. It may occur pathologically in conditions which damage the germinal epithelium, the interstitial cells remaining intact or becoming hyperplastic (p. 615). It is also seen in male pseudo-hermaphroditism (p. 587) and in testicular tumours which produce an excess of oestrogens or of chorionic gonadotrophin, such as chorion-epithelioma, interstitial cell tumour or Sertoli cell tumour. It is also a prominent feature of Klinefelter's syndrome (p. 583). (3) The oestrogen may be derived from exogenous sources, as in workers in the pharmaceutical industry, in children who take their mothers' tablets, and in the treatment of sexual offenders and patients suffering from acne, carcinoma of the prostate or coronary artery disease. (4) Chronic liver disease or impairment of liver function by malnutrition may result in failure to inactivate oestrogens. (5) Recovery from malnutrition may result in gynaecomastia, despite the absence of this symptom during the period of malnutrition, probably because the restoration of a normal diet increases the secretion of oestrogens. (6) Malignant adrenal or bronchial tumours occasionally cause gynaecomastia. (7) The condition has been reported as a result of intoxication with digitalis, whose structure is similar to that of steroid hormones.

Principles of tests and measurements

The investigations commonly carried out are in principle designed to assess (*a*) the functional adequacy of the gonads, (*b*) the functional adequacy of pituitary gonadotrophin secretion, and (*c*) the responsiveness of the end-organs to sex hormones.

VAGINAL SMEARS

A careful examination of a vaginal smear gives a relatively simple qualitative index of the concentration of biologically effective circulating oestrogen. In the relative absence of oestrogenic activity the vaginal epithelium is thin and the cells contain very little glycogen. When oestrogenic activity increases the vaginal epithelium proliferates and becomes transformed into stratified, squamous epithelium, the cells of which contain much glycogen. A further increase of oestrogenic output is associated with an increasing proportion of cornified cells with an increased production of lactic acid. As progesterone secretion rises during the luteal phase of the menstrual cycle, the proportion of cornified cells falls again, the cells shrink and the epithelium becomes infiltrated with leucocytes.

THE BASAL BODY TEMPERATURE

Measurements of the daily basal body temperature for one or more menstrual cycles is often used to decide whether ovulation has occurred.

At the time of ovulation the secretion of progesterone increases as the corpus luteum becomes established. Progesterone is metabolized to pregnanediol and related compounds which, in common with other C-19 and C-21 steroids having a 5β-H configuration (p. 521), are 'thermogenic'. The early morning temperature therefore rises about 1° F when these metabolites accumulate under the influence of progesterone from the corpus luteum. It stays up for the rest of the cycle and if pregnancy occurs, it persists at this higher level for the whole of gestation.

ENDOMETRIAL BIOPSY
An endometrial biopsy is essential for the diagnosis of dysfunctional uterine bleeding, but it can also be useful as a reliable means of deciding whether menstruation is ovulatory or not. If ovulation has occurred, a biopsy taken a few days before the next menstrual period will show a histological picture typical of the secretory phase (p. 607).

URINARY OESTROGENS
These can be estimated to provide an index of oestrogen output which is more quantitative than the appearance of a vaginal smear. But it should be remembered that the rate of urinary excretion of any hormone is not necessarily directly related to the actual secretion rate of the hormone, particularly in pathological conditions. Nor does it necessarily reflect the net result of oestrogenic activity in the whole individual. Any disorder affecting either the pathways of oestrogen metabolism or the renal clearance of oestrogens will distort the normal relationship between glandular secretion and urinary excretion. Furthermore, the adrenal gland contributes a small but variable amount of oestrogen to the urine. Nevertheless, useful but laborious quantitative chemical assays are now available for the measurement of urine oestrone, oestriol and oestradiol-17β. Chemical methods have largely replaced older techniques based on bio-assay, which are notoriously prone to error. In any case, bio-assay is barely more quantitative than using vaginal smears of the patient herself to measure her own endogenous oestrogen.

Figures of oestrogen output are of little value during the menstrual cycle, or during pregnancy, unless serial estimations are made.

URINARY PROGESTERONE METABOLITES
The estimation of the metabolites of progesterone in the urine is important as an index of progesterone secretion. Measurement of pregnanediol, the principal urinary metabolite of progesterone, can be

useful to detect ovulation if pelvic sepsis is present because infection makes the interpretation of vaginal smears, endometrial biopsy specimens and basal temperature readings very difficult. The urinary pregnanediol excretion may also be valuable for assessing the functional adequacy of the corpus luteum and the placenta in pregnancy. Normally pregnanediol excretion increases from about 10 mg. per day at the first missed period to 60 to 100 mg per day near term. In the first 6 to 8 weeks of pregnancy progesterone is secreted chiefly by the corpus luteum, but thereafter the placenta is the main source. In patients with threatened or habitual abortion who may be suspected of having a functional deficiency of the corpus luteum or placenta, estimation of the urinary pregnanediol may help in deciding whether to give, continue or stop treatment with exogenous progesterone. The urinary output of pregnanetriol which is the chief urinary metabolite of 17-hydroxyprogesterone, is a very useful test in the diagnosis of congenital adrenal hyperplasia (p. 529).

URINARY 17-OXOSTEROIDS

These provide a rough index of the secretion rate of androgens, but since the adrenals secrete considerable quantities of androgen, the total 17-oxosteroid excretion is a poor index of *testicular* androgen production.

URINARY GONADOTROPHINS

Pituitary gonadotrophins are usually estimated collectively by bio-assay of urine extracts, using the uterine weight of the immature female mouse. The excretion of gonadotrophins is increased in cases of primary failure of the gonads, or after castration or the menopause. Little or none can be detected in cases of hypogonadism due to pituitary failure.

The detection of chorionic gonadotrophin in the urine is used in the diagnosis of pregnancy. It depends upon the fact that chorionic gonadotrophin is predominantly luteinizing in type, though it is synergistic with FSH from the hypophysis. When injected into amphibia it results in extrusion of eggs by the female or of sperms by the male animal. Immunological tests are now available which are simpler, and equally accurate. The hormone can usually be detected in the urine and serum after the twenty-first to twenty-fifth day of pregnancy, that is to say about 2 weeks after the first missed period.

EFFECTS OF HORMONES ON UTERINE BLEEDING

The responsiveness of the uterus to exogenous oestrogen and its subsequent withdrawal can be used to test the integrity and adequacy of the 'end-organ' response. In a patient with amenorrhoea the ability to induce oestrogen withdrawal bleeding provides a rough indication that the endometrium is capable of responding adequately and that pregnancy does not exist. Furthermore, the occurrence of withdrawal bleeding after the administration of progesterone or one of its analogues is evidence not only for the integrity and responsiveness of the endometrium but also for the presence of adequate levels of circulating oestrogen. This is because the action of progesterone on the endometrium depends on previous oestrogenic influence.

Practical assessment

IN FEMALES

CLINICAL OBSERVATIONS
Menstrual history; appearance of external genitalia and vagina; presence and size of internal genitalia (by palpation); body hair and other secondary sexual characteristics. Isolated failure of breast development suggests local resistance to circulating oestrogens. Similarly, failure to menstruate (primary amenorrhoea) with normal secondary sexual characteristics suggests lack of uterine development (or imperforate hymen). Cessation of menstruation indicates ovarian failure, whether primary or secondary.

ROUTINE TESTS
Daily basal morning temperature or an *endometrial biopsy* in the week preceding menstruation may show that ovulation is occurring, but not all cycles are necessarily ovulatory. A vaginal smear should give a rough index of oestrogen activity. In patients with infertility, *examination of the cervical mucus after coitus* gives an indication of the motility of the sperms. A quantitative or qualitative deficiency of sperms in the post-coital test between about the tenth and sixteenth day of the menstrual cycle suggests 'hostility' of the cervical fluid. Normally sperms are actively motile in the cervical fluid at this time.

A measurement of the *daily output of urinary 17-ketosteroids* will help differentiate between pseudohermaphroditism due to adrenal hyperplasia and that due to other forms of intersex.

The *urinary chorionic gonadotrophin concentration* provides an excellent test for pregnancy within the first 12 weeks of pregnancy.

SPECIAL TECHNIQUES

Direct chemical estimation of *urinary oestrogens* and *progesterone metabolites* are at present only research procedures. As described under 'principles' (p. 622), they only give information about the urinary output of ovarian or placental hormones and, in any case, the adrenal cortex may contribute a considerable amount whereas the clinical and routine tests provide a means of assessing the net result of hormonal activity and its effect on the organism as a whole.

Other techniques include *tubal insufflation* and *hysterosalpingography* to demonstrate obstruction of the Fallopian tubes and *culdoscopy* to obtain a view of the ovaries without a formal laparotomy.

Urethroscopy is sometimes needed in cases of pseudohermaphroditism in order to demonstrate the existence of a vagina when the latter is fused at its lower end with the urethra in the form of a persistent urogenital sinus. Lipiodol may be injected at the same time in order to determine radiographically the presence of a uterus and tubes. *Laparotomy* is occasionally necessary to establish the sex of the gonads.

During the reproductive phase of life a *high urinary pituitary gonadotrophin output* is a clear indication of a reduced level of circulating oestrogen. Thus hypogonadism or amenorrhoea associated with a high urinary gonadotrophin output suggests a primary failure of the ovaries. Current techniques, however, are hardly quantitative.

IN THE MALE

CLINICAL OBSERVATIONS

Age at puberty; sexual potency; appearance of external genitalia, particularly the consistency and size of the testes; body hair; breast development. Undescended testes may be normal ('retractile testes') or less commonly they may indicate a true failure of pituitary gonadotrophin. Isolated failure of beard growth or of deepening of the voice suggests end-organ resistance to testosterone. This also occurs in male pseudohermaphroditism (p. 587).

ROUTINE METHODS

Spermatogenesis can be assessed by examination of seminal fluid, collected by masturbation after 5 days' abstinence. Criteria employed are: (1) the volume of the specimen, (2) the concentration of spermatozoa per unit volume of fluid, (3) the degree of motility of the spermatozoa, (4) the morphology of the spermatozoa. The most important of these criteria are the concentration and motility of the spermatozoa. A count of 20 million/ml is considered adequate, provided that motility is unimpaired. The volume of the seminal specimen tends to increase in inverse proportion to the sperm count and the percentage of abnormal forms tends to increase when the total count is low, but these probably only represent sperms which survived unduly long and have become degenerate. The specimen must be examined in a warm, fresh state and must be collected in a dry container and not in a sheath, since cooling, moisture and rubber tend to kill the sperms. The variability of the sperm count in any individual may be considerable; at least three specimens need to be examined if the first count is low.

Estimation of 17-*oxosteroids in the urine* is of limited value in the assessment of androgen secretion by the testis. Values may be normal in the total absence of functioning testes if the adrenal cortex compensates for the testicular deficiency. Very low values for urinary 17-oxosteroids are found when the function of both the adrenal cortex and the gonads are deficient, as in hypopituitarism (see p. 540), when Addison's disease occurs in a female, or as a result of general ill-health. Low values are not usually found in male hypogonadism without adrenal insufficiency, or in primary adrenal insufficiency without hypogonadism in males. Abnormally high values occur in the presence of adrenal cortical tumour or hyperplasia, and in the rare instances of adenoma of the interstitial cells of the testis. Precocious puberty of constitutional origin or resulting from hypothalamic disturbance is associated with an output of 17-oxosteroids proportional to the sexual age of the child, but the normal adult range is never exceeded.

SPECIAL TECHNIQUES

Testicular biopsy: needle biopsy of the testes is often performed in cases of hypogonadism and the characteristic findings in the various types of disordered function have already been described. The procedure adds little to the assessment of gonadal function. Spermatogenesis is more easily assessed by examination of the seminal fluid, though this may be misleading in cases in which sperms fail to pass from the epididymis into the seminal fluid as a result of obstruction of the vasa deferentia. Interstitial cell function is more readily assessed by clinical observation of the secondary sex characters.

Response to chorionic gonadotrophin. Injections of chorionic gonadotrophin may increase the output of testosterone in the urine in patients with testicular deficiency due to pituitary gonadotrophic failure and may result in some clinical improvement. Those with primary testicular failure show no response. Patients with pituitary infantilism develop secondary sex characters and show a spurt of growth. The response continues only as long as the treatment is maintained. On the other hand, those with constitutional stunting of growth and delayed puberty continue to improve spontaneously after an initial course of treatment lasting up to six months.

The *urinary output of testosterone* helps to distinguish primary from secondary hypogonadism in males.

TESTS IN EITHER SEX

Bone age
This can be estimated from radiographs of various epiphyses whose time of appearance and fusion is compared with that of average individuals. Bone age is a more reliable index of gonadal function during adolescence than is height-age.

Measurement of body proportions
This is a useful test in the assessment of primary failure of the gonads, or selective gonadotrophic failure, especially in males. Owing to the failure of epiphyses to mature under the influence of androgenic hormones (p. 309), growth of the long bones persists unduly because the secretion of pituitary growth hormone continues. The span of the outstretched arms exceeds the total height, and the distance from floor to pubis exceeds that of pubis to vertex.

Pituitary function
Pituitary gonadotrophins are detectable in the urine by biological methods from the age of 11 years in girls and 12 to 13 years in boys. Several years after the expected age of puberty the output of gonadotrophins in the urine may distinguish primary gonadal failure from pituitary gonadotrophic failure, being increased in the former and immeasurable in the latter. Other endocrine deficiencies point to a pituitary origin.

TABLE 19. Some normal values

(See Table 16, p. 543, for normal values for glucocorticoids)

URINARY OESTROGENS

	μg/24 hr		
	Oestriol	Oestrone	Oestradiol
Onset of menstruation	0–15	4–7	0–3
Ovulation peak	13–54	11–31	4–14
Luteal peak	8–72	10–23	4–10
Late pregnancy	16 000–41 000	290–1800	280–900

URINARY PREGNANEDIOL

	mg/24 hr
Male:	0·38–1·42 (Mean 0·92)
Female: proliferative phase	0·78–1·50 (Mean 1·12)
luteal phase	2·1–4·2 (Mean 3·3)
post-menopausal	0·28–0·86 (Mean 0·63)
pregnancy	Up to 100 (maximal between 32nd and 36th weeks)

PLASMA PROGESTERONE

	μg/100 ml
Male:	0·014–0·055
Female: proliferative phase	0·04–0·20
luteal phase	0·50–1·60

URINARY 17-OXOSTEROIDS

		mg/24 hr
Male:		10–20
Female:		5–15
Children (both sexes):	< 3 years	< 1
	3–8 years	1–5
	8–12 years	5–8

After 12 years values increase more in boys than in girls.

URINARY TESTOSTERONE

	μg/24 hr
Male:	35–200
Female:	2–15

PLASMA TESTOSTERONE

	μg/100 ml
Male:	0·3–0·9
Female:	0·015–0·050

References

WILKINS, L. (1957). *The diagnosis and treatment of endocrine disorders in childhood and adolescence.* (2nd ed.). Oxford: Blackwell.

HARRIS, G.W. (1955) Neural control of the pituitary gland. London: Arnold.

SOHVAL A.R. (1961) *Hormonal factors in male sex development and function.* In Modern trends in endocrinology. (2nd series). Ed. H. Gardiner-Hill. London: Butterworths.

MILLS I.H. (1961). *Endocrine changes during pregnancy and with foetal pathology.* In Modern trends in endocrinology (2nd series). Ed. H. Gardiner-Hill. London: Butterworths.

Some hormonal aspects of pregnancy and parturition (Joint meeting of the Society for Endocrinology and the Section of Endocrinology of the Royal Society of Medicine). *J. Endocr.* (1961), **22** (Proc.) IX–XXIV, and *Proc. Roy. Soc. Med.* (1961), **54**, 743–747.

LLOYD C.W. & WEISZ J. (1966). Some aspects of reproductive physiology. *Ann. Rev. Physiol.* **28**, 267–310.

EIK-NES K.B. & HALL P.F. (1965). Secretion of steroid hormones *in vivo. Hormones and Vitamins,* **23**, 153–208.

ROTHCHILD I. (1965). Interrelations between progesterone and the ovary, pituitary and central nervous system in the control of ovulation and regulation of progesterone secretion. *Hormones and Vitamins,* **23**, 209–327.

GROLLMAN A. (1964) Clinical endocrinology and its physiologic basis. Pitman Medical Publishing Co. Ltd.

BROOKS R.V. (1967). *Ovarian steroid biosynthesis and its clinical implications.* In Modern Trends in Endocrinology. Ed. Gardiner-Hill, H. London: Butterworths. Chap. 7, 127–51.

PRUNTY F.T.G. (1967). Hirsutism, virilism and apparent virilism and their gonadal relationship. *J. Endocr.* **38**, 85–103 (Pt I), 203–227 (Pt II).

Index